Readings in Community Health Nursing

Readings in
Community
Health Nursing

5TH EDITION

EDITED BY

Barbara Walton Spradley, RN, MN

Associate Professor Emeritus
School of Public Health
University of Minnesota
Minneapolis, Minnesota

Judith Ann Allender, RN,C, EdD

Professor
Department of Nursing
School of Health and Human Services
California State University
Fresno, California

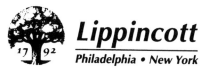

Lippincott
Philadelphia • New York

Acquisitions Editor: Susan Glover
Project Editor: Sandra Cherry Scheinin
Production Manager: Helen Ewan
Production Coordinator: Patricia McCloskey
Art Director: Susan Hermansen
Indexer: Vicki Boyle

Edition 5th

9 8 7 6 5 4 3 2 1

Library of Congress Cataloging in Publication Data
Readings in community health nursing / edited by Barbara Walton
   Spradley, Judith Ann Allender. — 5th ed.
        p.   cm.
   Reprinted from various sources.
   Includes bibliographical references and index.
   ISBN 0–397–55436–2 (alk. paper)
   1. Community health nursing.   I. Spradley, Barbara Walton.
   II. Allender, Judith Ann.
   [DNLM: 1. Community Health Nursing—collected works.   WY   106R283
1997]
   RT98.R4   1997
   610.73′43—dc20
   DNLM/DLC
   for Library of Congress   96–31654
                                                               CIP

To our wonderful grandchildren
Ryan
Nathan
Andy
Jackie
Danny
Christopher
Kevin
Emelie
Justine
Erica
Kevin Neil
and
Zachary
Kristen
Jeremy
Sydny
Nicolas
Nicole
Samuel

CONTRIBUTORS

CATHY ADEN, MS, RN
Director of Comprehensive Intermittent
    Services
Visiting Nurse Association of Omaha
Omaha, Nebraska

ELIZABETH ANDERSON, DrPH, RN, FAAN
Professor
University of Texas School of Nursing
Galveston, Texas

MILA A. AROSKAR, EdD, RN, FAAN
Associate Professor
Health Management and Policy
University of Minnesota School of Public
    Health
Minneapolis, Minnesota

DONELLE BARNES, MS, RN, (doctoral
    student)
Department of Mental Health, Commu-
    nity, and Administrative Nursing
University of California School of Nursing
San Francisco, California

PETER L. BEILENSON, MD, MPH
Commissioner of Health
Baltimore City Health Department
Baltimore, Maryland

JO ANNE BENNETT, PhD, RN
HIV Clinical Specialist/Community Health
    Consultant
New York, New York

ANDREA BERNE, MPH, CPNP
Associate Staff Analyst
Office of Child Health Planning
New York City Department of Health
New York, New York

CAROL E. BLIXEN, PhD, RN
Assistant Professor
Case Western Reserve University
Cleveland, Ohio

MAUREEN E. BRAGG
Health Educator
Central Valley Indian Health Service
Clovis, California

PAMELA J. BRINK, PhD, RN, FAAN
Associate Dean of Research
Faculty of Nursing
University of Alberta
Edmonton, Alberta, Canada

JACQUELYN C. CAMPBELL, PhD, RN, FAAN
Professor
Johns Hopkins University
Baltimore, Maryland

LEANNE KAISER CARLSON
Editor, *Healing and Healthcare*
Denver, Colorado

JANICE CAVANAUGH, MPA, RN, CNA
Director of Quality Management
In Home Health Services
Sparta, New Jersey

KATHLEEN CHAFEY, PhD, RN
Associate Professor
Montana State University College of
    Nursing
Bozeman, Montana

KAREN I. CHALMERS, BN, Msc(A), PhD
Associate Professor, Faculty of Nursing
University of Manitoba
Winnepeg, Manitoba, Canada

CANDY DATO, RN, CS, MS
Administrative Coordinator
St. Luke's Roosevelt Hospital Center
New York, New York

CAROLYNE K. DAVIS, PHD, RN, FAAN
Former Administrator of the Health Care
  Financing Administration
U.S. Department of Health and Human
  Services
Washington, DC

LISA DEAL, BS, RN
Graduate Student
Community Health Care Systems
University of Washington School of
  Nursing
Seattle, Washington

CHRISTOPHER DEGRAW, MD
Coordinator of Children and School
  Programs
Office of Disease Prevention and Health
  Promotion
Washington, D.C.

MARLENE A. DEHN, PhD, PHN
Professor, Department of Nursing
School of Health and Human Services
California State University
Fresno, California

LIZBETH A. DRURY-ZEMKE, MS, RN, PHN
Former Director of Nursing
Central Valley Indian Health Service
Clovis, California

MARY E. DUFFY, PhD, RN
Associate Professor
College of Nursing
University of Utah
Salt Lake City, Utah

MICHELE J. ELIASON, PhD, RN
Assistant Professor of Nursing
College of Nursing
University of Iowa
Iowa City, Iowa

CARMEN ERIBES, MS, RN, (doctoral
  student)
Department of Mental Health, Commu-
  nity, and Administrative Nursing
University of California School of Nursing
San Francisco, California

NAOMI ERVIN, PhD, RN
Clinical Assistant Professor and Acting
  Head
Department of Public Health Nursing
University of Illinois at Chicago College of
  Nursing
Chicago, Illinois

MYCHELLE FARMER, MD
Medical Director for Contraceptive
  Services
Baltimore City Health Department-STD
  Clinics
Johns Hopkins University Hospital
Baltimore, Maryland

LORNA FINNEGAN, RN,C, MS
Instructor
School of Nursing
St. Xavier College
Chicago, Illinois

BEVERLY C. FLYNN, PhD, RN, FAAN
Professor, Indiana University School of
  Nursing
Director, Institute of Action Research for
  Community Health
Head, WHO Collaborating Center in
  Healthy Cities
Indianapolis, Indiana

SUSAN A. FONTANA, PhD, RN, CS-FNP
Associate Professor
University of Wisconsin School of Nursing
Milwaukee, Wisconsin

LINDA FRANK, PhD, RN
Assistant Professor, Graduate School of
  Public Health and School of Nursing
Senior Project Director, Pennsylvania
  AIDS Education and Training Center
University of Pittsburgh
Pittsburgh, Pennsylvania

SARA FRISCH, PhD
Director of Nursing Research
Montreal General Hospital
Montreal, Quebec, Canada

TERRY L. FULMER, PhD, RN, FAAN
Formerly School of Nursing
Columbia University
New York, New York

LAINA M. GERACE, PhD, RN
Associate Professor
Department of Psychiatric Nursing
University of Illinois College of Nursing
Chicago, Illinois

SHIRLEY GIROUARD, RN, PhD, FAAN
Director, Child Health Planning and
  Evaluation
National Association of Children's
  Hospitals and Related Institutions
Alexandria, Virginia

DEANNA E. GRIMES, PhD, RN
Associate Professor, School of Nursing
Health Science Center
University of Texas
Houston, Texas

RICHARD M. GRIMES, PhD
Director, AIDS Education and Training
  Center for Texas and Oklahoma
Associate Professor, School of Public
  Health
Health Science Center
University of Texas—Houston
Houston, Texas

BETHANY A. HALL-LONG, PhD, RN,C
Assistant Professor, Center for Health
  Policy
College of Nursing and Health Science
George Mason University
Fairfax, Virginia

MARSHELLE HENRY, BSN, RN
Graduate Student
School of Nursing
University of California
San Francisco, California

ELIZABETH HOWZE, ScD
National Center for Chronic Disease
  Prevention and Health Promotion
Centers for Disease Control and
  Prevention
Atlanta, Georgia

LAURIE E. JACKSON, MSN, RN
Community Health Coordinator
Asian Mutual Assistance Program
Toledo, Ohio

RUTH ANN JACOBSON, RN, MPH
Vice President, EVERCARE
St. Paul, Minnesota

MELINDA L. JENKINS, PhD, RN-CS
Assistant Professor in Primary Care
School of Nursing
University of Pennsylvania
Philadelphia, Pennsylvania

TERESA JUARBE, MS, RN
Doctoral Student
Department of Mental Health, Commu-
  nity, and Administrative Nursing
University of California School of Nursing
San Francisco, California

REBECCA KANG, PhD, RN
Department of Community Health Care
  Systems
University of Washington School of
  Nursing
Seattle, Washington

CAROLINE KENNEDY, MSc(A), RN
Staff Nurse
CLSC Metro
Montreal, Quebec, Canada

MARCIA KILLIEN, PhD, RN, FAAN
Professor and Chair
Department of Parent and Child Nursing
University of Washington
Seattle, Washington

DUSHANKA V. KLEINMAN, MD
Deputy Director National Institute for
  Dental Research
Department of Health and Human Services
Washington, D.C.

C. EVERETT KOOP, MD
The C. Everett Koop Institute at
  Dartmouth
Hanover, New Hampshire

EDWIN W. KOPF
Formerly with Metropolitan Life Insurance
  Company
Former Member of American Statistical
  Association

LINDA J. KRISJANSON, BN, MN, PhD
Assistant Professor
Faculty of Nursing
University of Manitoba
Winnipeg, Canada

RICHARD LAUZON, PhD
(Former) Director, Public Education
Canadian Heart Foundation
Ottawa, Ontario, Canada

GARY LEAK, PhD
Associate Professor
Creighton University
Omaha, Nebraska

KAREN MARTIN, MSH, RN, FAAN
Director of Research
Visiting Nurse Association of Omaha
Omaha, Nebraska

MIRIAM E. MARTIN, PhD, RN
Professor and Director
Department of Nursing
Goshen College
Goshen, Indiana

DIANA J. MASON, RN,C, PhD
Associate Dean and Professor
Lienhard School of Nursing
Pace University
Pleasantville, New York

BEVERLY McELMURRY, EdD, RN, FAAN
Public Health Nursing
University of Illinois
Chicago, Illinois

CATHY McKILLIP, BA
Operations Manager
In Home Health Services
Sparta, New Jersey

AFAF IBRAHIM MELEIS, PhD, RN
Professor
Department of Mental Health, Commu-
  nity, and Administrative Nursing
University of California School of Nursing
San Francisco, California

MARGARET K. MILLER, RN, MS, CAC
Executive/Clinical Director
Danbury Center for Adolescent Treat-
  ment, Inc.
Danbury, Connecticut

ELIZABETH S. MIOLA, PNP, MSN
Instructor
The Johns Hopkins University School of
  Nursing
Baltimore, Maryland

LOIS MONTEIRO, PhD, RN
Department of Community Health
Division of Biology and Medicine
Brown University
Providence, Rhode Island

ADA CATHERINE MONTESSORO, PhD
Nursing Candidate at Case Western Re-
  serve University
Cleveland, Ohio

NORMA J. MURPHY, MSN, RN
Assistant Professor of Nursing
Dalhousie University School of Nursing
Halifax, Nova Scotia

MARTHA NELSON, MSN, RN (doctoral
  candidate)
Department of Mental Health, Commu-
  nity, and Administrative Nursing
University of California School of Nursing
San Francisco, California

CATHERINE NOONE, MS, RN, CNA
Administrator
In Home Health Services
Sparta, New Jersey

ANTONIA C. NOVELLA, MD
Surgeon General of Public Health Service
U.S. Public Health Service
Washington, D.C.

DEBORAH O. OAKLEY, MPH, PhD
Associate Professor, School of Nursing
University of Michigan
Ann Arbor, Michigan

DONNA AMBLER PETERS, PhD, RN, FAAN
Director
Clinical Systems IQ Technologies, Inc.
Bala Cynwyd, Pennsylvania

LYNELLE PHILLIPS, RN, MPH
Nurse Consultant
Epidemiology and Surveillance Division
National Immunization Program
Centers for Disease Control and
  Prevention
Atlanta, Georgia

CASSY D. POLLACK, MSN, RN, MPPM
Assistant Professor of Nursing
Associate Dean for Students and Masters
  Studies
Chairperson, Non-Nurse College Graduate
  Program
Yale University School of Nursing
New Haven, Connecticut

MICHAEL PRATT, MD, MS, MPH
National Center for Chronic Disease
  Prevention and Health Promotion
Centers for Disease Control and
  Prevention
Atlanta, Georgia

SUSAN PROCTOR, RN, MPH (doctoral
  candidate)
Department of Mental Health, Commu-
  nity, and Administrative Nursing
University of California School of Nursing
San Francisco, California

BEVERLY RAFF, PhD, RN, FAAN
Director, Division of Education and Career
  Pathway in Nursing
Mt. Sinai Hospital
New York, New York

MARGARET RAFFERTY, RN, MA, MPH
Instructor
Long Island College Hospital
School of Nursing
Brooklyn, New York

CHERIE RECTOR, PhD, RN,C
Associate Professor
Department of Nursing
School of Health and Human Services
California State University
Fresno, California

LINDA REUTTER, BSc, BA, MS, RN
Assistant Professor
Faculty of Nursing
University of Alberta
Edmonton, Alberta, Canada

ANN RHEAUME, MSc(A), RN
Research Assistant
Department of Nursing
Montreal General Hospital
Montreal, Quebec, Canada

ELAINE RICHARD, RN, MS
Director of Occupational Health
Health Line
St. Joseph's Hospital
Tampa, Florida

JANICE MAE RYAN, MS, RN
Assistant Professor
Community Health Nursing
Capital University
Columbus, Ohio

MARLA E. SALMON, RN, ScD, FAAN
Director, Division of Nursing
Public Health Service
Department of Health and Human
  Services
Rockville, Maryland

JUDITH M. SAUNDERS, DNSc, RN, FAAN
Assistant Professor
College of Nursing
University of Iowa
Iowa City, Iowa

LINDA SAWYER, MS, RN (doctoral
  student)
Department of Mental Health, Commu-
  nity, and Administrative Nursing
University of California School of Nursing
San Francisco, California

THOMAS L. SCHMID, PhD
National Center for Chronic Disease
  Prevention and Health Promotion
Centers for Disease Control and
  Prevention
Atlanta, Georgia

MURIEL SHAUL, MS, RN (doctoral
  candidate)
Department of Mental Health, Commu-
  nity, and Administrative Nursing
University of California School of Nursing
San Francisco, California

ANNE SMITH, BSc, RN
Nurse Manager
Montreal General Hospital
Montreal, Quebec, Canada

GLORIA R. SMITH, PhD, RN, FAAN
Acting Vice President
Program Coordinator of Health Programs
Program Director, W.K. Kellogg Founda-
  tion
Battle Creek, Michigan

JULIE A. SOCHALSKI, MS, RN
Nurse Educator
Michigan Diabetes Research and Training
  Center
University of Michigan
Ann Arbor, Michigan

KAREN L. STARR, RN, MSN, MAC
Associate in Psychiatry, Division of Alcohol
  and Substance Abuse
Vanderbilt University
Nashville, Tennessee

MARYFRAN McKENZIE STULGINSKY,
  MS, RN
Staff Nurse
Bon Secours Home Health and Hospice
Baltimore, Maryland

EILEEN M. SULLIVAN-MARX, PhD, RN
Assistant Professor and Director
Primary Care Adult Nurse Practitioner
  Program
School of Nursing
University of Pennsylvania
Philadelphia, Pennsylvania

MARIE L. TALASHEK, EdD
Department of Public Health Nursing
University of Illinois College of Nursing
Chicago, Illinois

JAYNE ANTTILA TAPIA, MS, RN
Director-Supervisor,
Arlington Visiting Nursing Association,
  Inc.
Arlington, Massachusetts

LINDA BETH TIEDJE, PhD, RN, FAAN
Associate Professor
Michigan State University College of
  Nursing
East Lansing, Michigan

TONI TRIPP-REIMER, PhD, RN, FAAN
Associate Dean and Professor
Lienhard School of Nursing
Pleasantville, New York

SUSAN NOBLE WALKER, EdD, RN, FAAN
Associate Professor and Chair
Gerontological, Psychosocial, and Commu-
  nity Health Nursing
University of Nebraska Medical Center
  College of Nursing
Omaha, Nebraska

MARY BOOSE WALKER, EdD, RN
Associate Professor and Assistant Dean for
  Graduate Studies
Widener University School of Nursing
Chester, Pennsylvania

CAROLYN A. WILLIAMS, PhD, RN, FAAN
Dean and Professor
University of Kentucky College of Nursing
Lexington, Kentucky

JOAN WOOD, PhD, RN
Assistant Professor
Michigan State University College of
 Nursing
East Lansing, Michigan

JOYCE V. ZERWEKH, EdD, RN
Assistant Professor
Community Health Care Systems
University of Washington
Seattle, Washington

PREFACE

Today's nurse faces unparalleled opportunities to serve the health needs of communities. With the turn of the century come demands made by changing life-styles and disease patterns, new and complex technologies, shifting demographics, global economics, dramatic health system changes, and sociobiological and environmental threats to health and safety that call for creative and effective population-based responses. Community health nursing offers today's practitioner the challenge and opportunity to meet these demands. This field of nursing practice specializes in combining nursing with applications of public health theory, philosophy, and principles to address the health needs of the public. It is the intent of *Readings in Community Health Nursing* to assist the nurse in understanding what community health nursing involves and how it can be most effectively practiced.

For nurses to understand the practice of community health nursing, they must be cognizant of (1) trends in nursing as a profession; (2) the effect of societal changes on health needs; and (3) changing patterns in health systems structure and delivery. Among the trends in nursing are the recognition of the need for higher levels of education, a stronger nursing research base, greater involvement in health system leadership and policy development, expanded sophistication and autonomy in practice, and salaries and status commensurate with worth. Nursing's voice is being heard on important health policy issues, and nursing is assuming a stronger leadership role in shaping the health system of tomorrow. These changes influence how community health nursing will be practiced in the future.

The second area, societal changes affecting health, is complex and multi-faceted. Many factors such as changing demographics with an aging population; shifting employment patterns; new developments in science and technology; increasing drug use, crime, and violence; and environmental health threats such as hazardous wastes all influence the public's health and dictate health needs. Nurses need to keep abreast of these changes and study their real or potential impact on community health. These changes call for creative and innovative community health nursing intervention and collaboration.

Changes in health systems structure and delivery is a third area affecting community health nursing practice. Among the variables influencing the structure of the health system are health care financing and insurance and the roles that health practitioners play in the delivery of services. As dissatisfaction mounts with a system that fails to provide equitable service or adequately fails to meet the needs of many populations at risk, the demand for a better system escalates. Community health nursing's role can be significant in shaping an improved system and in responding to population health needs.

Within the context of these challenges and opportunities, community health nursing needs to be clearly defined. Nurse educators have a monumental task in keeping up with the expansion of knowledge and conveying this knowledge in an understandable form to nursing students. Community health nursing instructors must often depend on their own experiences to assist them in defining this field; so, too, the practicing community health nurse may define the field in terms of her or his own experience. Like the proverbial blind men describing the elephant, each practitioner may perceive a single facet of community health nursing as the whole field.

Why is it important to understand the meaning of community health nursing? Concepts specific to this field are the essential fibers in the fabric of all good nursing practice. They should be woven into each nurse's experience throughout the preparatory period and during the nurse's entire professional life. Concepts such as wellness, prevention, culture, family, and the community need particular emphasis because of their importance to client health and improved nursing practice. That is, nurses practicing in any setting should apply these concepts at a basic level. Those who go on to specialize in community health nursing will broaden and deepen their understanding and skill in this field, expanding their expertise in epidemiologic investigation, the use of biostatistics, the application of management sciences, and population-based practice. Graduating nursing students need more than basic preparation in these areas; they need a clear understanding of the career choices that lie before them, including the option of aggregate-level practice in community health nursing.

This book forms an anthology of articles that provides the reader with a clearer understanding of the nature of community health nursing in the context of today's world. *Readings in Community Health Nursing*, fifth edition, is designed for undergraduate and graduate nursing students and their instructors, as well as for practicing community health nurses. It seeks to present important contemporary aspects of health services and community health nursing in an interesting and comprehensive manner. The chapters, 43 of them (or 75%) new to this edition, have been carefully selected for pertinence and readability, while the remaining 14 have been retained as classic articles germane to the study of the field. All have been arranged to provide a framework for more clearly understanding this nursing specialty.

The book has eight parts, each examining a different aspect of the context or content of community health nursing practice. Unit I, "Health and Health Services: Issues and Trends," presents timely topics that influence the future of health services delivery and nursing practice. Leaders discuss trends in public health policy; health care reform; the need for a nursing role in environmental health; serious public health threats such as human immunodeficiency virus (HIV), violence, substance abuse, and tuberculosis, and forecasts for the future of health care and nursing practice. It is imperative to understand these issues and trends because they profoundly affect the current and future practice of community health nursing.

Unit II, "Community Health Nursing: Articulating Its Mission," describes the nature of community health nursing. Several classic articles have been retained in this section to clarify its mission: What is community health nursing in business to do? To answer this question, various chapters address different perspectives of community health nursing's definition, history, effective interventions, ethical issues, roles in environmental and occupational health, and describe innovative practice models in the field (original to this edition).

Unit III, "Assessing and Building Healthy Communities," emphasizes how to create healthier communities. The chapters in this section describe how to assess community health, clarify the meaning of primary health care, discuss ethical paradigms for serving communities, show how to promote community capacity for health promotion, provide a case study in health planning, and apply marketing concepts to health promotion with vulnerable groups.

Unit IV, "Tools for Community Health Nursing Practice," presents selected means for enhancing the nurse's practice in community health. These include epidemiology and biostatistics. New to this edition are chapters on quality outcomes, case management, clinical partnerships, computer documentation, and use of the Omaha system for decision making.

Unit V, "Family Nursing," continues the fourth edition's focus on family health assessment and intervention with selected types of families and family problems. Topics include assessing family health, using the nursing process in family health, a family caregiving model, single mothers, child abuse, and preventive work with families.

Unit VI, "Community Health Nursing With Populations and Groups," describes ways to work with a variety of community populations. All of the eight chapters in this section are new to this edition and discuss such populations as healthy children, pregnant adolescents, support groups (original to this edition), people with acquired immunodeficiency syndrome (AIDS), homeless families, well elders, and home health clients.

Unit VII, "Cultural Influences on Community Health Nursing," emphasizes the importance of assessing and understanding cultural differences. Four of the six chapters in this section are new to this edition and provide the community health nurse with important tools for serving multicultural groups. Topics include cultural assessment, an empowerment approach (original to this edition), cultural relativity and poverty, ethics and transcultural nursing, multicultural health beliefs, and cultural self-care issues (original to this edition).

Finally, Unit VIII, "Community Health Nursing Leadership and Effecting Change," emphasizes community health nursing's role in influencing public policy and providing leadership in health services. Six of the eight chapters in this section are new to this edition. Topics include nursing leadership in health policy decision making, nursing's experience in politics, expanding nursing's influence on health policy, implementing policy changes with contraceptives use, cardiovascular disease prevention, school health, and a healthy cities model for community change.

In this fifth edition of *Readings in Community Health Nursing*, the topics selected for inclusion provide the reader with a basic grasp of the breadth and depth of this dynamic field of nursing practice. At the same time, we have shortened the total number of articles to keep the book a manageable size. The eight sections parallel the organization and complement the content of our text, *Community Health Nursing: Concepts and Practice*, fourth edition, so that this book of readings can be used as a supplement to that text, other texts, or stand alone to be used as a text by itself.

We are grateful to the many individuals who have helped in the completion of this book; their suggestions, contributions, assistance, and support have been wonderful. We especially want to thank Mila Aroskar, Janet Hagberg, Elaine Saline, Barb Schommer, Bob Veninga, and Lois Yellowthunder from Minnesota and Avo's Custom Photo Lab in Fresno, California, Maureen Bragg, Marlene Dehn, Harry Dulan, Liz Drury-Zemke, Betty Garcia, Grace Hernandez, and Cherie Rector from California. We are grateful to the many students and colleagues in our respective universities and communities whose ideas have guided the development of the manuscript. Our special thanks go to our editor, Susan Glover, at Lippincott–Raven Publishers, as well as to her assistant, Gene Bender, for their encouragement, ideas, and invaluable assistance. Finally, we thank our families and, once again, especially our husbands, Neil Kittlesen and Gil Allender, for being true partners in the process.

Barbara Walton Spradley, RN, MN
Judith Ann Allender, RN,C, EdD

CONTENTS

▬ UNIT 8
COMMUNITY HEALTH NURSING LEADERSHIP
AND EFFECTING CHANGE

Unit 1
Health and Health Services: Issues and Trends

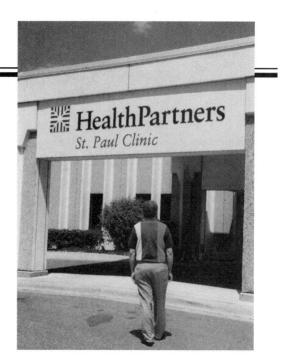

Community health nursing practice is strongly influenced by the issues and trends occurring in health and the health system. The ongoing debates over health care reform in the 1990s leave many questions unanswered and pose new challenges to community health nursing. An example is the question of how to contain health care costs and not compromise quality of services. Another is how to achieve universal health care coverage when 40 million Americans are either uninsured or underinsured. Health problems such as HIV/AIDS, environmental issues such as pollution, social problems such as homelessness, economic policies that restrict health care re-imbursement, and limited resources for prevention all help to shape community needs and to determine the resources available to meet those needs. As we move into the 21st century, nursing is in a prime position to respond to the demands of the present and, even more important, to help shape the future.

To respond with wisdom and compassion to community health needs, nurses must be informed. The ability to make wise decisions is directly proportional to the amount of information one possesses. What are the issues and trends affecting community health and health services delivery? Nurses must know these in order to effect change and assume a proactive role in protecting populations and promoting healthy communities.

Today's health system is complex and ever changing. We are reminded daily by the media of numerous health-related issues at local, national, and global levels and the literature abounds with research reports on health problems and potential solutions. To absorb this vast amount of information seems impossible. Yet, from the summarizing work of health care leaders as well as social forecasters such as John Naisbitt and Patricia Aburdene and Alvin and Heidi Toffler, one can distill this information into manageable areas for study. Six major forces continue to influence the future for community health, health services, and community health nursing: 1) globalization; 2) concern for the environment; 3) technologic advances; 4) privatization; 5) individual impact; and 6) concern for quality.

Globalization. We live in an era when no nation or continent functions inde-pendently. Expanded travel, global telecommunication, and the growing exchange of goods and services among countries have produced a global economy. Political events in one country affect the rest of the world; witness the democratization of Eastern Europe and Russia. The economic stability—or instability—of a nation in-fluences its neighbors, affecting the price of goods, wages, and the value of local currency. Diseases such as AIDS or social problems such as drug abuse quickly cir-cle the globe and require international resources to combat them. We cannot ig-nore our increasing world interconnectedness. Consequently, health policies and community health programs require constant monitoring to maintain their respon-siveness to global changes.

Concern for the environment. We also face the urgent need to preserve and re-store the environment. Pollution from industrial chemicals, nuclear radiation, pesti-cides, and household waste knows no boundaries. It crosses national borders, en-ters common seas, and threatens the quality of air, land, and water for plant, animal, and human existence. The indiscriminate use and abuse of natural re-sources is no longer acceptable. The time has come for a healing of the ravages in-flicted by civilization on the environment.

The trend toward restoration and preservation of the environment should have a long-term positive influence on public health. In the meantime, community health workers must be vigilant in identifying present and future health problems that re-sult from an unhealthy environment. Community health nurses in particular can help by reporting hazards, noting the frequency of similar health problems in a community, and educating the public to demand a safer and more healthful envi-ronment in which to live and work.

Technologic advances. Technology is a revolutionary force influencing almost every aspect of life: business, industry, national defense, health care, medicine, communications, agriculture, education, space exploration, and much more. Thanks to advanced technology, our ability to disseminate information and communicate with one another is staggering. Scientists are developing the capability to grow more nutritious and cost-effective food products. Genetic engineering has made it possible to clone the embryos sired by prize bulls for better breeding and to make implanted sheep and goats produce milk that contains vital drugs for human use, such as blood-clotting chemicals. Genetic engineering will also revolutionize the use of vaccines. In addition, technologic advances are making it possible to detect health risks in people earlier, to monitor the progress of health interventions, and to organize work patterns more efficiently for better delivery of health services.

Such technologic capabilities raise an increasing number of moral and ethical questions. How long should life be sustained artificially? How far can we go with genetic manipulation? Will such applications of technology as short-term chemical solutions for food production and environmental cleanup have long-term negative consequences? Community health professionals not only face the challenge of gaining skill in the use of technology for such purposes as conducting needs assessments, planning programs, delivering services, and monitoring the environment, but they also must wrestle with difficult ethical decisions that affect resource allocations and technologic applications.

Privatization. The recent failures of socialism and communism in various parts of the world represent a political trend of returning power to the people. Great Britain's remarkable redirection in the 1980s away from socialism and toward private enterprise provides a prime example as does the dissolution of the Soviet Union. Governments cannot afford the escalating costs of publicly subsidized programs. Bureaucratic red tape and rigidity has hampered the ability of state-controlled business and industry to respond creatively and improve productivity. State-owned enterprises, such as banks, insurance and telecommunication companies, utilities, railroads, and airlines are being sold to private owners. Expensive welfare systems are being replaced by systems in which individuals assume more responsibility for selecting their own services. Public-private partnerships may provide solutions to problems such as health insurance coverage for those who are unable to afford it. The phenomenon of privatization is shifting more power to the private sector and to individuals. For health care providers, this will mean changes to new structures, such as managed care organizations, and different sources of funding for delivery of services. Providers' roles will better facilitate client autonomy.

Individual impact. In the midst of globalization, individuals are gaining importance and power. Responsibility for decision-making and for the consequences of those decisions lies more and more with individuals. Gone is the socialist collective where the individual has no power and can hide from responsibility. Instead, Naisbitt and Aburdene propose in *Megatrends 2000* that the collective is being replaced with the community—the free association of individuals, each contributing, each responsible, each powerful.

The power of the individual is evident worldwide and extends to politics and foreign policy. Jesse Jackson, a private citizen, negotiated for the release of political prisoners in the Middle East; Samantha Smith, an eleven-year-old American girl, promoted better relations with the Soviet Union. Politics in the United States has become more decentralized and entrepreneurial. Candidates run as individuals and people vote as individuals, not as party members. Increasingly, individually owned small businesses are competing successfully with multinational corporations. Technology is making much of this possible because it facilitates information dissemination, and informed individuals are empowered individuals.

The trend toward individualization has increased consumerism. No longer do institutions dictate what people do or buy. Instead, consumers demand unique products and services. Evidence of consumer-driven products is everywhere: automobile designs, home conveniences, fashions for comfort, prepared foods for working people, day care, elder care, and leisure products. In health care, consumer demand drives decisions about corporate maternity policies, home-care equipment, insurance coverage, fitness programs, smoke-free environments, and more. In community health, we work with communities of individuals whose concerns need to be addressed. We can encourage these individuals to assume responsibility for their own health. We can provide the information that will empower them to create a healthier future for themselves and their children.

Concern for quality. This force for change embodies a dramatic shift in values. As we become a global community with less need for defense and a greater need for positive alliances, and as individuals become more powerful and demand a better world in which to live, there is increasing concern for quality. Evidence of this is the feminization of work and leadership. Workers are insisting on more humanitarian work environments. Controlling managers are being replaced by facilitating leaders, whose goal is to bring out the best in people. This kind of leadership (by men who share these values as well as women) shows respect for people and encourages self-management. It inspires commitment and creative productivity. This humanitarian shift in values promotes more women into leadership positions, a point that is evident in health services as well as other businesses.

An increasing interest in religion and a renaissance in the arts provide more evidence of the quest for quality. People are looking inward for spiritual answers to cope with the stress caused by rapid change. They are reexamining the meaning of life through the arts. Affluence, leisure time, and increasing numbers of retired persons who seek meaningful activity are all factors that further influence the quest for quality.

A value-driven society will affect health care in a number of ways. Health care consumers expect more humanitarian services. Health care providers, responding to the need for greater accountability, are promoting quality improvement programs, developing standards for such places as day-care centers and nursing homes, and monitoring community health services. Nursing's essence of caring and promoting holism can uniquely address the quest for quality.

Moving into the 21st century offers a remarkable opportunity for community health nurses. To understand the nature of community health needs, to assume a major role in shaping community health services, to effect changes such as nursing reimbursement policies, and, more important, to promote public health, nurses must stay informed. The chapters in Unit I provide critical insights into the issues and trends affecting decision-making for the future of community health.

Chapter 1

Public Health Policy: Creating a Healthy Future for the American Public

MARLA E. SALMON

What does it take to make and keep people healthy? The American health system has attempted to address this question but for many reasons has not been successful. The 1990s have been a decade of seeking answers through health system reform; perhaps the most crucial element of needed reform is effective public health policy to assure the health of the public. In this chapter Dr. Marla Salmon discusses determinants of health, problems with the current health system, and proposes a policy framework for enhancing the public's health. She describes eight essential elements of a satisfactory health system and challenges health professionals to work together to create a healthy future for the American public.

Never before in the history of the United States has the relationship between public policy and the health of the American people been more apparent or more important. As the nation enters an era of health system reform, prompted by the widespread recognition that the "system" of health services is too costly in both human and financial terms, the knowledge that policy is a major determinant of health must not be lost. Perhaps less well recognized—though no less significant—is the relationship between public health policy and the health of the people of this country. The symptoms of long-term neglect are obvious: Preventable communicable diseases have yet to be contained, new diseases are emerging, and the serious impact of environmental hazards must be faced. This country is rich in knowledge and technology but currently poor in the public health policies that mobilize these assets on behalf of the public's health. As the nation faces the ongoing challenge of health system reform, it is clear that the policies adopted must include comprehensive, intentional public health

The views expressed in this article are solely those of the author and not necessarily those of the Health Resources and Services Administration, the Public Health Service, or the US Department of Health and Human Services.

From *Family and Community Health* 18(1):1–11, 1995. Reprinted by permission of Aspen Publishers, Inc.

policy. A system that addresses personal care alone simply will not be capable of assuring the health of the people of this country. This article proposes the type of national public health policy approach that is necessary to genuinely reform the nation's health care system.

▬PUBLIC HEALTH POLICY AND NATIONAL HEALTH CARE REFORM

The Clinton administration's commitment to achieving universal insurance coverage, containing costs, enhancing access to care, and strengthening the foundations of public health is explicitly detailed in the President's proposed health system reform measures.[1] Throughout the administration's approach to health care reform, there is widespread recognition that the goals of universal coverage, cost reduction, and enhancement of access simply cannot be accomplished without the help of an efficient and effective public health system. The success of health system reform requires a public health system that works hand-in-hand with the personal care system to optimize early intervention, including widespread health promotion and disease prevention activities, as well as ensuring cost-effective health care services. It is only with such a coordinated, health-driven, savings-producing approach that this country can really afford and actually accomplish the health goals for the nation.

The health goals of increasing the span of healthy life for Americans and reducing health disparities among Americans are not foreign to most public health professionals. What is lacking now, however, is a system that can operationalize these values in a comprehensive, cost-effective manner. In other words, a system is needed in which public health is the foundation—unlike the current system in which illness, individual medical care, and technology are the cornerstones.[2]

How does one produce such a system? The key to both policy and implementation is to make certain that the personal care and public health systems share a common sense of direction and that the roles, responsibilities, and accountabilities of each are clearly delineated. Future national policy must recognize that the strength of each of these systems relies heavily on the extent to which they are interwoven and benefit from one another. Future policy must also recognize that an orientation toward health and the support of population-based strategies are essential to both systems.

▬FRAMING NATIONAL PUBLIC HEALTH POLICY

The development of a common vision and a common set of goals for the public health system and its counterpart personal care system requires a policy framework that is built on identification of areas of greatest concern and points for cross-system intervention. At a national policy level, this framework necessitates the articulation of a clear, well-documented view of the health (status) of the nation and its determinants and the establishment of goals that are relevant and measurable and that reflect conscious setting of national priorities. Such a framework also requires conceptualizing the system-level changes necessary to address these goals and move the national agenda forward.

Determinants of Health: The Policy Targets

Constructing national public health policy that is truly based on the health of the nation requires much more than a clear understanding of what the current health issues are that the country faces. It also demands that the constructs used to design both interventions and systems be built on solid recognition of what actually determines health. The current health care system, which focuses heavily on the interface between biology and medical technology, has limited usefulness in addressing the health problems of today. Although this framework has virtually guided modern medicine and the "health" care systems for the greater part of this century, a much more useful framework has emerged over the past three decades.

First widely articulated as national policy in 1979, *Healthy People: The Surgeon General's Report on Health Promotion and Disease Prevention*[3] proposed an alternative health policy framework that came to be called the "healthy people" framework consisting of three key categories of determinants of major risks relating to health: inherited biologic, environmental, and behavioral risks. This framework began to take hold as the basis for policy formulation and action with the subsequent publication of *Promoting Health, Preventing Disease: Objectives for the Nation.*[4]

The healthy people framework reflects a number of crucial studies and social policy statements over the past 25 years. One key study was the medical outcomes study,[5] which described five dimensions of health and its indicators: (1) clinical status, (2) physical functioning and well-being, (3) mental functioning and well-being, (4) social role functioning and well-being, and (5) general health perceptions. The healthy people framework also drew from the growing awareness both within and outside the United States that human behavior, the environment, and the ways in which health services are organized and delivered are key factors in determining the health of people. Fundamental to this evolution, of course, was the World Health Organization's definition of health, which clearly articulates a vision of health and its determinants that moves well beyond a biologic focus.[6]

Another landmark occurred in 1974 when the Canadian Department of National Health and Welfare proposed the "health field concept" as a basis for health policy.[7] This concept sectored health into four major elements: human biology, environment, lifestyle, and health care.

In 1977, Dever[8] proposed an epidemiologic model for health policy that also incorporated broader concepts of health. This model's four elements were (1) the system of health care organization, (2) lifestyle (particularly self-created risks), (3) environment, and (4) human biology. Of particular concern to Dever was the apparent mismatch of public resources and factors contributing most prominently to morbidity and mortality. He noted that the United States focused most of its health resources on health care despite the major role that lifestyle played in the morbidity and mortality of people.

Determinants of Health and the Nation's Health Agenda

Dever's[8] framework was significant both as an underpinning for the healthy people framework and as a link between policy and epidemiology as two fundamental tools for achieving the health of the people. Without recognition of the importance of both, Dever would not have had the basis for pointing out that although the majority of health-related resources in the United States were poured into personal health care, it was the lifestyle component that was the major contributing factor to present disease patterns. He concluded that "based on current procedures for reducing mortality and morbidity, little or no change in our present disease patterns will be accomplished unless we dramatically shift our health policy."[8(p453)]

Although nearly two decades have passed since Dever's[8] groundbreaking work, his conclusions continue to hold true. Despite major advancements in medical technology and increases in numbers of health professionals, the overall strategies for intervention remain largely the same. As a result, Americans continue to suffer from a national profile of preventable, premature mortality not unlike that of 20 years ago.

In a more recent analysis of causes of death in the United States undertaken in 1990, McGinnis and Foege[9] found that the role that lifestyle played in mortality had not changed greatly since 1977. Half of all deaths could still be attributed to tobacco, diet and activity patterns, alcohol, microbial agents, toxic agents, firearms, and sexual behavior, motor vehicles, and illicit drug use. With health resources continuing to be focused on personal health care, and lifestyle still playing the prominent role in causes of death, it is clear that the mismatch between resources and health determinants continues.

Clearly, the framework of health determinants applied to US populations has been extremely useful in developing an awareness of both the importance of factors beyond biology and the influences of medical technology. The framework has also provided the foundation for current goals for the nation's health. However, there is one significant national health goal that is not specifically stated in *Healthy People 2000*[10]: This goal is to reorient the health care system of this country. When one considers the framework of determinants of health and reviews the goals for the health of the nation, it is clear that Dever[8] was correct in his analysis. Without major changes in the policies that shape the ways that the nation delivers services, any hope for reaching those major causes of premature morbidity and mortality is futile.

■POLICIES FOR A NEW PUBLIC HEALTH

Despite increasing clarity in the agenda for the nation's health, the barrier to achieving this goal—the current system of services—remains intact. As discussed earlier, this system has been built largely on the notion that health is created by the interface between human biology and medical technology. A system built on the more expanded concepts of what determines health would be one in which personal care and public health are balanced in both resources and impact.

The public health system has suffered not only from a serious imbalance of resources, but also from the underlying policy assumptions on which favoring medical care is based. Public health, until recently, has been "policy invisible." That is, public health has not been in the forefront of public concern, resulting in many decades of deterioration in the nation's public health infrastructure and movement away from some of its central functions. The seriousness of this erosion was most vividly captured in the 1988 Institute of Medicine report that declared public health to be "in disarray."[11]

The American Public Health Association, in its 1993 report, *Public Health in a Reformed Health Care System: A Vision for the Future,*[12] echoed the Institute of Medicine's concerns. This report also confirmed that reform of the nation's health care system simply will not work without a vital public health system. A vital public health system, however, is one in which public health serves as the basis for the overall system.[13] However, when one considers that in 1993 less than 1% of the aggregate amount for all health care in the United States was spent on population-based public health activities, it is clear that much distance remains between the present state and true vitality.

What will it take to move toward a revitalized public health system— and, through it, to a genuinely reformed overall system of services? Such movement will require a policy framework that recognizes what actually determines health for both individuals and populations and where and how to intervene at all levels. Such a policy framework must view the entire health services system as a health determinant—something that either enhances or detracts from the health of people. Within this construct, then, a policy framework must contain the "levers" or elements that are necessary to make the health services system work in a genuinely cost-effective manner. While there are many such elements, eight of these are essential.

▬EIGHT ESSENTIAL ELEMENTS OF A SATISFACTORY HEALTH SYSTEM

The eight essential elements that provide a satisfactory health system constitute a blueprint for policy and action at both the national and state level.[14] They provide not only overall policy guidance but also a means for assessing the current system and measuring its development throughout the ongoing process of health care system reform.

The first element is universal coverage for comprehensive benefits, without any cost sharing for clinical preventive services. This element is fundamental to ensuring that the health system encompasses all people— and that it expands coverage that has been traditionally illness related into the critical domains of health promotion and disease prevention.

The second element is a payment system that rewards health plans for keeping their populations healthy. This element recognizes the importance of fiscal incentives and the need to focus their reward potential on promoting and maintaining health whenever possible. By reversing the current incentive system, which encourages later, more technologically intense intervention, the chances of actually promoting health and preventing diseases are greatly increased.

The third element is a national system of performance monitoring and report cards that focuses the attention of health plans on achieving healthy outcomes for their enrollees and that monitors how well they are accomplishing these goals. A particularly important feature of this element is that it requires the health services system to focus its attention, its resources, and ultimately its results on achieving established goals. A system that requires measures of performance is ultimately one in which goals are taken seriously.

The fourth element is an integrated health information system that reduces reporting burdens while providing participants with information to define health problems, assess performance, and take timely actions to protect and improve health. Clearly aimed at achieving efficiencies while enhancing effectiveness, this element recognizes the need to ensure that information systems are appropriate, nonduplicative, and of genuine assistance to all involved.

The fifth element, a properly educated, trained, and geographically distributed work force, is one for which national policies have been frequently unclear and contradictory. Certainly, one of the most important components of a functional health care system is a responsive work force. However, if the nation is to move its system of services into new, more appropriate ways of providing care, then policy must be used to shape a work force that is prepared and available to make such a system work.

The sixth element is support for health-related research, especially prevention research, health services research, behavioral and social science research, and epidemiologic research. As the changing health services system seeks to enhance its impact across all of the determinants of health, new knowledge about health and approaches to its enhancement must be developed. What this element means is that research cannot be an activity that is viewed somehow as apart from the delivery of services. Rather, research must be seen as the foundation of service delivery.

The seventh element is the organizational capacity to deliver coordinated, comprehensive health services to underserved populations. In the process of health system reform, careful attention must be paid to underserved populations and to ensuring that new categories of underserved populations do not emerge. Thus, design, delivery, and assessment of services must be based on the ability to serve all people adequately.

The eighth element, aimed at ensuring a strong foundation for the entire health care system, is developing a vital web of population-based, core public health functions that strengthen the capacity of the federal government, states, and communities to identify and address high priority health problems. This element both reaffirms the fundamental roles played by public health in the past and ensures that reform of the system is jump-started and guided by a vital public health infrastructure.

▀ COORDINATING PERSONAL AND PUBLIC HEALTH SYSTEMS

Application of the eight essential policy elements for health care necessarily focuses on three dimensions of the health care system: public health, personal care, and the interface and coordination between the two. While it is important to view each as a dimension of the overall system, they should also be understood within the context of public health—the entire system of personal health care services needs to be seen as resting firmly on the foundation of the public health infrastructure. Consequently, the public health system must be strengthened and redirected to give the providers of direct, personal care services the necessary critical support to protect and improve the public's health in a targeted, cost-effective manner. Clearly, specific systems changes must be made to coordinate the personal and public health systems as part of an overall strategy for achieving public health objectives.

Strengthening the Public Health System

To genuinely strengthen the public health system and its agencies, this nation will need to increase the investments it makes in three broad areas. First, increased investments must be made to provide both the knowledge-base (fundamental biomedical research, health services research, behavioral and social science research, epidemiologic research) to provide a properly educated and trained work force and the health information systems necessary to monitor the health status of the population, identify problems, and assess the performance of both the personal health care system and the public health system in achieving improved health outcomes in a cost effective manner.

The second area for increased investment in public health is removing barriers to care and facilitating the transition to a single-tier system in which all Americans have an adequate choice of culturally sensitive providers and health plans. Universal health insurance will not, in and of itself, guarantee that all Americans will have access to and receive necessary health care services. This limitation is particularly true for people living in rural areas; for the poor population in urban, inner-city areas; for disabled people; and for those who face language or other barriers to access. Policies to build the infrastructure needed to ensure access should include

- continuing current safety net programs in the early years of reform;
- increasing the supply of appropriately trained practitioners in rural and urban underserved areas;
- increasing the capacity to provide care through the development of community practice networks;

- providing federal support for enabling services such as transportation, translation, child care, and outreach;
- meeting the health needs of adolescents and young adults through school-based and school-linked programs; and
- providing funds to ensure that low-income, hard-to-reach individuals are made aware and take advantage of mental health and substance abuse treatment benefits, as well as other personal health services.

The third area for increased investment in public health is supporting population-based core public health functions that strengthen the capacity of the nation, states, and communities to identify and address high priority health problems. Emerging and existing health plans alone simply cannot be expected to contain their health care costs or address many of their enrollees' pressing health problems (eg, chronic disease, teenage pregnancy, lead poisoning, tobacco and drug abuse, and violence) unless the capability of state and local public health agencies to protect and improve the health of individuals in their communities is strengthened.

Public health agencies can support health plans and other providers in eight major ways:

1. Surveillance of communicable and chronic diseases will enable public health professionals to identify the magnitude, source, and trends of health problems so that they can direct the limited public health resources to populations at greatest risk.
2. Monitoring of communicable diseases, chronic diseases, and injuries ensures that public health agencies identify new problems early and that sources of infectious, environmental, or other exposure risks are removed.
3. Environmental protection safeguards the physical and social environment. For example, protecting the water and food supply, ensuring a safe workplace, and ensuring adequate housing all serve to protect against important causes of or contributions to disease.
4. Through public education and community mobilization, public health agencies can help prevent major causes of premature death and disability that are behavioral and societal.
5. Quality assurance activities protect consumers from medical and health services that do more harm to health than good. In addition, assurance activities enhance the likelihood of continuously improving health services.
6. Public health laboratory services can aid in the diagnosis of major infectious and environmental threats to health.
7. Through training and education of public health professionals, public health agencies ensure a work force capable of carrying out public health functions.
8. Leadership, policy development, and administration will enable public health agencies to set health objectives and to direct resources toward achieving those goals.

Strengthening the Personal Health System

The personal health care system must be moved into the larger framework of public health and population-based, systemwide approaches to services. Clearly, the achievement of universal coverage is a part of this approach. As part of this coverage, however, a greatly increased focus on health promotion, disease prevention, and early intervention should be incorporated throughout the system of services. All Americans should have access to comprehensive services, including clinical preventive services without deductibles or co-payments. To reinforce this orientation, health plans should receive a fixed, risk-adjusted annual premium to cover total patient care. These changes will alter the incentives in the health system and focus attention on outcomes and quality. To the extent enrollees are kept healthy, both health care costs paid by the plan and premiums paid by individuals and employers will be lower.

While fixed annual premiums can reward plans for keeping their populations healthy, they can also create incentives for plans to forgo providing necessary services, particularly to socioeconomically disadvantaged groups. To make sure consumers have access to the covered services, performance monitoring should hold health plans accountable. Performance monitoring should also focus attention on achieving healthy outcomes for enrollees and accomplishing population health goals. In addition, to enhance the ability of every consumer to make informed choices about his or her health provider and plan, report cards should be made available. Measures should include consumer satisfaction, access to care, appropriate use of medical care, and success in outcomes.

In addition to performance monitoring and report cards, to ensure that medical care is comprehensive and continuous, care should be provided, not so much by individual practitioners practicing in separate office-based practices on a fee-for-service basis, but by groups or networks of physicians working together with other health care professionals, including clinical advanced practice nurses, social workers, pharmacists, psychologists, dentists, physical and occupational therapists, and others. The approach should be that of teamwork and collaboration, ensuring that care is given by the most appropriate individuals, whether a neurosurgeon or a home health aide.

Performance monitoring and report cards, coupled with financing and payment system reforms, will reward health plans for keeping their populations well. Health plans will emphasize keeping people healthy and providing appropriate care for sick, injured, and disabled people. The nation should move away from a system based on insurers that simply pay bills for each medical service and sustain profits by selecting healthy enrollees to a system based on integrated personal health care delivery from plans that actively coordinate care and have the incentive to keep their enrolless healthy. By changing the incentive, health plans and public health agencies will have similar goals to protect and improve the health of their populations. With similar goals, increasingly close cooperation between the two should be evident.

Coordinating Personal Health Care and Public Health

By working closely with providers and health plans, public health agencies can be far more effective than they are now in achieving communitywide improvements in health. Health plans in states that are moving toward integrated health care systems, including Minnesota, Washington, and Hawaii, have already become advocates for public health agencies at the state and local levels. Common goals have been defined in a number of areas such as tobacco use, communicable disease control, chronic disease control, health education and community mobilization, maternal and child health, and reproductive health. In these areas public health agencies work through health plans to inform and educate individual patients and providers. In so doing, they reinforce the efforts of health plans and providers by protecting communities against environmental hazards, identifying and controlling community outbreaks of infectious diseases, and instituting communitywide education programs.

By providing the incentives to link public and personal health, health system reform can move the nation to a system that emphasizes primary, secondary, and tertiary prevention as well as treatment services. Emphasis will be on continuity and coordination of total patient care rather than on episodic, fragmented care provided by practitioners in independent practices. Populations, as well as individuals, will be considered patients. Both long-term and short-term objectives of a health system will be considered. And health professionals will work together as teams and be held responsible and accountable for keeping patients healthy. As these changes take place, health care costs will rise more slowly and resources will continue to be available to provide all medically necessary and appropriate care at the primary, secondary, and tertiary care levels. Consumer satisfaction and benefits will be maximized. The result will be a healthier population.

The health of every American is determined by many factors. These determinants are the foundation for a national health agenda and are crucial to developing cost-effective interventions. However, the health of the people will not be greatly improved without major attention to one key determinant: the system of health care. Of particular importance to this system is the public health infrastructure. Without a vital and broad-reaching infrastructure, attempts to improve the healthy life span of the American people simply will not succeed. National health goals, while crucial, are not enough. The challenge now and in the future of health system reform is to develop the national and state policy approaches that have been described. The outcome of such action will be a healthy future for the American public.

■ REFERENCES

1. *American Health Security Act of 1993.* Washington, DC: Bureau of National Affairs, Inc; 1993.
2. Smith DR. Porches, politics and public health. *Am J Public Health.* 1994;84:725–726.
3. Public Health Service, US Dept of Health, Education, and Welfare. *Healthy People: The Surgeon General's Report on Health Promotion and Disease Prevention.* Washington DC: US Dept of Health, Education, and Welfare; 1979. DHEW publication PHS 79-55071.

4. Public Health Service, US Dept of Health and Human Services. *Promoting Health, Preventing Disease: Objectives for the Nation.* Washington, DC: US Dept of Health and Human Services; 1991. DHHS publication PHS 91-50212.

5. Stewart A. Ware J. eds. *Measuring Functioning and Well-being: The Medical Outcomes Study Approach.* Durham, NC: Duke University Press; 1992.

6. World Health Organization. *Basic Documents.* 35th ed. Geneva. Switzerland: WHO; 1985.

7. Lalonde M. *A New Perspective on the Health of Canadians.* Ottawa, Ontario, Canada: Ministry of Health; 1974.

8. Dever GEA. Epidemiological model for health policy analysis. In: *Social Indicators Research.* Dordrecht, Holland: D. Reidel Publishing Co; 1976:2.

9. McGinnis J. Foege WH. Actual causes of death in the United States. *JAMA.* 1993;259:2207–2212.

10. Pubic Health Service, US Dept of Health and Human Services. *Healthy People 2000: National Health Promotion and Disease Prevention Objectives.* Washington, DC: Government Printing Office; 1991. DHHS publication PHS 91-50214.

11. Institute of Medicine. *The Future of Public Health.* Washington, DC: National Academy Press; 1988.

12. American Public Health Association. *Public Health in a Reformed Health Care System: A Vision for the Future.* Washington, DC: APHA; 1993.

13. Public Health Service, US Dept of Health and Human Services. *For a Healthy Nation: Returns on Investment in Public Health.* Washington, DC: US Dept of Health and Human Services; 1994.

14. Lee PR. Remarks presented at the 50th Anniversary Celebration of the 1944 Public Health Service Act; July 12, 1994; Washington, DC.

Chapter 2

A Personal Role
in Health Care Reform

C. EVERETT KOOP

As health care reform issues are debated and health system changes occur across the United States, health problems persist. Dr. C. Everett Koop, former Surgeon General of the United States, convincingly argues that problems in our society are major contributors to poor health. Among them he cites poverty, public apathy, the need for social justice, and the failure to practice preventive measures. This brief article provides a challenge to nurses and other health professionals to lead the way in reforming the health system to emphasize disease prevention and health promotion.

Following the failure of the Democrat-controlled Congress to enact significant health care reform legislation in 1994, and following the shift in political clout to the Republicans, the pundits have proclaimed that the great health care reform juggernaut has simply come to naught.

But that is not true. Congressional inaction notwithstanding, health care reform continues all across the country, in all sectors of the health care system. The federal government may have been done nothing, and state governments may have done little, but the private sector is reforming—even revolutionizing—health care every day. The countenance of medicine has been changed as insurance companies, health maintenance organizations, private practice physicians, nurses, health-care worker unions, hospitals, consumer advocates, drug companies, and a host of other vested interests fight furiously in a free-for-all struggle to come out on top. The patient may end up on the bottom.

Too much of the debate about health care reform has focused on questions of how we finance health care reform and on the economic and political dimensions of reform. This puts the cart before the horse. More important than the economic and political pressures is the ethical imperative for health care reform. We must realize that American health problems stem less from problems with our health care system that they do from problems in our society, especially the shameful prevalence of poverty in this rich country. In our efforts to provide health care for all Americans,

From *American Journal of Public Health* 85(6):759–780, 1995. Reprinted by permission of American Public Health Association.

we must remember that health care is not the same thing as health, and that health care expenditures that take away from our efforts to reduce overall poverty may not result in greater health.

All of us who are committed to enacting some form of comprehensive health care reform for all Americans face one big, simple problem: not all Americans want health care reform. In spite of all the talk about the need for health care reform, many Americans—maybe most Americans, that is, between 50% and 60% of our fellow citizens—have dug in their heels and said they do not want their own health care altered. National health care reform poses the greatest political challenge to a democratic republic because each of us is being asked to do something for all of us, and many of us feel that what might be best for all of us is not best for each of us. The challenge is simple. To meet and surmount it is not.

Before we can enact the sweeping reform we need in health care, we should agree on the basic values and ethics on which our health care system—and our society—is based and from which it derives its moral power. If we could reach an ethical consensus, many of the economic and political problems of health care reform would be solved easily.

At the heart of the ethical issues is the need for all of us, for each of us, to adopt the ethic of prevention in our personal lives and to encourage others to practice personal health promotion and disease prevention. We need a new American revolution, a revolution more important than the needed revolution in the structure of health care or in the financing of health care, a revolution that changes everyday individual behavior.

Some analysts claim that disease prevention and health promotion can postpone up to 70% of all premature deaths, whereas the traditional curative and reparative approach of medicine can postpone no more than 10% to 15% of such deaths. We incorrectly assume that high-tech medicine means high quality, when actually timely, low-tech, low-cost preventive measures can often do more to improve health and cut costs.

This is nothing new. Although in our day we have become accustomed to the dramatic life-saving miracles of high-tech medicine, our greatest strides in prolonging life have come not from medical miracles of the late 20th century, but from the public health accomplishments of the late 19th and early 20th centuries: vaccination and safer water, food, and housing. The great killers of humanity for most of our history, infectious diseases, have largely been eliminated, with some significant exceptions, such as acquired immunodeficiency syndrome (AIDS).

Throughout history, most premature deaths came from things people did not choose—work, war, and infectious disease—but now the old epidemics of infectious disease have been replaced by new epidemics of self-induced degenerative disease. Now, most premature deaths come from choices people make, from recreational accidents, from highway accidents without seat belts, from smoking, drinking, and poor choices in diet and exercise.

In other words, diseases are of two types: those we develop inadvertently and those we bring upon ourselves by failure to practice preventive measures. Preventable illness makes up approximately 70% of the burden of illness and associated costs. This has major implications for our debate on health care reform and for the use of our health care resources.

A recent study attributed the leading causes of death in the United States to only three factors: tobacco, diet and activity patterns, and alcohol.[1] Of total deaths in 1990 (n = 1,083,000), half were caused by nine factors: tobacco (18%), diet and activity patterns (13%), alcohol (4%), microbial agents (4%), toxic agents (3%), motor vehicles (2%), firearms (2%), sexual behavior (1%), and illicit use of drugs (1%). Other risk factors linked with death were poverty and lack of access to primary care. In other words, many of the reasons for death, especially premature death, are largely preventable.

True, we have made some strides in health promotion, as in the anti-smoking campaign, in which the percentage of the adult smoking population has declined from over 50% in 1964 to 25% in 1992. (However, it has jumped back up to 30%, with the tobacco companies mounting a new offensive.) And although many Americans seem to be more concerned about diet and exercise, the portion of the population reaping the rewards of that concern is rather small: more than 33% of Americans are overweight. We also now have hard evidence that being overweight is a leading contributor to disease and premature death.

The plain fact is that we Americans do a better job of preventive maintenance on our cars than on ourselves. (And we do not expect our car insurance to cover preventive maintenance on our cars.)

The needed emphasis on the ways that low-tech health promotion can prevent the need for high-tech medicine does not mean that we should assume a Luddite stance against technology. On the contrary, cutting-edge technology, especially in communication and information transfer, will enable the greatest advances yet in public health. Real health care reform will come only from demand reduction, as individuals learn to take charge of their health. Communication technology can work wonders for us in this vital endeavor. Eventually, personal home telemedicine links could provide every home with access to health information 24 hours a day, 7 days a week, encouraging personal wellness and prevention, and leading to better informed decisions about health care. A generation of children raised on video games will probably be more attuned to health messages coming from interactive videos than from lectures by the school nurse.

High-tech medical communication can join the public health campaigns with the practice of medicine, as high-performance computers, high-resolution television and video, and fiber-optic information pathways can put the entire world of medical science at the fingertips of even the most isolated rural family doctor. By linking telecommunication technology with medical education, health care reform, and personal health promotion, we can use high-tech methods to provide the low-tech and personal kind of health care and health we all enjoy. Although we have good reason to view costly high-tech medical gadgetry as a major cause of escalating health care costs, we can make high-tech cut the other way by investing dollars wisely in medical information technology that will provide better and more accessible health care at a lower cost for all of us. This will be true population medicine.

During the course of the last year's intensive debate about health care reform, I was dismayed by how little the health professions were able to make their voices heard. Too often, members of the health professions simply reacted to proposals advanced by political policymakers. We in the health professions need to assume a greater role of leadership, on the local level and on the national level, in forging the future of health care in the United States, and we need to improve the interface between public health and medicine. Those of us in public health know the importance of social justice in health care, and we need to ensure that social justice be part of any reform of the health care system.

The failure of Congress to pass sweeping health care reform legislation has provided us with a new opportunity to regroup, rethink, and revitalize our vision for a health care system, a health care system that starts with disease prevention and health promotion, a health care system that truly improves the health of the American people, rather than one that merely reacts to their diseases.

▬ REFERENCE

1. McGinnis JM, Foege WH. Actual causes of death in the United States. *JAMA.* 1993;270:2207–2212.

Chapter 3

Sensitizing Nurses for a Changing Environmental Health Role

LINDA BETH TIEDJE AND JOAN WOOD

> A fact often minimized in the delivery of health services is the impact of the environment on people's health. Important factors such as clean air, clean water, safe food, adequate housing, proper waste disposal, and many more make up the field of environmental health which is a crucial part of public health practice. In this chapter Drs. Tiedje and Wood describe the expanding role that community health nursing needs to play in promoting environmental health and thus the health of communities. They discuss seven key strategies that are included in nursing's role in environmental health.

■ BACKGROUND AND SIGNIFICANCE

Person, environment, health, and nursing generally are agreed upon as being the relevant phenomena for the discipline of nursing (Fawcett, 1995). The importance of environment, in particular, has been emphasized since Nightingale (1859) as a central tenet in community health nursing (see also Salmon's public health nursing model in White, 1982). Texts in community health nursing have reconceptualized the narrow traditional environmental focus from air, water, sewage, and restaurant inspection to an enlarged focus on the health effects of exposure to environmental pollutants and of global environmental change (Stanhope & Lancaster, 1992; Clemen-Stone, Eigsti, & McGuire, 1994; Clark, 1992; Wold, 1990). Environmental health is one of the 21 priority areas for the year 2000 health objectives (U.S. Public Health Service, 1990). This evolved focus on the environment also reflects the growing proportional contribution to mortality by environmental factors, which was estimated at 15%–20% in 1985 (Yoder, Jones, & Jones, 1985). Recent studies examining the relationship of pesticides in the environment to breast cancer provide evidence of a substantial link between environment and health (NCI, 1994). Indeed, environment may be the "single most important determi-

From *Public Health Nursing* 12(6):356–365, 1995. Reprinted by permission of Blackwell Scientific Publications, Inc.

nant of health in the very near future" (Salmon & Vanderbush, 1991, p. 173).

As textbooks have enlarged the focus of the environmental health role for nurses, the practice of nursing in the past several decades has also slowly changed, especially in the recognition and treatment of toxic exposures (Worthington & Cary, 1993). Yet to be explored in practice is the part of the role dealing with larger ecological phenomena, such as ozone depletion and climate change. Nursing education, in varying degrees, has responded by including broader environmental issues in coursework for community health nursing. Community health nursing educators are in a unique position to sensitize students to this evolving environmental role put forth in texts and partially practiced. Nurses as citizens and professionals are also in a unique position to incorporate the broader, evolved environmental role in their lives and practices.

The purpose of this paper is to: 1) review the changing role of environmental health as reflected in selected community health nursing texts over the past several decades; 2) examine the implementation of an expanded role for the community health nurse in promoting environmental health; and 3) describe a survey used to facilitate sensitization to this broader environmental role.

▬ THE COMMUNITY HEALTH NURSE
AND ENVIRONMENTAL HEALTH

The history of community health nursing is replete with references to the significance of the role of the community health nurse in the identification and resolution of environmental issues. Florence Nightingale (1859) was the first nurse to identify the role of the environment in influencing health. She also provided environmental strategies to be implemented by nurses based on physical elements affecting health such as unsanitary environmental conditions. By the late 1800s and the early parts of this century environmental issues of particular interest were typically those related to communicable disease control, improper food handling, inadequate sanitary disposal, and unsafe water supplies. By the late 1970s, due in part to a growing environmental consciousness that culminated in Earth Day, 1972, this biological/microbial perspective had broadened significantly to include physical hazards (radiation, lead, and noise) and chemical hazards (poisons and air pollution). The evolution of these environmental issues is reflected in community health nursing texts.

Thirty years ago Freeman's text (1963) defined environment in terms of location: family, work, school, and the community. All environments included aspects of protection from dangerous dusts or fumes, extremes of temperature or noise, communicable diseases, and insurance of water supplies, waste disposal, fire, and accidental hazards. In general, this conceptualization of environment continued until approximately five years ago when an expanded concept of the environment as the total habitat including the economy and society began to emerge (Wold, 1990). One of the precipitating factors in these expansion of the definition was the increase in chronic diseases, which required recognition of environmental factors as etiological—e.g., environmental carcinogens/toxins, altered food systems, and undesirable climatic changes.

In Spradley's text (1991), environmental preservation was advanced as a significant health care issue and a trend of global magnitude. Environmental issues of concern to community health nurses were expanded to include "the disposal of hazardous waste; acid rain; urban lead poisoning; inadequate solid waste disposal; noise pollution; air pollution; and water pollution" (p. 173). More global concerns included ozone depletion and the threat of thermonuclear war. Finally, by 1992, Stanhope and Lancaster presented the environment from a more ecological perspective as a "multi-faceted system made up of biophysical and sociocultural components" (p. 295). They further posited that the interaction between people and environment enhanced the well-being of both.

Three texts have identified categories of specific environmental hazards (Clark, 1992; Stanhope & Lancaster, 1992; Swanson & Albrecht, 1993). While there was some overlapping of items included in the categories, there was no universal consensus on what qualified as an environmental hazard. Biological, physical, and chemical were the most widely identified categories of environmental hazards. Stanhope and Lancaster also identified a psychosocial category and Swanson and Albrecht (1993) included the not previously mentioned categories of work risks, living patterns, housing, and violence risks.

In summary, it is evident that within the past five years a broader conceptualization of the scope of environmental issues is being reflected in community health nursing texts. Although the organizational framework used by the authors of these texts may differ, the authors agree that environmental threats to health and survival come primarily from two sources: 1) toxins or carcinogens posing immediate health risks; and 2) global hazards resulting from ozone depletion and climate changes posing larger ecological risks. The texts also maintain that global ecological risks pose threats in two areas: health effects and ultimate survival. For example, ozone depletion ultimately affects health by associated increases in skin cancer and glaucoma rates. Another ecological risk, global climate change, affects ultimate survival through food shortages resulting when fertile farmland is reduced to a desert environment (Harriss, 1989; Prinn, 1994; Vitousek, 1994).

▄ NURSING'S ROLE

A sampling of several community health nursing texts (Benson & McDevitt, 1980; Clark, 1992; Clemen-Stone et al., 1994; Freeman, 1963; Hall & Weaver, 1977; Hanchett, 1988; Saucier, 1991; Spradley, 1991; Stanhope & Lancaster, 1992; Swanson & Albrecht, 1993; Wold, 1990) reveals varying degrees of emphasis on the role of the nurse in the identification and reduction of environmental risks and hazards. In general, texts printed prior to the 1980s focused primarily on describing the nurse's role in educating the public to deter the transmission of communicable diseases through the securing of immunizations and the proper handling and storage of food. Also stressed was assessment for appropriate waste disposal and the case-finding and follow-up of children with high lead levels. Clark (1992) and Stanhope and Lancaster (1992) further refined environmental assessment, proposing two aspects: 1) examination of the existence of a hazard; and 2) determination of the effects of the hazard on the individual, family, group, or community. In addition to education and assessment, Freeman (1963) extended the nurse's role to the work place as one of enforcing safety rules and regulations and insuring the use of safety devices. Finally, prior to the 1980s the environmental nursing role was primarily linked with sanitation or public health engineers (Freeman, 1963). Although this linkage continues to be important, today's nurse has a more autonomous role in environmental health.

Spradley (1991) expanded the education and assessment role, contending that nurses must also take the initiative to educate themselves about the environment. Formal and continuing education is essential with environmental data, as research is constantly generating new information. To this end, the Nurses Environmental Healthwatch provides updated environmental information for nurses (Swanson & Albrecht, 1993). Formal education on environmental health across the country (e.g., curriculum and student clinical experiences) has not been surveyed.

The role of the nurse in environmental health legislation was described most clearly by Clemen-Stone et al. (1994) and Swanson and Albrecht (1993). Being informed about legislation because of its potential impact on natural resources and working with the public to implement more stringent environmental legislation are two role strategies proposed. Spradley further maintained that nurses must be participants in environmental policy debates integral to regulation formulation.

Although Saucier (1991) included chapters that described the role of the nurse in occupational and school health, reference to the role of the nurse in broader environmental issues was included in the chapter on leadership and change by Salmon and Vanderbush (1991), who concluded that "the nursing literature on environmental health and the role of . . . nurses . . . is alarmingly sparse" (p. 173).

Swanson and Albrecht (1993) added a critical process component to the nurse's role in environmental health. They argued that the nurse must involve the community in defining environmental issues, "listening to what the community defines as problematic and helping to raise consciousness about environmental danger" (p. 569). They proposed that this community involvement process was essential in bringing about change.

In summary, the new broader nursing role in environmental health is both proactive (primary prevention) and reactive (after the problem exists). The nursing role in environmental health includes seven key strategies (ICN, 1990): 1) to assess and detect hazards when they exist; 2) to provide information to individuals and aggregates on the health effects of environmental toxins and more global hazards; 3) to report serious environmental threats to appropriate agencies; 4) to develop and implement school based and work site wellness programs; 5) to aid in the formulation of public policy and legislation involving the environment; 6) to help prevent excessive exposure to immediate toxins and larger, global hazards; and 7) to help facilitate behavior change in people. Behavior changes related to the environment, such as using mass transit, recycling, and planting CO_2-absorbing trees, superficially seem less directly related to human health than do behavior changes nurses are more accustomed to facilitating, e.g., encouraging clients to exercise or to adopt low-sodium diets. However, behavior changes related to broader environmental issues ultimately affect human health and survival as well (see Table 3-1 for examples of these environmental role strategies). Finally, role strategies of the CHN involve *working with* 1) the community residents, 2) experts like environmental sanitarians, and 3) policymakers.

TABLE 3-1   Environmental Health: Community Health Nursing's Role

TYPE OF STRATEGY	EXAMPLE
Assess and detect hazards	Furnace fumes (CO) and ill child Cyanosis in infants and need for water testing Lack of curbside recycling in neighborhoods Detection of lead in environment
Provide information to individuals/groups	Disposal of paint and other chemicals CFCs[a] and ozone depletion
Report environmental threats to proper agency	Industrial air pollutions Improper auto air conditioning disposal (CFCs)
Occupational health nursing[b]	School and work site wellness programs
Public policy and legislation	Write position papers Write letters and testify at hearings
Help prevent exposure and causes of exposure	Protection of asthmatics from air pollution Smoking cessation programs for parents
Facilitate behavior change related to environment	Self-assessment Self-awareness Change self Enable change in others

[a]Chlorofluorocarbons.
[b]In occupational health nursing there are currently 14 centers, sites of graduate and continuing education programs (Worthington & Cary, 1993).

■ THE EVOLVING ENVIRONMENTAL ROLE IN COMMUNITY HEALTH NURSING PRACTICE

Although a broader role for nursing that includes relating to the environment is evolving, the actual practice of this role is only partial. Nurses have begun to address the health risks of environmental carcinogens and toxins, by, for example, assessing for lead and radon exposure and identifying the effect of air pollution on asthma prevalence (Cartmel, Loescher, & Villar-Werstler, 1992; Worthington & Cary, 1993). Harder to address are the global ecological hazards affecting human survival. These ecological hazards are harder to address in part because they are so large and far removed and in part because they are rooted in recalcitrant human behaviors. For example, the behavior changes needed to reverse global climate change include decreasing automobile use, which is neither convenient, pleasing, nor profitable (see Stern, 1993 for an overview of human behavioral causes of environmental change). The belief has persisted that global environmental hazards could be reduced with bigger and better technological interventions. But "technology has limitations" (Wold, 1990). Even though "much of the public believes the causes—even the existence—of global change to be uncertain and contentious topics," there are specific, scientifically established components of global environmental change (Vitousek, 1994, p. 1862). The causes of environmental problems like deforestation, loss of biodiversity, pollution, climate change, and ozone depletion are rooted in human behaviors (National Research Council, 1992). Further, scientists suggest that the time for altering the course of climate change and global environmental hazards is growing short (Brussard, 1992) and that the next one hundred years may be one of the most dangerous periods of the environment since the origin of life on earth (Weiner, 1990). In summary, the challenge is for the practice of nursing to change to be congruent with a role already reconceptualized in texts—a role which addresses health risks from environmental toxins and global ecological hazards.

■ A SENSITIZING SURVEY

The survey described here can be used to sensitize either students or practicing nurses to the new and broader environmental health role described above. Use of the survey can help move the nurse from a passive observer to an active participant in this expanded role through the assessment of her/his environmental attitudes and behaviors. Using awareness of her/his attitudes and behaviors, the nurse can then focus on her/his professional role in creating attitude and behavior change in clients and communities.

Because generally people view environmental issues as external, they are passive observers and not active participants in environmental activities. This makes them more susceptible to inappropriate apathy and anxiety in responding to environmental risks (McCallum, Hammond, & Covello, 1991). The survey potentially is a vehicle for personalizing and internalizing environmental issues. Once nurses or nursing students have assessed their attitudes and behaviors and have put themselves in the role of client/citizen/consumer, they become more self-aware. They may even attempt needed behavior changes in recycling or mass transit use and thus better anticipate problems others may have in making changes for the environment. Such self-assessment potentially creates empathy and a more open-minded attitude toward environmental behaviors. In summary, the survey provides for self-assessment of environmental attitudes and behaviors, creates self-awareness, and potentiates personal behavior change and an appreciation for needed environmental behavior changes in individuals and communities (see work of Langer, 1989 on the ways in which helping professionals must change personal perceptions of behavior before expecting change in others).

The survey described here was used as a means of introducing the broader environmental role to senior nursing students enrolled in a community health nursing course. The 29 questions addressed: 1) attitudes about the environment; 2) attitudes about environmental regulations; 3) specific behaviors underlying environmental problems; and 4) intentions related to cleaning up the environment (see Table 3-2 for selected questions from the survey). The survey was based on an environmental poll conducted in March, 1990 by the Gordon S. Black Corporation among a nationwide sample of 850 adults (Kalette, 1990).

One hundred students completed the survey over six terms (1990–1992), a number which largely reflects the number of students present at

TABLE 3-2   Selected Questions from the Environmental Survey[a]

CATEGORY	QUESTION[b]
Attitude	People in the United States contribute more to pollution than people in other parts of the world. The environment can be kept clean and safe without making drastic changes in lifestyle. There is not much one person can do to help the environment.
Regulations	I favor mandatory recycling of newspapers, bottles and cans. How do you feel about regulations that would require us to use mass transit and limit the use of cars?
Behaviors	How often do you use mass transit (bus, train, etc.)? I recycle newspapers, bottles or cans. I turn off water when brushing my teeth.
Intentions	I would be willing to pay 15% more for groceries if they were packaged for recycled use. I would be willing to pay an additional 15% in taxes to reduce pollution significantly. I would be willing to pay $50 more per month for electricity.

[a]Questions did not appear by category on the survey.
[b]Response to questions were either Likert or True/False in format. Response format is not included here due to space limitations.

lecture (100) vs. the number of students enrolled in the course (144), for a 69% response rate. The survey was done in class before the environmental health lecture. The lecturer was the same and instructions were given identically at all six administrations of the survey.

The students ranged in age from 20 to 45 years with 83% between 20 and 23 years of age. Students were mainly from a large urban area adjacent to a state university in the Midwest. Survey responses were examined according to age and year of enrollment in the class. No differences were noted, so data described are for the total group of students. The survey was not given again as a post-test after instruction.

Although the survey was a sensitizing strategy and not a research survey, it soon was evident from the students' in-class discussion that the survey enabled students to see connections between their attitudes and behaviors, as well as to reflect on the relationship between their attitudes and behaviors and those of the residents in the communities in which they would reside and practice. In addition, the survey results revealed the collective position of the participating students on environmental issues, which will be reported here.

Hazardous waste (85% of students said this was a concern to them), landfills (58%), and acid rain (47%) do not appear on the Environmental Protection Agency (EPA) list of most important environmental concerns (Reilly, 1990). Further, global warming and climate change, prominent on the EPA list, were low on the list of student concerns (44%) (see Table 3-3). This student survey is but one example of conflicting perspectives between the lay public and professional environmental scientists on how to

TABLE 3-3   Environmental Concerns

EPA'S TOP CONCERNS[a] (NOT IN RANK ORDER)	STUDENT CONCERNS (IN RANK ORDER) $N = 100$
Ecological Risks Global climate change Stratospheric ozone depletion Habitat alteration Species extinction and biodiversity loss **Health Risks** Criteria air pollutants (e.g., smog) Toxic air pollutants (e.g., benzene) Radon Indoor air pollution Drinking-water contamination Occupational exposure to chemicals Application of pesticides Stratospheric ozone depletion	1. Water pollution (85%) 2. Hazardous waste (82%) 3. Ozone (73%) 4. Cancer-causing materials in the environment (64%) 5. Air pollution (63%) 6. Landfills (58%) 7. Wilderness (disappearance) (56%) 8. Rainforests (disappearance) (51%) 9. Acid rain (47%) 10. Global warming (44%)

[a]From Reilly (1990).

interpret environmental threats (Brown, 1992). This incongruity troubles scientists, especially because of lay people's influence on public policy. This is of concern to scientists who typify the last 20 years of federal policy-making as piecemeal, because politicians respond to ever-changing public concerns rather than to input from the scientific community on environmental risks. Since the political process in the United States is in part a response of politicians to constituents and special interest groups, the need to educate students and practicing nurses on environmental concerns based on scientific data is especially important.

Students in general were very concerned about the environment and believed that the United States contributes to pollution more than does the rest of the world. But they generally engaged in non-environment-friendly behaviors, e.g., rarely using campus mass transit. Further, they were reluctant to change their behaviors and believed their environment could be clean and safe without such changes. These attitude and behavior discrepancies are familiar to health care providers and are important in understanding keys to behavior change (for further reading in attitudes intention, and behavior connections see Fishbein & Ajzen, 1975).

▬CONCLUSION

This paper has traced a reconceptualized version of the environment in community health nursing and a strategy used to sensitize students and, potentially, other health care providers about that evolving environmental role. Implications for research indicate post-testing to examine whether students and other nurses exposed to the survey altered their personal behaviors or performed differently in their professional environmental role.

Practicing nurses are only beginning to address health risks related to toxic environmental exposures for their clients and communities. The evolving role of the community health nurse addresses health risks from environmental exposures and global ecological changes, as well as needed behavior changes. Enlarging the vision of practitioners of this reconceptualized role is essential. This paper is a beginning step in that direction.

▬ACKNOWLEDGMENTS

The first author gratefully acknowledges the assistance of the Social Science Research Institute (SSRI) at the University of Hawaii provided during a recent sabbatical while this manuscript was being prepared.

The authors wish to thank Barbara Given, R.N., Ph.D., FAAN, Suzanne Budd, R.N., Ph.D., and Rachel Schiffman, R.N., Ph.D. for their helpful comments on an earlier version of this manuscript.

▬REFERENCES

Benson, E.R., & McDevitt, J.Q. (1980). *Community health and nursing practice* (2nd ed.). Englewood Cliffs, NJ: Prentice-Hall Inc.

Brown, P. (1992). Popular epidemiology and toxic waste contamination: lay and professional ways of knowing. *Journal of Health and Social Behavior, 33,* 267–281.

Brussard, P.F. (1992). Book review. *Science. 258,* 1506.

Cartmel, B., Loescher, L., & Villar-Werstler, P. (1992). Professional and consumer concerns about the environment, lifestyle, and cancer. *Seminars in Oncology Nursing, 8* (1), 20–29.

Clark, M.J. (1992). *Nursing in the community.* Norwalk, Conn.: Appleton & Lange.

Clemen-Stone, S., Eigsti, D.G., & McGuire, S.L. (1994). *Comprehensive family and community health nursing.* St. Louis: Mosby Year Book.

Fawcett, J. (1995). *Analysis and evaluation of conceptual models of nursing* (3rd ed.). Philadelphia, Penn.: F.A. Davis.

Fishbein, M., & Ajzen, I. (1975). *Belief, attitude, intention, and behavior: an introduction to theory and research.* Reading, Mass.: Addison-Wesley.

Freeman, R. (1963). *Public health nursing practice* (3rd ed.). Philadelphia, Penn.: W.B. Saunders.

Hall, J.E., & Weaver, B.R. (1977). *Distributive nursing practice: a systems approach to community health.* Philadelphia, Penn.: J.B. Lippincott.

Hanchette, E.S. (1988). *Nursing and frameworks: community as client.* Norwalk, Conn.: Appleton & Lange.

Harriss, R.C. (1989). Experimental design for studying atmosphere-biosphere interactions. In M.O. Andreae & D.S. Schimel (Eds.). *Exchange of trace gases between terrestrial ecosystems at the atmosphere* (pp. 291–301). Chichester, England: John Wiley & Sons.

International Council of Nurses. (1990). *Nurses and the environment.* Geneva, Switzerland: International Council of Nurses.

Kalette, D. (1990, April 13). Poll finds waste fears are piling up. *USA Today,* 10a.

Langer, E. (1989). *Mindfulness.* Reading, Mass.: Addison-Wesley.

McCallum, D.B., Hammond, S.L., & Covello, V.T. (1991). Communicating about environmental risks: how the public uses and perceives information sources. *Health Education Quarterly, 18* (3), 349–361.

National Cancer Institute. (1994). *The Northeast/Mid-Atlantic Study: cancer facts.* Washington, D.C.: National Institute of Health.

National Research Council. (1992). *Global environmental change: the human dimensions.* Washington, D.C.: National Academy Press.

Nightingale, F. (1859). *Notes on nursing: what it is and what it is not.* London: Harrison. Reprint ed., Philadelphia, Penn.: J.B. Lippincott, 1946.

Prinn, R.G. (1994). The interactive atmosphere; global atmospheric-biospheric chemistry. *Ambio, 23*(1), 50–61.

Reilly, W. (1990). Counting on science in EPA. *Science, 249,* 616.

Salmon, M.L., & Vanderbush, P. (1991). Leadership and change in public and community health nursing today. The essential intervention. In K.A. Saucier (Ed.). *Perspectives in family and community health* (pp. 169–175). St. Louis: Mosby Year Book.

Saucier, K.A. (1991). *Perspectives in family and community health.* St. Louis: Mosby Year Book.

Spradley, B.W. (1991). *Readings in community health nursing* (4th ed.). Philadelphia, Penn.: J.B. Lippincott.

Stanhope, M., & Lancaster, J. (1992). *Community health nursing: process and practice for promoting health* (3rd ed.). St. Louis: Mosby Year Book.

Stern, P.C. (1993). A second environmental science: human-environment interactions, *Science, 260,* 1897–1899.

Swanson, J.M., & Albrecht, M. (1993). *Community health nursing: promoting the health of aggregates.* Philadelphia: W.B. Saunders.

U.S. Public Health Service. (1990). *Healthy people 2000.* Washington, D.C.: Author.

Vitousek, P.M. (1994). Beyond global warming: ecology and global change. *Ecology, 75*(7), 1861–1876.

Weiner, J. (1990). *The next 100 years: shaping the fate of our living earth.* New York: Bantam.

White, M.S. (1982). Constructs for public health nursing. *Nursing Outlook, 30,* 527–530.

Wold, S.J. (1990). *Community health nursing: issues and topics.* Norwalk, Conn.: Appleton & Lange.

Worthington, K., & Cary, A. (1993). Primary health care: environmental challenges. *The American Nurse, 25*(10), 10–11.

Yoder, L.E., Jones, S.L., & Jones, P.K. (1985). The association between health care behavior and attitudes. *Health Values, 9*(4), 24–31.

Chapter 4

HIV/AIDS: An Imperative for a New Paradigm for Caring

MARY BOOSE WALKER AND LINDA FRANK

A major threat to the public's health and therefore of great concern to community health nurses is the epidemic of HIV/AIDS. As the disease spreads and remains without cure, Drs. Walker and Frank in this chapter eloquently argue for revolutionary new perspectives and creative solutions in health services. They call for a shift to a new community-based paradigm in which communities are acknowledged as resources and partners in service and nurses actively collaborate with community members and professionals to address the epidemic. They describe steps that must be taken in both nursing education and practice to operationalize the paradigm of caring with community as partner.

Cindy is a young mother with acquired immunodeficiency syndrome (AIDS), infected by her now-deceased, drug-injecting husband. She is dying and afraid: not only of pain and death, but for her soon-to-be-orphaned children who are affected but not infected.

HIV/AIDS is a global epidemic for which there is not yet a cure, only care (Wardrop, 1993). Worldwide, 40 million people will be infected with HIV by the year 2000, and over a million people in the United States will have AIDS (Center for Disease Control, 1992). Women are the fastest growing population of people with HIV disease, which disproportionately affects those from racial and ethnic minorities and from economically disadvantaged backgrounds. By the turn of the century, as many as 126,000 American children may be motherless because of this one disease: AIDS (Collins, 1994).

The HIV/AIDS epidemic has been described as three distinct, yet intertwined challenges: infection with HIV; the disease AIDS; and the social, cultural, political, and economic responses to HIV/AIDS (Wardrop, 1993; Zerwekh, 1992). Its visibility and urgency compel nursing to address all three simultaneously. Providing expert care within the context of these challenges should be one of the highest priorities for the nursing profession as it plans for health care and nursing reform. It is also a formidable task.

From *N&HC: Perspectives on Community* 16(6):310–315. Reprinted with permission. Copyright 1995 National League for Nursing.

"We all have AIDS" is more than a political slogan (Fedor, 1992, p. 65): AIDS has permeated every aspect of our world—political, social, economic, cultural, and educational—to become part of the fabric of contemporary society. HIV/AIDS is rapidly changing our world even as the nursing profession is engaged in conversations for its transformation to a community-based care paradigm—including the inevitable changes in education associated with it (deTornyay, 1992; Shoultz, Hatcher, & Hurrell, 1992; Tri-Council for Nursing, 1991). But nursing is not alone in facing this lethal epidemic; other disciplines are also realizing that the preparation of health care practitioners for the future begins with today's reality—a future with HIV/AIDS. Even now, as those conversations occur and questions are asked about the necessary skills and competencies needed for community-focused practice in the next millennium (Shugars, O'Neil, & Bader, 1991), nursing no longer has the luxury of pondering evolutionary perspectives. Cindy and her children, representing this high-stakes threat to global health, have arrived at the table, demanding revolution, not evolution. Caring for them has highlighted every imaginable deficiency in the present health care delivery systems, which are based upon treatment and cure. It has also highlighted our antiquated educational systems (Shoultz et al., 1993; Wardrop, 1993; Frank & Walker, 1993). Fedor (1993) further reminds us that, by merely tinkering with present systems, we are basing our reforms on a past that no longer exists. Although progress has been made over the past decade toward understanding the epidemiology of HIV/AIDS and its clinical management, there remains no cure. It is our contention that a commitment is essential now to prepare practitioners for a world with HIV/AIDS.

The HIV/AIDS epidemic is forcing nursing care and education to have greater relevance to societal needs, requiring that nursing recognize diversity in both caregivers and those for whom they care. It calls upon nursing to engage directly in the health problems of both individuals and defined populations, including those women like Cindy, who are hopeless, vulnerable, disenfranchised, and often marginalized (Lacey, 1993). It also presents nursing with a unique opportunity to address reform in bold, new ways, to move beyond the existing paradigms for care and education, and to acknowledge that those like Cindy (who are living with the epidemic) are not only consumers of care, but also expert partners in caring.

Khun (1970) has posited that the paradigm is a central concept of scientific progress and that paradigm shifts are scientific revolutions. While he applied the concept to the natural sciences, it is valid today for nursing reform, since a shift of the magnitude demanded by HIV/AIDS calls for revolutionary new perspectives and creative solutions. Public health, epidemiology, and nursing paradigms must be blended into a new metaparadigm for health (Clark, Beddone, & Whyte, 1993). Links must be forged among health care professionals, faculty, students, and communities. These links must cross boundaries: historical, institutional, cultural, professional, and national. For, as Moccia (1992) and Reverby (1993) have reminded us, boundaries of fear and ignorance, traditional power and authority relationships between patients and providers, individuals and nations must be obliterated if we are to form the new connections and linkages needed for finding creative solutions. Above all, new ways of preparing tomorrow's practitioners must always be framed in the language of caring (Tri-Council for Nursing, 1991).

To that end, in a quest to articulate new and emerging knowledge and meaning relative to HIV/AIDS, a statewide Nursing Faculty Institute was developed by the Pennsylvania AIDS Education and Training Center (PA AIDS ETC), one of 17 federally funded programs charged with preparing practicing primary care practitioners (nurses, physicians, and dentists, among others) for the management of HIV disease in all its dimensions and complexities (Frank, et al., 1993). The Institute is an endeavor directed at preparing faculty now by providing them with research-based knowledge while awakening them to the realities of HIV/AIDS practice and its curriculum implications in the face of consumer needs and demands. It is an effective forum for sharing "stories from the field" and the lessons they teach, as well as for moving beyond ad hoc change by isolated faculty to a collective, creative response to HIV disease now and in the future.

■HOW WILL COMMUNITY-BASED CARE PARADIGMS PROVIDE THE NECESSARY CHANGE?

Globally, the focus of health care over the past decade has undergone important changes—a topic of great interest to nursing, as it has planned its own response to meeting the needs of a rapidly changing world. The major elements of primary care, initially defined in 1978 by the Alma-Ata Conference as "Health for All, 2000" (World Health Organization, 1978a, b), have been reaffirmed. The Canadian approach to achieving "health for all" was to focus on the public health through health promotion and disease prevention initiatives (Labonte, 1987), while the United States' intent to change the acute care dominated medical paradigm to one where primary health care is a priority was articulated in the federal mandate *Healthy People 2000* (U.S. Department of Health and Human Services, 1991). The goal is to improve the health of individuals and populations, not just to improve health care delivery (World Health Organization, 1978a, b). All of these commitments point to a global health care paradigm shift to one that is community-based and oriented to health promotion and disease prevention, providing a balance to technological advances directed at cure. But with the newest epidemic, there is no cure, so how will community-based care paradigms provide the necessary change? Communities must be acknowledged as resources and partners in care and nursing must actively collaborate with all its sectors as well as other health care professionals if we are to overcome barriers to addressing this lethal global epidemic in all its dimensions. Shoultz et al., (1992) remind us that the health of the nation stems from the health of communities, and therefore, the health of communities as well as individuals must be addressed. This reasoning holds true for HIV/AIDS. There will need to be emphasis on promoting the public health through identification of risk factors in the social and physical environment, promotion of health, and teaching of disease prevention in addition to knowledge of epidemiology, the management of chronic illness and disabilities within the context of HIV infection and, finally, the acute, life threatening illness AIDS. Furthermore, care will need to be reconceptualized to accommodate sensitivity to alternative lifestyles and culturally diverse practices and customs in the new global arena. There will be informed consumer participation in shared decision making at both the individual and aggregate levels, with care delivered by multidisciplinary teams in nontraditional sites. Care delivery, including different ways to accommodate or maintain health, will move outside the walls of institutions with emphasis on cost-effective, coordinated, high quality, comprehensive, and accessible services for the consumer, delivered by practitioners sensitive to the needs of diverse populations (deTornyay, 1992; Hegyvary, 1992; Leininger, 1994). HIV/AIDS—the wild card introduced into an already turbulent health care reform environment—will demand ingenious responses, for its problems are complex, the ground is less familiar, and the answers must be found within the larger societal context.

As problems highlighted by the three challenges of HIV/AIDS are identified and addressed, recurring questions imbedded in them swirl around a central issue: How do we ready nurses for practice in the world of today where vulnerable populations, including those with HIV/AIDS, are not being adequately cared for, and at the same time prepare for the practice of a tomorrow with massive global populations infected with HIV, whose needs are not yet clear? The emerging call is to fundamentally change how we prepare nurses—for reappraisal of not only technical skills and role preparation, but also of attitudes, values, and the needed analytical skills. Directions for change will be dichotomous. While great knowledge and technical competence will always be required in dealing with individual patients who are critically and terminally ill with AIDS, nurses also need to be prepared for roles that address the welfare of the aggregate. Neither direction can be ignored. Nurses must function in concert with those in the fields of public policy, business, and social welfare, as well as medicine and public health, tempering stark realities with humanity: Where previously, nurses rarely dealt with orphaned children either in acute care or community settings, they will in the future seek solutions to potentially staggering numbers of children worldwide who have been orphaned by AIDS. How will nurses facilitate the collaborative decisions for providing care to these aggregates? Finding a balance to caring for sick individuals while promoting the health of communities will not be easy, but it must be sought, for either without the other will not meet societal needs. Herein lies the strength of our century old public health nursing legacy—caring with community as partner.

PUBLIC HEALTH LEGACY: THE PAST AS PROLOGUE

Early public health nurse leaders, including Lillian Wald, looked at the realities of their communities and challenged the status quo (Backer, 1993; Buhler-Wilkerson, 1993). They combined care with social activism, mobilizing community resources for health promotion and disease prevention as well as the treatment of plagues and epidemics (Reverby, 1993; Wald, 1934; Zerwekh, 1993). Just as diversity of population and culture has become part of the fabric of contemporary culture, so has HIV disease (Mullen, 1989). Nurses will need to be central to health care delivery in our inner cities, which have become the new battlefront of health and social problems. As in the past, they will go where others refuse to go. They will take responsibility for care for the physically and mentally disabled and the vulnerable and socially devalued. They will battle not only physical and psychological wounds but also epidemics, infectious diseases, sexually transmitted diseases, and tuberculosis—the most common HIV-related, opportunistic disease in the world. They will do so against a backdrop of antiquated medical and outmoded social systems (Frank & Walker, 1993). In many ways, the HIV/AIDS epidemic has worsened the crisis in communities already reeling from substance abuse, poverty, teen pregnancy, illiteracy, unemployment, homelessness, and hopelessness (Lacey, 1993). The adversary in the 1990s, HIV infection and its ally tuberculosis, have again placed nursing on the front lines of battles that will be fought publicly and politically, within local, national, and global arenas. The urgent realities and the magnitude of today's HIV/AIDS epidemic mandate that solutions be sought by turning again to the larger societal context from which the problems and the questions key to their solutions emanate. The health of communities may depend on the rapid response of the nursing profession to the challenges of HIV/AIDS, looking to its public health legacy for insight into addressing the epidemic in all its dimensions—from leadership in innovative care delivery to educational reformation.

HOW RESPONSIVE WILL NURSING EDUCATION BE TO SOCIETY?

Within the societal context, perspectives on education also provide a dichotomy, just as they did for service. First, the view from outside is impatient with the inadequacies (and perceived rigidities) of the present system, especially for clinical experiences. For example, is caring for individuals with AIDS integrated into the curriculum? Second, do nurse educators reach out to populations, especially vulnerable populations such as women and children with HIV disease, whether or not they seek care? If, the answer is yes, then is it by curriculum design, or as a pilot project which may be transient? Who will fund the innovations, and at what cost? The devil lies in the details. There are practical matters enmeshed in the educational dichotomy, but the key question remains: How responsive will nursing education be to society—balancing needs of sick individuals with health needs of populations? Even change involves a dual challenge: that of breaking new ground and its potential clash with traditional values as education and care move outside the walls of our institutions (Backer, 1993; Fahy,1993; Walker & Doherty, 1994). Nursing educators should view universities and colleges as societal institutions with a strong obligation to society. There are forces that will resist change because the need is not seen, or because self interest is at stake, or because existing individual or system values are in question, or because the price is too high. But meaningful change will occur depending on the redefinition of education based on the needs of society (deTornyay, 1992; Shugars et al., 1991).

Educational reform calls upon nursing to equip nursing students with the knowledge and skills necessary to practice in community-based environments as well as institutional settings (deTornyay, 1992; Flynn, 1993). In the new practice arena, students recruited from diverse populations will be prepared as new kind practitioners by working collaboratively and in partnership with faculty mentors, consumers, and other health professionals (Clark et al., 1993; Flynn, 1993). Students will learn to deliver nursing care to diverse groups, including culturally diverse and vulnerable populations: the elderly, new immigrants, the homeless, women and children, and those with HIV/AIDS (Wardrop, 1993). The boundaries of practice will broaden and blur for both faculty and students as they work together in schools, the workplace, homeless shelters, and the streets, seeking ways to empower consumers to participate in making informed health care choices, while preserving the public responsibility for health. But faculty must have the support of their institutions if they are to creatively find new methods and approaches for serving as community-based mentors. In return, faculty must support students in becoming more self directed and in taking responsibility for their own learning as well as empowering those for whom they care in this problem based, interactive learning environment (Clark et al., 1993; deTornyay, 1992; Flynn, 1993; Walker & Doherty, 1994). Already developed models such as the Healthy Cities (HC) approach can be a resource for change (Flynn, Rider, & Ray, 1991; Flynn, 1993). Here, a broad definition of health is used that incorporates concepts of social justice, political action, and ethical decision making within a health promotion framework. Nurse faculty can embrace all the Healthy Cities strategies, including community development, mass communication, self-help through community empowerment, public policy development, financial management, and organizational change within the educational process applied to HIV/AIDS. Community and political activities become part of the professional role development while consumers learn individually and collectively to make informed health decisions and to be responsible for their own health (Clark et al., 1992; Wardrop, 1993). In addition, opportunities for consumer collaboration are not as limited in community settings. Most traditional health care settings are often inaccessible to those most vulnerable and frequently socially stigmatized groups (Frank, et al., 1994).

A major emphasis in this new faculty practice environment must be outcomes research, for it provides the data for retrospective evaluation of the effectiveness of care delivered, as well as prospective planning. Using research-based findings as a conceptual base, nurse educators and their students have the freedom to try new strategies that are relevant for consumers like Cindy who are experts through practical wisdom gained by living with AIDS. Collaboration and dialogue between nurse faculty, students, and consumers foster a process of discovery where all are simultaneously teachers and learners. Students learn the interrelationship between health and its social determinants, such as housing, employment, child care, nutrition, education, literacy, and poverty, that impact the quality of life of a community and its residents (Shoultz et al., 1992; Walker & Doherty, 1994). Using problem-based and interactive learning opportunities within nontraditional settings (such as refugee centers, hospices, HIV clinics, substance abuse treatment centers, and homeless shelters), students learn that health and well being are interconnected. They learn that consumers must participate in developing locally relevant solutions in order to improve the health of the community as well as its residents (Flynn, 1993).

The HIV epidemic, due to the many complexities of the disease itself and the required supports and services needed, is both catalyst and mandate for shifting the care paradigm to a community base. The types of services needed and the nature of the care require increased emphasis on the need for more links with community. The health care community, including medicine and nursing, will have little success with HIV initiatives unless other community sectors such as business, education, the creative and performing arts, the media, and the social, political, and economic systems work in partnership.

▬NURSING FACULTY INSTITUTE DEVELOPED TO ENCOURAGE CREATIVE SOLUTIONS BY USING COLLECTIVE FACULTY WISDOM

The Nursing Faculty Institute is a forum in which to consider the many dimensions of the mandate, including but not limited to:

- curriculum renewal,
- clinical and epidemiology updates,
- population-based learning,
- faculty mentoring roles in an interactive learning process,
- ethics and health policy development, as well as
- the research base.

The Pennsylvania AIDS Educational Training Center (PA AIDS ETC), Nursing Faculty Institute was developed to encourage creative solutions by using collective faculty wisdom to resolve common dilemmas for caring where there is yet no cure. Pennsylvania has more cases of AIDS than 38 other states, with all counties reporting cases (Frank, et al., 1993). Just as many practicing nurses were prepared before the epidemic, so also were faculty. Yet, since they will be on the front lines, with direct interaction on a daily basis with people with AIDS, their families and partners, faculty need the most current knowledge and skills. Nurse educators, along with practicing nurses and students of the future must be prepared to give quality, comprehensive, and compassionate HIV/AIDS care in a variety of settings. Therefore, the PA AIDS ETC, with input from its advisory committee as well as from nurses attending the PA AIDS ETC educational programs, developed the Nurse Faculty Institute. Representatives from all levels of education were included in the planning process. Content areas were identified. The first was curriculum development on HIV disease, the second, development of a nursing policies on HIV disease, and third, the role of nursing research.

Through a curriculum needs assessment, specific content areas were identified, including constantly changing treatment and care issues, innovative nursing interventions, and strategies for prevention-focused consumer education. The changing epidemiology of HIV disease requires that considerable attention be focused on this aspect in order for faculty to have the information necessary for implementing needed curriculum redesign. The crucial role of nursing on the care team was also acknowledged as an area of special emphasis as were professional standards and codes of conduct that delineated legal and ethical expectations for both faculty and students caring for persons with HIV/AIDS. Topics addressed relative to nursing school policies included:

- policies for the HIV infected student,
- the HIV infected faculty member,
- requirements for students to care for persons with HIV disease, and
- ways of managing students who refuse or are reluctant to care for a person with AIDS.

Finally, in the area of nursing research, the topics addressed included:

- successful methods for the development of nursing research activities both at the undergraduate and graduate level,
- research innovation,
- the use of models and conceptual frameworks for nursing research,
- development of community ties for the conduct of nursing research, and
- the acquisition of funding for research projects.

The faculty were recruited from Pennsylvania schools of nursing, as well as leading nursing experts in HIV disease from across the country. It was acknowledged that the two-day annual Nursing Faculty Institute, now in its third year, provides an effective vehicle for faculty to acquire current state-of-the-art information necessary for curriculum development. It also provides a forum in which faculty can explore concerns and dilemmas from a multi-institutional perspective. The research focus encouraged faculty to share their ideas, approaches, and interventions. Topics discussed in addition to the development, enhancement and funding of research included collaboration between health professions disciplines and between nurse researchers and practice-based nurses. The caring imperative was a unifying theme throughout the institute for, while nursing has always considered "caring" at the centerpiece of practice, HIV/AIDS places caring squarely in the center of all aspects of education for nursing and health care.

HIV/AIDS is both mandate and catalyst for a new paradigm for nursing. This new paradigm will make important differences in the lives of individuals and communities by using a caring tradition that embraces all—including those that society does not. In that world, Cindy will not be the forgotten face of the women with AIDS, nor her children a forgotten legacy of HIV.

■REFERENCES

Backer, B. (1993). Connecting caring with activism. *Nursing and Health Care, 14*(3), 122–129.

Buhler-Wilkerson, K. (1993). Bringing care to the people—Lillian Wald's legacy to public health nursing. *American Journal of Public Health, 83*, 1778–1786.

Centers for Disease Control, Public Health Service (1992, June). *HIV/AIDS Surveillance Report.*

Clark, H., Beddone, G., & Whyte, N. (1993). Public health nurses' vision of their future reflects changing paradigms. *Image*, 305–310.

Collins, H. (1994, March 29). AIDS orphans in U.S. may total 175,000 by end of decade. *Philadelphia Inquirer*, pp. A1, 13.

deTornyay, R. (1992). Reconsidering nursing education: The report of the PEW Health Professions Commission. *The Journal of Nursing Education 37*(7), 296–301.

Fahy, E. (1993). The scholarship of application (editorial). *Nursing and Health Care, 14*(8), 395.

Fedor, M. (1992). AIDS: Advocacy and activism. *Nursing and Health Care, 13*(2), 65.

Fedor, M. (1993). My AIDS education, part II: Political realities. *Nursing and Health Care, 14*(9), 453–454.

Flynn, B. (1993). Healthy cities: the future of public health. *Health Care Trends and Transitions, 4*(3), 14–18, 80.

Flynn, B.C., Rider, M., & Ray, D.W. (1991). Healthy Cities: The Indiana model of community development. *Public Health Education Quarterly, 18*, 331–347.

Frank, L., Donnelly, G., & Lopez, I. (1994). *HIV Nursing Faculty Institute: Impacting nursing education. Proceedings of the second national AIDS Education and Training Centers Workshop.*

Frank, L., Ricksecker, A., Spence, M., & Ho, M. (1993). *The AIDS Education and Training Centers: Impacting health professionals and HIV care* (paper presented at International Conference on AIDS, Berlin, Germany, June 6–11).

Frank, L., & Walker, M.B. (1993). *Impact of HIV on nursing: Historical implications for nursing practice and education* (unpublished paper, delivered at the Pennsylvania Public Health Association Conference, Pittsburgh, PA, March).

Hegyvary, S. (1992). Nursing education for health care reform. *Journal of Professional Nursing, 1*(8), 3.

Khun, T.S. (1970). The structure of scientific revolutions. *International Encyclopedia of Unified Science.* Chicago, IL: University of Chicago Press.

Labonte, R. (1987). Community health promotion strategies. *Health Promotion, 26*(1), 5–10, 32.

Lacey, B. (1993). Definition of poverty needs rethinking. *Nursing and Health Care, 13*(2), 59.

Leininger, M. (1994). Transcultural nursing education: A worldwide imperative. *Nursing and Health Care, 15*(5), 254–257.

Moccia, P. (1992). A nurse in every school. *Nursing and Health Care, 13*(1), 14–18.

Mullen, F. (1989). *Plagues and politics: History of the United States Public Health Service*, New York, NY: Basic Books.

Reverby, S. (1993), From Lillian Wald to Hillary Rodham Clinton. What will happen to public health nursing? *American Journal of Public Health, 8*(12), 1662–1663.

Shoultz, J., Hatcher, P., & Hurrell, M. (1992). Growing edges of a new paradigm: The future of nursing in the health of the nation. *Nursing Outlook, 40*(2), 57–61.

Shugars, D.A., O'Neil, E.H., & Bader, J.D., (eds). (1991). *Healthy America: Practitioners for 2005: An agenda for action for U.S. health professional schools a report of the PEW Health Professions Commission.* Durham, NC: Duke University Medical Center.

Tri-Council for Nursing. (1991). *Nursing's agenda for health care reform.* Washington, DC: American Nurses Association.

U.S. Department of Health and Human Services. (1991). *Healthy People 2000.* Washington, DC: U.S. Government Printing Office.

Wald, L.D. (1934). *Windows on Henry Street.* Boston, MA: Little, Brown and Company.

Walker, M.B. & Doherty, A. (1994). Healthy cities: Empowering vulnerable populations for health through partnerships. *Journal of Family and Community Health, 17*(2), 78–81.

Wardrop, K. (1993). A framework for health promotion; a framework for AIDS. *Canadian Journal of Public Health,* [Supplement I], 59–63.

World Health Organization. (1978a). *Report of the International Conference on Primary Health Care, Alma-Ata, USSR.* Geneva, September 6–12.

World Health Organization. (1978b). The Alma-Ata Conference of Primary Care. *WHO Chronicle, 3*(11), 409–430.

Zerwekh, J.V. (1992). Public health nursing legacy. Historical practical wisdom. *Nursing and Health Care, 13*(2), 84–91.

Chapter 5

Violence as a Nursing Priority: Policy Implications

JACQUELYN C. CAMPBELL   ELIZABETH ANDERSON

TERRY L. FULLMER   SHIRLEY GIROUARD

BEVERLY McELMURRY   BEVERLY RAFF

Another major threat to the public's health is violence. The incidence and prevalence of homicides, assaults, rapes, and other forms of violence are staggering. The authors of this chapter comprised an American Academy of Nursing expert panel on violence. They studied the issue, and describe policy changes that have been occurring relative to violence and discuss nursing's role with respect to these policy changes. They cite various nursing research studies on violence, including research on women and elder abuse, and suggest responses to address the problem of victimization, especially for women and children.

Violence has become a major health care problem, costing the American society thousands of lives, millions of dollars, and untold physical and psychologic morbidity. Homicide is the seventh leading cause of premature death in this country and the leading cause of death for young black men and women, aged 15 to 35.[1] It is also the leading cause of death in infants under 2 after the first 6 weeks. The rate of homicide in this country is by far the highest of any westernized country not at war. The incidence of assault injuries in adults is 11.1 per 1,000 population—almost one and a half times as high as the rate of accidental injuries. At least 30 of each 1000 women are severely physically abused by their male partner each year, and 25 of every 1000 children are physically, sexually, or emotionally abused or neglected each year by their parents. Abuse of the elderly is a national disgrace, affecting between 700,000 to 1 million of our elderly population annually.[2] Of every 1000 women, 108 are raped each year, and it is estimated that 1 of every 4 women and at least 1 of every 10 men will be sexually assaulted by age 21.[1] Perpetrators of rape and child sexual assault are most often a family member or friend of the victim. The established statistics are horrifying, but the totality of ramifications for the health care system are only beginning to be tabulated.

From *Nursing Outlook* 41(2):83–92, 1993. Reprinted by permission of Mosby-Year Book, Inc.

In recent research we are finding that not only is the health care system dealing with the physical injuries from assault, but that many of the chronic health problems we struggle with are related to violence. For instance, the most common physical complaint of abused women in the health care system is chronic pain.[3] Irritable bowel syndrome, arthritis, pelvic inflammatory disease, and neurologic damage in women are also associated with years of physical assault from male partners. Chronic pelvic pain, headache, asthma, and alcoholism are all sequelae for women sexually abused in childhood.[4,5] A significant proportion of women with diagnosed psychiatric illness have been identified as having a history of sexual or physical abuse.[6,7] Abused children are often first identified because of stress-related illnesses.[8] The most current nursing research is finding a 15% prevalence of partner abuse during pregnancy, and low birthweight has been associated with this form of violence.[9,10] Incest and date rape accounts for a significant proportion of adolescent pregnancy.[11] The children of battered women are at risk for health, school, and emotional problems, as well as for increased aggressiveness, which may continue into adult violence.[12] Children are often the witnesses of other forms of violence, including homicide, in today's world. The effects of this exposure are relatively unstudied, but significant according to mental health clinicians.

▬POLICY CHANGES

Only recently has the role of the health care system as being equally important as the judicial system in dealing with violence been articulated.[13-15] This is a significant change in national policy. Instrumental in making that policy change has been the work of Burgess, whose work was the earliest and is still one of the most influential programs of nursing research in the area of violence. Her initial article on the rape trauma syndrome is considered a classic in the area of rape research and is cited in nearly every article on the subject.[16] Her program of research has gone on to establish a model of how children respond emotionally to sexual abuse that explains their ongoing and delayed symptoms, and she has explored rape victims' concerns about AIDS.[17,18] She is frequently an advocate for child victims of sexual assault as an expert witness in courts and works regularly with the Federal Bureau of Investigation to formulate policy related to violence. The most influential policy component of Dr. Burgess' work was her participation as one of only nine national experts on violence on the Department of Justice Task Force on Family Violence, formed in 1983. The report from that commission clearly indicated that the health care system needed to be involved in the national efforts to address the problem of violence.

Shortly after that report was issued, Surgeon General Everett Koop organized a workshop to formulate the responsibilities of the health care system in that regard. Dr. Burgess and Dr. Hartman cowrote the background paper on rape and sexual assault for that conference. Twenty other nurses joined Dr. Burgess, among the 150 invited national experts on violence at the workshop, and held an informal caucus to make sure nursing's voice would be heard in the resulting policy initiatives. Among those nurses was Joyce Thomas, whose long advocacy for abused children has been and continues to be an important influence on national policy in the family violence arena.

As an outgrowth of the surgeon general's conference, official health care policy for the U.S. Public Health Services has been to consider violence as a critical public health problem. The change in policy was formalized by inclusion of a set of objectives on Violent and Abusive Behavior in the new *Healthy People 2000* guidelines for national health care in the next decade (Table 5-1).[15]

TABLE 5-1   Objectives from Healthy People 2000

7. Violent and Abusive Behavior Health Status Objectives

7.1   Reduce homicides to no more than 7.2 per 100,000 people. (Age-adjusted baseline: 8.5 per 100,000 in 1987)

SPECIAL POPULATION TARGETS

	Homicide Rate (per 100,000)	1987 Baseline	2000 Target
7.1a	Children aged 3 and younger	3.9	3.1
7.1b	Spouses aged 15–34	1.7	1.4
7.1c	Black men aged 15–34	90.5	72.4
7.1d	Hispanic men aged 15–34	53.1	45.1
7.1e	Black women aged 15–34	20.0	16.0
7.1f	American Indians/Alaska Natives in reservation states	14.1	11.3

Baseline data source: National Vital Statistics System.

7.2   Reduce suicides to no more than 10.5 per 100,000 people. (Age-adjusted baseline: 11.7 per 100,000 in 1987)

SPECIAL POPULATION TARGETS

	Suicides (per 100,000) Among:	1987 Baseline	2000 Target
7.2a	Youth aged 15–19	10.3	8.2
7.2b	Men aged 20–34	25.2+	21.4
7.2c	White men aged 65 and older	46.1	39.2
7.2d	American Indians/Alaska Natives men in reservation states +1986 baseline	15	12.8

Baseline data sources: National Vital Statistics System; Indian Health Service Administrative Statistics.

(continued)

TABLE 5-1   Objectives from Healthy People 2000 (*continued*)

7.3   Reduce weapon-related violent deaths to no more than 12.6 per 100,000 people from major causes. (Age-adjusted baseline: 12.9 per 100,000 by firearms; 2 per 100,000 by knives in 1987)

Baseline data source: National Vital Statistics System.

7.4   Reverse to less than 25.2 per 1,000 children the rising incidence of maltreatment of children younger than age 18. (Baseline: 25.2 per 1,000 in 1986)

TYPE-SPECIFIC TARGETS

Incidence of Types of Maltreatment:	*1986 Baseline*	*2000 Target*
7.4a Physical abuse	5.7/1,000	<5.7/1,000
7.4b Sexual abuse	2.5/1,000	<2.5/1,000
7.4c Emotional abuse	3.4/1,000	<3.4/1,000
7.4d Neglect	15.9/1,000	<15.9/1,000

Baseline data source: Study of the National Incidence of Child Abuse and Neglect.

7.5   Reduce physical abuse directed at women by male partners to no more than 27 per 1,000 couples. (Baseline: 30 per 1,000 in 1985)

Baseline data source: National Family Violence Survey.

7.6   Reduce assault injuries among people aged 12 and older to no more than 10 per 1,000 people. (Baseline: 11.1 per 1,000 in 1986)

Baseline data source: National Crime Survey.

7.7   Reduce rape and attempted rape of women aged 12 and older to no more than 107 per 100,000 women. (Baseline: 120 per 100,000 in 1986)

SPECIAL POPULATION TARGET

Incidence of Rape and Attempted Rape (per 100,000)	*1986 Baseline*	*2000 Target*
7.7a Women aged 12–34	250	225

Baseline data source: National Crime Survey.

7.8   Reduce by 15% the incidence of injurious suicide attempts among adolescents aged 14 to 19. (Baseline data available in 1991)

Risk Reduction Objectives

7.9   Reduce by 20% the incidence of physical fighting among adolescents aged 14 through 17. (Baseline data available in 1991)

7.10 Reduce by 20% the incidence of weapon-carrying by adolescents aged 14 through 17. (Baseline data available in 1991)

7.11 Reduce by 20% the proportion of weapons that are inappropriately stored and therefore dangerously available. (Baseline data available in 1992)

(continued)

TABLE 5-1   Objectives from Healthy People 2000 *(continued)*

Services and Protection Objectives

7.12   Extend protocols for routinely identifying, treating, and properly referring suicide at-tempters, victims of sexual assault, and victims of spouse, elder, and child abuse to as least 90% of hospital emergency departments. (Baseline data available in 1992)

7.13   Extend to at least 45 states implementation of unexplained child death review systems. (Baseline data available in 1991)

7.14   Increase to at least 30 the number of states in which at least 50% of children identified as physically or sexually abused receive physical and mental evaluation with appropriate follow-up as a means of breaking the intergenerational cycle of abuse. (Baseline data available in 1993)

7.15   Reduce to less than 10% the proportion of battered women and their children turned away from emergency housing due to lack of space. (Baseline: 40% in 1987)

   Baseline data source: Domestic Violence Statistical Survey

7.16   Increase to at least 50% the proportion of elementary and secondary schools that teach nonviolent conflict resolution skills, preferably as a part of quality school health education. (Baseline data available in 1991)

7.17   Extend coordinated, comprehensive violence prevention programs to at least 80% of local jurisdictions with populations over 100,000. (Baseline data available in 1993)

7.18   Increase to 50 the number of states with officially established protocols that engage mental health, alcohol and drug, and public health authorities with corrections authorities to facilitate identification and appropriate intervention to prevent suicide by jail inmates. (Baseline data available in 1992)

Those who oppose this policy direction speak of the inappropriateness of "medicalizing social problems." However, the problem of violence in this country is clearly beyond the capabilities of any one system to solve. So long as the end result of this problem is detrimental to the health of the nation and the health care system is affected in such magnitude by it, health care professionals must become involved. New impetus is also being directed toward women's health issues in this country, and violence toward women is clearly a significant women's health problem that affects women of all ages and in all areas of health and well-being.[19,20]

■ROLE OF NURSING IN THE POLICY CHANGE

Nurses are seeing both victims and perpetrators of violence in all health care settings and every diagnostic category. Nursing always has been part of the clinical team in identifying child abuse and taking care of abused children. They have always given excellent physical care to gunshot victims, battered women, victims of sexual assault, and anyone else physically injured by another person. The new direction for nursing is to be on the forefront of the development of knowledge in this area and to use that knowledge to provide leadership for change in health care policy. If nursing can generate the information necessary about how to better identify victims of violence early and provide interventions that lessen the likelihood for them to be victims or perpetrators again, there is potential to change the quality of life in this country.

Important nursing research has been conducted in the area of violence, and there is recognition both within and outside the discipline of the legitimacy and importance of nursing having this critical role in the effort to ameliorate the effects and perpetration of violence. This legitimacy has been formalized by significant funding of nursing research in the area of violence by the National Center for Nursing Research, the Centers for Disease Control, the American Nurses' Foundation, and by the National Institutes of Mental Health. The American Nurses Association national convention has been having major sessions on violence for almost 10 years and did so again in 1992. Surgeon General Koop and the current *Healthy People* objectives on violence and abuse have made clear that the nursing role is considered to be crucial in the national policy change. There is a formalized Nursing Network on Violence Against Women that had official input into the formation of the *Healthy People* objectives and is consulted on an informal basis by national, state, and local legislatures and grassroots organizations.

One example illustrates the impact nursing has had on the current changes in health care policy; it began with clinical nursing concerns, then moved to research, and finally to professional and policy change. In 1984 a student in the graduate (MSN) nursing program at Texas Women's University became interested in the problem of abuse during pregnancy. She was inspired in this endeavor by her faculty advisors, Elizabeth Anderson and Judith McFarlane, and the then recently published *Nursing Care of Victims of Family Violence,* by Campbell and Humphreys. At that point, the only research that had identified abuse during pregnancy as a problem was retrospective studies of battered women who reported abuse often starting or getting worse during pregnancy (e.g., Walker[21]). Between 15% and 45% of samples of battered women report to researchers that they were abused during pregnancy; however, this kind of finding is subject to recall bias and is limited to women identifying themselves as battered. Helton[22] conducted one of the two first prevalence studies of abuse during pregnancy, which helped validate the findings of the first, conducted by Hillard,[23] a physician. Together, the two studies helped establish that at least 8% of pregnant women are abused during pregnancy and that an additional 15% are abused before pregnancy, making them highly at risk to be abused again.

On the basis of this study a program of research was begun and has continued under the direction of Dr. McFarlane with the assistance of Linda Bullock.[9,24,25] Some of the important findings from that research have included the establishing of a link between abuse during pregnancy and low birthweight and an 8% abuse prevalence rate in a primary care setting of women not pregnant. The Centers for Disease Control is currently funding Drs. McFarlane and Parker in a major cohort study of patterns of abuse during pregnancy and associated infant outcomes.[10]

As well as the research component of this program, funding was secured from the March of Dimes for training nurses in the identification and treatment of women abused during pregnancy. This program was carefully designed for maximum impact by training the nurses to train others in their local communities. In conjunction with this program, a videotape, *Crimes Against the Future*, was produced and is available through the March of Dimes. The March of Dimes has subsequently officially recognized abuse during pregnancy as a major contributor to adverse birth outcomes. An additional outcome of the integral advocacy and policy influence aspect of this program of research since its inception has been the official recognition of abuse during pregnancy as a major health problem for pregnant women by former Surgeon General Everett Koop and the American College of Obstetrics and Gynecology.

▀UNIQUE PERSPECTIVE OF NURSING RESEARCH

Other forms of violence are appropriate areas for nursing inquiry in terms of the resulting significant health problems, the holistic responses to violence experienced by those victimized, the potential for further morbidity and mortality because of the escalating nature of all forms of abuse, and the chances for significant primary and secondary prevention efforts. Nursing research adds a unique perspective to the knowledge development in the field because of its holistic perspective. Medical research concentrates on the physical injury with the parallel emphasis in psychiatry on pathology. The literature on victims in psychology, sociology, and even victimology and women's studies tends to concentrate on documenting emotional effects and sociologic and psychologic causative factors. The nursing research to date has been more concerned with responses to and characteristics of victims of violence than causation and has examined a combination of physical injury and physical responses with emotional and behavioral reactions. This is reflective of nursing's Social Policy Statement definition,[26] and this allows an easily comprehensible identification of nursing's unique body of knowledge in this field.

A women's health orientation—either using an overtly feminist framework or at least avoiding the androcentric biases of much early research and some of the continued research in other fields—is also apparent in the nursing research on violence against women. Nursing studies have avoided the victim blaming and the emphasis on pathologic characteristic of much other research that has served to encourage a distancing perspective of women victimized by violence as a deviant group.[27–29] There have also been connections with the grassroots sexual assault and battered women's movement by most nursing authors in the field. In the area of wife abuse, there has been a general avoidance of the controversies surrounding the extent and nature of female violence against male partners. Nursing has concentrated—and rightly so—on the threat that wife abuse poses for women's health, rather than obscuring the issue under such labels as "spouse abuse" or "domestic violence."

Nursing research on victimization has also approximated a critical theory approach,[30] in that the published reports have almost always had an emancipatory component, either in terms of the clinical prescriptions derived for nursing care or in the way the study itself was conducted (e.g., Hoff[31]). Those victimized by violence are most often of disenfranchised groups, of a minority ethnic group, or women and children. Research has shown that health care professionals contribute to the further subjugation of these people. For instance, health care professionals are more likely to report poor and minority parents for child abuse than middle-class white couples whose children have comparable injuries.[32] Health care professionals are more likely to derogatorily label, tranquilize, and give inappropriate care to battered women in the emergency department than other patients.[33,34] Battered women have identified health care professionals as the least helpful category of professionals they have gone to for assistance.[35] One of the reasons that health care professionals may try to distance themselves from victims of violence, and the problem of violence in general, is the perception that it is a problem of "the other," or a deviant group. It is encouraging to have research demonstrate that at least in one area of violence, wife abuse, practicing nurses are less believing than physicians of the myths that blame victims for the violence directed against them.[36]

Nursing research has also begun to explore cultural issues related to violence (e.g., Torres[37]), and most studies have been ethnically heterogeneous. In addition, there has been a variety of philosophic and methodologic approaches to the study of violence in nursing, including both qualitative and quantitative analysis of data. This has supported the validity of similar findings from contrasting methodologies and has enriched the knowledge base generated.

The findings from at least one nursing study were used for emancipation through a state legislative change to make marital rape no longer exempt from prosecution.[38] Nurse researchers almost always provide interventions when they work with those victimized by violence, either directly with the women or by providing staff training. They also almost always make clinical suggestions in research reports. These nursing implications often go beyond what has been found in the study, but reflect the nurses' concern and rich clinical background with those affected by violence that they bring to their research. These additions are not usually deliberately guided by a theoretic or philosophic premise of emancipation but probably reflect the clinical grounding of all our research plus the recognition of survivors' need for empowerment, both in the health care system and in their lives.

Nurses who conduct research in this area usually have worked closely with survivors and have grown to know them well, in contrast to many of the other scientists in the field. Nursing research has generally grown out of clinical concerns rather than a deductive theoretical testing approach. Thus our research is, in general, congruent with the calls for an "activist research agenda" being proposed by those who align themselves with the grassroots sexual assault and battered women's movement, afrocentric theory, feminist theory, and critical theory.[39] These researchers and activists want to make sure that the primary agenda for future research in this area is to empower the men, women, and children involved (rather than further blaming or pathologically labeling them) and to put the onus of responsibility on the social system to change, rather than the individual. Nurse researchers' knowledge of and ability to influence the health care system, in combination with their social consciousness and clinical concerns, gives them a unique and crucial part in that agenda. At least one consortium, the Nursing Research Consortium on Violence and Abuse, has been formed with clearly articulated purposes of advocacy and policy change based on a scientific body of knowledge.

■STATE OF NURSING SCIENCE IN VIOLENCE RESEARCH

The majority of nursing research into the responses to violence and related issues has been in the area of wife abuse. There have also been important studies in the spheres of homicide, children of battered women, child abuse, child sexual abuse, elder abuse, and sexual assault. Research is beginning in such important areas as appropriate interventions for spinal cord–injured patients who are gunshot victims, a different group than the majority of rehabilitation patients.[40] The same issues are involved in the nursing care of patients with stomas who are gunshot victims.[41] The editors of the 1992 *Annual Review of Nursing Research* contained a research review covering data-based inquiries related to battering of female partners and the effects on their children.[42] They plan a future chapter on nursing research covering the other forms of family violence, rape, and child sexual assault.

Nursing Research on Woman Abuse

Nurse researchers have investigated many different aspects of woman abuse, and the body of knowledge accumulated is beginning to be impressive. One of the most useful trends is beginning programs of research (e.g.,McFarlane, Campbell) and research that builds on prior work by other nursing investigators. Similar inquiries in terms of research questions—but using disparate methods and samples and both identical and different instruments for measuring similar concepts in different samples—are extremely important in building a knowledge base. There is a Nursing Research Consortium on Violence and Abuse, consisting of 14 nursing researchers from around the country who are working collaboratively to do exactly this kind of work and who have two extramurally funded investigations in process so far. Nursing is approaching a point where this base may be generalized, or at least used as a starting point, for nursing interventions in multiple settings.

The findings accumulated thus far that may be said to be trustworthy include that at least 8% of women in prenatal and primary care settings have been abused by a male partner and that approximately 20% of women in emergency rooms have a history of abuse.[3,9,25,43] There is evidence that one-to-one interviews of women by nurses yields the highest rates of disclosure of woman abuse, but even including as few as five assessment questions on a nursing history form prompts many battered women to disclose.[44]

Obviously, this prevalence data—coupled with consistent findings of the danger of homicide and suicide in battering relationships, other significant health problems, lack of medical record documentation, and abused women's perceptions of poor care by health care professionals— indicates a need for nursing continuing and basic education in all settings.[35,38,42,45-48] Tilden and Shepherd[49] have provided evidence of the effectiveness of an emergency training program, and further studies like theirs are needed in other arenas.

Nursing research has also documented a consistent finding of low self-esteem in battered women, perhaps especially those also sexually abused.[50-53] In addition to other findings of emotional problems, nursing studies have identified significant strengths of battered women, indications of normal processes of grieving and recovering, and cultural and social support influences on responses to battering.[31,54] These findings, taken cumulatively, are beginning to indicate data-based nursing interventions that will in many cases duplicate the clinical suggestions already in the literature. Many of the studies have very small samples or unsophisticated methodologies; however, the findings from those studies in many cases support more advanced research, both inside and outside nursing. Most exciting is the emphasis on strengths, rather than pathology, and the implications for interventions that empower rather than patronize.

Nursing Research on Elder Abuse

The mistreatment of elderly persons afflicts between 700,000 to 1.2 million people annually in this country. Nursing research in this area has served to form the bulk of what we know about elder mistreatment. Mandatory reporting laws on elder abuse have compelled a number of nurse researchers to study this field. While much progress has been made over the past decade, there is much that is needed to improve the body of science in this area. Most studies today have been conducted on small, nonrandom convenient samples and are not generalizable to other populations.[55] The information that has been generated relates to instrumentation, theory development, and clinical decision making. Phillips and Rempush-eski[56,57] have conducted work related to decision-making models for diagnosing and intervening in elder abuse and neglect. Phillips[58-60] has also done extensive work in care of the frail elderly at home that looks at abuse and neglect for those individuals. Quinn[61] wrote a text on the causes, diagnoses, and intervention strategies related to clinical care of victims of elder mistreatment. Capezuti[62] studied the issue of dependency as a relevant factor in elder abuse and neglect. The program of research conducted by Fulmer and Ashley[63,64] developed instruments for detecting and assessing elder mistreatment and has also studied the concept of neglect extensively, with emphasis on indicators which might lead to diagnosed neglect. Dr. Fulmer has also been active in influencing public policy in regards to elder abuse and neglect.[65,66] Hudson[55,67] has provided research related to definitional issues related to elder mistreatment and has conducted extensive expert panel reviews to determine ways in which clinicians define elder mistreatment.

▬OBJECTIVES ON VIOLENT AND ABUSIVE BEHAVIOR

Based on the accumulated body of nursing knowledge and individuals and groups of nurse advocates already in position in the area of violence and abuse, the discipline is poised to make a substantive contribution to achievement of the objectives outlined in *Healthy People 2000*. There are 18 objectives in the violence area (see Table 5-1), including eight addressing the reduction of rates of homicide, suicide, assault, child maltreatment, abuse of female partners, rape and attempted rape, and adolescent suicide attempts (7.1–7.8). By increasing nursing identification and interventions with those at risk for these intentional injuries, these objectives have a greater chance of being reached. A start has already been made, as discussed, in terms of abuse during pregnancy, but increased coordination is needed between such organizations as NAACOG, the American College of Nurse-Midwives, and the March of Dimes. To further increase nursing awareness and expertise in terms of violence and abuse, the Nursing Network on Violence and Abuse (NNVAW) has advocated systematic inclusion of appropriate material, beyond child-abuse information, in basic nursing curricula, as well as increased inservice education on these topics. Part of this effort has included collection and dissemination of information on courses, protocols, and training materials available through the regular NNVAW conferences and in the NNVAW column in the journal, *Response to the Victimization of Woman and Children* (Guildford Press).

Response to the Victimization of Women and Children

Another aspect of this policy work has been consulting with congressional staff to include nursing education in a bill introduced to mandate the inclusion of wife abuse in the curricula of health care professional education in schools receiving federal funds, similar to the law that passed in the 1960s mandating the inclusion of child abuse. Similarly, nursing has begun to work with the coalition of activists, including the NOW Legal Defense and Education Fund, to help with the final shaping and passage of the Violence Against Women Act before Congress.

NNVAW members have also worked with the National Coalition on Domestic Violence and state coalitions, NOW, local shelters, state and local health departments, and many schools of nursing. They have also given presentations at several regional and national conferences, including ANA, NLN, NAACOG, the National Emergency Nurses' Association, and

Sigma Theta Tau. What is needed is more systematic national activity through coordination, directives, bulletins, and board-level action from these and other national nursing organizations.

Also needed is increased coordination between nursing and our national allies on these issues as they affect women—organizations such as the Black Women's Health Network and the National Women's Health Network. Coalitions such as these can be helpful in advocating for more stable funding and expansion of wife abuse shelters throughout the country. Such development will help bring to fruition the objective to reduce to less than 10% (from 40% currently) the proportion of battered women and their children turned away from emergency housing due to lack of space (7.15).

A similar coordinated effort inside nursing and with pertinent consumer health organizations also will help address the separate Year 2000 objectives on increasing the number of identified child abuse victims receiving appropriate care and the extending protocols for identifying all assault and abuse victims to 90% of emergency departments (7.12 and 7.14). Thanks in part to the efforts of NNVAW, in conjunction with the National Coalition Against Domestic Violence and especially the Pennsylvania Coalition Against Domestic Violence, the 1992 Joint Commission on the Accreditation of Hospitals Organization standards include a stipulation for just such protocols (Table 5-2). Individual efforts by NNVAW members are underway in such states as California, Connecticut, Illinois, Massachusetts, Michigan, and Pennsylvania to work in conjunction with the state coalitions against domestic violence and emergency departments to make sure those new protocols include a feasible, legitimate, and appropriate outline for nursing interventions as well as identification. Taylor and Campbell[68] have presented an updated list of already developed protocols and training manuals available to hospitals and other health care settings along with a "model" protocol that can be adapted to any setting. What is needed is systematic coordination at the national level, including the ANA and National Emergency Nurses Association, along with the NNVAW. For elder abuse identification and treatment issues, gerontologic nursing organizations are already active and will be part of these coalitions.

The remaining objectives include several that need to be implemented through our school systems. The objectives on reducing physical fighting and weapon carrying among adolescents (7.9, 7.10) may perhaps be best addressed through the separate objective on increasing to 50% the number of primary and secondary schools teaching conflict resolution, ideally as part of quality school health education (7.16). Such education needs to include gender-specific conflict resolution information and discussion so that issues of power and control in male-female relationships, date rape, other forms of dating violence, and attitudes toward women are addressed, as well as the more common gender neutral or male-male forms of conflict resolution curriculum materials. The Community Health practice council of the ANA, the National Association of School Nurses, the Public Health Nursing Section of APHA, and the U.S. Public Health Service would be the possible nucleus of a working coalition to help advocate and shape such

TABLE 5-2   Accreditation Manual for Hospitals, 1992 Hospital-Sponsored Ambulatory Care Services

HO.3.2.15 The handling of adult and child victims of alleged or suspected abuse or neglect.

    HO.3.2.15.1 Criteria are developed for identifying possible victims of abuse:

        HO.3.2.15.1.1 The criteria address at least the following types of abuse:

            HO.3.2.15.1.1.1 physical assault;

            HO.3.2.15.1.1.2 rape or other sexual molestation; and

            HO.3.2.15.1.1.3 domestic abuse of elders, spouses, partners, and children.

    HO.3.2.15.2 Procedures for the evaluation of patients who meet the criteria address:

        HO.3.2.15.2.1 patient consent;

        HO.3.2.15.2.2 examination and treatment;

        HO.3.2.15.2.3 the hospital's responsibility for the collection, retention, and safeguarding of specimens, photographs, and other evidentiary material released by the patient; and

        HO.3.2.15.2.4 as legally required, notification of, and release of, information to the proper authorities.

    HO.3.2.15.3 A list is maintained in the ambulatory care services department of private and public community agencies that provide, or arrange for, evaluation and care for victims of abuse, and referrals are made as appropriate.

    HO.3.2.15.4 The medical record includes documentation of examination, treatment given, any referral(s) made to other care providers and to community agencies, and any required reporting to the proper authorities.

    HO.3.2.15.5 There is a plan for education of appropriate staff about the criteria for identifying and the procedures for handling possible victims of abuse.

Accreditation Manual for Hospitals, 1992 Emergency Services

ES.5.1.2.10 the handling of adult and child victims of alleged or suspected abuse or neglect.

    ES.5.1.2.10.1 Criteria are developed for identifying possible victims of abuse.

        ES.5.1.2.10.1.1 The criteria address at least the following types of abuse:

            ES.5.1.2.10.1.1.1 physical assault:

            ES.5.1.2.10.1.1.2 rape or other sexual molestation; and

            ES.5.1.2.10.1.1.3 domestic abuse of elders, spouses, partners and children.

    ES.5.1.2.10.2 Procedures for the evaluation of patients who meet the criteria address:

        ES.5.1.2.10.2.1 patient consent;

        ES.5.1.2.10.2.2 examination and treatment;

        ES.5.1.2.10.2.3 the hospital's responsibility for the collection, retention, and safeguarding of specimens, photographs, and other evidentiary material released by the patient; and

        ES.5.1.2.10.2.4 as legally required, notification of, and release of information to, the proper authorities.

    ES.5.1.2.10.3 A list is maintained in the emergency department/service of private and public community agencies that provide, or arrange for, evaluation and care for victims of, abuse, and referrals are made as appropriate.

    ES.5.1.2.10.4 The medical record includes documentation of examinations, treatment given, any referrals made to other care providers and to community agencies, and any required reporting to the proper authorities.

    ES.5.1.2.10.5 There is a plan for education of appropriate staff about the criteria for identifying, and the procedures for handling, possible victims of abuse.

curricula. The National Coalition Against Domestic Violence has dating violence curriculum materials that may be used. The same combination of organizations would be appropriate for working to meet the objective to extend coordinated, comprehensive violence-prevention programs to at least 80% of jurisdictions with populations of more than 100,000.

Objectives specifically concerning child maltreatment may be addressed by coalitions of maternal-child nursing organizations, interdisciplinary child abuse associations, and the Children's Defense Fund. As Joyce Thomas is currently the President of the American Professional Society on the Abuse of Children, the basis for an important coalition is already in place. These coalitions can increase attention to violence-prevention initiatives carried out through parental education, such as addressing the objective on proper storage of weapons in the home (7.11). Nurses can have valuable input into the unexplained child-death review systems that are recommended to be implemented in at least 45 states (7.13). Nurses should also be an integral part of all existing hospital child abuse and neglect "teams," interdisciplinary professional groups that were organized in almost all hospitals to monitor child abuse and neglect cases and issues in the 1970s but which have lost impetus in many hospitals in the last decade.

Finally, the objectives on reducing the number of weapon-related deaths (7.3), reducing weapon carrying by adolescents (7.10), as well as reducing inappropriately stored weapons (7.11) all can be best addressed by nursing taking a more active stand on handgun regulation. A national law outlawing handguns would also do more to decrease the incidence of homicide and suicide, and address the objectives under the unintentional injuries section on decreasing head and spinal cord injuries, than any other single measure we could take.[69] For years, the *New England Journal of Medicine* and the APHA have been calling for far stricter handgun regulation, and it is time for nursing to take a similar stand. The ANA resolution on violence has called for support of the "Brady Bill," proposing a mandatory waiting period before handgun purchase so that records of the purchaser may be checked. This is an excellent and courageous step, and it is hoped that the ANA will take a prominent role in the congressional debate on this bill. However, it is time for nursing to consider taking an even firmer stand, to work visibly and diligently to make handguns illegal in this country.

Thus, programs of nursing research, nursing organizations, and individual nurses have already helped change national policy on the prevention of violence and abuse. Policy now includes the health care system as a major contributor to the solution of this national horror. With systematic and coordinated efforts and leadership from within nursing, this foundation can be enlarged to become more influential.

▬ REFERENCES

1. United States Department of Health and Human Services. Education about adult domestic violence in U.S. and Canadian medical schools, 1987–88. Morbidity and Mortality Weekly MMWR 1989;38(2):17–19.

2. Fulmer T, Ashley J. Clinical indicators which signal neglect. Appl Nurs Res 1989;2:161–7.
3. Goldberg WG, Tomlanovich MC. Domestic violence victims in the emergency department. *JAMA* 1984;251:3259–64.
4. Cunningham J, Pearce T, Pearce P. Childhood sexual abuse and medical complaints in adult women. Journal of Interpersonal Violence 1988;3(2):131–44.
5. Miller BA, Downs WR, Gandoli DM, Keil A. The role of childhood sexual abuse in the development of alcoholism in women. Violence and Victims 1987;2:157–72.
6. Carmen EH, Ricker PP, Mills T. Victims of violence and psychiatric illness. Am J Psychiatry 1984;151:378–83.
7. Gelles RJ, Harrop JW. Violence, battering, and psychological distress among women. Journal of interpersonal violence 1989;4:400–20.
8. Gilbert CM. Psychosomatic symptoms: implications for child sexual abuse. Issues Ment Health Nurs 1988;9:399–408.
9. Bullock L, McFarlane J. Higher prevalence of low birthweight infants born to battered women. Am J Nurs 1989;9:1153–5.
10. McFarlane J, Parker B, Soeken K, Bulluck L. Assessing for abuse during pregnancy. JAMA 1992;267:3176–8.
11. Butler JR, Burton LM. Rethinking teenage childbearing, is sexual abuse a missing link? Family Relations 1990;39:73–80.
12. Humphreys JC. Children of battered women: worries about their mother. Pediatr Nurs 1992;17:342–5.
13. United States Surgeon General. Surgeon General's workshop report on violence and public health. Washington: Public Health Service, U.S. Dept. of Health and Human Services, 1985.
14. Mercy JM, O'Carroll P. New directions in violence prediction: the public health arena. Violence and Victims 1988;3:285–301.
15. United States Department of Health and Human Services, Public Health Service. Healthy people 2000: national health promotion and disease prevention objectives, (DHSS Publication No. (PHS) 91-50212). Washington: US Government Printing Office, 1990.
16. Burgess AW, Holmstrum LL. Rape trauma syndrome. Am J Psychiatry 1974;131:981–6.
17. Baker TC, Burgess AW, Brickman E, Davis RC. Rape victims' concerns about possible exposure to HIV infection. Journal of Interpersonal Violence 1990;5:49–60.
18. Hartman CR, Burgess AW. Information processing of trauma. Journal of Interpersonal Violence 1988;3:443–57.
19. McBride AB. Violence against women: overarching themes and implications for nursing's research agenda. In: Sampselle CM, ed. Violence against women. New York: Hemisphere, 1992:83–9.
20. Stern PN. Woman abuse and practice implications within an international context. In: Sampselle CM, ed. Violence against women. New York: Hemisphere, 1992:143–52.
21. Walker LE. The battered woman. New York: Harper & Row, 1979.
22. Helton AS. The pregnant battered woman. Response 1986;9(1):22–3.
23. Hillard PJ. Physical abuse in pregnancy. Obstet Gynecol 1985;66:185–90.
24. Bullock L, McFarlane J, Bateman LH, Miller V. The prevalence and characteristics of battered women in a primary care setting. *Nurs Pract 1989;*14(6):47–55.
25. Helton AS, McFarlane J, Anderson ET. Battered and pregnant, a prevalence study. Am J Public Health 1987;77:1337–9.
26. American Nursing Association. Nursing: a social policy statement. Kansas City: American Nurses' Association, 1980.
27. Campbell JC. Public health conceptions of family abuse. In: Knudson D, Miller J, eds. Abused and battered. New York: Aldine de Gruyter, 1991:35–47.
28. Schur ME. The politics of deviance, stigma contests and the uses of power. Englewood Cliffs, New Jersey: Prentice-Hall, 1980.
29. Wardell L, Gillespie DL, Leffler A. Science and violence against wives. In: Gelles RJ, Hotaling GT, Straus MA, Finkelhor D, eds. The dark side of families. Beverly Hills, California: Sage, 1983:69–84.
30. Allen RB. Measuring the severity of physical injury among assault and homicide victims. Journal of Quantitative Criminology 1986;2:139–56.
31. Hoff LA. Battered women as survivors. London: Routledge, 1990.

32. Newberger EH, Newberger CM, Hampton RL. Child abuse, the current theory base and future research needs. J Am Acad Child Psychiatry 1983;22:262–8.
33. Kurz D. Emergency department responses to battered women: resistance to medicalization. Social Problems 1987;34:501–13.
34. Stark E, Flitcraft A. Medicine and patriarchal violence: the case against the patriarchy. Social Problems 1979;9:461–93.
35. Brendtro M, Bowker HL. Battered women: how can nurses help? Issues in Mental Health Nursing 1989;10:169–80.
36. Saunders GD, Rose K. Attitudes of psychiatric and nonpsychiatric medical practitioners toward battered women: an exploratory study. Unpublished doctoral dissertation, University of Wisconsin, Wisconsin, 1987.
37. Torres S. Hispanic-American battered women why consider cultural differences? Response 1987;10(3):20–1.
38. Campbell JC. Nursing assessment for risk of homicide with battered women. Adv Nurs Sci 1986,8(4):36–51.
39. Dobash RE, Dobash R. Research as social action: the struggle for battered women. In: Yllo K, Brograd M, eds. Feminist perspectives on wife abuse. Beverly Hills, California: Sage, 1988:51–74.
40. Wesley RL. Psychosocial adjustment of spinal cord injured who are victims of gunshot wounds. Unpublished manuscript, Wayne State University, College of Nursing, Detroit, Michigan.
41. Pieper B. Persons who have stomas: violent injury versus disease. J ET Nurs 1992;19(1):7–11.
42. Campbell JC, Parker B. Battered women and their children. In: Fitzpatrick J, Taunton R, Jacox A, eds. Annual review of nursing research, Vol. 10. New York: Springer, 1992:77–94.
43. Stark E, Flitcraft A, Zuckerman D, Grey A, Robison J, Frazier W. Wife abuse in the medical setting. Domestic violence monograph of the National Clearinghouse on Domestic Violence, (Series No. 7). Rockville, Maryland: National Clearinghouse on Domestic Violence, 1981.
44. McFarlane J, Christoffel K, Bateman L, Miller V, Bullock L. Assessing for abuse: self-report versus nurse interview. Public Health Nurs 1991;8:245–50.
45. Drake VK. Battereed women: a health care problem in disguise. Image 1982;14:40–7.
46. Foster LA, Veale CM, Fogel CI. Factors present when battered women kill. Issus Ment Health Nurs 1989;10:273–84.
47. Ryan J, King MC. A study of the health care needs of women experiencing violence in their lives. In: Proceedings of the Third Nursing Network on Violence Against Women. Concord, California, 1989.
48. Stuart EP, Campbell JC. Assessment of patterns of dangerousness with battered women. Issues Ment Health Nurs 1989;10:245–60.
49. Tilden VP, Shepherd P. Increasing the rate of identification of battered women in an emergency department: use of a nursing protocol. Res Nurs Health 1987;10:209–15.
50. Campbell JC. A test of two explanatory models of women's responses to battering. Nurs Res 1989;38(1):18–24.
51. Campbell JC. Women's responses to sexual abuse in intimate relationships. Health Care Women Int 1989;8:335–47.
52. Trimpey ML. Self-esteem and anxiety: key issues in an abused women's support group. Issues Ment Health Nurs 1989;10:297–308.
53. Ulrich Y. Women's reasons for leaving abusive spouses. Women's Health Care International, 12.
54. Landenburger K. A process of entrapment in and recovery from an abusive relationship. Issues Ment Health Nurs 1989;10:209–27.
55. Hudson MF, Johnson TF. Elder neglect and abuse: a review of the literature. In: Annual review of gerontology and geriatrics. Vol. 6. New York: Springer, 1986:81–134.
56. Phillips LR, Rempusheski VF. A decision-making model for diagnosing and intervening in elder abuse and neglect. Nurs Res 1985;34:134–9.
57. Phillips LR, Rempusheski VF. Making decisions about elder abuse. Social Caseworker 1986;67(3):131–40.

58. Phillips LR. Elder abuse—what is it? Who says so? Geriatr Nurs 1983;4:167–70.
59. Phillips LR. Abuse and neglect of the frail elderly at home: an exploration of theoretical relationships. J Adv Nurs 1983;8:379–92.
60. Phillips L. Theoretical explanations of elder abuse: competing hypotheses in unresolved issues. In: Pillemer KA, Wolf RS, eds. Elder abuse: conflict in the family. Dover, Massachusetts: Auburn House, 1986:197–217.
61. Quinn MJ. Elder abuse and neglect. San Francisco: San Francisco Court System, 1986.
62. Capezuti L. Commentary on the debate over dependency as a relevant predisposing factor in elder abuse and neglect. Journal of Elder Abuse and Neglect 1990;2:(1&2):63–5.
63. Fulmer T, Ashley J. Neglect: what part of abuse? Pride Institute Journal 1986;5(4):18–24.
64. Fulmer T, Ashley J. Toward the development of a social policy statement on elder abuse. Oasis 1988;5(3):1, 3.
65. Fulmer T. the debate over dependency as a predisposing factor in elder abuse and neglect. Journal of Elder Abuse and Neglect 1990;2(12):51–8.
66. Fulmer T. Elder mistreatment: progress in community detection and intervention. Fam Community Health 1991;14(2):26–34.
67. Hudson MF. An analysis of the concepts of elder mistreatment, abuse and neglect. Journal of Abuse and Neglect 1989;1:5–25.
68. Taylor WK, Campbell JC. Treat protocols for battered women. Response to the Victimization of Women and Children 1992;14(4):16–21.
69. Kellerman A, Reay D. Protection or peril? An analysis of firearm related deaths in the home. N Engl J Med 1986;314:1557–60.

Chapter 6

The Substance Abuse Pandemic: Determinants to Guide Interventions

MARIE L. TALASHEK   LAINA M. GERACE   KAREN L. STARR

Substance abuse poses yet another major threat to the public's health. As community health nurses address the needs of communities, their responsibilities include detecting and preventing substance abuse. To enhance nurses' effectiveness in serving this population, the authors of this chapter propose a comprehensive model to serve as an organizing framework for understanding and intervention. They describe four key determinants that affect substance abuse: biologic, sociocultural, medical–technologic–organizational, and environmental factors. They also discuss appropriate interventions relative to each determinant.

Substance abuse continues to be one of the most devastating problems faced by our society, despite the downward trend in drug abuse and alcohol consumption during the 1980s. It is estimated that 10.5 million adults in the United States show symptoms of alcohol dependence (National Institute on Drug Abuse, 1991a), and that 103,232,000 persons over age 12 years have used alcohol during the past month (National Institute on Drug Abuse, 1991b). Seventy-five and a half million Americans have used an illicit drug at least once. Monthly use of selected drugs includes 1.89 million using cocaine, 479,000 using crack, and more than 3 million using psychotherapeutics (National Institute on Drug Abuse, 1991b). Consequences such as failing personal health, decreased work productivity, family distress and violence, fatal and serious accidents, and fetal alcohol and drug syndromes are staggering and complex, costing the United States billions of dollars each year.

The nursing profession is beginning to make increasingly important contributions to dealing with these health care problems. Funded programs and projects have been developed to upgrade nursing curricula and practice skills in screening, assessment, intervention, and referral of substance-abusing clients (Gerace et al., 1992). These and other developments are beginning to prepare nurses to deal more effectively with such clients in a variety of settings.

From *Public Health Nursing* 11(2):131–139, 1994. Reprinted by permission of Blackwell Scientific Publications, Inc.

Public health nurses have a critically important role in detecting and preventing substance abuse because their primary focus is the welfare of the community. To enhance effectiveness, they require a comprehensive model from which to organize the vast array of knowledge necessary for practice in the community. Such a model has been proposed that provides an organizing framework for assessing, diagnosing, planning, and implementing care and evaluating trends in use, abuse, and addictions (Salmon, Talashek, & Tichy, 1988; Talashek, Tichy, & Salmon, 1989). Public health nurses historically look beyond the essential nursing determinants of human biology and lifestyle, and consider the key determinants of environment and health care delivery in their practice. The model provides a framework for organizing factors that affect health status into four determinants—biologic, sociocultural, medical–technologic–organizational, and environmental—that provide focus for the development of preventive and treatment interventions targeted toward improving community health status (Fig. 6-1). We used the model to organize the body of knowledge related to alcohol and substance use.

■BIOLOGIC DETERMINANTS

Biologic determinants of substance use have been studied for many years, but only recently are they being widely accepted by the health care community. The genetic component of alcoholism was cited for the first time in 1990 (National Council on Alcoholism and the American Medical Society on Addiction Medicine, 1990). Increased attention is being given to the association of genetics to substance addiction, the psychophysiology of tolerance, the adverse physical effects of substance use, and the progression of addiction.

Presently, there are four major research areas in the genetics of alcoholism: familial transmission, association and linkage with biologic markers, vulnerability studies, and characterization of alcohol-metabolizing enzymes (Merikangas, 1990). Findings on familial transmission indicate an average sevenfold increase in the risk of alcoholism among parents and siblings of alcoholics compared with controls. The risk of illness is consistently greater in male than female relatives. This may be attributed to environmental determinants such as exposure and genetic differences, or biologic components such as hormonal factors specific to women (Merikangas, 1990). Research indicated a fourfold increase in rates of alcoholism among grandfathers of male alcoholics (16%) compared with those of nonalcoholic males (5%) (Reich et al., 1980).

Several potential trait markers of vulnerability have been identified. One in particular is decreased intensity of reaction to ethanol. For example, sons of alcoholics have decreased intensity of intoxication and smaller decrements in cognitive and psychomotor performance than matched controls despite similar blood levels of ethanol (Schuckit, 1985). Reactions to low doses of ethanol by sons of alcoholics indicate that these individuals have more difficulty discerning when they are becoming drunk at moder-

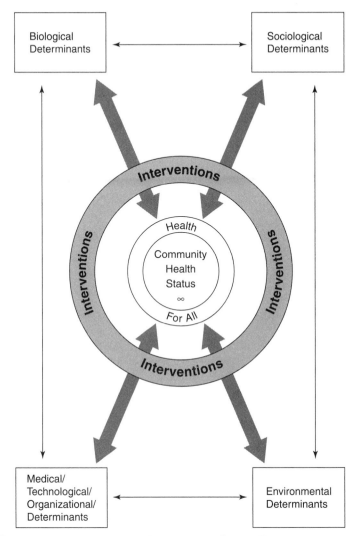

FIGURE 6-1 Health for all: A model for nursing's contributions.

ate doses, thus increasing the difficulty in knowing when to quit before be-coming too drunk (Schuckit, 1985). In addition, two types of brain waves were tentatively indicated as markers associated with a predisposition to al-coholism (Schuckit, 1986).

Research in the biologic area led to a definition that distinguishes be-tween primary and secondary alcoholism. In primary disease severe life problems associated with heavy and persistent drinking develop in individ-uals with no major preexisting psychiatric illness (Schuckit, 1983, 1984). Secondary alcoholism is associated with life problems related to alcohol use after the emergence of a psychiatric illness such as bipolar affective disorder (manic-depressive illness). Both primary and secondary disorders may have a genetic component. Research usually excludes secondary alcoholics from investigation, however, because genetic factors influencing the psychiatric disorder may obscure the genetic factors that predispose the subject to alcoholism.

Research related to genetic vulnerability to drug abuse is limited, although genetic factors are implicated in certain personality traits preceding the onset of chemical dependency. Three central behaviors are impulsivity, failing to inhibit behavior that previously led to negative consequences, and placing more value on immediate drug effects such as intoxication than on long-term consequences such as liver damage (Khantzian & Treece, 1985). Evidence does suggest a pattern of inheritance for drug abuse similar to that for alcoholism, and high rates of alcoholism are found among relatives of drug abusers (Pickens & Svikis, 1988). Alcohol and drugs in the chemically dependent population are frequently interchangeable; rarely is abuse or addiction limited to one agent. Genes do not act independently in determining whether a person will become alcoholic or drug dependent, and thus the need for a biopsychosocial model of addiction.

Many theories have been postulated concerning the neurochemistry of addiction. In the 1970s and 1980s hormonal neurotransmitters were first implicated in the etiology of alcoholism, and other data suggested a deficiency of naturally produced encephalins in the brains of alcoholics (Blum & Frachtenberg, 1987). Others hypothesized an inborn deficiency of catecholamines or hyposensitive neuron receptor sites (Cohen, 1988). Part or all of these may contribute to vulnerability, but since research is in the early stages the definitive answer is pending.

More clearly understood is the psychophysiology of tolerance that contributes to addiction. The liver and other organs deal with repeated use either by metabolizing a drug more efficiently or adapting target cells to its presence, perhaps by down-regulation (Schuckit, 1984). Another factor is the organism's capacity to adjust to the effects of the drug by behavioral adaptation. Individuals are able to tolerate large amounts of a substance without being inebriated; however, over time, alcohol adversely affects every organ system in the body. Subsequently, tolerance diminishes and the individual is unable to metabolize as efficiently or adapt behaviorally to the drug.

Biologic differences between men and women are demonstrated. Men with chronic alcoholism and women in general have less alcohol dehydrogenase activity than do nonalcoholic men. This enzyme detoxifies alcohol, and thus deficiency results in higher bioavailability of alcohol. Therefore, women suffer the long-term effects of alcohol intake at much lower doses in a shorter time span, and are generally sicker than men (Schenker & Speeg, 1990).

Alcohol adversely affects nutrition as a result of deficiencies in folic acid, pyridoxine, thiamine, iron, zinc, and vitamins A, D, and K (Stein, 1991). The skin, lungs, heart, and bone marrow also are adversely affected. Many gastroenterologic problems such as esophageal and gastric varices, peptic ulcer disease, duodenitis, pancreatitis, malabsorption syndrome, alteration in intestinal motility, and structural changes in the upper gastrointestinal tract are associated with ethanol use. The central nervous system is affected, resulting in disordered thought processes, decreased coordination, respiratory depression, problems with thermoregulation, and polyneuropathy. Alcohol abuse is responsible for Wernicke-Korsakoff psychosis and dementia, in addition to numerous other psychiatric problems. Chronic use increases liver size and contributes to jaundice, hepatitis, and cirrhosis. Normal systemic hormone balances and carbohydrate metabolism are affected, and alcohol interferes with adrenocortical, adrenomedullary, thyroid, gonadal, and pituitary function (Stein, 1991).

Chronic use of drugs such as cocaine causes appetite suppression and interference with absorption of water-soluble vitamins B and C, creating malnutrition and severe weight loss in a few weeks (Weiss & Mirin, 1987). Smoking drugs such as cocaine and marijuana causes local irritation of the mucous membranes, which leads to increased secretions, chronic bronchitis, lung inflammation, and lung degeneration. With intravenous cocaine use, particulates can cause emboli. Cocaine is a powerful vasoconstrictor that increases heart rate and may cause arrhythmias, ventricular tachycardia, ventricular fibrillation, aneurysms, and hemorrhage (Weiss & Mirin, 1987).

Marijuana impairs specific intellectual and psychomotor tasks, and interferes with transfer of data to long-term memory storage, thus impeding acquisition of knowledge. The drug impairs driving ability and perspective, increases paranoia and anxiety, and interferes with sperm production and the luteal phase of the menstrual cycle. Many drugs slow reaction time, cause drowsiness, decrease eye-hand coordination, depress respirations, and severely affect the central nervous system (Mann, 1985).

The progression of addiction occurs differently depending on sex, age, metabolism, tolerance, and patterns of use. Quantity of intake does not necessarily indicate early, middle, or late stage of disease, as people are affected individually. In the early stages, experimentation for effect occurs, tolerance develops during the middle stage (more and more of the same drug to achieve the same effects), and the late stage of addiction is associated with a decrease in tolerance signaling the body's inability to clear toxins.

Interventions

The biologic determinants give direction for nursing care through current knowledge of the genetic link in alcoholism and drug abuse, as well as information concerning the association of alcohol and/or drug use with many common health care problems. Diagnosis and interventions will be more timely once nurses routinely gather relevant family and personal data. When nurses begin to identify those at potential risk for alcoholism or substance use, patient education can be directed toward prevention. Interventions can be guided by the stage of disease. Patients in the early stage can best be approached with education, with emphasis on the specific effects of alcohol and drug use on emotional, physiologic, spiritual and family well-being. An invitation to attend Alcoholics Anonymous (AA) or Narcotics Anonymous (NA) meetings can be extended. Patients in the middle stage who have good support systems and who have not failed out-patient treatment are candidates for continued outpatient treatment. Hospitalization is generally the treatment of choice for patients in the late stage of the disease (Secretary of Health and Human Services, 1990). Routine substance use histories will enable nurses to counsel or refer patients for treatment as necessary.

▬ SOCIOCULTURAL DETERMINANTS

Attitudes, beliefs, and behaviors related to substance use are influenced by sociocultural contexts. Important determinants are social systems, special populations, and family systems, all three of which operate within the constraints of cultural norms. Substance use patterns may either distinguish a cultural group's identity, such as abstinence in certain religious groups, or they may bind groups together, such as in ceremonial use (Hill, 1989; Westermeyer, 1980). The importance of sociocultural determinants is reflected in the commonly accepted definition of substance abuse: excessive use that differs from accepted social practice.

Elements in our American society contribute to developing and maintaining alcohol and drug abuse. This is a predictable consequence of a culture that emphasizes consumerism, immediate gratification, and a pain-free, pleasurable life. Drinking, smoking, and drug taking are supported through advertising, public policies, and ready availability. To compound the problem, our society sends mixed messages that lead to confusion about how to control what we use (Mosher, 1990; Lorion, 1990).

Historically, these problems prevail less in cultures where substances are less readily available and use patterns are rigidly prescribed. Today, however, most cultures are loosening social controls, and substances are more easily obtained. For example, over much of the world the relatively low cost of alcoholic beverages, adolescents' easy access to money, and loosening of adult supervision have influenced greater alcohol experimentation and abuse in teenagers (Westermeyer, 1989). In poor urban neighborhoods, alcohol and drug use must be viewed in the context of socioeconomic conditions: poverty, crime, unemployment, lack of male role models, family disruptions, teen pregnancy, and substandard housing (Arkin & Funkhouser, 1990).

The role culture plays in determining substance use patterns is reflected in data about per capita consumption and alcohol-related problems (drunk driving arrests, accidents, family disruption) in various groups. For instance, in the Italian culture where consumption of alcohol is high, but alcohol-related problems are low, children are introduced early to drinking small amounts of wine mixed with water at family meals. Drinking is associated with daily life in the context of eating, not with the purposes of relaxation, relieving stress, or becoming drunk and engaging in high-risk behaviors, such as drunk driving (Heath, 1989). In contrast, among Irish men, drinking rates are often high, as are alcohol-related problems. In this culture, excessive drinking among men is not unusual and is thought to relate to the tight social controls over sexual behavior and marital roles. In addition, because many Irish men socialize with each other in local bars, drinking is associated with stress relief and companionship (Bennett, 1989).

Currently, research in substance abuse emphasizes specific populations, especially in terms of etiology, treatment, and prevention. For some populations a great deal of information is available, and for others less is known. Each population group studied can be considered a culture. Included as special populations of concern are women, the elderly, ethnic minorities, gays and lesbians, and adult children of substance abusers (Lawson & Lawson, 1989; Lex, 1985). Others are adolescents (Logan, 1991; Smart & Jansen, 1991) and pregnant women and their growing fetuses (Lindenberg et al., 1991). Certain aspects of substance abuse are common across these populations, but other aspects are specific and warrant further study.

The public health nurse must beware of sociocultural stereotyping. Differences exist, but it is important to avoid drawing simplistic conclusions about populations and cultural patterns. Cultural influences are never static. The types of substances most commonly used change constantly, as do societal attitudes toward them and patterns of their use. The important issue is how we can change cultural norms and meet the needs of special populations to prevent substance abuse and addiction. Prevention and treatment programs have to be based on cultural understanding.

The family is a social unit within a larger culture. Family systems theory provides a framework for understanding how substance abuse affects its structure, roles, and functions. A family operates through subsystems that guide members' behavior and communication patterns. It is important to recognize that substance abuse is not necessarily an outcome of dysfunctional family roles and boundaries. Often, the opposite is true; having a substance-abusing member creates so much stress in the family that dysfunctional patterns result. Roles and boundaries are altered when children fill in for parents weakened by substance abuse, or spouses compensate for an addicted partner (Silvia & Liepman, 1991).

Today, we hear much about codependency. This concept grew out of clinical observations that family members who live with the chaos created in the family by an addicted member are significantly affected by that person's use of alcohol or drugs (Gomberg, Nelson, & Hatchett, 1991). Codependency is defined as stress-induced preoccupation with the addicted person's life, leading to extreme dependence and excessive concern with the addict (Carruth & Mendenhall, 1989). The family member may take on the same coping style (rationalization, denial) as the addicted person. As a result, the individual has a poor sense of interpersonal boundaries and often behaves in ways that help to maintain addiction. Codependency is a popularized concept that tends to encompass too broad a spectrum of meanings and implications; however, it helps shed light on how family members shield the addicted person from experiencing the consequences of substance abuse.

Interventions

Public health nurses can base interventions on sociocultural determinants in several ways. First, they can help raise public awareness about the social complexities underlying substance use and abuse. Second, they can influence institutions and agencies to work together to solve these in the community. Third, nurses must support public policies designed to modify cultural attitudes and practices, such as promoting the practice of designated drive as a way to avoid drunk driving, or encouraging workplaces to be free of smoking, drugs, and alcohol.

Knowledge of sociocultural determinants can be used therapeutically in substance abuse treatment. In effect, the treatment milieu for addicted individuals has some aspects of a subculture. Treatment programs and self-help follow-up groups (AA, NA) are predicated on the idea that recovery necessitates a new drug- and alcohol-free community with which addicts can identify. In these communities, recovering individuals find support and new cultural norms that help them reenter society to live substance-free, productive lives (Yablonsky, 1989).

Finally, the implications of family systems enter into both prevention and treatment. Children of substance abusers are themselves at higher risk for developing addiction and anxiety disorders, and must be targeted for primary prevention (Haack & Alium, 1991). Public health nurses have to encourage family members to take part in treatment programs so that codependent patterns can be identified and healthier patterns reestablished. Familiarity with the philosophy as well as availability of self-help groups for adult children and other family members is necessary, because these are excellent referral sources. With regard to substance abuse prevention and treatment, public health nurses can, and should, make a difference in the social systems and with the special populations and families served.

▬MEDICAL, TECHNOLOGIC, AND ORGANIZATIONAL DETERMINANTS

Medical, technologic, and organizational determinants are related to accessibility, availability, acceptability, and accountability of health care services. Detecting alcohol and other drug abuse or addiction is difficult, because direct physical evidence may not be available until late in the disease progression (Stein et al., 1991). Therefore, clinicians must rely on indirect methods such as patient history, screening questionnaires, and laboratory analysis of body fluids. A combination of methods is preferable because of differences in sensitivity (the ability to detect those with the condition) and specificity (the ability to rule out those who do not have the condition) of each screening tool (U.S. Preventive Task Force, 1989).

All practitioners can question patients about the quantity and frequency of substance use. This remains an important method for identifying patterns that are or have the potential to become abusive or addictive. However, there is no cohesive body of research indicating the level of accuracy related to self-report. Some studies consider patient self-reports to be accurate (Sobell & Sobell, 1975), whereas others cite low levels of sensitivity (Cyr & Wartman, 1988; Persson & Magnusson, 1988). Thus efficacy must be considered in light of the client, the health practitioner, and the circumstances under which the interview takes place (U.S. Preventive Task Force, 1989).

The use of questionnaires as screening methods for alcohol abuse has been extensively evaluated. The Michigan alcoholism screening test (MAST) has reported sensitivity from 84% to 100% and specificity from 87% to 95% (Selzer, 1971; Pokorny, Miller, & Kaplan, 1972; Moore, 1972). The four-item CAGE questionnaire asks the following questions:

C   Have you ever felt a need to *C*ut down on your drinking/drug use?

A   Have you even been *A*nnoyed at criticism of your drinking/drug use?

G   Have you ever felt *G*uilty about something you've done when you've been drinking/high from drugs?

E   Have you ever had a morning *E*ye-opener—taken a drink/drugs to get going or treat withdrawal symptoms?

It is used routinely in primary care settings, and has reported sensitivity as high as 85% to 89% and specificity between 79% and 95% (Dean & Poremba, 1983; Bernadt et al., 1982; Bush, Shaw, & Cleary, 1987). However, other studies reported sensitivity as low as 49% to 68% (Hayes & Spickard, 1987). The drug abuse screening test (DAST) for identifying drug abuse in general lacks empirical data about instrument sensitivity and specificity. Results from these screening tests must be considered in light of the individual patient's background data and the circumstances under which the data are gathered.

Laboratory analysis of body fluids is another method of detecting substance abuse. Long-term alcohol use is often associated with elevated hepatic enzymes and/or elevated erythrocyte mean corpuscular volume. These are not good screening methods, because positive findings are not consistently present with long-term drinking and may be indicative of other problems. The most sensitive (30–60%) laboratory test for alcohol is the serum gamma-glutamyltransferase. However it has poor specificity (50%) because drugs, trauma, diabetes, and heart or kidney disease can cause false positive results (U.S. Preventive Task Force, 1989). Therefore, one must look beyond these tests for more definitive indicators of abuse.

The physical examination can reveal signs, such as spider angiomata, jaundice, track marks, epigastric tenderness, hepatomegaly, and body odors. Many of these manifestations occur late in the disease process; therefore practitioners have to employ client report, laboratory findings, and screening questionnaires in addition to the physical examination to identify substance abuse or addiction.

Interventions

Initially, patients identified as abusive of or addicted to alcohol and other drugs do not have to want help to receive help, nor do they have to hit bottom before beginning recovery. Intervening for these patients is as appropriate as any other medical decision the health care team makes. Nurses can be effective in screening and referring patients into treatment, because they spend more time with patients in health care settings than do other practitioners. They also are generally effective communicators, thus enhancing the chance for patient disclosure and willingness to act on the referral.

Comprehensive chemical dependency programs are designed for inpatient or outpatient treatment, and admission is based on individual needs. Inpatient treatment ranges from 3 days of nonmedical detoxification in a free-standing facility to 30 days of hospital-based care. It is usually the treatment of choice for individuals who lack support systems, whose home environments are not conducive to recovery, or who require intensive medical management. Referral is sometimes made to a halfway house to continue treatment in a less structured environment but with provisions for continuing support during recovery. Comprehensive outpatient chemical dependency programs are becoming more widely accepted for certain patients because of cost containment and the salutary effect of remaining with a positive support system during treatment.

A multidisciplinary team of nurses, social workers, physicians, dietitians, spiritual counselors, and chemical dependence therapists should be available in the treatment setting. The goal is to meet the client's physiologic, psychosocial, and chemical dependence needs. Treatment cites are located in major medical centers, social service agencies, and university hospital settings.

Most widely recognized are treatment programs based on the 12-step philosophy of AA. This is based on 12 traditions and was founded over 50 years ago by two recovering alcoholics. Adaptations of the program have been made for NA, Cocaine Anonymous, and Double-Trouble Recovery Meetings (for those with a diagnosis of chemical dependence and a psychiatric diagnosis). The overall goal of these programs is to provide an intensive setting that encourages abstinence and supports the long-term recovery of individuals and families. Treatment assists the individual and family members to understand the disease of addiction, and the impact of alcohol and other drugs on every area of life. Public health nurses should familiarize themselves with such options in their communities, thus enhancing ability to match patients' needs with treatment modalities.

Financial considerations are of primary concern to public health nurses attempting to make referrals. Finding treatment slots (beds) for uninsured individuals is difficult, as so few "indigent" or "free" beds are available and waiting lists are usually long. Locating treatment for Medicaid and/or Medicare clients depends on individual states' services and should be investigated before referral. Insurance benefits are frequently very restrictive for psychologic, psychiatric, and chemical dependency treatment. Public health nurses who are familiar with admittance criteria of local facilities can provide more efficient referrals. This will allow matching patient needs, including social support and financial resources, with preventive and treatment resources.

▄ENVIRONMENTAL DETERMINANTS

Environmental determinants are those things over which an individual has little or no control. Public attitude is an important variable in legislative and regulatory actions directed toward limiting access to harmful substances and enforcing legal sanctions for substance abusers. Preventing substance use and alcohol abuse are important agendas for the nursing profession. Empirical evidence indicates that communities can limit substance use problems by controlling the availability of alcohol. This is done by implementing zoning that limits the number of establishments that can sell alcohol, as well as the hours for sales. Imposing federal and state taxes on alcohol is another effective environmental change that limits heavy use (Cook, 1981) and decreases fatal vehicular mortality (Saffer & Grossman, 1987). Restrictions limiting sales to those over 21 years of age is also effective in decreasing motor fatalities among youth (General Accounting Office, 1987).

The federal government has markedly increased funding ($9.48 billion in 1990) for supply-reduction efforts since the passage of the Anti-Drug Abuse Act of 1986 (White House, 1990). Major emphasis has been placed on enforcement actions that increase the risks and costs for drug traffickers. The role of the military and U.S. intelligence forces has been expanded allowing for multiagency approaches to halting trafficking. According to a presidential national security directive, the international drug trade is a national security concern for the United States. Therefore, the State Department has increased foreign assistance to drug-enforcement activities including crop eradication. These increased resources and new initiatives have had a positive impact on the accomplishments of federal agencies responsible for reducing the supply in the United States (General Accounting Office, 1988).

Efforts to decrease the supply can work only when the demand is reduced. Federal demand-reduction strategies target prevention and treatment. The Anti-Drug Abuse Act of 1988 created a cabinet-level Office of Drug Control Policy to coordinate federal activities, and elevated the federal Office for Substance Abuse Prevention to institute status (General Accounting Office, 1988). The Office for Substance Abuse Prevention was directed to develop a demonstration grant program to facilitate the development of effective models for the prevention, treatment, and rehabilitation of drug abuse and alcohol abuse among high-risk youth. These efforts have the potential for identifying effective prevention strategies for youth, because programs with strong evaluation components are given funding priority. Public health nurses who practice in the school can play an instrumental role in prevention programs in addition to intervening with high-risk youth to refer them for counseling and treatment.

Workplace interventions have potential for demand reduction, because 70% of current users of illicit drugs are employed (National Institute on Drug Abuse, 1990). Employee assistance programs (EAPs) are expanding their focus to include identification and referral of employees with drug and/or alcohol problems. More than half of all states mandate that insurers offer substance abuse coverage in their policies, whereas only 30% workplaces have access to an EAP (Office for Substance Abuse Prevention, 1990). Components of an EAP can include employee education about alcohol and other drugs, training of employees to act as referral agents, case consultation, problem assessment, employee referral for counseling or treatment, follow-up cases referred, and feedback to management of services rendered. Some high-risk industries have also instituted mandatory routine employee drug screens as components of their EAP. All of these efforts can be effective for demand reduction. Public health nurses employed in the occupational setting can assume major responsibilities for planning, implementing, and evaluating EAPs. They can guide the process so that workers who have alcohol and drug problems can be identified and referred for treatment while making certain their civil rights are protected.

Interventions

The nursing profession must have policies that give guidance for programs targeted at preventing abuse within the profession as well as their client populations. Public health nurses with school and work site practices can encourage policies and programs to prevent alcohol and substance use and to intervene in a timely fashion to refer individuals who require treatment. They can support funding for prevention programs, especially those with a strong evaluation component. All public health nurses can work in their communities to encourage a positive public attitude about laws, zoning, and education directed toward preventing substance use and abuse.

■SUMMARY

Although the body of knowledge in alcohol and drug abuse is large and complex, the health for all model consisting of four major determinants provides a framework for organizing this vast array of information. Determinants provide focus for the development of preventive and treatment interventions targeted toward improving community health. By becoming familiar with key findings within each determinant, public health nurses can develop intervention strategies that match the needs of individual families and communities.

■REFERENCES

Arkin, E.B., & Funkhouser, J.E. (1990). *Communication about alcohol and other drugs: Strategies for reaching populations at risk.* OSAP Prevention Monograph 5. Rockville, MD: U.S. Department of Health and Human Services.

Bennett, L.A. (1989). Family, alcohol, and culture. In M. Galanter (Ed.), *Recent developments in alcoholism* (Vol. 7). *Treatment research.* New York: Plenum Press.

Bernadt, M., Mumford, J., Taylor, C., et al. (1982). Comparison of questionnaire and laboratory tests in the detection of excessive drinking and alcoholism. *Lancet, 1*, 325–328.

Blum, K., & Frachtenberg, M. (1987). New insight into the causes of alcoholism. *Professional Counselor, 433*(3), 30–34.

Bush, B., Shaw, S., & Cleary, P., et al. (1987). Screening for alcohol abuse using the CAGE questionnaire. *American Journal of Medicine, 82*, 231–235.

Carruth, B., & Mendenhall, W. (1989). *Co-dependency: Issues in treatment and recovery.* New York: Haworth Press.

Cohen, S. (1988). *The chemical brain: The neurochemistry of addictive disorders.* MN: CompCare.

Cook, P. (1981). The effect of liquor taxes on drinking, cirrhosis and auto accidents. In Moore & Gerstein (Eds.), *Alcohol and public policy: Beyond the shadow of prohibition* (pp. 255–285). Washington, DC: National Academy Press.

Cyr, M., & Wartman, S. (1988). The effectiveness of routine screening questions in the detection of alcoholism. *Journal of the American Medical Association, 259,* 51–54.

Dean, J., & Poremba, G. (1983). The alcoholic stigma and the disease concept. *International Journal of Addiction, 18,* 739–751.

General Accounting Office. (1987). *Drinking-age laws: An evaluation synthesis of their impact on highway safety.* Washington, DC: Author.

General Accounting Office. (1988). *Controlling drug abuse: A status report.* Washington, DC: The White House.

Gerace, L., Sullivan, E., Murphy, S., & Cotter, F. (1992). Faculty development and curriculum change in substance abuse. *Nurse Educator, 17*(1), 24–27.

Gomberg, E.S., Nelson, B.W., & Hatchett, B.F. (1991). *Family and Community Health, 13*(4), 61–71.

Haack, M.R., & Alim, T.N. (1991). Anxiety and the adult child of an alcoholic: A co-morbid problem. *Family and Community Health, 13*(4), 49–60.

Hayes, J., & Spickard, W. (1987). Alcoholism: Early diagnosis and intervention. *Journal of General Internal Medicine, 2,* 420–427.

Heath, D.B. (1989). Environmental factors in alcohol use and its outcomes. In H.W. Goedde & D.P. Agarwar (Eds.), *Alcoholism: Biomedical and genetic aspects* (pp. 312–332). New York: Pergamon Press.

Hill, A. (1989). Treatment and prevention of alcoholism in the native American family. In G.W. Lawson & A.W. Lawson (Eds.), *Alcoholism and substance abuse in special populations.* Rockville, MD: Aspen.

Khantzian, E., Treece, C. (1985). DSM III psychiatric diagnosis of narcotic addicts: Recent findings. *Archives of General Psychiatry, 34,* 1022–1027.

Lawson, G.W., & Lawson, A.W. (1989). *Alcoholism and substance abuse in special populations.* Rockville, MD: Aspen.

Lex, B.W. (1985). Alcohol problems in special populations. In Mendelson & N. Mellow (Eds.), *The diagnosis and treatment of alcoholism.* New York: McGraw-Hill.

Lindenberg, C.S., Alexander, W.M., Gendrop, S.C., Nencioli, M., & Williams, D.G. (1991). Review of the literature on cocaine abuse in pregnancy. *Nursing Research, 40*(2), 69–75.

Logan, B.N. (1991). Adolescent substance abuse prevention: An overview of the literature. *Family and Community Health, 13,* 25–36.

Lorion, R.P. (1990). Creating drug-free environments: Beyond and back to the individual. In H. Resnik (Ed.), *Youth and drugs: Society's mixed messages.* OSAP Prevention Monograph 6. Rockville, MD: U.S. Department of Health and Human Services.

Mann, P. (1985). *Marijuana alert.* New York: McGraw-Hill.

Merikangas, K. (1990). The genetic epidemiology of alcoholism. *Psychological Medicine, 20,* 11–22.

Moore, R. (1972). The diagnosis of alcoholism in a psychiatric hospital: A trial of the Michigan alcoholism screening test (MAST). *American Journal of Psychiatry, 128,* 1565–1569.

Mosher, J.E. (1990). Drug availability in a public health perspective. In H. Resnik (Ed.), *Youth and drugs: Society's mixed messages.* OSAP Prevention Monograph 6. Rockville, MD: U.S. Department of Health and Human Services.

National Council on Alcoholism and the American Medical Society on Addiction Medicine. (1990). Editorial: The disease of alcoholism. VIII. Is alcoholism really a disease? *Medical/Scientific Advisory, 5*(4), 7.

National Institute on Drug Abuse. (1990a). Research on drugs and the workplace. *NIDA Capsules, 24.*

National Institute on Drug Abuse. (1990b). *National household survey on drug abuse: Main findings.* Washington, DC: Author.

National Institute on Drug Abuse. (1991a). *National household survey on drug abuse; Population estimates 1991.* Washington, DC: Author.

National Institute on Drug Abuse. (1991b). *Drug abuse and drug abuse research: The third triennial report to Congress from the Secretary, Department of Health and Human Services.* Rockville, MD:

Office for Substance Abuse Prevention. (1990). Employee assistance contracts are available in every state. *The Fact Is . . .* , MS373.

Persson, J., & Magnusson, P. (1988). Comparison between different methods of detecting patients with excessive consumption of alcohol. *Acta Medica Scandinavica, 233,* 101–109.

Pickens, R., & Svikis, D. (1988). Genetic vulnerability to drug abuse, Division of Clinical Research, National Institute on Drug Abuse. *NIDA Research Monograph, 89,* 1–8.

Pokorny, A., Miller, B., & Kaplan, H. (1972). The brief MAST: A shortened version of the Michigan alcoholism screening test. *American Journal of Psychiatry, 129,* 342–345.

Reich, T., Rice, J., Cloninger, C., & Lewis, C. (1980). The contribution of affected parents to the pool of affected individuals: Pathological analysis of the segregation distribution for alcoholism. In L.N. Robins, P.J. Clayton, & J.K. Wing (Eds.), *The social consequences of psychiatric illness.* New York: Brunner/Mazel.

Saffer, H., & Grossman, M. (1987). Drinking age laws and highway mortality rates: Cause and effect. *Economic Inquiry, 25,* 403–417.

Salmon, M., Talashek, M., & Tichy, A. (1988). Health for all: A transnational model for nursing. *International Nursing Review, 35*(4), 107–112.

Schenker, S., & Speeg, K. (1990). The risk of alcohol intake in men and women: All may not be equal. *New England Journal of Medicine, 322*(2), 127.

Schuckit, M. (1983). Alcoholism and other psychiatric disorders. *Hospital and Community Psychiatry, 34,* 1022–1027.

Schuckit, M. (1984). *Drug and alcohol abuse: A clinical guide to diagnosis and treatment* (2nd ed.). New York: Plenum Press.

Schuckit, M. (1985). Studies of populations at high risk for alcoholism. *Psychiatric Developments, 3,* 1022–1027.

Schuckit, M. (1986). Biological vulnerability to alcoholism. *Journal of Consulting and Clinical Psychology, 55*(3), 301–309.

Secretary of Health and Human Services. 1990. *Seventh special report to the U.S. Congress on alcohol and health.*

Selzer, M. (1971). The Michigan alcoholism screening test: The quest for a new diagnostic instrument. *American Journal of Psychiatry, 12,* 1653–1659.

Silvia, L.Y., & Leipman, M.R. (1991). Family behavior loop mapping enhances treatment of alcoholism. *Family and Community Health, 13*(4), 72–83.

Smart, R.G., & Jansen, V.A. (1991). Youth substance abuse. In H.M. Annis & C.S. Davis (Eds.), *Drug use by adolescents: Identification, assessment and intervention* (pp. 25–52). Toronto, Canada: Alcoholism and Drug Addiction Research Foundation.

Sobell, L., & Sobell, M. (1975). Outpatient alcoholics give valid self reports. *Journal of Nervous and Mental Disorders, 161,* 32–42.

Stein et al., (Eds.). (1991). *Internal medicine* (3rd ed.). Boston: Little, Brown.

Talashek, M., Tichy, A., & Salmon, M. (1989). The AIDS pandemic: A nursing model. *Public Health Nursing, 6*(4), 182–188.

U.S. Preventive Task Force. (1989). Screening for alcohol and other drug abuse. In *Guide to clinical preventive services: An assessment of the effectiveness of 169 interventions* (pp. 277–286). Baltimore: Williams & Wilkins.

Weiss, R., & Mirin, S. (1987). *Cocaine.* Washington, DC: American Psychiatric Press.

Westermeyer, J. (1989). Cross-cultural studies on alcoholism. In H.W. Goedde & D.P. Agarwar (Eds.), *Alcoholism: Biomedical and genetic aspects* (pp. 305–311). New York: Pergamon Press.

White House. (1990). *National drug control strategy.* Washington, DC: Author.

Yablonsky, L. (1989). *The therapeutic community.* Bridgeport, CT: Gardner Press.

Chapter 7

Tuberculosis: What Nurses Need to Know to Help Control the Epidemic

DEANNA E. GRIMES   RICHARD M. GRIMES

Tuberculosis, once nearly eradicated, is now a serious threat to public health. Nurses must understand why this is so and what can be done if they are to effectively serve the community. In this chapter Drs. Deanna and Richard Grimes provide a thorough discussion of tuberculosis—its etiology, signs and symptoms, case finding, treatment, and prevention. They describe the roles of both public health and institutions, such as hospitals and nursing homes, in tuberculosis control and challenge nurses to assume leadership in controlling the epidemic.

Historically, tuberculosis (TB) has been one of the great scourges of humankind. In the United States it was a leading cause of death until the 1940s. With the advent of antibiotic therapy the occurrence of the disease began a precipitous decline—until the mid-1980s. Beginning in 1984 the downward slope in the incidence curve flattened and began to reverse itself. The Centers for Disease Control and Prevention (CDC) estimates that between 1984 and 1992, 51,700 more cases of TB occurred than would have been expected if the historic downward trend had continued.[1]

Several reasons are given for this current epidemic. First, there has been a co-epidemic of HIV infection. HIV-infected persons are far more susceptible to acquiring new TB infections, and their infections are more likely to convert to active disease. In addition, if an HIV-infected person has a preexisting, latent TB infection that person is at far higher risk of the infection becoming active disease. For example, immunocompetent persons newly infected with the TB bacilli who do not receive prophylactic treatment have about a 1% to 5% chance of active TB developing within the next 2 years. If the infected person receives appropriate prophylaxis, there almost is no chance that active disease will develop. Of the 95% who do not have active TB during this time frame and do not receive prophylaxis, 5% to 10% will have active disease develop at some time during their lives.[2,3] In contrast, persons infected with HIV who are newly infected with

From *Nursing Outlook* 43(4):164–173, 1995. Reprinted by permission of Mosby-Year Book, Inc.

the TB bacilli and are not treated have a 50% chance of having active TB develop within 60 days of infection and a 7% to 10% annual risk for having active disease develop from a latent infection.[2-4] The high prevalence of active TB in the population infected with HIV also means that those who are in contact with persons infected with HIV will also have a higher probability of acquiring TB infection. This includes those in the infected person's social networks, who also may be HIV infected and susceptible to converting to active disease. This, of course, sets up a reinforcing epidemic that will grow as the HIV epidemic expands and as HIV-infected persons survive longer.

A second reason that is given for the change in TB incidence is the increase in immigration from countries where TB is prevalent. Several million immigrants have entered the United States in the past decade, and most have come from countries where TB is prevalent. Although no one with active TB can be legally admitted to this country, those with latent infection can immigrate. In addition, not all immigration is done through legal channels. As a result, substantial numbers of persons with latent infection and an unknown number of persons with active TB have entered this country. The rate at which imported latent infection converts to active disease is unknown, but it certainly is as frequent as in the native born. The potential effect of immigration can be seen by looking at the rates of TB by ethnicity. Asians and Pacific Islanders have active TB at a rate that is 10 times higher than that of non-Hispanic whites. Similarly, Hispanics have a risk of active disease that is five times higher than that of non-Hispanic whites.[4]

Immigration does not account for all of the increase in TB. TB is a disease of poverty as much as it is a disease of place of birth. This is demonstrated by the TB rates among Native Americans and African-Americans. The former have active TB develop at five times the rate of non-Hispanic whites; the latter contract it at a rate that is eight times higher.[4] Thus much of the excess in TB rates among immigrants may merely reflect that immigrants, as minority groups, are more likely to live on the economic margins of society.

A final explanation for the increases in TB may be the cavalier attitude toward this disease on the part of politicians and health professionals. Both groups have seemingly equated reduced levels of the disease with elimination of the disease. Lack of vigilance in preventing, detecting, and treating this disease and lack of funding for comprehensive control programs may have fueled the current epidemic.

■ NURSES ARE AT RISK

This emerging epidemic has implications for nursing, the most important of which is that nurses and their fellow health care workers are at increased risk for becoming infected with TB. The risk for an individual nurse is proportionate to the amount of exposure that he or she has to patients or coworkers who have active TB. This has always been the case for nurses. A classic study done in the 1930s showed that, while 28% of nursing students were infected at the start of their training, 100% were infected at graduation 3 years later.[5] Those high infection rates reflected the fact that nursing students in that era were in contact with large numbers of patients with active, communicable TB. Nurses today have not experienced anything near those rates of infection, not because they are less susceptible to TB than their predecessors but because they do not encounter as many infected patients. Therefore the rising rates of TB in the population should be of concern to nurses because higher rates mean that a nurse is more likely to encounter a patient with active disease and thereby increase the likelihood of the nurse becoming infected. The literature documents this. There have been multiple reports of nosocomial outbreaks of TB in health care workers,[6-9] prison employees,[10] and homeless shelter workers.[11] These epidemics have involved both conventional strains of TB bacilli and multidrug-resistant strains.

▰BASICS OF TB TRANSMISSION, INFECTION, AND DISEASE

Nurses should be aware of the changes in the extent of TB, but the changes need not cause panic. Transmission of TB can be prevented. TB disease, to a large degree, can be prevented, and the disease is treatable and almost always curable. This statement may best be understood in the context of the natural history of the infection.

Transmission

The organism responsible for TB is *Mycobacterium tuberculosis*. The bacilli are transmitted by airborne droplets expelled from the airways of a TB-infected person who has open, active lesions containing TB bacilli in the lungs, pharynx, or larynx. The infectiousness of the person with TB correlates with the number of organisms that are expelled in the air. For the infection to be transmitted to another person, the droplets containing viable bacilli must be inhaled and the bacilli must invade and begin replicating in the lung, pharynx, or larynx of the new host. Unchecked bacilli then invade the lymphatic system and disseminate, creating inflammatory lesions at multiple body sites.

The probability of inhaling the exhaled air from another person is proportional to the amount of time spent in the same air space with the person, the proximity of the person, and the degree of ventilation. Not all patients are equally infectious; the number of bacilli being shed seems to be related to severity of the case, the extent of the cavitation, the location of lesions, and the presence of cough. Patients who simply cover their mouths when they cough or laugh are much less likely to transmit bacilli. Patients who are receiving anti-TB therapy are rendered increasingly less infectious as their therapy progresses and generally are not infectious after 1 month of appropriate anti-TB therapy.

Infection

TB infection is different from active TB disease. *Infection* refers to the successful colonization of *M. tuberculosis* in a host. Pathogenic processes may not be present. *M. tuberculosis* is a relatively slow-growing organism, which generally allows the body to mount defenses against the infection before the infection becomes pathogenic. The principal defense is a cell-mediated (T lymphocyte) immune response that produces a granuloma around the colony of TB bacilli. Once this has occurred, the bacilli cease to multiply but remain viable within their granulomatous cocoons. As long as the TB bacilli remain encapsulated in the granuloma, the infection is considered to be in a latent state and noninfectious. The organism continues to be viable, however, even though it is not replicating, causing pathologic changes, or being shed. The immune system is remarkably effective in containing this organism. Persons with intact immune systems will create an encapsulating granuloma before disease occurs in 95 of 100 cases. This granuloma will remain intact and prevent pathologic changes from occurring for the rest of a person's life in all but 5% to 10% of cases.[2]

Active Disease

Active TB describes the pathogenic process associated with infection with *M. tuberculosis*. The organism replicates, disseminates, causes caseating necrosis in infected tissue, and may be transmitted. Progression to active disease, either immediately after initial infection or after a period of latency, is generally associated with failure of immune mechanisms. In the event of immunosuppression due to HIV infection, aging, nutritional deprivation, use of corticosteroids, or other reasons, the granuloma may never form or may break down and allow the bacilli to replicate again. Without treatment, the pathologic changes associated with active TB will then occur.

Therefore for a health care worker to become infected and for active TB to develop, several conditions have to prevail. The bacilli must: (1) be expelled from the site of infection in the patient, (2) remain viable outside of the patient, (3) be inhaled by the health care worker, (4) colonize in the airway of the worker, and (5) overcome the cell-mediated immune response or wait many years for a breakdown in the health care worker's general physical health, which will allow the bacilli to escape the granuloma.

Each of these steps is difficult to accomplish. Continuous exposure to an individual with active TB seems to be necessary for transmission to occur. Most health care workers who work with TB patients do not get infected with the TB bacilli. Most household contacts of persons with active disease do not get TB infection. The reasons for this are not clear. It may be that frequency of infected droplets being coughed is low, or it may be that the volume of bacilli in droplets is so low that the organism fails to colonize. The generalized body defenses (e.g., nasal hairs, antiseptic character of saliva, coughing, mucillary clearance) of the potential host may prevent infection. Even if these barriers are overcome, there is only a 5%

chance of the bacilli defeating a competent cell-mediated immune system and progressing to active disease. Nurses do have a low risk of infection, when exposed, and the risk increases as the length of exposure increases. The risk for active disease is also very low. Concrete steps may be taken to reduce the risk of transmission and eliminate the chance of active disease once infection has occurred.

■ HOW TO PREVENT TRANSMISSION OF INFECTION

Transmission of TB can be prevented by: (1) early identification of cases of active disease, to be treated until they are noncommunicable, (2) isolating known and suspected cases of TB until they are determined to be not infectious, and (3) establishing environmental controls that deter transmission.

Case Finding

Health care professionals must seek out those in the active stage of the disease. The key is to become vigilant in looking for it—to think *TB!* Almost all patients with active TB will have symptoms, and many will seek care to alleviate these symptoms. Nurses must be alert for patients with symptoms that could be TB related. While relatively nonspecific, the presence of any of the symptoms listed in Box 7-1 should raise one's suspicion of the presence of TB.

Knowledge of the epidemiology of TB also helps identify potential cases. The populations listed in Box 7-2 are more likely to be infected with *M. tuberculosis.*[12] Those with HIV infection, immigrants from countries with a high prevalence of TB, certain ethnic and low-income populations, and persons with altered immune status from any cause have increased risk. Other high-risk groups include those whose living conditions or life-styles increase their chance of being exposed to infection or progressing to ac-

---

BOX 7-1   *Signs and Symptoms of TB*

- Weight loss
- Anorexia
- Generalized weakness and fatigue
- Continual slightly elevated temperature
- Night sweats, with or without chills
- Persistent cough, nonproductive in early infection but usually progressing to mucopurulent; may become bloody in later stages (hemoptysis). Productive coughs lasting more than 2 weeks should raise the suspicion of potential TB.
- Dyspnea, particularly on exertion, in more advanced disease
- Pain with respiratory movement if pleural involvement
- Rales over apex of lungs
- Hoarseness if larynx is involved
- Dysphagia if pharynx is involved

BOX 7-2   *Population Groups at Higher Risk for TB*

- Persons infected with HIV
- Close contacts of persons known or suspected to have TB, sharing the same household or other enclosed environments
- Persons with medical risk factors known to increase the risk of disease if infection has occurred (see Box 7-3)
- Foreign-born persons from countries with high TB prevalence (particularly countries in Asia, Africa, Latin America, and the Caribbean)
- Medically underserved low-income populations, including high-risk racial or ethnic minority populations (e.g., African-Americans, Hispanics, and Native Americans) and persons who are homeless
- Alcoholics and injection drug users
- Residents of long-term-care facilities, correctional institutions, mental institutions, nursing homes/facilities, and other long-term residential facilities
- Any other populations identified by local health authorities as being at high risk

From the Centers for Disease Control[12]

---

tive disease. This includes those institutionalized in prison, nursing homes, or mental hospitals and those from shelters for the homeless. The homeless have multiple risk factors because of poverty, compromised immune function due to substance abuse, and exposure to persons with inadequately treated TB who are frequently crowded together in shelters or other makeshift living conditions. Many older adults also possess a combination of risks. They lived when TB was far more prevalent and, therefore, are more likely to have latent infection. Advanced age is also associated with declining immune function so latent infection may convert to active disease.

Certain medical conditions predispose individuals with a latent TB infection to progress to active TB (Box 7-3).[12]

The probability of a patient having active, infectious TB is based on symptoms, personal characteristics, life experiences, and medical conditions. The most important is symptoms. While TB symptoms are nonspecific, their presence requires that TB be ruled out. As the number of symptoms increases in a patient, the index of suspicion should be raised. Single symptoms in persons in high-risk populations have more significance than in persons from low-risk groups, but single symptoms should not be ignored in the latter group.

M. tuberculosis is an equal opportunity infector. A person's present state in life means nothing; a latent infection may have been acquired at an earlier, less favored time.

Nurses who suspect, for any of the previously stated reasons, that a person has TB must refer that person for immediate diagnosis and treatment. In general, persons who are thought to have active TB and those with confirmed TB should be considered infectious if cough is present, if cough-

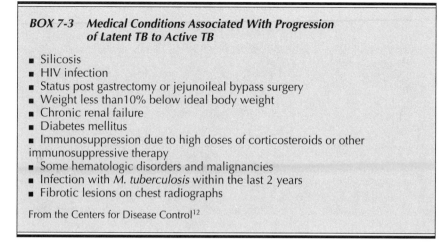

BOX 7-3   Medical Conditions Associated With Progression of Latent TB to Active TB

- Silicosis
- HIV infection
- Status post gastrectomy or jejunoileal bypass surgery
- Weight less than10% below ideal body weight
- Chronic renal failure
- Diabetes mellitus
- Immunosuppression due to high doses of corticosteroids or other immunosuppressive therapy
- Some hematologic disorders and malignancies
- Infection with *M. tuberculosis* within the last 2 years
- Fibrotic lesions on chest radiographs

From the Centers for Disease Control[12]

inducing procedures are performed, or if sputum smears are known to contain acid-fast bacillus (AFB), and if these patients are not receiving anti-tubercular therapy, have not completed at least 3 to 4 weeks of therapy, or have had no change in their symptoms since starting therapy. In addition, those diagnosed with active disease should be considered infectious until three consecutive sputum specimens, each taken 1 day apart, are negative for AFB.[13]

Isolating Known and Suspected Cases

By using knowledge of symptomology, risk factors, and patient physical condition, nurses can assign risk of TB infection to patients to prevent their transmitting infection to others in the health care setting. When a known case of active TB is encountered or when the nurse's clinical judgment suggests TB, immediate efforts should be taken to isolate the person from other patients and to protect health care workers. Until infectiousness has been ruled out, diagnosed and suspected cases should be kept separate from other patients in both outpatient and inpatient settings. Nurses can and should take the initiative to isolate both known and suspected cases.[13]

In an outpatient setting these patients may be assigned to wait in a separate room that is directly ventilated to the outside of the building. Nurses can train other staff, including the receptionist, about the signs of TB. These staff can then alert the nurse of a potential TB case in the clinic. Once alerted, the nurse can make the judgment on whether segregation is necessary. In most circumstances the professionals may not encounter a patient until other patients and staff have been sharing the same air for extended periods. An alert and well-trained receptionist may be key to good TB control in the outpatient setting.

Anyone who is known to have active TB must be placed in AFB isolation as soon as possible after admission to the inpatient facility (Box 7-4).[13] If

---

BOX 7-4   AFB Isolation

Acid-fast bacillus (AFB) isolation is an isolation category for patients with pulmonary or laryngeal TB who have a positive sputum smear or a chest radiograph that strongly suggests active TB. Specifications:

1. Private room with "negative" ventilation (air flows into the room but is ventilated to the outside and away from other patient care area; door to room remains closed).
2. Respiratory protection is to be worn by health care worker when with patient who is considered to be infectious and not covering mouth adequately when coughing and by health care worker performing cough-inducing procedures. Disposable particulate respirators with a tight-fitting facial seal are preferred over most surgical masks.
3. Gowns are indicated only if necessary to prevent soiling of clothing.
4. Gloves are indicated for handling blood, body fluids, mucous membranes, nonintact skin, and all secretions (as in universal precautions).
5. Hands must be washed after touching the patient and potentially contaminated articles and before caring for other patients.
6. Articles are rarely involved in transmission of TB. However, contaminated articles should be thoroughly cleaned and disinfected or discarded.

From Grimes and Grimes[14]

---

the admitting physician has not ordered such accommodations, the nurse must arrange for transfer of the patient to an AFB isolation room and ensure that the proper AFB isolation procedures are followed. In the event that such action is opposed, the nurse should file an incident report and contact appropriate hospital authorities, including the infection control committee. Failure to isolate an infectious patient is irresponsible and endangers staff, other patients, and visitors.

When the nurse's clinical judgment is that TB is possible, his or her actions will depend on the situation and the policies of the facility. The first step is generally to consult with the patient's physician about AFB isolation while the patient is being evaluated for active TB. If the physician does not order isolation, the nurse should consult the policies of the hospital. At some institutions nursing can order AFB isolation. At other institutions there may be a complex process of appeals, consultations, and involvement of other authorities. If nursing cannot independently order isolation, the appropriate hospital officials should be contacted. Depending on the institution, this may include nursing supervisory personnel, hospital administration, infection control personnel, the infection control committee, or some combination of these groups. It is important to be assertive in these circumstances to protect other staff, patients, and visitors from possible exposure.

AFB isolation is one method of reducing the spread of infectious droplet nuclei into the general air circulation by controlling them at their source. The most effective "source control" method is for patients to wear a correctly fitted surgical mask or valve-less respirator when sharing the same air space with others and to cover their mouth when coughing, sneezing, or laughing.[13] Nurses have a responsibility to educate patients about isolation procedures, particularly how and when to wear a mask. Teaching strategies that involve patients as participants in the learning process are generally the most effective. For example, a lecture on wearing a mask is not as useful as having patients demonstrate proper methods of wearing a mask, ensuring that it is tightly fitted around the mouth to minimize broadcasting aerosols. An adequate supply of masks and tissues must be made available to patients.

▄PERSONAL RESPIRATORY PROTECTION

There has been much debate about the appropriate method of filtering out infectious droplet nuclei from the air being inhaled by health care workers. The ideal mask is one designed to have a tight face seal and to filter out particulates in the droplet nucleus size range (1 to 5 μm). Standard surgical masks may not meet these specifications. The mask must also be comfortable enough to be worn when needed. The best filtration device is useless if it is removed constantly because of heat or difficulty breathing. According to the CDC, "The precise level of effectiveness of respiratory protection in protecting health care workers from transmission of *M. tuberculosis* in health care settings cannot be determined with currently available data."[6] Nevertheless, the CDC continues to recommend the use of disposable personal particulate respirators. These respirators are similar to the cup-shaped surgical masks in appearance, but they provide a better facial fit and filtration capability. They should be worn by persons in the same room with a patient whose signs and symptoms suggest a high potential for infectiousness and by those performing procedures that are likely to produce bursts of droplet nuclei (Box 7-5).[13]

BOX 7-5   High-Risk Employment Activities for Nurses

- Administration of aerosolized pentamidine or other aerosol treatments
- Sputum induction
- Bronchoscopy
- Endotracheal intubation/suctioning
- Cough-inducing procedures, including spirometry
- Caring for patients with TB and other pulmonary diseases
- Caring for patients who are immunosuppressed for any reason, including HIV-infected patients
- Working in ambulatory care areas that see many patients who are at high risk for TB (see Boxes 7-2 and 7-3)
- Working in areas that share air space where any of the above procedures are performed or where any of the above patients are provided care

Modified from the Centers for Disease Control[13]

Environmental Controls

The best defenses against TB transmission have already been discussed. They are active case finding, isolation of known or suspected cases, prophylactic treatment of latent infection, together with treatment of active TB and use of personal particulate respirators when in close or prolonged contact with an infectious patient. However, there are also environmental measures that may be taken.[13] Rapid exchange of air in clinics or units with high-risk patients will reduce the concentration of infected droplets in the ambient air. The air cannot, however, simply be more rapidly flowing air that has been recirculated from the same high-risk clinic or unit. The air replacing the contaminated air must come from an uncontaminated source. In addition, the potentially droplet-containing air that is removed from the high-risk area cannot be circulated to other areas of the institution. It should be exhausted to the outside. If, because of building design, air must be recirculated, then some reduction of airborne bacilli may be achieved with the use of filters in the ventilation system and by passing the recirculated air through ultraviolet light. The degree of efficacy of these procedures is not established, but they are believed to be at least partially effective.

Dealing with air circulation is a complicated engineering problem that is beyond the scope of nursing. Nevertheless, nursing can initiate requests for studies of air flow and request consultation on solving air-flow problems.

Again, it must be emphasized that nursing need not rely on environmental controls to prevent transmission. These approaches are expensive, have unproven efficacy, and require constant maintenance. Nurses will not be well protected if they fail to carry out the effective actions over which they have control.

▬HOW TO PREVENT ACTIVE DISEASE

Active TB disease may almost always be prevented by early treatment of the infection. The key is to detect the infection so that prophylactic treatment may be instituted. Therefore periodic skin testing of health care workers must be done.

Skin Testing

The recommended skin test is the Mantoux test. The test is performed by intradermal injection of 0.1 mm purified protein derivative tuberculin containing 5 tuberculin units into either the volar or flexor surface of the forearm. Improper administration will lead to false-negative results; therefore the test should be administered according to procedures well documented in the literature.[14–16]

The test detects the cellular T-lymphocyte immune response to infection with mycobacteria, including *M. tuberculosis*. Reactions may be detected within 2 to 10 weeks of infection with mycobacteria in immunocompetent persons. The reaction must be read 48 to 72 hours after the injection. Test readings before 48 hours frequently yield false-positive results by measuring the diffuse inflammatory responses associated with the injection rather than the reaction to the purified protein derivative.

The result is ready by measuring the size of the induration (raised hardened tissue) at the injection site. Only the induration is measured and not the erythema (the red, inflamed area). The measurement should be made on the transverse diameter and not on the lengthwise diameter. An easy method for measurement is to mark each of the outside points of the induration with a ballpoint pen and then use a ruler to measure the distance between the pen marks. The size of the induration is recorded in millimeters and interpreted as positive for TB infection in adults according to criteria that are based on the differential risk for infection in certain populations.[17] The classification criteria for test results are as follows:

- >5 mm: positive for persons with known or suspected HIV infection; close contacts of known TB cases; and persons with chest radiographs consistent with old, healed TB lesions.
- >10 mm: positive for high-risk persons including persons with other medical risk factors known to substantially increase the risk of TB once infection has occurred (Boxes 7-2 and 7-3).
- >15 mm: positive for all others.

Negative results do not exclude the possibility of TB infection or disease. False-negative results may occur if the test was administered improperly, if the infection is too recent to have elicited an immune response, or if the cell-mediated immune system is suppressed, a phenomenon called *anergy*. Cell-mediated responses may be suppressed for many reasons, including severe or febrile illness, HIV infection, live virus vaccination, Hodgkin's disease, sarcoidosis, overwhelming miliary or pulmonary TB, or use of corticosteroids and other immunosuppressive drugs.

Interpreting skin test results is complicated by the "booster" phenomenon. The cellular immune reaction that develops in response to mycobacterial infection gradually wanes over time in some persons. One TB skin test administered years after the initial infection may elicit negative results, while restimulating, or "boosting," the quiescent immune system, creating a delayed, hypersensitivity reaction. A second TB test administered after a few weeks will elicit a large, positive (hypersensitivity) reaction, falsely suggesting that the person was recently infected. A hypersensitivity reaction is more likely in persons over 55 years old whose initial mycobacterial infection occurred some time in the past. The CDC recommends that when tuberculin skin testing of adults is to be repeated periodically, an initial two-step testing procedure should be used for anyone who has not been recently tested.[17] If the first test result is classified as negative, a second test should be performed a week later. If the reaction to the second test is negative, the person may be considered to be uninfected. A second test result that is positive probably represents a boosted reaction, unless there are symptoms that suggest active TB.

Prophylaxis

If the infection is recent or if latent infection is present, the recommended approach to treatment is to use isoniazid prophylactically for 6 months (extended to 9 to 12 months if the person is coinfected with HIV).[12] This regimen is believed to make a person free of *M. tuberculosis* infection, thus removing the opportunity for new infection to develop into active disease or for latent infection to develop into active disease later in the person's life. The availability of effective prophylactic treatment is the reason for the emphasis that is placed on TB skin test screening for health care workers, which is discussed below in the presentation on institutional control of TB. The CDC criteria for determining the need for preventive therapy is reproduced in Box 7-6.[12]

Treatment

Treatment of active TB is complicated. *M. tuberculosis* is an organism that rapidly mutates in response to antiinfective drugs. Therefore multiple drug therapies are utilized in treating active disease. By using several drugs, the patient will receive an effective drug for each likely mutation. In effect, active TB is treated as a multiple organism infection that necessitates multiple drugs to treat each organism. Current recommendations suggest beginning therapy with four drugs (isoniazid, rifampin, pyrazinamide, and ethambutol or streptomycin) and increasing, decreasing, or changing the regimen on the basis of sensitivity testing and the patient's

---

BOX 7-6   *Criteria for Determining Need for Preventive Therapy for Persons With Positive Tuberculin Reactions, by Category and Age*

Category	<35 Years Old	>35 Years Old
With risk factor*	Treat at all ages if reaction to PPD >10 mm (or >5 mm and patient is recent contact, HIV-infected, or has radiographic evidence of old TB)	
No risk factor High-incidence group†	Treat if PPD >10 mm	Do not treat
No risk factor Low-incidence group	Treat if PPD >15 mm‡	Do not treat

*Risk factors include HIV infection, recent contact with TB, recent skin-test conversions, abnormal finding on chest radiograph, injection drug use, and medical risk factors.

†High-incidence groups include foreign-born persons, medically underserved low-income populations, and residents of long-term care facilities.

‡Lower or higher cut points may be used for identifying positive reactions, depending on the relative prevalence of *M. tuberculosis* infection in the population.

Modified from the Centers for Disease Control[12]

response to therapy.[18] Antitubercular drugs initially act to suppress the organism, thus allowing time for the body to mount an effective immune response. Together, they eradicate the organism. Because of the expected mutations in *M. tuberculosis* it is important that the antimycobacterial regimen be followed to the letter and that patients be monitored closely for their response to the therapy. Deviations from the recommended drugs, dosages, or frequency of administration encourages development of resistant strains that necessitate treatment with even more complicated and lengthy drug regimens.

▬MULTIDRUG-RESISTANT TB

There have been several recent reports of strains of TB bacilli resistant to one or more anti-TB drugs.[18,19] Using the term in its broadest meaning, multidrug resistance to anti-TB drugs is not a new phenomenon. Active TB is treated with multiple drugs because of the potential for the bacilli to mutate into drug-resistant forms. This has been true since the 1940s, when the first anti-TB drug, streptomycin, was heralded as the cure for TB (until it was found to lose its effectiveness within a few months). Additional drugs had to be added to streptomycin therapies to cure TB. Since then new drugs have been introduced that were first promised as a cure but that were later shown to be ineffective against some strains of TB. Over the years these drugs have been employed in various combinations of two-drug, then three-drug, and now four-drug therapies.

Development of resistance is hypothesized to be caused when individuals do not complete their anti-TB therapy in the prescribed manner. That is to say, the infected person ceased taking his or her drugs before the organism was eradicated. The surviving organisms then include types that have developed resistance to a given drug. If therapy had been continued as prescribed, one of the drugs in the combination therapy would have destroyed this strain. When active TB recurs in the incompletely treated person, the dominant type of organism is resistant to the drug. This resistant type, when transmitted to others, becomes part of the community's flora. Bloch et al.[19] provided evidence for this in their study of all TB isolates discovered by all the state health departments in the first quarter of 1991. They found that TB in individuals with no history of TB were resistant to isoniazid 8.1% of the time, whereas resistance was found in 21.5% of recurrent cases. Similar drug resistance was found in recurrent cases originally treated with other first-line anti-TB drugs such as rifampin, pyrazinamide, streptomycin, and ethambutol. The study also showed that, of the 472 isolates that were drug resistant, 41.5% were resistant to more than one drug. Four percent were resistant to five drugs.

So, while the term *multidrug resistant TB* could be applied to a significant portion of TB infections, a specific meaning has been attached to it in recent years. It has come to mean strains of TB bacilli that are resistant to both isoniazid and rifampin or these two drugs and any other anti-TB drugs.[19] Resistance to these drugs is significant because they have been the

most effective drugs for treating *M. tuberculosis.* They are also well tolerated, cheap, easily administered oral drugs that have proved ideal for outpatient use, particularly when used in combination with other, less effective drugs. When resistance develops, therapy becomes more complicated,
more expensive, and more uncomfortable for the patient. Thus noncompliance is more likely, raising the specter of even more drug-resistant
strains.

Experience with multidrug-resistant TB is limited but sobering. In the
several reported outbreaks fatality rates have been high, ranging from 70%
to 90%.[9,19] These outbreaks have occurred mainly in persons who were im-
munocompromised (for example, those with HIV infection or undergoing
cancer chemotherapy). Therefore it is not clear whether these new strains
pose a significant threat to those with intact immune systems. The strains
are, however, a significant threat to a number of patients who are being
seen in health care facilities. The appearance of these strains certainly
raises the specter of their mutating into even more complicated, universally pathologic, deadly organisms.

▬PUBLIC HEALTH ROLE IN TB CONTROL

The rise in TB cases and the appearance of MDRTB strains have posed significant challenges to an already stressed public health system. Because of
the concern about making certain that every person on anti-TB medications is complying with the appropriate regimen for the complete length
of the prescribed course of treatment, public health workers are increasingly carrying out what is called *directly observed therapy.* This involves going
into the community and finding the person under treatment each time
they need to take a medication and then directly observing the person taking the drug. If because of drug resistance the regimen calls for an in-
jectable drug to be used along with the oral drugs, then the intramuscular
drug is given by the nurse at the same time. This is difficult and occasionally dangerous work.

Carrying out directly observed therapy has been added to the traditional task of case finding. Each time a case of active TB is discovered, public health practice requires that the close contacts of the individual, including health care workers, be examined for TB infection. The person with
active disease probably has a relatively recently acquired infection so that it
is likely that someone in his or her social circle has active TB. Even if the
present disease is a conversion of latent infection to active disease, it is possible that the patient's contacts have acquired a recent infection from the
identified case. Failure to follow up on all contacts of an active TB case
raises the probability that active cases will remain untreated and continue
to transmit the infection.

Investigation of patient contacts and arranging for them to receive TB
diagnostic services and making certain that they receive and take their
anti-TB medications are complex tasks that are usually performed by public health nurses. For this part of TB control to be accomplished at all, TB
cases must be reported to the local health department.

Reporting is not only a proper professional nursing behavior, it is an action required by law. In all political jurisdictions in the United States, every known or suspected case of active disease must be reported to health department authorities.[20] Nurses should see that cases are reported as rapidly as possible to ensure rapid investigation (and, it is hoped, a speedier end to the current epidemic). This is also a professional courtesy to the public health nurse who must track contacts, a job that becomes difficult as the trail gets less distinct with time. Professional duty also requires that patients and health care workers who may have been exposed to the active TB case are identified, screened, and treated.

▬INSTITUTIONAL CONTROL OF TB

Hospitals, clinics, nursing homes, and other health care facilities are the places where infectious and other diseases are centralized in society. There are two implications to that statement: First, patients in these facilities are likely to be debilitated and, therefore, susceptible to acquiring infectious disease. Second, they are likely be infected with diseases that can be transmitted to others. Thus health care facilities are excellent breeding grounds for the acquisition and dissemination of TB. This, of course, implies that anyone who works in these facilities is much more likely to become infected with *M. tuberculosis*.

Any health care worker who has active TB is a serious infection control problem. They will be having regular contact with patients who, because of their conditions, will be prone to infection and development of active disease. In addition they will be spending many hours per day with fellow workers who will share the same air with them during that time. So, a real potential exists for the worker with active disease to infect patients and coworkers. The latter group then can infect other patients and become a reinforcing element of a preventable nosocomial epidemic.

The best method of preventing this kind of epidemic is to regularly perform skin tests to discover changes in the infection status of health care workers.[13] All health care workers should have the results of a purified protein derivative skin test on file. If that test result is positive, then no further skin testing is necessary. However, anyone who has a recently converted positive skin test result should have been offered the opportunity to have received prophylactic treatment. If the employee did not receive a full course of appropriate prophylaxis, he or she should be considered to be infected with *M. tuberculosis*. Such persons have the potential for converting to active TB. These employees should be educated as to the signs and symptoms of TB so that they can seek diagnostic evaluation if symptoms appear. These individuals should also be monitored by employee health personnel to make certain that infection does not become active disease.

If employees have a negative skin test finding, then they should be tested periodically to see if the skin test has become reactive. If a formerly negative employee becomes positive, then the employee is considered to be infected with *M. tuberculosis*. Because the chances of the infection becoming active are highest in the first 2 years, any newly positive person should be strongly encouraged to complete prophylactic drug therapy. If an employee refuses drug prophylaxis, he or she must be closely monitored for onset of active disease. Monitoring should include regular review of symptoms and, perhaps, acid-fast bacillus examinations of sputum specimens. Employees who refuse to comply with the regimen should be either placed in jobs with little interpersonal contact or fired.

The frequency at which employees should be tested is still being debated. At the minimum, all health care workers should be tested at least annually.[13] Nurses who engage in high-risk employment activities or who work in high-risk areas of the health care facility should be tested more frequently (Boxes 7-5 and 7-7).[6] The present standard is for these higher risk employees to be tested every 6 months. While some changes are being proposed in this schedule,[6] it is certainly reasonable to follow this standard.

Recommendations recently proposed by the CDC suggest that regardless of task or location, testing should be done more frequently in any group of workers who have worked in an area of known or expected TB transmission.[6] Evidence of transmission includes patient-to-patient transmission, more than one member of the work group converting from negative to positive for the purified protein derivative test in a 3-month period, or the work group having a significantly higher purified protein derivative conversion rate than other work groups. In these circumstances, employees should be tested every 3 months until there is no further evidence of transmission.[6] An additional proposed change is that employees who work in areas that have cared for more than five active cases of TB in a 12-month period should be tested every 6 months. A prudent nurse manager

---

BOX 7-7   *Risk Ratings for Health Care Settings*

High Risk: Skin test every 3 months

Areas that see patients from multiple physical areas in the facility (e.g., x-ray) that:

   Have had a significantly higher TB skin test conversion rate among its employees than other patient care areas or groups

   Have had two or more skin test conversions within 3 months

   Care for patients in an area where there is evidence of patient-to-patient transmission of TB

Medium Risk: Skin test every 6 months

Areas that have had more than five active TB cases in their patient populations during the previous 12 months

Low Risk: Skin test yearly

Less than six TB patients in area per year

From the Centers for Disease Control[6]

might want to combine these approaches—that is, test everybody in the high-risk groups (shown in Box 7-7) every 6 months, and if these or any other employees meet the criteria for suspected transmission or contact with active cases, then test them more frequently.

Nursing's role in skin testing is not just one of putting policies in place; it is one of actively supporting infection control and occupational health personnel in carrying out the testing. Active support includes giving release time for testing, supporting these departments in their efforts to locate and test those who do not comply, and, if necessary, removing noncompliant employees from their jobs until they have undergone their skin tests. Senior management must also show leadership by complying as well. In-service education time could be devoted to periodic review of TB and the steps for self-protection.

Professional nursing must demonstrate leadership for controlling the epidemic of TB. Nurses who take TB seriously will discover that their coworkers will take the disease seriously as well. As a result, everyone's risk of becoming infected will be reduced. Treating the disease as a nonproblem, ignoring one's own or a patient's symptoms, and failing to cooperate in skin testing will only help reinforce the growth of this epidemic and increase everyone's risk of becoming infected.

▄ REFERENCES

1. Centers for Disease Control. Tuberculosis morbidity—United States 1992. MMWR 1993;42:696–704.
2. Benenson AS. Control of communicable diseases in man. 15th ed. Washington: American Public Health Association, 1990:457–65.
3. Berkow MD, ed. The Merck manual of diagnosis and therapy. Vol. 1, 16th ed. Rahway, New Jersey: Merck Research Laboratories, 1992:109–12.
4. Hinman AR. Overview. In: Tuberculosis symposium: emerging problems and promise. J Infect Dis 1993;168:537–9.
5. Catanzaro A. Nosocomial tuberculosis. Am Rev Respir Dis 1982;125:559–62.
6. Centers for Disease Control and Prevention. Draft guidelines for preventing the transmission of tuberculosis in health-care facilities. 2nd ed. Federal Register 1993; 58:52810–54.
7. Perri GD, et al. Transmission of HIV-associated tuberculosis to healthcare workers. Infect Control Hosp Epidemiol 1993;14:67–72.
8. Haley CE, McDonald RC, Rossi L, Jones WD, Haley RW, Luby JP. Tuberculosis epidemic among hospital personnel. Infect Control Hosp Epidemiol 1989;10:204–10.
9. Dooley SW. MDR-TB-Epidemiology. In: Tuberculosis symposium: emerging problems and promise. J Infect Dis 1993;168:539–41.
10. Centers for Disease Control. Probable transmission of multidrug-resistant TB in a correctional facility in California. MMWR 1993;42(3):48–51.
11. Centers for Disease Control. Prevention and control of tuberculosis among homeless persons: recommendations of the Advisory Council for the Elimination of Tuberculosis. MMWR 1992;41(RR-5):13–21.
12. Centers for Disease Control. Screening for tuberculosis and tuberculosis infection in high-risk populations and the use of preventive therapy for tuberculosis infection in the United States: recommendations of the Advisory Committee for Elimination of Tuberculosis. MMWR 1990;39(RR-8):9–12.
13. Centers for Disease Control. Guidelines for preventing the transmission of tuberculosis in health-care settings, with special focus on HIV-related issues. MMWR 1990;39(RR-17):1–29.

14. Grimes DE, Grimes RM. AIDS and HIV infection. St. Louis: Mosby–Year Book, 1994:91.
15. Grimes DE. Infectious diseases. St. Louis: Mosby–Year Book, 1991:45.
16. Avey MA. TB skin testing: how to do it right. Am J Nurs 1993;93(9):42–4. Errata: 1994;94(1).
17. Centers for Disease Control and the American Thoracic Society. Core curriculum on tuberculosis. Atlanta: The Centers for Disease Control, 1991.
18. Centers for Disease Control. Initial therapy for tuberculosis in the era of multidrug resistance: recommendations of the Advisory Council for the Elimination of Tuberculosis. MMWR 1993;42(RR-7):108.
19. Block AB, et al. Nationwide survey of drug-resistant tuberculosis in the United States. JAMA 1994;271:665–71.
20. Centers for Disease Control. Tuberculosis control laws—United States, 1993. MMWR 1993;24(RR-15):1–28.

Chapter 8

Lessons Learned: Challenges For the Future

GLORIA R. SMITH

We live in an era of revolutionary change, not only in health care but in society, and not only in the United States but globally. How will these changes affect the health of present and future generations? How will they influence the practice of public health and health services generally? How will they affect nursing practice? Citing well-known futurists, Gloria Smith in this chapter offers a provocative and helpful discussion of trends affecting society, health care, and nursing. She challenges nursing to see the positives—the opportunities—that lie in these trends and seize them in partnership with communities to shape a healthier world.

Nursing is a profession that historically has rendered unique and significant service to society. As we approach the new millennium, knowledge generated through nursing research and practical study will be in increased demand. Globally, populations with increased life expectancies will draw on nursing knowledge for information and techniques on living healthier, happier, productive lives. Evolving more humanistic, cost-effective health delivery systems also increasingly will be informed by nursing knowledge. Current trends in reconfiguration of health care delivery worldwide and future projections suggest health care systems that are more community responsive and consumer friendly. Though nursing as a profession is preeminently qualified to be the midwife in assisting the paradigm shift, there are opportunities that the profession must seize to be better prepared for the future.

Futurists have described major global trends from which some sectors, such as agriculture, business, and the military, have drawn frameworks to guide future development. Current restructuring in health care delivery appears to be market-driven and present-directed. While it is evident that some future trends, such as the telecommunications revolution, have informed health care restructuring, other major forecasts seem to have been ignored. Fueled by the telecommunications revolution, wealth generation and work are being transformed. Knowledge is the new global basis of wealth creation, the new capital (Naisbitt, 1993; Toffler, 1981).

From *N&HC: Perspectives on Community* 16(4):188–191. Reprinted with permission.
Copyright 1995 National League for Nursing.

Coupling with the preeminence of knowledge will be an emphasis on human talent—individual initiative and the value added by individual knowledge. "Workers will become less and less interchangeable" (Toffler, 1990, p. 239).

Toffler cites the new military as an example of the future requirement for smart workers: "The Gulf War was fought and won by a military that took ten years to prepare . . . soldiers who use their brains, can deal with a diversity of people and cultures, who can tolerate ambiguity, take initiative, and ask questions even to the point of questioning authority" (Toffler, 1993, p. 74). One might ask what are the parallels in the health care sector? If the military and business require "smart workers" for the future, what are the implications for the organization of health care, health care workers, and nursing?

▬WHAT THE FUTURISTS CAN TELL US

Let me report on two principal trends we may translate into concrete possibilities and use to build up an imaginative picture of the nursing practice of the future. The first trend is a fundamental shift in the nexus of power in organizations. The second is the formation of new resources through relationships.

In speaking of a fundamental shift in the nexus of power in organizations I am drawing on the ideas of the futurists Heidi and Alvin Toffler and John Naisbitt. In *Powershift: Knowledge, Wealth, and Violence at the End of the 21st Century* Alvin Toffler (1990) identifies as "[t]he central powershift of our time" that knowledge "has now become the dominant source of both economic wealth and military strength" (p. 452). The knowledge inside the head of the individual worker has become wealth-producing capital and the worker, thereby, "own[s] a critical, often irreplaceable, share of the 'means of production'" (p. 239). Workers attain much more autonomous roles in decision-making and, to speed decision-making within organizations "[h]ierarchy is flattened or eliminated" (p. 239). "The new hero[ine] is no longer a blue-collar worker, a financier, or a manager, but the innovator (whether inside or outside a large organization) who combines imaginative knowledge with action" (p. 239). "Producer and consumer, divorced by the industrial revolution, are reunited in the cycle of wealth creation. . . . Consumer and producer fuse into a 'prosumer'" (p. 239). In *War and Anti-War: Survival at the Dawn of the 21st Century* Heidi and Alvin Toffler (1993) say, "In the Third Wave military, exactly as in the Third Wave corporation, decisional authority is being pushed to the lowest level possible" (pp. 77–78). Forecaster John Naisbitt adds another dimension to the phenomenon identified by Alvin Toffler in which "[s]low-moving bureaucracies are replaced by small . . . work units, temporary . . . teams, . . . complex alliances . . ." (Toffler, 1990, p. 239). In the 1994 book, *Global Paradox*, Naisbitt describes a paradoxical trend in the world economy: "The bigger the world economy, the more powerful its smallest players" (p. 12).

Another trend is of the formation of new resources through relationships. The implication from which it derives is that economies of scale are out and small or mid-size, manageable, and fast are in. Big businesses are forming strategic alliances with competitors in order to avoid getting bigger. Naisbitt describes the unarticulated rationale for these alliances as follows: "Forming an alliance rather than merging or making an acquisition means that *you gain added muscle without getting any bigger* (emphasis supplied)" (p. 19). What can be learned from this is that relationships give strength, not raw resources or power, and these relationships may be highly counter-intuitive.

This lesson is important in an era of dwindling resources. In education, in health care, and in other sectors it is necessary to multiply the impact of resources. The paradox is that this means giving up part of the territory and control in order to gain impact. In the old way of thinking—where resources make up a fixed pie and allocation of them is a zero-sum game in which any gain is someone else's equal loss and any loss is someone else's equal gain—giving up something cannot mean a gain. Working in multidisciplinary teams can be seen as an illustration of the nurse's both receiving and giving up territory in order for the work of the whole team to be more powerful than isolated work by the members.

Flattening of hierarchy in military and industrial organizations is a result of pressures to survive, compete, and win. It is not a result of a commitment by the leaders of powerful organizations to humanize the conditions in which we live and work. An issue is whether those, like nurses, whose purpose is to humanize, can turn the trend to that purpose.

Flattening of hierarchy and the holding by workers of wealth-producing capital, namely knowledge, operate to devolve greater responsibility and decision-making autonomy onto the individual. This broad trend, when taken in combination with community-based practice, gives rise to the possibility of freedom and space in which the power of nursing's principles and practice really take hold of and transform how care is delivered and how patients experience care.

Some of the world's most forward thinking organizations have identified the characteristics of the workplace of the future. One dominant characteristic is better educated workers who challenge management and share power in the workplace. This seems obvious: the more educated the work force, the more democracy it demands. Asking questions and challenging assumptions become part of everyone's job. In the knowledge-based organizations into which transition is occurring, the knowledge levels and decision levels are being redistributed. Managers cannot expect to know everything, to carry the entire knowledge load for organizations. Knowledge and decision making must be diffused throughout the work force (Toffler & Toffler, 1993).

Because of this diffusion, the nurse's workplace of the future, the non-inpatient setting, affords the opportunity to redirect change occurring for one purpose to a nobler end. The National League for Nursing's 1993 *Vision for Nursing Education* refers to a "growing consensus between consumers and the nursing community regarding health care reform . . . to serve the health needs of . . . people . . ." (p. 5) and to the role of the consumer as an "informed participant in decisions affecting . . . care" who replaces "hospitals and other institutions" as "the central focus or dominant influence" (p. 6) in the health care system. The shift to ambulatory care may increase the chance that the health care system may reorient toward the needs of people, but the envisioned consensus between nursing and consumers is not the reason for the shift. The reason is cost-containment. The issue is, then, whether a trend arising for an economic reason can be turned to the purpose of humanizing care and practice.

■COMMUNITIES ON THE MOVE

In our grant making at the W.K. Kellogg Foundation, we are seeing communities in many parts of the world engage in redefining health and designing new approaches to organizing health care services. Comprehensive community-based care and primary care are ascending in importance. We are seeing nursing strive to develop partnerships with consumers and communities.

The trend to deliver care outside the hospital is a force for nursing's return to practice in neighborhoods. However, so much transformation of both nursing and neighborhoods has occurred since neighborhood practice was central to our mission that nurses cannot say we are going back on the path we came down. I think it is more useful to imagine nursing's path as U-shaped, with the years of nursing's transformation corresponding to the letter's bottom curve. We were drawn in by the institutions to help provide the intensive high-technology care that soared in the 1970s and 1980s. It is my hope that during these intervening years we have gained the experience, the strength and the savvy to now pull the institutions behind us as we return to community, as well as the sophistication to facilitate the formation of community-institutional partnerships.

In the intervening years, some communities have become unrecognizable and unpleasant. No one can chide a nurse who thinks the outlook for communities is bleak or dreads going out to help people living in domestic hells or local war-zones. Fortunately, a new way of looking at communities, one that is congruent with nursing's *Vision,* is emerging in America. John McKnight, of the Center for Urban Affairs and Policy Research at Northwestern University, contrasts mapping communities in the traditional way that profiles needs, problems, and deficits with a new way of mapping. In the new way, strengths, resources, assets and capacities are profiled (Kretzmann & McKnight, 1993). Dr. McKnight has been documenting community initiatives that pursue the positives and has begun to edge his way into the mainstream by being retained to retrain the thinking of United Way executives.

The shining gift of nursing is to be able to see the positives, not just the problems, in communities. We will enhance this gift should we succeed in diversifying the composition of nursing student-bodies. The Kellogg Foundation thinks partnerships between the community from which a student comes and training institutions will help achieve such diversification by supporting the student's academic success.

Worldwide, Healthy Cities and Healthy Communities movements are evolving to create new visions of communities that support the best quality of life in all citizens—movements that combine the practical and conceptual. A number of communities around the globe, both large and small, are planning or undertaking initiatives under these rubrics. Other significant efforts may work toward the same end but not carry the label. The Foundation has embarked on a major effort in Michigan to assist three communities to look at how they would structure health care in their locales if they could wipe the slate clean and reallocate available resources. One lesson learned from the project, Comprehensive Community Health Models of Michigan (CCHMs), is that the public values a broadened concept of health. A national study, *What Creates Health? Individuals and Communities Respond,* was carried out by the Healthcare Forum Leadership Center (1994) with partial support by the Foundation and the Healthcare Forum's Healthier Communities Partnership. The study included a nationally representative telephone survey and revealed several important emerging trends among which two are pertinent to this discussion:

1. "The public has a *new concept of what creates health* . . . that moves away from defining health as the avoidance of disease and embraces active pursuit of wellness and an appreciation for the influence of more broad, non-medical quality of life factors" and

2. "People are *discouraged about the health of their own communities*" (Healthcare Forum, 1994, p. 1).

Support for a *healthy communities/healthy cities* initiative may come from government, business, civic organizations, and foundations, including community foundations, which are an important resource for local action.

The new way of conceptualizing health in the community and the nature of the community action it takes to achieve community health are worthy objectives. These trends open opportunities in the United States and other western countries to apply some of the lessons learned from experiences of developing nations, which by necessity have been driven to adopt community development approaches to meeting health needs.

STRATEGIES FOR BUILDING INTEGRATED, COMPREHENSIVE HEALTH CARE SYSTEMS

The W.K. Kellogg Foundation's Health Goal is to help people improve their health and that of their communities by building comprehensive, integrated health systems. In these systems four sectors come together: communities and institutions, services, and education. The Foundation has adopted a series of strategies designed to work together to bring models of comprehensive, integrated health systems into being.

We have drawn on lessons learned under a 1986 goal that had been devised to shift the paradigm to communities and away from institutional dominance. In 1986. we thought communities that solved high-priority health problems of the underserved and vulnerable would build upon that success and go on to resolve other issues.

Our evolving paradigm is the community-institutional partnership. Three lessons from programming under the 1986 goal matured our thinking into the partnership paradigm and the concept of integrating the sectors of communities, institutions, educations, and services.

First, we saw that some community-based projects evolved into greater comprehensiveness of service or inclusiveness of those served. This capacity suggested the potential for movement on a continuum from a single- or problem-focus to system-building.

Second, we learned that, while the distance between communities and institutions is immense, communities need the institutions' resources and expertise. The chasms are wide, but partnerships can build bridges. An East Baltimore pastor who once asked a Johns Hopkins University researcher recruiting subjects for a study, "Why should we help you when Hopkins just uses neighborhood people as guinea pigs in experiments?" more recently said, "Hopkins was used to coming out in the community and telling us. Now they realize that the community has something to share" (Cohen, 1992, p. 13).

Third, we learned that strong community-based health services projects did not, on their own, reach the stage of integrating health professions education into service delivery, although they needed to. Our Community Partnerships for Health Professions Education (CP-HPE) initiative grew out of this realization. Health professionals are needed for new models of delivering services through multidisciplinary teams in community sites. For professionals to be available to *practice* in new models, new models have to be available to them to *train* in. The Community Partnerships is an initiative to build replicable models for core tasks in transformation of the work force. It funds seven local consortia in the United States comprising community health services organizations, community members in the neighborhoods served, and health professions.

▬NURSING IN PARTNERSHIP WITH COMMUNITIES

Professional nursing has already begun forming alliances with consumers for shaping the health care system of tomorrow. One example is the American Nurses Association/Foundation and the National Consumers League, who have developed a partnership to promote and coordinate nationwide coalition-building between nurses and consumers. The two organizations undertook the Community-Based Health Care Project with a three-year grant from the W.K. Kellogg Foundation. Among the project's accomplishments have been, first, that more than 800 consumer and nurse leaders have been successfully trained to assume active roles in the changing health care system and, second, that eleven pilot sites have built coalitions and used a bottom-up approach to addressing local needs for access to care. The independent project evaluation shows, I believe, the ability of nursing in action to value and nurture the decision-making capacities of communities and consumers. The evaluators say that for the pilot sites, "the lack of highly prescriptive guidance for the formation and operation of the sites has enabled 1) the development of local sites that appear to be truly responsive to local needs; and 2) the fostering of a variety of strategies that are adaptive to community needs for improved access to health care" (Teitelbaum & Bieg, 1994, p. iii).

▬THE CHALLENGES AHEAD

One of the most outstanding issues for nursing is whether the field has been adequately informed by trends and projections of the future to envision new approaches to nursing education. Clearly, there has been a response to the demand for increased numbers of primary care providers. Impressive plans have been crafted to increase the numbers of nurse practitioners, nurse midwives, and other advanced practice nurses. Curricula are being reassessed for content relevant to primary care. The field has also responded to the trend of delivery of more care outside the hospital. There is evidence of increased student clinical practice in community-based sites. I am confident that our educational programs will achieve the appropriate balance of community-based experience. The Tofflers' image of the new "smart soldier" still nags, however; I am less certain that our training program holds the image of a new "smart nurse" who, aided by 21st century technology (e.g., personal intelligent-communicators), taps into databases anywhere in the world.

During the early 1970s, Dr. Lawrence Weed, a guru of the problem-oriented medical record was extraordinary in his grasp of the future. He foresaw the potential for clinical practice and health care services in the coming together of communication technologies: computers, consumer electronics, communications, and information. While many during this period focused on the method of the problem-oriented medical record for gathering and organizing data, Weed emphasized the potential of linking clinical data with what he called artificial intelligence, which could enhance clinical judgment and expand the diagnostic skills of clinicians.

I do not feel that we are yet cresting the wave of the future that Weed enabled me to see. In that future the telecommunications revolution has changed the way that health professionals are educated; integrated clinical data and related information systems necessitate collaboration and shared decision making among health professionals; and consumers have increased access to their own clinical data and databases that increase their capability to manage their own health and emerging health problems. In such a future, both health professionals and consumers have expanded knowledge and roles.

For maximum functioning, the more integrated health services and health information systems of the future will require increased collaboration among health professionals and between health professionals and consumers. Health professions education must find ways to enable students to understand the premises and language systems of the various disciplines. Health professionals in collaboration with each other and in alliance with consumers and communities will be best able to define and solve the persistent health problems in the world.

Let me return to the *Vision* statement for a closing word to the reader on remembering ourselves, our strengths, our value, our capacities. Nursing is up against a very tough task. It is not just a matter of shaping the new or of reaching out to grasp the essence of a future trend. It is a matter of countering forces that would shape the new in nonbenign ways and of countering our own habits and what we may have been insidiously taught to think of ourselves. New thoughts will not think themselves. *We* have to think them. But when we do, our leading thoughts bring new forces into the world to shape it. It is *our power to shape the world* that we must be conscious of and courageously carry forward for the sake of the human. We must cultivate our inner resources, however untested and undeveloped when we begin, to build up the strength for the task in reforming health care globally the *Vision* statement reminds us nurse providers must undertake: "to radically redefine their clinical practice, loyalties, political allies, and power dexus" (pp. 6–7).

▬REFERENCES

Cohen, M. (1992, October). And a neighborhood shall lead them. *Baltimore Magazine, 13.*

Healthcare Forum. (1994). *What creates health? Individuals and communities respond.* San Francisco, CA: Healthcare Forum.

Kretzmann, J.P., & McKnight, J.L. (1993). *Building communities from the inside out: A path toward finding and mobilizing a community's assets.* Evanston, IL: Northwestern University.

Naisbitt, J. (1994). *Global paradox.* New York, NY: William Morrow and Co.

National League for Nursing. (1993). *A vision for nursing education.* New York, NY: NLN Press.

Teitelbaum, M., & Bieg, K. (1994). *Evaluation of the community-based health care project, final report.* Bethesda, MD: Abt Associates.

Toffler, A. (1990). *Powershift: Knowledge, wealth, and violence at the edge of the 21st century* (paperback ed., 1991). New York, NY: Bantam Books.

Toffler, A. (1981). *The Third Wave.* New York, NY: Bantam Books.

Toffler, A., & Toffler, H. (1993). *War and anti-war: Survival at the dawn of the 21st century.* Boston, MA: Little, Brown and Co.

Unit 2
Community Health Nursing: Articulating Its Mission

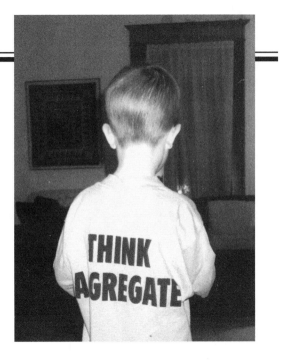

With an increasing volume of health services being offered in the community, it is easy to confuse community or public health with community-based care and community health nursing with community-based nursing. There are important differences.

To understand this field of nursing, one must first clarify its mission: What is community health nursing in business for? What is its purpose? Community health nursing combines the knowledge and skills of nursing with those of the public health sciences to preserve, protect, and promote the health of specific populations, aggregates, and communities. Community health nursing is a specialized field of practice. Its unique contribution to the health system lies not in where it is practiced but in the nature of its practice. It seeks to prevent illness, promote health, and identify persons and specific populations who have an increased risk of illness or disability. It assesses the needs of a population and develops and implements interventions intended to optimize health and decrease the risk of illness, disability, or premature death. It then evaluates these interventions by comparing current health levels with preintervention assessment levels. To clarify community health nursing's mission further, consider its distinctive nature.

Community health nursing has six salient features. First, it is a specialty field of nursing that maintains a commitment to provide quality nursing service—ethically based, accessible, holistic, caring. Nursing theory and principles form a fundamental base for its practice.

Second, community health nursing combines public health and nursing. This means understanding and applying the philosophy of public health practice, incorporating concepts from, for example, the measurement and analytical sciences of epidemiology and biostatistics into nursing practice to solve community health problems. It means understanding the concept of community—how to assess needs and provide service at the aggregate or population level. It means applying principles of leadership, management, and social change to a situation to influence health policy and promote community health.

Third, community health nursing is oriented to populations. This field of nursing shares with public health practice the mission of improving the personal and environmental health of populations and communities. A population or larger group, such as a community, is composed of people who share a common feature such as geography, age, a social concern, or a health problem. Even when working with individuals and families, the community health nurse must maintain this population focus and see these people as parts of larger systems. One can learn from individuals about the health needs of the larger group(s) of which they are a part.

Fourth, community health nursing emphasizes health. Although addressing health problems is a part of community health nursing, its larger mission is to prevent those problems and promote optimal health. This specialty field concentrates on the wellness end of the wellness–illness continuum. Community health nurses must understand the causes of community health problems in order to help prevent them. The use of epidemiologic approaches, then, becomes an essential part of the nurse's practice in establishing an accurate data base and in determining appropriate interventions.

Fifth, community health nursing involves interdisciplinary collaboration. Community health nurses work as full members of a professional health team. To serve population groups, such coordination and cooperation is essential. Individualized efforts and specialized programs, when planned in isolation, can lead to fragmentation and gaps in health services. Certainly, service to families and groups is enhanced by drawing on resources and expertise from other disciplines. Such interdisciplinary collaboration is needed even more for serving populations and communities.

Sixth, community health nursing promotes clients' participation in determining their own health. Only when people assume responsibility for their own health, learn self-care, and become involved in determining health care policy can nursing begin to achieve the goal of optimal health for communities. Ivan Illich, in his classic book *Medical Nemesis,* berates the health care system for creating a passive, dependent clientele. Community health nurses can help to reverse this dependency because first, their emphasis is on wellness and self-care and, second, they have the opportunity and the responsibility to engage clients as full partners in creating a healthy public.

How can community health nurses carry out the mission of preserving, protecting, and promoting the health of populations and communities? The answer lies in incorporating these six features into their practice. Community health nursing can be practiced on a home visit to an elderly couple, for example, when the nurse assesses them as part of a population of elderly persons who may be isolated, lonely, and in need of meaningful activity and companionship—a group for aggregate intervention. Community health nursing can be practiced in a school with a group of pregnant teenage girls among whom the nurse promotes self-care responsibility, even while she or he views them as part of a larger aggregate of pregnant adolescents in the community. With this perspective, the nurse can assess needs and can plan and evaluate health interventions for that larger group in collaboration with other public health professionals, thereby moving the nurse's practice to the population level. This is community health nursing. The chapters in Unit II further articulate the mission of community health nursing and the nature of its practice.

Chapter 9

Community Health Nursing— What Is It?

CAROLYN A. WILLIAMS

A number of years ago, confusion over the definition of community health nursing led Dr. Williams to restate and clarify its meaning. Today these emphases continue to be true and to elucidate our understanding of this field. In this chapter Carolyn Williams presents a strong, logical case for defining community health nursing in terms of its amalgamation with public health theory and practice. Community health nursing, drawing on a public health orientation and commitment, focuses primarily on the health of aggregates and population groups. This aspect distinguishes it from other kinds of nursing practice and makes it a specialty within the profession.

When we talk about community health nursing today, what do we mean? Many nurses in both education and service seem to be in a conceptual and semantic muddle about the nature of community nursing practice: What it is or should be, whether it constitutes or should constitute a specialty, and—if it is a specialty—how it is distinct from other specialties. Even community health nurses have some trouble with the concept; while there is evidence of renewed interest in increasing the amount and types of personal health services provided by community-based agencies, it is questionable whether such services are being planned, delivered, and assessed in a manner consistent with public health philosophy.

One way, perhaps, to diminish some of this confusion and ambivalence is to look again at those fundamental concepts and approaches that have traditionally been a part of public health practice and note their contemporary relevance. Although such a review may not resolve the dilemma, it may stimulate thinking about skills and approaches to bring about more responsible and effective participation by nurses in decision making related to health care delivery.

At present, there are three key barriers to effective integration of preventive and therapeutic community health services and to the planning,

From *Nursing Outlook* 25(4):250–254, 1977. Reprinted by permission of Mosby-Year Book, Inc.

delivery, and evaluation of nursing services that are in touch with community needs, include appropriate consumer participation, and give attention to the natural history of the problems being addressed. Two of the barriers are conceptual ones: first, defining public health nursing practice solely in terms of *where* care takes place and/or whether or not the provider functions in a family-oriented fashion; and second, failing to understand the distinction between the respective foci of clinical nursing and medicine, on the one hand, and public health practice, on the other. The third barrier, in part a legacy of the first two, is an organizational one: paucity of service settings in which the individualistic clinical approach of nursing and medicine and the basic public health strategy of dealing with aggregates are effectively merged and practiced.

▬WHY SUCH BARRIERS?

Many nurses tend to view care settings other than inpatient hospital units as community settings and to define the nursing care which takes place there as community nursing. Some even consider community nursing so defined as a specialty! Such distinctions are less than helpful, and for several reasons.

First, a very narrow definition of community results when one leaves acute care institutions and meaningful articulation between such institutions and other delivery systems out of the picture. Second, although such distinctions may once have enjoyed some validity, other specialty areas in nursing are now preparing students to consider family factors and to practice in extrahospital situations. The result is a blurring of specialties and the emergence, particularly in graduate education, of confusion about the focus of community nursing. Finally, and most important, the distinctions cited do not appropriately reflect the essence of public health practice, its relationship to other specialty areas, and its relevance in addressing health-related problems in a rational manner.

Further, in viewing direct care services provided outside of institutional settings as community health practice, those responsible for education and service programs have either completely neglected or seriously deemphasized the distinction between the foci of clinical nursing and medicine, on the one hand, and public health practice, on the other. *And they are different.* In clinical nursing or medicine the individual patient or family is the unit of care, whereas the central feature of public health practice, according to Sidney Kark is, ". . . focus on the health of population groups (aggregates) such as . . . [those in a defined] community."[1]

Both nursing and medical education focus primarily on preparing professionals to make decisions at the individual patient level. Students are taught to assess the health status of individuals, to make appropriate decisions regarding the care each patient or client should receive, and to see that such care is provided through their own efforts or those of others. Considerably less attention is given to defining problems and proposing solutions at the group or aggregate level, and the transition to this kind of approach may be difficult.

While the integration of community health concepts into basic nursing programs might have been expected to facilitate such thinking, the teaching has frequently emphasized individualistic approaches as opposed to methods of defining problems and assessing impact at aggregate levels. As a result, the graduates are not familiar with group-level decision making, nor are they explicitly aware of the relationship between decisions made at the aggregate level and those made at the patient-provider encounter level.

DISTINGUISHING AGGREGATES OR GROUPS

Group, as defined here, is not limited to an interacting entity—a sociological term—although in some cases it may be. Rather it refers to an aggregate of individuals who have in common one or more personal or environmental characteristics. Some of these characteristics may mean that a group is at high risk of developing specific health problems: for instance, those with hypertension and thereby at greater risk of developing a stroke or coronary heart disease, or those persons living alone who are discharged from an institution to home and may therefore have a lower potential for dealing with a variety of circumstances. Other characteristics may be positively associated with specific problems—that is, black males have a higher prevalence rate of hypertension than white males.

Aggregates can be determined at many levels. Thus, for certain health-related decisions (Medicare), individuals over 65 years throughout the country can be grouped. Locally, decisions about aggregates are made by community agencies in establishing criteria for admission to service and for the types of services which will be offered.

Such a focus on groups or aggregates, however, is not reflected in movements such as the development of expanded roles for nurses and training programs in family medicine. Instead, these developments represent efforts to strengthen the clinical aspect of *personal* health service programs. While they have often resulted in more available, accessible, and acceptable structures for health care delivery at community health centers, rural satellite clinics, and health maintenance organizations, they have also tended to perpetuate the episodically oriented, patient demand, provider response approach to care.

In such situations, patients *select themselves* into the care system, and the provider's role is to deal with what the patients bring to them. No one worries about the relationship between the individual patient's problems and the problems within the community as a whole or within select subpopulations. As the clinical components of these programs are strengthened, individualistic and, less frequently, family-oriented approaches seem to be emphasized to the detriment of a population (aggregate) or community orientation, which would serve to put the clinical services into proper perspective. Although individual or even family-oriented clinical services are necessary for dealing with the personal health service needs of populations, they are not enough!

In 1974, Sheps commented:

It is difficult to find an official or unofficial health agency which is clearly taking on the tasks of monitoring, protecting, and restoring the health of the population; it is not a simple matter to find one that is placing proper emphasis on prevention, and reflects, in its program, the understanding that there are major forces in the way people live that affect their health. These are the problems which public health must address in the future by encompassing the whole area of the environment, patterns of living, and opportunities for the full development of human beings both physically and mentally.[2]

Obviously, Sheps was sketching in broad terms a mandate for the entire field of public health, while the focus of nursing is primarily on two of its components—the promotion of health-related behaviors and the provision of personal health services to members of populations or communities. His comments, however, raise several questions: Why is it unusual to see evidence of public health practice? How would a personal health program that is consistent with a public health philosophy differ from one that is not? And, finally, why isn't there more evidence of personal health programming in which clinical and community dimensions have been appropriately merged?

Despite the fact that it is not easy to change or improve the environment, such efforts may be easier to conceptualize at the community level than are personal health service programs. The need, the relevance—indeed, the potential—in personal health service programs for obtaining group-level data—by conducting a community diagnosis, for instance, or monitoring the health status over time of those receiving care in a particular program—appears to be less obvious. Yet, if the concept of public health practice is to have meaning in the area of personal health care services, it must be operationalized in relevant and viable practice terms which are clear to all.

One approach is to develop an epidemiology in practice orientation similar to that described by Kark.[3] Such an orientation stresses the need to anticipate and estimate the extent of personal health problems at the community level, without limiting the problem definition to only those subgroups seeking care. Such programs, it is suggested, should have a scientific basis and thus reflect what is known about the natural history of the problems being addressed. Further, such an approach demands a continuing surveillance of the delivery system—the types of services given, to whom, and at what points in the natural history of the problem—just as the status of an individual patient would be monitored. And it also suggests that the relationship between services provided and health status changes, both in those served and in the overall target population, should be assessed.

That it *is* possible to take an aggregate approach with personal health service programs is attested to by the following examples.

Many agencies have difficulty in estimating the relationship between those who need a service and those who are already receiving the service. Unfortunately, most agencies simply accept those who are referred to them, without considering the biases operating in the referral system which may bring to attention only a subset of those in need. Another difficulty lies in obtaining an estimate of the need for prevention or for help in maintaining function, rather than an estimate of the requirements for care after an illness event.

In order to deal with these problems, a county health department in the Midwest conducted a community diagnosis as a first step in restructuring its nursing services.[4] Through a systematic, rigorous survey of a sample carefully chosen to be representative of community residents 65 years and older, staff were able to document the status of this population in terms of health conditions as reported, physical functioning, social isolation, and accessibility of medical care. On the basis of these diagnostic data, they projected that their services were reaching only about 25 percent of the people in that age group who could potentially profit from them. And because of other data gathered, they were able to estimate where those in greatest need could be found. These data are being used in restructuring and refocusing the nursing program.

■ POPULATIONS AT RISK

In another county health department, the focus was on a school population.[5,6] The services provided to school children were a responsibility of the department's public health nursing staff. Because of time limitations, however, and with the exceptions of hearing and vision programs, the nurses' school-related responsibilities were frequently limited to one-time episodic encounters with individual children referred by teachers or principals or occasionally self-referred. Response to such service needs may be necessary; however, persisting in these activities would result in an unbalanced program, with insufficient preventive services. Further, children with problems unidentified by the teacher, principal, or themselves often did not come to the attention of the nurse at all. Aware of this fact, the health department decided to continue the usual services provided to the schools while also conducting a pilot program that was preventive in nature and directed to a defined group of children.

How could children with needs or at risk of developing problems be identified? Industrial studies have shown that a small proportion of persons are responsible for the majority of illness in work groups.[7] Further, a recent school study indicated that a good predictor of a pupil's future absences is his previous year's absence record.[8] The significant point here is that at least 80 percent of school absences have been found to be for health reasons.[9,10] It was therefore decided that identification of children with a high record of absences would be a reasonable way of defining a group who would be at high risk for future episodes of illness and absence and who, as a group, might have more basic health problems than children with a history of low absence. And it was further decided that this was a group to whom nursing services could be profitably directed.

In order to evaluate the services, the design of the program called for a comparison of results in one population to those in a control population.

Two groups of high absence children comparable in factors thought to be associated with absence experience were therefore selected. One group received professional nursing services, the control group did not, and the results were documented in terms of change in absence status.

At the beginning of the school year, the nurses assigned to the experimental groups made a family-centered assessment of each high absence pupil as soon as possible. In the process, the nurses were expected to assess and identify possible explanations for the previous year's absence, determine the child's current health status, and assist the family in recognizing and coping with problems or situations which might result in future difficulties.

On completion of the study, it was found that (1) children with high absence records had many needs for preventive and corrective action; (2) the difference in absence experienced between the two groups had meaning both statistically and practically; and (3) while about 99 percent of the 302 children in the experimental group actually received services, only 12 or 3.9 percent of the 302 children in the control group ever came to the attention of the nurse. In other words, if one accepts the notion that high absence children are a group with either problems or potential problems, it is interesting that where there was not an explicit attempt to identify such children, only a small proportion came to the attention of the nurse.

Clearly, the preceding examples demonstrate movement toward systematic community health practice in the area of personal health services. In both cases there was a conscious focus on aggregates or subpopulations, which served to direct clinical care services.

An example of the benefits derived from targeting services to a specific group is suggested from data generated in a midwifery project.[11] The project, which served the segment of a community who contributed greatly to the community's overall prematurity and infant mortality rates (those who utilized the county hospital in which the program was based), reported important favorable changes in rates for those who delivered at the county hospital. However, a year after termination of the nurse-midwifery services, the county neonatal mortality rate showed a dramatic increase to 30.0 (per 1,000 live births) from 17.6 during the last year of the program. This shift in county-level rates suggests that the subpopulation in the county contributing the most to high rates is the subpopulation the program served.

In summary, such more attention needs to be given to the distinction between diagnosis, treatment, and evaluation at the individual patient level (the focus of clinical nursing) and at the aggregate level (the focus of public health). And, after acknowledging the distinction, we need to consider carefully what it means to think in aggregate terms and how clinical and aggregate approaches interrelate.

Such thinking is not only the route to more effective service, which is directed to those most likely to benefit, but it is necessary if we are to implement appropriate priorities for clinical practice. In addition, this type of thinking is necessary for the development and effective use of a knowledge base for practice—that is, the appropriate generation and application of research findings. Finally, such an approach is essential to meaningful collaboration with other disciplines and to the actualization of leadership in health care delivery.

▬COMMUNITY HEALTH PRACTICE SKILLS

Although a group orientation is an essential feature of public health, other characteristics also distinguish community health practice from clinical orientations. For instance, careful consideration must be given to the health status of *many* aggregates. These aggregates may be defined in various ways—infants during their first year, expectant mothers, children of school age, the older population, or those who have just experienced the death of a spouse. A public health orientation demands attention to multiple and sometimes overlapping aggregates as opposed to concern for only one or two specific subgroups, as in the case of clinical specialities such as midwifery or pediatrics.

Further, if practice is to be consistent with public health philosophy, attention must be given to the influence of environmental factors (physical, biological, and sociocultural) on the health of populations, and priority must be given to preventive and health maintenance strategies over curative strategies.

The skills necessary to deal with aggregates, particularly multiple aggregates, are different from those needed for clinical practice. Although some persons may be prepared to function effectively at both levels, it is questionable how realistic such an expectation could be. In the past, failure to recognize this distinction has led to neglect or merely superficial development of skills for dealing with decision making at the aggregate level. Learning these skills is as demanding and time-consuming as developing advanced clinical skills. Therefore, within service settings, it seems reasonable to have both types of skills represented on the staff. Since it may be impossible to have both types of skills in the same person, then communication and collaboration among the staff should be emphasized.

The examples used in this paper focused on the application of selected analytical and measurement skills in both epidemiology and biostatistics to programming for the delivery of personal health services. However, as the following recommendation on higher education for public health points out, such skills represent only one of several deemed essential for public health practice.

In order to produce professional personnel with the appropriate knowledge, skills, and perspective so that they might deal effectively with the new challenges in public health, all institutions providing higher education for public health should build their educational programs on the unique knowledge base for public health. This combines the three elements central and generic to public health with content from many related fields such as medicine and other patient care disciplines; economics, political science, and sociology; biology and the physical sciences. The elements central to public health are the measurement and analytic sciences of epidemiology and biostatistics; social policy and the history and philosophy of public health; and the principles of management and organization for public health. This knowledge base may be modified and expanded with changes in the nature and scope of health problems and the techniques used to deal with them, but an appropriate mix of its central elements with selected related fields is crucial to the effectiveness of any program of higher education for public health.[12]

From a service perspective, it is clear that if nurses are going to have a meaningful role in making policy decisions that deal with aggregates and thus share in determining the boundaries within which direct care providers shall function, nursing educators must give attention to turning out graduates with skill in one of three areas central to public health practice. Historically, graduate nursing programs in both schools of nursing and of public health have offered programs in nursing administration and nursing supervision. Yet it can be argued that those programs have not given sufficient attention to such matters as policy analysis and development and the use of epidemiology in making practice decisions.

What about the future? Although I did not intend to carve out a specialty area for community health nursing, the potential of approaches long associated with public health practice indicate a need for a broader perspective in the preparation of nurses at the graduate level. In addition to programs to prepare direct care providers, such as nurse practitioners, much more attention must be given to the preparation of nurses at the master's and doctoral level whose focus will be on aggregate level decision making. Although not completely separate, the two types of skills are different.

Further, just as direct care clinicians may concentrate on the care of one type of patient defined in terms of age or problems, those preparing for aggregate decision making may focus on developing one of the variety of skills necessary at that level. In addition, there is a serious need for (1) providing core content in the aggregate level skills for those focusing on preparing for specific clinical roles, and (2) developing practice models which clearly demonstrate effective collaboration between clinical approaches and strategies for dealing with aggregates. This is necessary if nursing is to prepare a cadre of professionals who have not only developed skill in their own areas of decision making but who appreciate the context of their practice and can work in a complementary manner with others.

■ REFERENCES

1. Kark, S. *Epidemiology and Community Medicine.* New York: Appleton-Century-Crofts, 1974, p. 319.
2. Sheps, C. G. Crisis in Schools of Public Health: The Issues. *The Body Politic* (School of Public Health at the University of North Carolina, Chapel Hill) 2:3, 1974.
3. Kark, *op. cit.*
4. Managan, D., et al. Older Adults: A Community Survey of Health Needs. *Nurs. Res.* 23:426, 1974.
5. Tuthill, R. W., et al. Evaluating a School Health Program Focused on High Absence Pupils: A Research Design. *Am. J. Public Health* 62:40, 1972.

6. Long, G. V., et al. Evaluation of a School Health Program Directed to Children with History of High Absence: A Focus for Nursing Intervention. *Am. J. Public Health* 65:388, 1975.
7. Hinkel, L. E., Jr., et al. Continuity of Patterns of Illness and the Prediction of Future Health. *J. Occup. Med.* 3:417, 1961.
8. Roberts, D. E., et al. Epidemiological Analysis in School Populations as a Basis for Change in School Nursing Practice. *Am. J. Public Health* 59:2157, 1969.
9. Rogers, K. D., and Reese, G. Health Studies—Presumably Normal High School Students: 2. Absence from School. *Am. J. Dis. Child* 109:9, 1965.
10. School Absenteeism. *Stat. Bull.* (Metropolitan Life) 31:4, 1950.
11. Levy, B. S., et al. Reducing Neonatal Mortality Rate with Nurse-Midwives. *Am. J. Obstet. Gynecol.* 109:53, 1971.
12. Milbank Memorial Fund. *Commission on Higher Education for Public Health.* Cecil G. Sheps, Chairman. New York. Produst, 1976, Recommendation No. 3, pp. 74-75.

Chapter 10

Florence Nightingale on Public Health Nursing

LOIS A. MONTEIRO

Public health nursing owes much of its early development and concern for the poor, for environmental health, and for disease prevention to Florence Nightingale (1820–1910). Eleven of her writings on public health nursing—spanning more than 30 years—have been summarized by Dr. Monteiro in this chapter. As a concerned professional, health care reformer, politically astute consumer advocate, researcher, statistician, and writer, Florence Nightingale serves as a significant role model for today's community health nurse.

■NIGHTINGALE AS SANITARIAN, REFORMER

The accomplishments of Florence Nightingale in identifying the need to educate women who were to work as hospital nurses and in establishing a school at St. Thomas' Hospital are readily acknowledged by the public and the nursing profession. Less well recognized are her efforts as a sanitarian and social reformer. She was especially concerned with the care of the sick poor in workhouses and workhouse infirmaries, as well as the quality of life in their homes and in the slums, and the problems of prostitution and crime that such conditions created. Her writing on nursing for the sick poor outside of hospitals—on what we would now call public health nursing—extend from her early work in 1861, throughout her productive years, and into her very late writing in 1897 when she was 77 years old. These eleven essays are scattered in diverse places such as government reports, a letter to the *London Times,* and a memorial essay for a deceased nurse, rather than appearing as a single definitive volume on the topic, as was the case with *Notes on Nursing* in which she consolidated her thoughts on care of the sick. The content of these essays, and the circumstances that

From *American Journal of Public Health* 75(2):181–186. Reprinted by permission of American Public Health Association.

prompted Nightingale to write them, provide an insight into her views on nursing in a wider context than nursing education.

Nightingale's initial public comments on the subject of public health nursing appear in a November 30, 1861, letter to William Rathbone about a "Proposed Plan for the Training and Employment of Women in Hospital, District, and Private Nursing, 1861," written in response to a request from Rathbone, a rich merchant from Liverpool. A member of the District Provident Society in Liverpool, Rathbone had employed a nurse to care for the sick poor of his district since 1859; in 1861, at his own expense, he tried to expand the services to other districts, but could not find trained nurses. He therefore wrote to Florence Nightingale, who in the previous year had been successful in starting the St. Thomas School to train nurses for hospital work. By 1861, however, Nightingale had already turned to a different project, a Sanitary Reform Commission for the British Colony in India, and was unable to give Rathbone's request her full attention. Nevertheless, she wrote him a long letter in which she "came to the conclusion that the only satisfactory solution was to train nurses specially" (for his project), and suggested that he should approach the Royal Liverpool Infirmary to open a training school that would prepare nurses both for the infirmary and for his district nurse group. He followed her advice and, with his financial support, a Training School was started in Liverpool the next year.[1]

■WORKHOUSE INFIRMARIES

Within a few more years (1864), Rathbone had another request. By that time, the Royal Infirmary was producing trained nurses for the infirmary and the Liverpool district, but the problem of sick paupers had not been addressed. Under the British Poor Laws, the most desperately poor of the large cities were gathered in large workhouses where, when ill, they were placed in crowded workhouse infirmaries. There were 1,200 sick paupers in the Liverpool Workhouse Infirmary, but none of the nurses being prepared in the Liverpool training school could be spared for the workhouse infirmary. He asked Nightingale to help him convince the supervisors of the Liverpool workhouse of the need for reform and to help a matron and a staff of nurses to do the work.

At the time, Nightingale's main attention was centered elsewhere. In January 1864, she had co-authored "Suggestions in Regard to Sanitary Works Required for the Improvement of India Stations," and was much involved in the dealings of the India Office and the War Office.[1] Nevertheless, stimulated by Rathbone's request, Nightingale became peripherally involved in the Workhouse Reform movement.

There had been a growing public awareness of the need for general reform in the workhouses in London as well. Since the 1850s, Lady Visitors, under the leadership of Louisa Twining, had been reporting on the sorry state of workhouse inmates, and some of the workhouse physicians had begun to protest the neglect of the sick poor.[2,3] In December 1864, there was a scandal following a newspaper report of the death "from filthiness caused by gross neglect" of a pauper in a workhouse. Nightingale, recognizing an opportunity, wrote to the head of the Poor Law Board, the overseers of the London workhouse, to suggest reform along the lines then being planned for Liverpool. She urged the Board President, Charles Villiers, to use the inmate's death to "initiate an investigation of the whole question of the sick poor."[1] Her contact with Villiers led to a plan to conduct a survey by means of a questionnaire ("Form of Enquiry") drafted in part by Nightingale and sent to each workhouse in the Metropolitan District to Determine the scope of the problem. Villiers reported to the House of Commons that the Poor Law Board had received communications "from Miss Nightingale who was now taking much interest in the matter."[1]

Nightingale and the others interested in reform recognized that it would be impossible to improve workhouse conditions without reforming workhouse administration, and that to do so would require a change in the Poor Law legislation. Although this was a much more formidable task and would take much longer than the project of producing nurses to work in the infirmaries, Nightingale faced the task with her usual determination, using her connections in Parliament and backing her plans with evidence from the workhouse survey, which "revealed facts so shameful that they could not be ignored." During 1865, she took the initiative to write a report for Parliament, entitled "Suggestions on the Subject of Providing, Training, and Organizing Nurses for the Sick Poor In Workhouse Infirmaries," detailing a three-part plan:

- To insist on separating the sick, the insane, the incurable, and the children in workhouse schools into four separate divisions separate from each other and from the usual population of paupers;
- To advocate a single central administration to ensure uniformity and economy in all workhouses; and
- To support the sick, the insane, and incurable through a Medical Relief Fund to be raised through general taxes.[4]

Nightingale' ideas were incorporated into a proposed bill that met with support from reformers. A formidable push toward change in the treatment of the sick poor, as it had been for earlier health reform, was the fear that disease would spread from the workhouses to the general population.[5] The bill met with opposition and delay, however. Villiers himself was afraid to introduce a controversial bill at a time when the Whig Government, then in power, was in trouble. Others in the opposition were concerned with the high costs of the proposed changes. Furthermore, the motivations of many reformers, while partly humanitarian, also stemmed from self-interest; medical officers, for example, stood to gain financially under the new regulations.

In June of 1866, there was a change of government, with Villiers replaced by a new President of the Poor Law Board, Gathorne Hardy, who shunned Nightingale and her offers of help. This change in leadership of the board caused further delay and led the impatient Nightingale to write,

"It was a cruel disappointment to me to see the Bill go just as I had it in my grasp." Hardy acted independently to investigate matters and eventually to introduce his own bill with many of the same features of the previous one, but under his name only. Hardy's Bill, which Nightingale felt was short of perfection because it did not emphasize nursing, was introduced in the House of Commons in February 1867 and passed on March 29, 1867. The act formed a Metropolitan Asylum District "for the treatment of insane, fever, and small pox cases formerly dealt with in the workhouses. Separate infirmaries were formed for the noninfectious sick . . . and dispensaries were established throughout the metropolis" and a Metropolitan Common Poor Fund was established for the financial support of these asylums.[4] The sick were separated from the paupers, and medical relief was made the responsibility of government. Nightingale, although angry that Hardy had not consulted her, assessed the gains and said, "This is a beginning; we shall get more in time."[4] That spring, Nightingale noted in a diary, "Easter Sunday. Never think that you have done anything effectual in nursing in London till you nurse, not only the sick poor in workhouses, but those at home."[4]

In the meantime, Rathbone's Liverpool experiment in district and workhouse nursing was progressing well. There were 18 districts, each with trained nurses; Agnes Jones, one of the St. Thomas' School nurses, had somewhat reluctantly taken on the leadership role of reforming the care of the workhouse sick, a situation likened by Nightingale to going "among lions," although she added that the paupers were "more untameable than lions."[6] In 1865, Superintendent Jones had 12 trained nurses to care for 1,200 inmates under impossible working conditions. Over the course of the next year, however, progress was made, the experiment received praise from Liverpool authorities, and the Liverpool Workhouse became the model for reform in workhouses in other British cities. The momentum of the reform continued even after Agnes Jones died, in 1868, of typhus contracted during an epidemic in the workhouse. In a dramatic essay entitled "Una and Her Paupers," Nightingale eulogized Agnes Jones' work as "Scutari over again." F. B. Smith, author of a revisionist biography of Nightingale, suggests that Nightingale had expected the Liverpool experiment to fail, but had changed her attitude after Jones died and opportunistically used the memorial essay for her own "wish-fulfillment" and "calculated pleading."[7] Whatever her motivation, the memorial piece served Nightingale's purpose in that it once again focused attention on the situation of nursing in the workhouses.

During those same years, Nightingale's work on Indian Sanitary Reform was progressing in parallel with her push for Poor Law reform in England. With the 1867 Poor Law victory, she turned her attention more fully to India, with all the political difficulties of reform facing her once again. By then 48 years old, she was beginning to feel her age, and to lose some of her fierceness, saying, "I am becoming quite a tame beast" in a letter to a friend in 1868.[1] Also, as her parents' health began to fail, she had to leave London to supervise their care at the country estate in Embly. During the next few years, because of her need to be out of London for months at a time, she limited her work to keeping her ties with the St. Thomas' School and its probationers.

DISTRICT NURSING

In 1874, William Rathbone approached her once more, this time with the idea of instituting district nursing in London. Although Nightingale's Easter Sunday 1867 note had made clear her intention to work for nurses to care for London's poor, Rathbone's request came at a time when, as her biographer notes, "she had to refuse—family difficulties prevented her from undertaking anything which required her to be in London. She could not personally organize but she did everything that could be done from a distance."[4]

Nightingale write in a notebook, "I had resolved to give myself to promoting District Nursing, and now that District Nursing comes it is too late for me to help."[4] The work that she could do from a distance consisted mainly of writing a report, "Suggestions for Improving the Nursing Service for the Sick Poor," and a public statement published in the *London Times,* entitled "On Trained Nursing for the Sick Poor," in which she stressed the need for "district" nursing and appealed for money to support such programs. Furthermore, her earlier efforts in getting public recognition of the need for trained nurses in hospitals and workhouses had changed the climate of public opinion. Rathbone's efforts met with success, and District Nursing, through the Metropolitan Nursing Association, was established in London in 1875 with Florence Lees, another Nightingale school graduate, as the superintendent. Nightingale's essay in the *Times* concluded with: "The object of the Association is: to give first-rate nursing to the sick poor at home (which they never have had)."[8]

In the remaining years of her productive life, Nightingale had two other occasions to help the cause of District Nursing through her writing. One of these was in 1893 when her paper on "Sick-Nursing and Health-Nursing" was read in the United States at the Chicago Exposition. The second, "Health Teaching in Towns and Villages," was written in 1894 to support the extension of district nursing into the rural areas of England. In both papers, she praised the success of district nursing and made a plea for its financial support.

Several recurrent themes are found in the various pieces that Nightingale wrote on the topic of nursing outside of hospitals—a type of nursing that she sometimes referred to as "health nursing" in contrast to "sick nursing." Among the most persistent of these themes are: the need to train the nurse; the nature of poverty and "pauperization"; the importance of preventing disease especially by teaching cleanliness and sanitation; and the nurse's role, particularly the difference between a nurse and a philanthropic visitor.

Her writing style, perhaps the secret of her success in furthering reform, was to hammer away at points, often with repetition in the same piece, and with repetition of certain points each time she approached the subject in different essays. Although the themes are interrelated and sometimes overlap, there is a hierarchy of importance to them, i.e., she insists on some points and will give way on others.

The point on which Nightingale was most adamant, and which she placed above all the others in importance, was that the nurse should be adequately trained. Her statement on district nurse qualifications, delineated in "On Trained Nursing for the Sick Poor,"[8] called for a month's trial in district work, a year's training in hospital nursing, and three to six months' training in district nursing. In that same essay, she wrote:

At home: it is there that the bulk of sick cases are. But where can nurses be trained for them? In hospitals: it is there only that skilled nurses can be trained. All this makes real nursing of the sick at home the most expensive kind of nursing at present.

The need for training was the main emphasis of her first response in 1861 to Rathbone's request for nurses for Liverpool, that is, she determined that what Rathbone needed was not a few nurses, but rather to start a school to train nurses so that they would be available for both homes and hospitals. Her philosophy was that before anything could be done, there had to be properly trained people to do it. This is one key to Nightingale's approach to reform. There is a logical progression in her approach to get things done. For example, she began the workhouse reform with a survey questionnaire to determine the state of existing conditions before she commented on how they should be changed.

Her point that enough nurses for workhouse infirmaries should be trained before reform could begin was repeated in the workhouse reform report of 1867 under the heading of "the present sources of supply of trained nurses, and method of improving the supply of trained nurses." She commented, "to put one trained nurse, however efficient, in an ordinary large workhouse infirmary of a large town, is very much like putting a needle in a bottle of hay. . . . I should discourage . . . the casting ashore of a nurse, here and there, like Robinson Crusoe, on a desolate island, for some overcrowded workhouses are *very* desolate islands."[8]

In addition to her insistence on the need to train nurses, she insisted that one could *not* substitute untrained women, even if educated and with good intentions, for trained nurses. "There is no such thing as amateur nursing" was her response to those who felt that any woman of the "better" classes could do nursing. She further emphasized her point with the comparison: "As if a woman could undertake hospital management, or the management of a single ward . . . without having learnt anything about it, any more than a man can undertake to be, for example, professor of mathematics without having learnt mathematics."[6] Even in her later writing, "Sick-Nursing and Health-Nursing," in 1893, when nursing schools had been in existence for over 30 years, she reiterated that nursing was an "art requiring an organized, practical and scientific training,"[8] and went on to specify the necessary elements of a good training school.

The second theme that permeates her willing on public health nursing builds on the need for training, and focuses on the role of the nurse. Before the advent of district nursing or trained nursing, there was a tradition of Christian charity in which women, to whom Nightingale once referred as "Lady Bountiful," would visit the poor to offer them relief. Ladies' Benevolent Societies or Missions were often involved in this activity. Nightingale held the view that these activities needed to be clearly separated from the distinctive role of the nurse:

> One may pretty safely say that, if district nurses begin by giving relief, they will end by doing nothing but giving relief. Now, it is utter waste to have a highly-trained and skilled nurse to do this: without counting the demoralising and pauperising influence on the sick poor.
>
> Nurses are nurses—not cooks, nor yet almoners, nor relieving officers. But if needed, things are procured from the proper agencies, and sick comforts made as well as given by these agencies. A District Nurse must first nurse.[8]

This separation of the nursing role from the philanthropic visitor role emphasizes the need for special training, and also delineates the specific nursing role. Nightingale had three points that she frequently repeated when specifying the District Nurses' work:

1. A District Nurse must be of a higher class and have fuller training than a hospital nurse, because she has no hospital appliances at hand at all; and because she has to make notes of the case for the doctor, who has no one but her to report to him. She is his staff of clinical clerks, dressers, and nurses.
2. A District Nurse must "nurse the room" as well as the patient and teach the family to nurse the room. To make the room one in which the patient can recover, to bring care and cleanliness into it, and to teach the inmates to keep up that care and cleanliness.
3. A District Nurse must bring to the notice of the Officer of Health, or proper authority, those sanitary defects, which he alone can remedy. Thus dustbins are emptied, water butts cleaned, water supply and drainage examined and remedied.

The two themes that have been discussed—the role of the nurse and the training of the nurse—were the most important points for Nightingale and were repeated in one way or another in most of her writings on the subject of nursing in the home. The remaining broader themes of poverty and sanitation also occur throughout her writing but, with the exception of her two articles specifically on pauperism in *Fraser's Magazine* 1869 and *Social Notes* 1878, these themes are usually incorporated into comments on nursing and are not the main thrust of the writing.

■ DEPAUPERIZING THE POOR

With regard to poverty, Nightingale saw the nurse as one means to "depauperize" the poor, for to her pauperism was not only being poor but also a state of mind, similar to that which Oscar Lewis in his contemporary work called the "culture of poverty." As the following quotes suggest, Nightingale felt that the nurse could change that state of mind and be an agent of societal and individual reform:

> *To set these poor sick people going again, with a sound and clean house, as well as with a sound body and mind, is about as great a benefit as can be given them—worth acres of gifts and relief. This is depauperizing them.*[8]
>
> *Trained nursing enabled the parish doctor to perform a very serious operation in the woman's own home, whereby the parish was saved a guinea a week, and the poor woman's home was saved from being broken up. And this saving of the home from being broken up is of inestimable benefit.*[8]
>
> *The trained district nurse (under the doctor) nurses the child or bread-winner back to health without breaking up the home—the dread of honest workmen and careful mothers who know the pauperising influence of the workhouse even if only temporary.*[9]

Her remarks on poverty were also often combined with comments on the theme of prevention and cleanliness, especially on the nurse's role in teaching cleanliness in the home. In her frequently repeated phrase, the nurse "must nurse the room," she refers to the need for the nurse to show the patient how to be clean, for as she put it, "The very thing that we find in these sick poor is that they lose the feeling of what it is to be clean. The district nurse has to show them."[8] In one essay she described district nursing as a "crusade against dirt and fever nests—the crusade to let light and air and cleanliness into the worst rooms of the worst places of sick London."[8] The themes of cleanliness and prevention are linked in the comments, "She shows them in their own home . . . how they can be clean and orderly, how they can call in official sanitary help to make their poor one room more healthy,"[9] and "The nurse also teaches the family health and disease-preventing ways."[9]

In addition to her insistence on cleanliness and its teaching as the basis for prevention, she made more sophisticated statements similar to those heard at present-day public health meetings:

> *We hear much of 'contagion and infection' in disease. May we not also come to make health contagious and infectious. (1890)*
>
> *Preventible disease should be looked on as a social crime. (1894)*
>
> *It is cheaper to promote health than to maintain people in sickness. (1894)*
>
> *Money would be better spent in maintaining health in infancy and childhood than in building hospitals to cure diseases. (1894)*
>
> *The life-duration of babies is the most delicate test of health conditions. (1893)*

And, in one summary comment, she demonstrated her sense of humor on the issue of prevention:

> *The work we are speaking of has nothing to do with nursing disease, but with maintaining health by removing the things which disturb it . . . dirt, drink, diet, damp, draughts, and drains.*[8]

This review of Nightingale's role in the initial development of the public health nursing field emphasizes the recurring themes of this body of Nightingale's work. Many other subjects of current interest are covered in these essays, including: costs of care, rural health problems, and the position of women in Victorian England. Further research into Nightingale's ideas through study of her published works and her letters and unpublished comments would illuminate her grasp of the complexity of public health problems. While Nightingale herself is famous, the depth of her knowledge and ability have been overshadowed by the public myth that surrounded her. Her importance as a scholar and public reformer has yet to be thoroughly appreciated.

■REFERENCES

1. Cecil Woodham-Smith: Florence Nightingale 1820–1910. London: Constable, 1950, pp. 460, 422, 463, 502, 539–40.
2. Brian Abel-Smith: The Hospitals 1800-1948. Cambridge: Harvard University Press, 1964, pp. 69–72.
3. ———.: A History of the Nursing Profession. London: Heinemann, 1975, pp. 37–38.
4. Edward T. Cook: The Life of Florence Nightingale. London: Macmillan and Co, 1914, v. 2, pp. 133, 139, 143, 253.
5. Gwendoline M. Ayers: England's First State Hospitals and The Metropolitan Asylums Board 1867–1930. Berkeley, CA: University of California Press, 1971, pp. 10–22 passim.
6. Una and Her Paupers, Memorials of Agnes Elizabeth Jones, introduction by Florence Nightingale. New York: George Routledge and Sons, 1872, pp. xv, xxxi.
7. F. B. Smith: Florence Nightingale: Reputation and Power. London: Croom Helm, 1982, p. 175.
8. Lucy Seymer: Selected Writings of Florence Nightingale. New York: MacMillan Co., 1954, pp. 318, 275, 357, 312, 314–7, 362.
9. William Rathbone: History and Progress of District Nursing, with introduction by Florence Nightingale. London: Macmillan and Co, 1890, pp. xv, xi.
10. W. J. Bishop, Sue Goldie: A Bio-Bibliography of Florence Nightingale. London: International Council of Nurses, 1962. (This bibliography is selected from the more comprehensive list compiled by these authors.)

Acknowledgment
An earlier version of this paper was presented at the American Public Health Association's 111th annual meeting in Dallas, 1983.

■APPENDIX:

A Chronological Bibliography of Florence Nightingale's Writings on Public Health Nursing[10]

1865—"Introduction: Organization of Nursing in a Large Town." *In:* An Account of the Liverpool Nurse's Training School, Its Foundations, Progress and Operation in Hospital, District and Private Nursing. London: Longman, Green, Reade and Dyer, 1865. (Miss Nightingale wrote the introduction to this account of the Liverpool plan to train nurses for hospital and home care.)

1867—"Suggestions on the Subject of Providing, Training, and Organizing Nurses for the Sick Poor in Workhouse Infirmities," January 18, 1867. *In:* Report of the Committee Appointed to Consider the Cubic Space of Metropolitan Workhouses presented to both Houses of Parliament. London: Her Majesty's Stationery Office, 1867, pp. 64–79. (In these remarks addressed to the parliamentary committee investigating Workhouse Infirmaries, Nightingale takes the opportunity to discuss "the relation of efficient infirmary nursing to training, organization, infirmary management, and infirmary construction," and makes suggestions for their general improvement and the separation of the sick from the paupers in workhouses.)

1869—"A Note on Pauperism." *Fraser's Magazine,* March 1869; 79:281–290. (In this general statement on issues of poverty, Nightingale urges the removal of the sick from workhouses and makes comments such as "the hungry should not be punished for being hungry" and "bad housing is at the root of much pauperism.")

1872—"Introduction." *In:* Una and Her Paupers, Memorials of Agnes Elizabeth Jones. New York: George Routledge and Sons, 1872. (Miss Nightingale wrote the introduction to this volume commemorating Agnes Jones, the Nightingale-trained nurse who was the first superintendent of the Liverpool Workhouse Infirmary. The comments, which first appeared as "Una and the Lion" in *Good Words,* June 1868, pp. 360–366, focus on the problems that Agnes Jones faced in workhouse reform. Nightingale appeals to women to become trained to work with the sick poor and includes a statement of the requirements and the training program at St. Thomas' Hospital.)

1876—"On Trained Nursing for the Sick Poor." *The London Times,* April 14, 1876, p. 6. (This is a letter that Nightingale wrote to *The Times* supporting the Metropolitan and National Nursing Association for providing nurses for the sick poor. She comments on "what a district nurse is to be" and "what a district nurse is to do.")

1878—"Who Is the Savage." *Social Notes,* May 11, 1879; 1: (10) 145–147. (This article on life in the slums of a large city suggests reforms such as improved housing, work with prostitutes, cooperative stores. She also proposes that nurses be the agents of reform, because nurses are the only people who have access to the people living in slums.)

1890—"Introduction to the History of Nursing in the Home of the Poor." *In:* Sketch of the History and Progress of District Nursing by William Rathbone. London: MacMillan and Co, 1890. (In this introduction to a book on nursing in Liverpool, Nightingale again describes what a district nurse can do: "Besides nursing the patient, she shows them in their own home how they can help in this nursing, how they can be clean and orderly, how they can call in official sanitary help to make their poor one room more healthy, how they can improvise appliances, how their home need not be broken up.")

1893—"Sick-Nursing and Health-Nursing." *In: Woman's Mission.* London: Sampson Low, Marston and Company, 1893, pp. 184–205. (This was also read as a paper at the Chicago Exposition in 1893. In an addendum she describes district nursing: "District nurses nurse the sick poor by visiting them in their own homes, not giving their whole time to one case, not residing in the house. They supply skilled nursing without almsgiving, which is incompatible with the duties of a skilled nurse, and which too often pauperizes the patient. . . . She may take, perhaps, eight cases a day, but must never mix up infectious or midwifery with others.")

1894—*Health and Local Government.* Aylesbury: Poulton and Co, Printers, Bucks Advertiser Office, 1894, two-page pamphlet. (A brief statement of some "laws of health" that include: "Preventible disease should be looked upon as a social crime"; "Money would be better spent in maintaining health in infancy and childhood than in building hospitals to cure disease"; and "It is much cheaper to promote health than to maintain people in sickness." These were presented at a Sanitary Conference held in Aylesbury, Bucks County, October 31, 1894.)

1894—*Health Teaching in Towns and Villages, Rural Hygiene.* London: Spottiswoode and Co, New Street Square, 1894, 27-page pamphlet. (This was originally prepared as a paper to be presented at a Conference of Women Workers on November 7, 1893. In it Nightingale reviews the problems of rural poor and the "dreadful" condition of sanitation (water, refuse, sewage). "We want a fully trained Nurse for every district . . . a water supply pure and plentiful; . . . School teaching of health rules." She also details a plan for Rural Health Missioners, nonnurse health visitors to instruct the "cottage mothers" in sanitation and hygiene.)

1987—*To the Nurses and Probationers Trained under the Nightingale Fund, London, June 1897.* London: Spottiswoode and Co, Printers, 1897, 17-page pamphlet. (Nightingale was 77 years old when she wrote this review of the developments in nursing over her adult lifetime. She discusses district nursing as "the Star of Bethlehem, the crown of good nursing, the modern civilizer of the poor." She says it is "not only the nursing of the patient, but in the nursing of the room, the teaching of the family or neighbors how to help the nurse, the teaching of how to keep in health. . . .")

Chapter 11

The Effectiveness of Community Health Nursing Interventions: A Literature Review

LISA W. DEAL

Community health nurses practice in many settings and provide a variety of types of services. Their interventions with community clients require special skill and creativity at a time when population-based health needs have been escalating while resources for public health have been diminishing. In this chapter Lisa Deal describes services provided by community health nurses—both home-based and community level interventions—and then documents the effectiveness of these interventions based on published research. She recommends convincingly that such documentation is necessary on an on-going basis for nurses to influence policy decisions and gain support for promoting a healthier society.

▆ INTRODUCTION

As the devastating impact of public health problems such as AIDS, infant mortality, adolescent pregnancy, child abuse, and domestic violence become more evident nationwide, a clear need exists for effective population-based health programs. Escalating health care costs and competing health care demands, however, severely limit resources available for public health services. Within this climate that threatens the demise of public health programs, it is imperative that community health nurses (CHNs) define their services and provide evidence supporting the effectiveness of interventions they offer (Oda & Boyd, 1987).

The purpose of this article is to describe the types of services provided by community health nurses and to document the efficacy of community health nursing interventions based on available literature. Policy recommendations supported by the documented effectiveness of CHN services are also offered. The interventions provided by CHNs are divided into two broad categories: home-based and community-level, depending on the clients being served. In home-based interventions, the family unit or indi-

From *Public Health Nursing* 11(5):315–323, 1993. Reprinted by permission of Blackwell Scientific Publications, Inc.

viduals within the family are the focus of CHN services. Community-level or population-based nursing interventions focus on the identified health needs of high-risk groups and promote behavioral or social change within a community in an effort to enhance the overall health status of community constituents.

Although these terms are used to distinguish two separate geographic domains, the effectiveness of community health nursing interventions relies on both an understanding of the daily struggles faced by individual clients or families and knowledge of the social, environmental, and economic conditions affecting health within the community where people live (Zerwekh, 1993). Hence, the specific conditions used by community health nurses are similar whether interventions occur in the home or in a community setting, and community-level interventions may contain a home-visiting element as illustrated in the examples provided.

Community health nursing interventions were selected for inclusion in this review based on two minimum criteria: (1) they focused on health-promotion or disease-prevention services offered to families or aggregate community groups; and (2) descriptive analyses or outcome evaluations documenting the efficacy of these interventions were found in a comprehensive literature search. Because the scope of CHN interventions is too broad to cover in a single article, programs were chosen within each category to reflect the breadth of community health nursing practice.

▄MODELS OF EFFECTIVE INTERVENTIONS
Home-Based Interventions

Although the delivery of population-based nursing services is advocated as the ideal community health nursing model (Williams, 1984), constraints imposed by our current health care system coupled with the complex emotional and physical health needs of disenfranchised families demand that the majority of community health nursing efforts focus at the level of the individual or family unit (Zerwekh, 1992a). A heightened understanding of the impact of social and environmental factors, including poverty, lack of maternal social support, family stress, and inadequate community resources on health makes community health nursing interventions with high-risk families imperative. Traditionally, CHNs advocate a family-centered approach to care by fostering responsibility and promoting self-help among socially high-risk clients during home visiting interventions (Zerwekh, 1992b). Discussion of specific strategies utilized by community health nurses working with vulnerable families includes advocacy, parental teaching, counseling and support, and case management.

Although early evaluations measuring the effectiveness of home visiting by public health nurses demonstrated only limited benefits, these interventions have been associated with increased birth weight and with increased utilization of prenatal care and support services (Baldwin & Chen, 1989). Inadequate study designs, small sample sizes, failure to provide an operational definition of the interventions being evaluated, and lack of data supporting the reliability of measures used were common methodological flaws that limit the usefulness of early evaluation efforts (Combs-Orme, Reis, & Ward, 1985; Baldwin & Chen, 1989). Furthermore, several studies did not target high-risk women (Yauger, 1972; McNeil & Holland, 1972; Hall, 1980; Stanwick, Moffatt, Robitaille, Emond, & Dok, 1982), and many were limited in the number and intensity of interventions aimed at improving maternal-infant outcomes (Lowe, 1970; McNeil & Holland, 1972; Hall, 1980; Stanwick et al., 1982; Barkauskas, 1983).

More recent studies of higher methodological quality indicate that home-based interventions by nurses are indeed effective at promoting maternal-child health when interventions begin prenatally, target women in high socio-demographic risk groups, and provide intensive services to meet comprehensive client needs (Barnard, Magyary, Sumner, Booth, Mitchell, & Spieker, 1988; Olds, Henderson, Tatelbaum, & Chamberlin, 1986a, 1988; Olds, Henderson, Chamberlin & Tatelbaum, 1986b; Starn, 1992). Two exemplary programs, in particular, support the effectiveness of nurse home-visiting interventions that are based on an ecological model incorporating health education with social-support interventions for socially disadvantaged women (Barnard et al., 1988; Olds et al., 1986a, 1986b, 1988). A third study, though smaller in number ($N = 30$), yielded similar results and will be discussed later in this review (Starn, 1992).

Results from a randomized investigation of nurse home visiting conducted in Elmira, New York, indicate that families benefit from extended prenatal and postpartum nursing interventions focused on educating mothers about pregnancy and infant caregiving, encouraging social support networks, and linking families with appropriate health and social services (Olds et al., 1986a, 1986b, 1988; Olds & Kitzman, 1990). In this study, prenatal nursing interventions resulted in less smoking, improved dietary intake, improved maternal health, enhanced social support, greater use of community services during pregnancy, and increased birthweight among infants born to smokers and young adolescents. The benefits associated with postpartum interventions, also most efficacious for children of adolescent mothers living in poverty, included enhanced mental development, less punishing behavior, a lower incidence of child abuse and neglect, and fewer emergency room visits by infants in the intervention groups.

Another component of the home-based interventions offered by nurses included life-skills training aimed at assisting the women in their decisions about pursuing further education, returning to work, and practicing family planning. Relying on the trusting relationships established with these vulnerable women, CHNs were successful in helping women with this cognitive process and teaching them effective life skills. Women receiving this intervention were more likely to obtain further education or employment, were less dependent on public assistance, and had fewer unplanned pregnancies as compared to women in control groups. As with previous outcomes, interventions proved most efficacious for women at greatest social risk (Olds et al., 1988).

The utility of home-based community health nursing interventions that consider the interaction between social environment, inadequate knowledge, and limited caregiving skills is illustrated in a study by Barnard and colleagues (1988). In this randomized investigation, maternal-infant outcomes in families receiving traditional public health nursing services including information giving, health education, and service referral were compared with those among families receiving more intense, comprehensive interventions reflecting an ecological approach to nursing care (Olds & Kitzman, 1990). Evaluated at one year post-delivery, mothers in the later group experienced more positive self-perception, lower levels of maternal depression, greater social support, and better maternal-infant interaction. As in the Elmira study, the beneficial effects associated with home-based CHN interventions were most evident among the least competent mothers.

In another, more recent investigation, the effectiveness of home-based CHN interventions was tested on a small sample of 30 socially disadvantaged pregnant women randomly assigned to a control group or one of two intervention groups (Starn, 1992). The study found that mothers in the intervention groups were more likely to return to work or school after delivery and more likely to report a decrease or elimination of drug use as compared with women in the control group. Mothers in both intervention groups had fewer perinatal complications as compared with controls, and mothers receiving both prenatal and postpartum nurse visits showed better maternal-infant interaction at six months post-delivery. These findings, consistent with those reported earlier, contribute to growing evidence supporting the need for postpartum follow-up to enhance long-term functioning among socially disadvantaged families.

The studies reviewed provide evidence that home-based CHN services produce the most beneficial outcomes measured by maternal and infant well-being when home visits are initiated early during pregnancy; interventions are longer in duration; an ecological model is the basis for interventions; and visits target families with multiple social risk factors. Through interactions with families in the home environment, CHNs gain insight about potential health concerns and are able to intervene before these escalate into serious health problems (Kristjanson & Chalmers, 1991). The high-risk families seen by CHNs are often ill-equipped to negotiate their way through the bureaucratic maze linking them to appropriate health and social service networks. Furthermore, families may be distrusting of "the system," causing them to avoid seeking needed health services. Consequently, suspicion, avoidance, and not knowing how to access services often require active case-finding by nurses to reach those families at greatest social risk.

The cost-effectiveness of preventive interventions that CHNs offer high-risk families is difficult to measure given the fee-for-service orientation of our health care delivery system (Shamansky & Clausen, 1980). It is believed, however, that the costs associated with these services can be offset by a reduction in medical complications, fewer foster care placements, a decrease in unnecessary emergency room visits, and a diminished need for child protective service workers (Olds et al., 1986b; Starn, 1992).

One randomized study has successfully quantified the cost-effectiveness of home-visit follow-up by expert neonatal nurses for infants with very low birthweights (Brooten, Kumar, Brown, Butts, Finkler, Bakewell-Sachs, Gibbons, & Delivoria-Papadopoulos, 1986). Results from this investigation support the cost-effectiveness of early discharge with intense home-based nursing follow-up for 18 months post-hospitalization among these high-risk neonates. By calculating cost savings based on reduced hospitalization and physician charges for infants in the early-discharge group, and factoring in the added cost of nursing services, the authors report a net savings of $18,560 per infant for those in the intervention group. Infants in the early-discharge group had fewer acute-care visits and a lower incidence of failure to thrive, were less likely to be abused, and were less likely to require foster care during the first year of follow-up.

The cost-effectiveness of home-based CHN services can also be evaluated indirectly by identifying positive outcomes and estimating the associated cost-savings. The impact of nurse home-visiting interventions on reducing the incidence of low birthweight illustrates this point. Based on an estimate by the National Commission to Prevent Infant Mortality (1988), preventing low birthweight in just one infant saves $14,000 to $30,000 in health care expenditures during an infant's first year of life. It is estimated that initial hospital costs per low-birthweight infant average $21,000, compared with approximately $2,900 for an infant of normal weight (Kent, 1992). This potential cost savings has major implications for community health nursing interventions that have been shown to reduce the incidence of low-birthweight deliveries.

Community-Level Interventions

Community health nurses face the challenge of moving beyond traditional family-centered interventions to utilize their expertise in population-based health efforts. A discussion of select programs illustrates the diversity of community health nursing expertise and reflects the magnitude of public health problems addressed by CHNs. These examples from the literature document CHN competencies in community assessment, collaboration and coordination, community empowerment, designing and implementing health programs for vulnerable populations, and participation in multidisciplinary practice. Although programs were initially selected for review based on the efficacy of measured outcomes, such evaluations have not been conducted on many community-based nursing interventions. Consequently, descriptive examples of community-level programs are also covered in this review. The absence of definitive outcome data associated with many community-based nursing interventions weakens statements about the effectiveness of these efforts. Rigorous outcome evaluations of community-level nursing strategies should be a major focus of future research efforts.

COMMUNITY PARTNERSHIPS IN MATERNAL-CHILD HEALTH. Improving access to prenatal care is an essential component of public health efforts aimed at reducing infant morbidity and mortality associated with low birthweight. Such efforts require community-level collaboration to overcome barriers that often keep women from initiating early prenatal care. Community health nurses have been effective at mobilizing communities to invest in this cause, and at building partnerships with communities to develop programs aimed at breaking down the barriers to women accessing early pregnancy care (Mahon, McFarlane, & Golden, 1991; May, McLaughlin, & Penner, 1991).

The Pregnancy Outreach Program of the Arizona Department of Health Services is one example of an effective partnership between public health nurses (PHNs) and neighborhood outreach volunteers (May et al., 1991). Using a social marketing framework, this program sought to assess the needs of women at risk for inadequate health care and develop an outreach model aimed at increasing early entry into prenatal care. Outreach workers assisted in case finding and coordination, working as liaisons between high-risk women and appropriate services. PHNs provided core leadership in program development; established community networks; intervened through case management of prenatal clients; and recruited, trained, and supervised community outreach workers. In this capacity, PHNs utilized both individual and community-level strategies to meet program objectives.

The limited time frame of this project precluded measuring outcome data associated with the program's impact on low birthweight, prematurity, or infant mortality, although other population-based programs incorporating intense nursing participation have proved successful at reducing the incidence of low-birthweight deliveries among high-risk women (Buescher, Meis, Ernest, Moore, Michielute, & Sharp, 1989). Despite these limitations, the Pregnancy Outreach Program was able to identify barriers to prenatal care in target communities, raise community awareness concerning problems associated with low birth weight, and increase access to prenatal-care services for socially high-risk women (May et al., 1991). These process-oriented outcomes are commendable given the informational focus of volunteer interventions and the limited time period secured for program funding.

A similar program, De Madres a Madres, was implemented in a Hispanic community in Texas in an effort to increase the number of women who begin early prenatal care (Mahon, et al., 1991). This program promoted the development of a partnership between the business community, the general public, and volunteer mother that was used to identify pregnant women unlikely to seek care, to enhance social support networks, and to disseminate community resource information. The community health nurse employed as project director conducted a community assessment, promoted community activism through networking, and trained volunteer mothers to work as advocates linking high-risk pregnant women with community resources and prenatal care.

A combination of quantitative and qualitative evaluation methods supports the effectiveness of De Madres a Madres. In the first year of De Madres a Madres, 2,000 Hispanic women were visited by volunteer mothers. Contact with volunteer mothers helped women access prenatal care and other community resources including food banks and shelters for battered women. As establishing community ownership is essential to the long-term success of community health programs, nursing activities focused on enhancing community involvement will be emphasized during phase two of De Madres a Madres (Mahon et al., 1991).

THE IMPACT OF FOLLOW-UP SERVICES. Cost-effective, community-based telephone follow-up has been shown to increase the utilization of targeted preventive health services among high-risk children. A quasi-experimental study conducted by Oda and Boyd (1988) evaluated the effectiveness of public health nursing interventions, in this case a telephone call or single home visit, at increasing utilization of Early and Periodic Screening, Diagnosis, and Treatment (EPSDT) services among a population of children from low-income families. During this intervention public health nurses utilized ". . . interviewing and communication skills, health education and counseling principles, and growth and development theory" (Oda & Boyd, 1988: 210). The intervention families who received either a telephone call or home visit ($N = 68$), and the control families not contacted by a public health nurse ($N = 68$) were followed for six months after the interventions to identify whether the target child received a health assessment through the EPSDT program. Results indicate that while nearly 21% of children in the intervention group received a health assessment, this was true for less than 5% of the control children ($p = 0.0005$).

An earlier study by Oda, Fine, and Heilbron (1986) also supports the cost-effectiveness of telephone follow-up by PHNs as a means of increasing the utilization of dental visits for necessary restorative care. In this study, 934 inner-city children identified based on their need for restorative dental services were randomized to either an intervention ($N = 462$) or control ($N = 472$) group. Intervention families received telephone follow-up from a public health nurse to educate them about the need for restorative services, while control families were not contacted by a nurse. Findings indicate a significant increase in the number of dental visits by children in the experimental group. The cost of public health nursing follow-up was calculated to be $8.92 per family contacted, suggesting this is a relatively low-cost intervention. Both of these investigations support the efficacy of community health nursing interventions at increasing appropriate health service utilization among low-income families and suggest strategies for improving the health status of disadvantaged children.

PROMOTING HEALTH IN DAY CARE CENTERS. As the proportion of women in the work force continues to rise, more families rely on day care facilities to assume responsibility for their children during working hours. Maintaining the health and safety of these children is a community-wide concern to which public health nurses respond by conducting site visits, providing health and safety education, conducting health screenings, and offering consultative services. Descriptions of innovative public health nursing programs developed to promote the health and safety of children in licensed day care facilities have been documented (Schmelzer, Reeves, & Zahner, 1986; Lie, 1992; Grayville, 1991; Carlin, Sabol, & Schloesser, 1986). Although outcome evaluations measuring the impact of these interventions have not been widely publicized, a discussion of two such programs illustrates the effective utilization of PHNs in day care settings.

Schmelzer and colleagues (1986) discuss the essential role of public health nurses in a health program developed for children enrolled in licensed day care centers in Madison, Wisconsin. Based on a public health nursing service model, the program was designed to promote healthy behaviors, provide health screening, offer guidance for health-problem management, and provide education about safety measures in the day care setting. The expert competencies of PHNs in collaboration, networking, coordination, screening, health education, and anticipatory guidance contributed to the program's success. Using these practice competencies, public health nurses were effective in the delivery of comprehensive, coordinated services.

Another model program providing public health nursing consultation and services to both center-based facilities and family day care homes was implemented at the Minneapolis Health Department, where a small team of PHNs offers phone consultation, home visits, and group training sessions to day care workers (Lie, 1992). This team also provides information and education about such issues as infection control, first aid, diapering procedures, and child stress. A randomized evaluation of the usefulness of these services found that 67% of day care providers surveyed had received PHN services, and many providers requested the expansion of existing services. These results support the efficacy of public health nursing interventions in promoting the health of children in day care settings.

PROGRAMS FOR VULNERABLE POPULATIONS. Although many community health nursing interventions focus on maternal-child health, CHNs also work with more inclusive high-risk populations. Programs developed for the homeless and people at risk of HIV/AIDS illustrate interventions not specific to certain age or gender groups.

As a major public health concern during the past decade, the AIDS epidemic has demanded intense collaboration between public health departments and other community organizations. As essential providers of individual and population-based health services, CHNs have played an integral role in the development and implementation of AIDS-related programs designed for specific communities and high-risk populations (Flaskerud, 1988; Goff & McDonough, 1986; Jones, 1988; Lyne & Waller, 1990). A case study of one such program illustrates the synthesis of community health nursing interventions at the individual, family, and aggregate levels (Kuehnert, 1991).

This study describes a program in which a community health nursing AIDS coordinator was hired to help design and implement a comprehensive community-wide AIDS program. In collaboration with various community agencies, the AIDS coordinator conducted a needs assessment; participated in policy-development activities; developed education strategies for high-risk groups; facilitated the development of a nonprofit AIDS organization; and provided individual health services, health education, counseling, and emotional support. This program demonstrates the expert competencies community health nurses have in working with individuals and families, and in developing effective program and policy strategies.

Homeless people in the geographic areas served by CHNs represent another high-risk group targeted for community-level interventions. Nurse-managed clinics serving the homeless are being implemented at the grass roots level (Bowlder & Barrell, 1987; Reilly, Grier, & Blomquist, 1992; Turner, Bauer, McNair, McNutt & Walker, 1989). Given the complex needs of the homeless, recent studies reporting community health nursing interventions have focused primarily on assessing the health needs of this population and developing a framework for effective interventions.

One study assessing the health needs among homeless people in Richmond, Virginia, concluded with recommendations for a nurse-managed health clinic targeting this population. Suggested interventions were grounded in the holistic approach to care promoted in community health nursing practice and included health assessment and treatment of minor acute health problems; the development of referral and outreach programs; counseling and health education; and community-level collaboration to ensure coordinated care. Evaluating the impact of community health nursing interventions on health outcomes in homeless populations should be the focus of further research in this area (Bowlder & Barrell, 1987).

MULTIDISCIPLINARY APPROACHES TO WORKING WITH HIGH RISK YOUTH. The need for community health nurses who are prepared to participate in interdisciplinary collaboration with other professionals is evident (Selby, Riportella-Muller, Legault, & Salmon, 1990). CHNs often work as part of a multidisciplinary team to develop and implement programs targeting complex social and health situations. Child-abuse prevention and teenage pregnancy are major social and public health problems that benefit from this collaborative approach. A model public health–social service partnership aimed at preventing child abuse has been successful in Brown County, Minnesota (Saunders & Goodall, 1985). A case history of the collaborative practice between nurses and social workers draws on the competencies of community health nurses in case identification, preventive interventions, and coordinating comprehensive family needs. With expertise in child development, child health, and health education strategies, CHNs are essential members of the cooperative child-protection team. The trusting relationships developed with clients provide a foundation for health-advocacy interventions used by CHNs and give nurses credibility as nonthreatening professionals, thus improving the effectiveness of their interventions.

A similar partnership between social work and public health nursing was developed in King County, Washington, to provide services for homeless and prostituting adolescent females, who are at substantial risk for adverse pregnancy outcomes and often have poor parenting skills (Deisher, Farrow, Hope, & Litchfield, 1989; Deisher, Litchfield, & Hope, 1991). In the collaborative model developed, PHNs conduct health assessments, provide health education and referral services, teach parenting skills, and offer other case-management services. Again, the success of these efforts depends on trusting relationships the PHN and social worker are able to establish with these vulnerable young women, who are often suspicious and lack trust (Farrow, 1991).

COLLABORATIVE APPROACHES TO CITY-LEVEL HEALTH PROMOTION. At a more global community level, CHNs develop partnerships to foster changes consistent with broad-based health promotion efforts, promote community collaboration to achieve these efforts, and assist in the development of effective health policies. These partnerships are grounded in an ecological approach to health promotion that emphasizes the effect of individual and social-environmental influences on health and illness (McLeroy, Bibleau, Steckler, & Glantz, 1988). Two examples from the literature reflect the efficacy of such interventions in situations where a city is identified as the target community (Scotts, 1991; Flynn, Rider, & Ray, 1991). In both cases, community participation and ownership in health-promotion efforts were essential to program success.

In an intervention utilizing public health nursing expertise to foster community collaboration and mobilization, a PHN specialist assisted two southwestern cities in an effort to promote citywide clean-air policies (Scotts, 1991). In one city where a community coalition of nonsmokers interested in the project developed rapidly, the PHN served as a resource on the detrimental effects of environmental tobacco smoke. In the second city, however, participation was limited, so the PHN assumed a more direct leadership role. In both cases, the community nursing model employed integrated illness-prevention, protection, and health-promotion components. The PHN worked with citizen groups to assess community needs and identify community diagnoses. As a result of this partnership process, clean-air ordinances were passed and community norms about smoking practices in public were altered. In a qualitative evaluation of the program, local leaders and community constituents voiced support for the new ordinances, which created a healthier environment (Scotts, 1991).

In a second city-level program known as Healthy Cities Indiana, community health nurses are involved in an interdisciplinary collaboration with public health professionals and six Indiana cities to promote community health and wellness (Flynn et al., 1991). Healthy Cities Indiana is based on a community development framework, whereby the impetus for change comes from the communities rather than from a formalized power structure. This process is achieved through consensus building, emphasizing self-help, nurturing the development of community leadership, and enabling community constituents to have a voice in health planning efforts.

With technical assistance from expert community health nurses and public health leaders, committees from each of the participating cities have identified priority health problems, initiated indepth community assessments, and promoted city-wide efforts aimed at strengthening healthy public policy. Although evaluation of Healthy Cities Indiana is a high priority, this process is in the early phases and evidence supporting the efficacy of the Healthy Cities model has not yet been substantiated. Preliminary findings, however, indicate that broad-based community involvement in leadership and assessment activities has facilitated action congruent with the goal of community health promotion (Flynn, Rider, & Ray, 1991).

As with home-based interventions, documenting the cost-effectiveness of population-based CHN services poses a challenging task given the qualitative nature of many services, the focus on health promotion rather than illness care, and the complex bureaucratic matrix of many programs involving the delivery of community-oriented nursing services (Oda & Boyd, 1987). Consequently, developing suitable criteria to evaluate the costs and benefits of all community health nursing interventions presents a major challenge that must be addressed by community health nurse leaders to secure funding for these services. Meanwhile, CHNs can use their experience, expertise, and knowledge to inform policy makers about the need for outreach to vulnerable families and underserved communities.

▬POLICY IMPLICATIONS

These examples of home-based and community-level interventions describe the diverse services offered by community health nurses and provide evidence supporting the efficacy of CHN interventions. In doing so, a broad spectrum of community health nursing competencies are illustrated as they apply to the care of high-risk families; the assessment, planning, and implementation of preventive-health programs; and the development of healthy public policies sensitive to the concerns of vulnerable populations. The examples selected are not meant to be all-inclusive but rather to reflect the diverse roles in which community health nurses can be effective at enhancing the health status of high-risk groups.

The recent shift toward health promotion and community-level interventions sets the stage for the expansion of community health nursing efforts. Although nationwide CHNs have actively worked to improve the health of communities, too often their work has gone unrecognized and community health nurses have been invisible in their efforts (Martin, White, & Hansen, 1989). With intimate knowledge about major public health problems and expertise in community-focused health interventions, CHNs are an essential resource in our rapidly changing health care system. Their ability to create positive change in the health of communities, however, requires support from legislators, policy makers, practice agencies, professional organizations, educators, and research institutions. Recommendations for supporting community health nursing practice include:

For legislators and policy makers, include funding to support community health nursing in state and local budget proposals; and increase funding for outcome-based research on the effectiveness of community health nursing practice.

For practice agencies and professional organizations, use qualitative information gathered by community health nurses in the assessment, planning, and evaluation phases of community health programs; promote interdisciplinary collaboration with other professional groups; and generate and disseminate data on outcomes of community health nursing interventions.

For educators and research institutions, develop appropriate criteria for evaluating the costs and benefits of community health nursing interventions; promote process and outcome research on the efficacy of community health nursing practice; and promote skills for developing client partnerships and interdisciplinary practice with paraprofessionals, professionals, and community leaders.

These recommendations provide guidelines for supporting and enhancing community health nursing practice. Joint support from policy makers, legislators, educators, research institutions, and practice agencies will provide a climate for recognizing the positive outcomes associated with community health nursing interventions. Historically, CHNs have been effective at addressing the health-promotion and disease-prevention needs of ever-changing communities. In the future, CHNs will undoubtedly play an integral role in the national effort to achieve a healthier society for all.

▬ACKNOWLEDGMENTS
This paper was prepared with support from the Washington State Public Health Association, Service Education and Research in Community Health Nursing, Washington State Public Health Nursing Directors, and the Washington State Nursing Foundation. The author gratefully acknowledges the careful review and suggestions of the following committee members who contributed to the development of this paper: Janet Lenart, A.R.N.P., M.N., M.P.H., Public Health Nursing Consultant, Washington State Department of Health; Judy Schoder, R.N., M.N., Public Health Nursing Consultant, Washington State Department of Health; Maura Egan, R.N., Ph.D., Associate Professor, St. Martin's College; Durlyn Finnie, R.N., M.P.H., Assistant Chief of Nursing Services, Seattle-King County Department of Public Health; Jan Dahl, R.N., M.A., Nursing Director, Whatcom County Health Department. The author would also like to thank the following faculty member at the School of Nursing, University of Washington for reviewing this manuscript: Marjorie Muecke, R.N., Ph.D.; Joyce Zerwekh, R.N., Ed.D., and Kathryn Barnard, R.N., Ph.D.

▬REFERENCES
Allen, C.E. (1991). Holistic concepts and the professionalization of public health nursing. *Public Health Nursing, 8,* 74–80.

Baldwin, K.A., & Chen, S.C. (1989). The effectiveness of public health nursing services to prenatal clients: An integrated review. *Public Health Nursing, 6,* 80–87.

Barkauskas, V. (1983). Effectiveness of public health nurse home visits to primiparous mothers and their infants. *American Journal of Public Health, 73,* 573–580.

Barnard, K.E., Magyary, D., Sumner, G., Booth, C.L., Mitchell, S.K., & Spieker, S. (1988). Prevention of parenting alterations for women with low social support. *Psychiatry, 51,* 248–253.

Bowdler, J.E., & Barrell, L.M. (1987). Health needs of homeless persons. *Public Health Nursing, 4,* 135–140.

Brooten, D., Kumar, S., Brown, L.P., Butts, P., Finkler, S.A., Bakewell-Sachs, S., Gibbons, A. & Delivoria-Papadopoulos, M. (1986). A randomized clinical trial of early hospital discharge and home follow-up of very low birth weight infants. *New England Journal of Medicine, 315,* 934–939.

Buescher, P.A., Meis, P.J., Ernest, J.M., Moore, M.L., Michielute, R., & Sharp, P. (1989). A comparison of women in and out of a prematurity prevention project in a North Carolina perinatal care region. *American Journal of Public Health, 78,* 264–267.

Carlin, J., Sabol, B. J., & Schloesser, P.T. Health of children in day care: Public health profiles. Kansas: Kansas Department of Health and Environment, December, 1986.

Chapman, J., Siegel, E., & Cross, A. (1990). Home visitors and child health: Analysis of selected programs. *Pediatrics, 85,* 1059–1068.

Combs-Orme, T., Reis, J., & Ward, L.D. (1985). Effectiveness of home visits by public health nurses in maternal and child health: An empirical review. *Public Health Reports, 100,* 490–499.

Deisher, R.W., Farrow, J.A., Hope, K., & Litchfield, C. (1989). The pregnant adolescent prostitute. *American Journal of Diseases in Children, 143,* 1162–1165.

Diesher, R.W., Litchfield, C., & Hope, K.R. (1991). Birth outcomes of prostituting adolescents. *Journal of Adolescent Health, 12,* 528–533.

Farrow, J.A. (1991, September). Homeless pregnant and parenting adolescents: Service delivery strategies. *Maternal & Child Health Technical Information Bulletin.* Seattle: University of Washington.

Flaskerud, J.H. (1988). Prevention of AIDS in blacks and Hispanics: Nursing implications. *Journal of Community Health Nursing, 5,* 4–58.

Flynn, B.C., Rider, M., & Ray, D.W. (1991). Healthy cities: The Indiana model of community development in public health. *Health Education Quarterly, 18,* 331–347.

Goff, W., & McDonough, P. (1986). A community health approach to AIDS: Caring for the patient and educating the public. *Journal of Community Health Nursing, 3,* 191–200.

Grayville, S. (1991, May/June). What can a health consultant do for you? *Family Day Caring,* 8–9.

Hall, L.A. (1980). Effect of teaching on primiparas' perceptions of their newborns. *Nursing Research, 29,* 317–322.

Jones, L.H. (1988). AIDS, education, and the community health nurse. *Journal of Community Health Nursing, 5,* 159–165.

Kent, C. (Ed.). (1992, May). Slow progress against infant mortality. *Medicine and Health Perspectives.*

Kuehnert, P.L. (1991). Community health nursing and the AIDS pandemic: Case report of one community's response. *Journal of Community Health Nursing, 8,* 137–146.

Krisjanson, L.J., & Chalmers, K.I. (1991). Preventive work with families: Issues facing public health nurses. *Journal of Advanced Nursing, 16,* 147–153.

Lie, L. (1992). Health consultation services to family day care homes in Minneapolis, Minnesota. *Journal of School Health, 62,* 29–31.

Lowe, M.L. (1970). Effectiveness of teaching as measured by compliance with medical recommendation. *Nursing Research, 19,* 59–63.

Lyne, B.A., & Waller, P.R. (1990). The Denver nursing project in huamn caring: A model for AIDS nursing care and professional education. *Family and Community Health, 13,* 78–84.

McLeroy, K.R., Bibleau, D., Steckler, A., & Glantz, K. (1988). An ecological perspective on health promotion programs. *Health Education Quarterly, 15,* 351–370.

McNeil, H.J., & Holland, S.S. (1972). A comparative study of public health nursing teaching in groups and in home visits. *American Journal of Public Health, 62,* 1629–1637.

Mahon, J., McFarlane, J., & Golden, K. (1991). De Madres a Madres: A community partnership for health. *Public Health Nursing, 8,* 15–19.

Martin, E.J., White, J.E., & Hansen, M.M. (1989). Preparing students to shape health policy. *Nursing Outlook, 37,* 89–93.

May, K. M., McLaughlin, F., & Penner, M. (1991). Preventing low birth weight: Marketing and volunteer outreach. *Public Health Nursing, 8,* 97–104.

National Commission to Prevent Infant Mortality (1988). *Death Before Life: The Tragedy of Infant Mortality.* Washington, D.C.: National Commission to Prevent Infant Mortality.

Oda, D.S., & Boyd, P. (1987). Document the effect and cost of public health nursing field services. *Public Health Nursing, 4,* 180–182.

Oda, D.S., & Boyd, P. (1988). The outcome of public health nursing service in a preventive child health program: Phase I, health assessment. *Public Health Nursing, 5,* 209–213.

Oda, D.S., Fine, J.I., & Heilbron, D.H. (1986). Impact and cost of public health nurses' telephone follow-up of school dental referrals. *American Journal of Public Health, 76,* 1348–1349.

Olds, D.L., Henderson, C.R., Tatelbaum, R., & Chamberlin, R. (1986a). Improving the delivery of prenatal care and outcomes of pregnancy: A randomized trial of nurse home visitation. *Pediatrics, 77,* 16–28.

Olds, D.L., Henderson, C.R., Chamberlin, R., & Tatelbaum, R. (1986b). Preventing child abuse and neglect: A randomized trial of nurse home visitation. *Pediatrics, 78,* 65–78.

Olds, D.L., Henderson, C.R., Tatelbaum, R., & Chamberlin, R. (1988). Improving the life-course development of socially disadvantaged mothers: A randomized trial of nurse home visitation. *American Journal of Public Health, 78,* 1436–1445.

Olds, D.L., & Kitzman, H. (1990). Can home visitation improve the health of women and children at environmental risk? *Pediatrics, 86,* 108–116.

Reilly, F.E., Grier, M.R., & Blomquist, K. (1992). Living arrangements, visit patterns, and health problems in a nurse-managed clinic for the homeless. *Journal of Community Health Nursing, 9,* 111–121.

Saunders, E.J. & Goodall, K. (1985). Social service—public health partnership in child protection: A rural model. *Public Health Reports, 100,* 663–666.

Schmelzer, M., Reeves, S.R., & Zahner, S. J. (1986). Health services in day care centers: A public health nursing design. *Public Health Nursing, 3,* 120–125.

Schorr, L.B. (1988). *Within Our Reach: Breaking the Cycle of Disadvantage.* New York: Doubleday.

Scotts, R.C. (1991). Application of the Salmon Model: A tale of two cities. *Public Health Nursing, 8,* 10–14.

Selby, M.L., Riportella-Muller, R., Legault, C., & Salmon, M.E. (1990). Core curriculum for master's-level community health nursing education: A comparison of the views of leaders in service and education. *Public Health Nursing, 7,* 150–160.

Shamansky, S.L., & Clausen, C.L. (1980). Levels of prevention: Examination of the concept. *Nursing Outlook, 28,* 104–108.

Stanwick, R.S., Moffatt, M.E.K., Robitaille, Y., Emond, A., & Dok, C. (1982). An evaluation of the routine postnatal public health nurse home visit. *Canadian Journal of Public Health, 73,* 200–205.

Starn, J.R. (1992). Community health nursing visits for at-risk women and infants. *Journal of Community Health Nursing, 9,* 103–110.

Turner, S.L., Bauer, G., McNair, E., McNutt, B., & Walker, W. (1989). The homeless experience: Clinic building in a community health discovery–learning project. *Public Health Nursing, 6,* 97–101.

Williams, C.A. (1984). Population-focused practice. In M. Stanhope & J. Lancaster (Eds.). *Community Health Nursing: Process and Practice for Promoting Health,* 805–815. St. Louis: C.V. Mosby.

Yauger, R.A. (1972). Does family-centered care make a difference? *Nursing Outlook, 20,* 320–323.

Zerwekh, J.V. (1993). Commentary: Going to the people—public health nursing today and tomorrow. *American Journal of Public Health,* 83(12), 1676–1677.

Zerwekh, J.V. (1992a). Community health nurses—A population at risk. (Editorial). *Public Health Nursing, 9,* 1.

Zerwekh, J.V. (1992b). The practice of empowerment and coercion by expert public health nurses. *Image Journal of Nursing Scholarship, 24,* 101–105.

Chapter 12

Ethical Issues in Community Health Nursing

MILA A. AROSKAR

Community health nursing practice is fraught with many ethical dilemmas. How do community health nurses decide between serving the elderly, the homeless, or pregnant teenagers when resources are limited and a program can only be developed for one population group in the area? Should cost of care, client needs, available resources, quality of service, or other ethical values determine decision making in health care delivery? In this chapter, Dr. Aroskar discusses three ethical approaches to dilemmas in community health nursing and describes their application to practice. Ethical solutions, she states, will not be found unless ethical dimensions are first considered in the decision-making process.

Much current discussion of ethical issues in nursing focuses on nurses in hospital bureaucracies caring for individual patients. While the majority of nurses are employed in hospital and other institutional settings, the majority of patients and clients are elsewhere in the health care system. They are in ambulatory care settings such as clinics, health maintenance organizations, physicians' offices, and work and school situations. Many patients are in their own homes and halfway houses. The moral concerns of nurses in all settings are similar, i.e., truth-telling, paternalism, coercion, self-determination, and allocation of scarce resources. The differences in setting do not make a difference per se in the ethical concerns confronting nurses and nursing administrators.

Nurses in the larger community, however, generally look at different dimensions starting with a wider context of concern than the individual patient, which is the predominant concern for the hospital-based nurse. Goals of community health nursing focus on the family and groups at risk in the larger community. Community health nursing is more pointedly concerned with the social dimension of ethics, if only because of the broader aspects and subsystems of society with which it deals.

From *Nursing Clinics of North America* 14(1):35–44. Reprinted by permission of W. B. Saunders Co.

▬COMMUNITY-ORIENTED NURSING

Some specific differences and variability that may be noted between hospital and community-oriented nursing are in areas such as: 1) boundaries of service, e.g., hospital unit versus community, as defined by an agency for purposes of delivering nursing service; 2) direct physician supervision and back-up, e.g., types of independent, dependent, and interdependent decision making; 3) control of patient behavior by the nurse on a hospital unit versus a home or ambulatory care setting; and 4) different types and levels of care coordination in a hospital versus the wider community, where such systems as education and social service are often directly involved.

Focus of Care

In community settings, there is generally a broader focus on both physical and mental health than on disease per se, and on the variables that affect health directly or indirectly, such as life-style, family interaction patterns, and community resources (public transportation and adequate housing). All these variables influence the kinds of ethical dilemmas identified by individual nurses and nursing agencies in making decisions about who should get nursing service and when and how these services are to be delivered. These issues are representative of problems of *distributive justice,* a core ethical problem for society. Distributive justice concerns the distribution of benefits and harms in society and what society and the state owe the individual.

Williams points out that orientation to the setting where care occurs is a somewhat limited definition of community health nursing, because this orientation still focuses primarily on individualistic clinical approaches to care of individuals and families.[5] It may overlook the health needs of aggregates of people or the arrangements for continuity of acute and non-acute care. Community-oriented nursing considers the health needs of population groups at risk, or aggregates, and ways of organizing the community to meet these identified needs. Aggregates have environmental characteristics in common; e.g., an aggregate may be composed of individuals with hypertension, university students, elderly persons who live alone, or pregnant teenagers.[5] The community itself is viewed as a system with a number of interacting subsystems, of which the health care system is one example. This subsystem is concerned with identifying and meeting health and illness needs. The values of a community are reflected in their identification of health needs and how they are met or not met based on some notion of rights to health and justice. These values in turn are reflected in health agency goals, objectives, and programs.

This community focus is often not employed in many community health nursing agencies, which perpetuate the episodic, individual patient-demand and provider-response approach to nursing and health care. In this approach, community group needs for nursing service are not identified by the agency initially. The necessary data base does not exist. This is an ethical dilemma in and of itself in terms of allocation of scarce resources, i.e., should nursing manpower resources be used for preventive or curative services? In order to gain a more coherent view of the health care system, individuals needing secondary and tertiary institutional services might also be broadly considered as another community aggregate. This broader view would change the way in which one considers the need for nursing services in a defined community, in terms of the types of services required and where they are needed.

The notion of community aggregates could expand the ways in which we look at primary, secondary, and tertiary services on a care continuum, rather than employing a mind-set that usually excludes the hospital as a community health resource or agency per se. Nurses in hospital settings should also have a community orientation, although their major focus is on the individual patient. After all, the patient comes from and generally returns to the larger community. Implementation of continuity of care might then become more of a reality than it is as a paper statement in the Patients' Bill of Rights.

Types of Communities

An additional dimension of the community health orientation is the fact that the concept of community itself is somewhat elusive. The term may be used to connote structural, emotional, or functional communities.[1] A *structural community* may be an aggregate of people or a geopolitical entity. An *emotional community* is one in which the individual has a feeling of be- longing, or it may be a special-interest community, such as a group that provides recreational opportunities for disturbed children. A *functional community* is viewed as a group of identifiable need, such as migrant work- ers or the mentally retarded living in the community. This last concept of community seems to be more congruent with Williams's concept of com- munity aggregates (discussed previously). Community health nurses must be aware of all these groups in order to provide effective health and nurs- ing services. Perhaps the major point is that nurses, patients, and clients not only are individuals acting alone on a principle of freedom and self- determination, but are also members of groups and a community in which it is recognized that one's activities and participation affect others, not only one's self.

Ethical dilemmas facing nurses and administrators in community set- tings other than hospitals include both the individualistic and aggregate approaches. This paper focuses on a selected dilemma that confronts com- munity health nursing agencies: providing services to population groups at risk in the larger community (i.e., nursing concerns in the context of a wider social ethic).

■ETHICAL APPROACHES TO DILEMMAS

Dilemmas are situations of ambiguity and conflict with equally unattractive alternatives for choice, decision making, and action. Although there are a variety of issues in health care ethics, it is usually the *dilemmas* involving the questions, "What is the right thing to do in this situation? Why?" that pro- voke the most agonized thinking and discussion. There is no dilemma when clearly identified goods and evils conflict; a conflict between competing values must exist. For example, the following questions are dilemmas: How should finite nursing, medical, and technical resources be allocated? Should these resources be used for preventive or curative efforts? For what groups in the community? How should those affected by a particular decision be involved in the decision-making process? The last question has been partially answered by the growth of consumer involvement in federally mandated health systems agencies. The allocation of scarce resources falls into the area of distributive justice—a most difficult point of social concern for individuals and communities.

Ethical theories, which all reflect values, neither solve ethical dilemmas per se nor provide us with decisions for action. They do, however, provide a basis for more open discussion, for clarifying and refining dilemmas for discussion, and for making judgments on the basis of reflective thinking rather than simply relying on gut-level feelings of rightness or wrongness (although these are, too, involved in dealing with ethical dilemmas).

Egoist Approach

The traditional ethical positions or theories of egoism, deontology (formalism), and utilitarianism can be used to discuss and clarify ethical dilemmas in health care generally and community health nursing specifically. In the *egoist position*, the individual nurse or agency would say that something was good because that is what the nurse or agency desires. In considering alternatives for action, the nurse or agency would only consider what is best for them. Others involved in or affected by the decision would not be considered. For example, in an issue of truth-telling, the nurse might decide to lie because it is simply easier to do so, regardless of the implications for a family or community group. The ethical egoist acts and judges by the standard of his own advantage in terms of differentiating right from wrong.

Deontologic Approach

The *deontologic approach* suggests that rightness or wrongness of decisions and actions depends on more than the nurse's or agency's own advantage or the consequences of a proposed action. Rightness or wrongness depends on the inherent moral significance of these decisions and actions, e.g., promise-keeping and truth-telling. Moral significance is also attached to certain relationships, e.g., the nurse–patient relationship, and forms the basis for duties and obligations. These duties and obligations would not necessarily be applicable if one were not in this relationship.

Similar obligations might be considered to hold for agencies that offer particular services to the community. In other words, it is wrong for an agency to say that it offers counseling services to pregnant unwed teenagers and then to make them available only to those who can pay. Obligations in relationships may be based on performing certain actions or following particular rules or moral principles. The values of the individual person or agency are all-important in this instance.

Kant, a philosopher in the deontologic tradition, suggests in his "categorical imperative" that one should act only on the maxim that one at the same time wills to be a universal law, e.g., the Golden Rule. It is one's duty to follow the imperative regardless of the consequences. Another rule based on this imperative is that persons should always be treated as ends, not simply as means. This has implications for the ways in which agencies deal with their employees in addition to implications for patients and client care. To champions of the deontologic position, certain actions such as lying or killing would be seen as wrong-making and could therefore never be advocated or carried out, regardless of the consequences or good to be achieved.

Utilitarian Approach

The *utilitarian position* generally defines "good" as happiness or pleasure and "right" as the greatest good and the least amount of harm for the greatest number of persons. This position assumes that one can calculate harms and benefits and thereby arrive at a decision that has the greatest possibility of insuring that good prevails over evil. This is a *consequentialist position*, which looks at how certain actions affect the general welfare of all in a given situation—a more community-oriented ethic. This is the ethical tradition often invoked in making decisions about allocation of health care resources. A basic question that still remains unanswered in this philosophy is whether we should seek total happiness for some or moderate happiness for all. How or whether this question is answered by the health care system has implications for all of us. This position is in direct conflict with the traditional medical ethic, which says that one should do all one can for the individual patient.

Each of these traditional positions has serious limitations when applied to specific ethical dilemmas in nursing and health care, but they do provide us with different perspectives from which to make thoughtful moral judgments and decisions.

"Justice as Fairness"

A contemporary theory that can be applied to dilemmas of distributive justice is proposed by Rawls, a philosopher, in his theory of "justice as fairness." Facets of the deontologic approach may be detected in this philosophy. The heart of Rawls's theory is the concept of the "original position," in which people come together under the "veil of ignorance" to negotiate the principles of justice, by which all are then bound to live.[3] The principles of justice concern what Rawls calls primary goods, i.e., income, wealth, liberty, opportunity, and the bases of self-respect. The negotiators have general knowledge about such areas as physics and economics but no specific knowledge about themselves or others, e.g., personal characteristics such as sex, social class, or age. It is therefore impossible for these negotiators in the "original position" to seek their own interest at the expense of others. They do not know what their own positions will be in society and must favor principles that include everyone's best interests.

Rawls's concept of justice as fairness is articulated in two basic principles of justice: 1) each person has an equal right to the liberty available to all, and 2) social and economic inequalities are to be distributed so that the least advantaged have benefits as well as the more advantaged in society, and offices and positions in that society are open to everyone under conditions of equal opportunity.[3] The liberty principle has priority if and when the two principles conflict. Inequalities are allowed only to improve the condition of the least advantaged in the community, e.g., the retarded, children, and the elderly. The least advantaged are in the normative position in society in terms of distribution of burdens and benefits. Basic rights and obligations are based on the notion of fairness for these disadvantaged groups. Justice as fairness to the least advantaged becomes the categorical imperative in the Kantian tradition.

Rawls makes no claim that his theory can be applied directly to problems of justice in contemporary society. Yet he has provided us with another way to look at problems of distribution in society generally and in health care specifically. How might the delivery of nursing services be structured if the needs of the least advantaged were considered first in making a policy decision regarding allocation of nursing resources?

Rawls also suggests that there are five criteria for determining the rightness of any ethical principle: 1) universality, i.e., the same principles must hold for everyone; 2) generality, i.e., they must not refer to specific people or situations, such as "my mother" or "your divorce"; 3) publicity, i.e., they must be known and recognized by all involved; 4) ordering, i.e., they must somehow order conflicting claims without resorting to force; and 5) finality, i.e., they may override the demands of law and custom.[3] By these criteria, ethical egoism as a valid moral position is ruled out as a standard for making ethical judgments. However, this does not rule out the possibility that decisions may still be made on this basis by individuals and groups in the health care system

One may find any one of these positions or a combination of them represented in health care settings, whether or not decision makers articulate the assumptions or value positions underlying particular decisions and actions. There are serious difficulties in appealing to any one theory for "the answer" to complex moral problems arising on the continuum from individual nurse-patient relationships to policy making for a neighborhood health center or the community at large. In summary, these are selected positions that can be and are used in clarifying and refining ethical issues and dilemmas in the decision-making process.

▬ETHICAL DILEMMAS CONFRONTING COMMUNITY HEALTH NURSING AGENCIES

The ethical approaches discussed briefly in preceding paragraphs will now be used to look at an ethical dilemma confronted by community health nursing agencies at both the individualistic level of care and the population-at-risk or aggregate level in relation to policy matters. The dilemma focuses on what kinds of nursing care shall be given to whom and in what order, i.e., allocation of scarce resources, since this is a dilemma inherent in, if not articulated by, community health nursing agencies. This is a basic ethical question that intersects all social, political, legal, and economic issues facing society, and nursing as a part of that society. Even the notion of identifying populations at risk for which nursing service is appropriate involves pertinent issues relevant to the ethical implications of social intervention.

Ethical Implications of Social Intervention

Two social scientists, Kelman and Warwick, place social intervention on a continuum from policy-making in neighborhood health centers and in experimentation with human subjects to national policy matters.[4] Their concept of social intervention is any planned or unplanned action that changes the characteristics of an individual or that changes the pattern of relationships between individuals. The notion of nursing intervention in identified aggregates of individuals is an example of this concept. Major ethical issues are raised in the following four aspects of any proposed social intervention: 1) the choice of goals for the proposed change, which maximizes certain values and minimizes others, e.g., a planned change from individualistic care to care of aggregates; 2) definition of the target of change, i.e., individuals or the environment(s); 3) the means chosen to implement the intervention; and 4) evaluation of the consequences of the intervention.[4]

One of the key issues in examining the goals of social intervention and the means for implementing the goals is the extent to which affected population groups have their values and interests represented, e.g., various socioeconomic groups, women, children, the unemployed, the healthy, the sick, providers, and consumers. Whose interests are being served by the proposed intervention—the agency proposing a community health nursing program or the target population(s)? Is the power of one group strengthened at the expense of another? To whom is the community agency morally accountable? Often, these concerns are not considered in social interventions because of the difficulty in discerning which values should predominate and the difficulty of predicting the consequences of particular actions for any selected value, e.g., the freedom of the individual or the welfare of society.[4] These questions should be considered in any policy change involving changes in relationships between individuals or groups.

In considering populations at risk in the community and plans for nursing intervention, one needs to keep in mind what the bottom line will be in making these decisions. For example, the bottom line currently is cost and cost containment. Some agencies are very straightforward in stating that cost of care is the first factor considered in whether or not a particular program will be offered. At the same time, one finds authors such as economist Victor Fuchs who suggest that values other than economic ones, i.e., ethical values, need to be taken into account in considering delivery of health care services.[2]

Allocation of Scarce Resources

A dilemma that occurs in many community health nursing agencies at the policy-making level is whether to use nursing manpower resources for identified community health needs, preventive or curative, or to provide these services on the demand of particular population groups, such as the elderly, for whom funding is provided for nursing service through Medicare. What should be the agency's community(ies) for nursing care if one has the chronically ill elderly, the deinstitutionalized mentally retarded, and unwed pregnant teenagers competing for these resources? With finite resources, what are the agency's moral obligations to each group? Should nursing service be provided to all groups on the moral principle of fairness and equity, a notion of justice? Alternatively, should the administrator evaluate the amount of "good" to be gained from providing services to selected groups according to a notion of the greatest good for some, but not all, at this point in time? Who should be involved in making these decisions? Should the actual or potential productivity of individuals in the groups at risk be considered in the decision-making process?

The alternatives in this policy situation seem equally unattractive in the sense that not everyone can obtain needed nursing service because of finite resources. Can an agency then justify providing care for some groups or segments of groups at risk and not others on the basis that funding is available only for care of some groups, which employ all the available resources? If economic aspects are not considered, the agency may not remain viable in the community to provide nursing care for anyone. The allocation of scarce resources readily demonstrates how economic, social, political, legal, and moral dimensions intersect in such a dilemma.

This represents a community problem, not simply a nursing problem. One cannot begin to solve this dilemma thoughtfully without a data base identifying the needs for nursing service of the defined community and its aggregates. Another factor is the definition of and values given health in a specific community. A community profile is an essential first step! Demand for service alone is not adequate as a basis for an ethically correct solution.

The ethical egoist would have no problem in choosing the alternative that is best for the agency without regard for groups with identified health needs. However, as mentioned previously, this is not a morally defensible stance. The strict deontologist would consider some moral principles or the inherent goodness or rightness of particular alternatives, regardless of the consequences. However, if one were to follow both a principle of need and a principle of equity in providing service, one finds that these two may be in conflict. How does one resolve the conflict? Philosophers have not provided a satisfactory resolution of this question. This approach, then, is not particularly helpful in dealing with a complex policy situation in which different conflicting values are brought to the decision-making situation.

A utilitarian would seek the greatest amount of service for the greatest number of groups at risk, at the same time bringing the least amount of harm to these same groups. This is sometimes known as "calculus morality." One also looks at the consequences of alternative suggestions for the general welfare of present and future generations. Probably, the use of a computer would be necessary in this approach, since it considers an extremely large number of complex variables, a kind of ethical cost/benefit analysis. Using the Rawlsian approach of justice as fairness, one might look at alternative solutions from the point of view of the least advantaged groups with identified needs for nursing service. Nobody would benefit from any particular alternative unless the least advantaged benefited. For example, the poor in these identified groups would have to receive services in order for anyone to receive services.

Consideration of various alternative solutions using these ethical approaches will not provide an agency with "the answer" concerning allocation of nursing manpower resources. It will, however, clarify and refine the dimensions of the dilemma, provide for articulation of the value bases according to which particular choices might be made, and bring reflective thinking to bear on the suggested alternatives in order to arrive at decision(s) for action.

There are a number of additional ethical issues faced by community health nurses and agencies in terms of the "right" use of nursing resources. A specific example is the kind of issue faced by nurse practitioners in neighborhood health centers who must decide between the delivery of a more comprehensive range of care and provision of a minimal level of physical care. Surfacing in discussions with community health nurses and administrators are a host of concerns that require community solutions, involving consumer, legal, political, economic, social service, and educational subsystems in addition to health care professionals. These subsystems are all competing for scarce resources.

Additional issues include recognition of inadequate health care received by the poor; care at home of individuals who do not have adequate housing, food, and other necessities; life-style-related health problems; identification of individuals with unacknowledged drug and alcohol abuse problems; and recognition of individuals whom the nurse believes do not have adequate medical supervision.

▬SUMMARY

Ethical solutions to these dilemmas will never occur if the ethical dimension is not an articulated part of the discussion of alternatives confronting individuals and agencies in decision making. This is a complex and difficult endeavor, but to refuse to include this dimension in policy making is to decrease the humanistic and caring aspects of policies relative to community health nursing services.

▬REFERENCES

1. Archer, S. E., and Fleshman, R. *Community Health Nursing: Patterns and Practice.* North Scituate, Mass.: Duxbury Press, 1975. pp. 18–22.
2. Fuchs, V. R. *Who Shall Live? Health, Economics and Social Choice.* New York: Basic Books, 1974.
3. Rawls, J. *A Theory of Justice.* Cambridge, Mass.: Harvard Univ. Press, 1971.
4. Warwick, D. P., and Kelman, H. C. Ethical Issues in Social Intervention. In G. Zaltman (Ed.), *Process and Phenomena of Social Change.* New York: Wiley, 1973.
5. Williams, C. A. Community Health Nursing—What Is It? *Nurs. Outlook* 25: 250, 1977.

Chapter 13

Chattanooga Creek: Case Study of the Public Health Nursing Role in Environmental Health

LYNELLE PHILLIPS

A healthy community requires a healthy environment. As community health nurses seek to promote health and prevent illness and injuries with community clients, they must expand their awareness of the environment and assess whether it is health-enhancing or health-threatening. In this chapter Lynelle Phillips demonstrates the important roles of assessment and communication that nurses can play in protecting a community from an environmental health threat—in this case hazardous waste. She describes a successful collaborative project in which environmental assessment and community health education led to reduction of an environmental health hazard in one community.

▬ INTRODUCTION

What do you do when you shatter a glass on the kitchen floor? I am sure everyone would say: Well, you clean it up, of course! Have you ever informed everyone in the household not to walk barefoot through the kitchen for a while, for fear you missed some pieces? I bet everyone has done that, too; yet since this "education" action is simple common sense to people, you hardly even think about it when you do it.

In environmental health today, scientists may not consider the importance of community health education. When hazardous wastes are present in a community, many may say the answer is obvious—clean them up! But community health education is also a fundamental part of protecting communities from hazardous waste releases. The Agency for Toxic Substances and Disease Registry (ATSDR) is a federal agency whose mission is to prevent exposure and adverse human health effects and diminished quality of life associated with exposure to hazardous substances from waste sites, unplanned releases, and other sources of pollution in the environment.

From *Public Health Nursing* 12(5):335–340, 1995. Reprinted by permission of Blackwell Scientific Publications, Inc.

144

ATSDR achieves its mission through working directly with communities potentially affected by a hazardous substance release. In some cases, this means recommending that a site be placed on the U.S. Environmental Protection Agency's (USEPA) National Priorities List (NPL), allowing the USEPA to allocate funds for remediating or removing contamination from a hazardous waste site.

As a public health nurse and environmental health scientist at ATSDR, I work with communities affected by a hazardous waste release. The following case study demonstrates the pivotal role nurses at both the federal and local levels may play in protecting the health of communities from hazardous waste. In this case study of a community in Chattanooga, Tennessee, a community assessment found that area residents were exposed to hazardous wastes in amounts that represented a public health hazard. Nursing actions included community health education, which empowered residents to minimize their exposures. The importance of a community assessment that includes environmental hazards, and collaboration with other disciplines in county, state, and federal agencies are also emphasized.

▬ THE SENTINEL EVENT

Members of a local activist group, Stop Toxic Pollution (STOP), contacted ATSDR, local nurses, and other health officials with concerns about a creek in their neighborhood, Chattanooga Creek. They reported that the creek was grossly polluted with dangerous industrial wastes. They were concerned because, despite posted warning signs, children and adults continued to play and fish in the creek. They felt that the pollution in the creek had endangered the health of their community. This activist group had also contacted one of their senators and the local media.

▬ COMMUNITY ENVIRONMENTAL ASSESSMENT

Nursing assessment skills were employed to conduct a community environmental assessment of the Chattanooga Creek area. Information was retrieved by contacting local, state, and federal agencies and other community members, and by visiting the site (ATSDR, 1993b).

Site Description

Chattanooga Creek is a medium-size tributary of the Tennessee River, about 23.5 miles long draining 75 square miles. The creek originates in northwest Georgia and flows 16 stream miles northward, through a mostly rural area in the Chattanooga Valley before entering Tennessee. The stream banks average approximately two to four feet except where artificially heightened. Periodic flooding occurs, as evidenced by trash entangled in the trees and bushes three to four feet above the normal stream level. The USEPA identified the Chattanooga Creek site as the 7.5-mile long section flowing north from the Georgia-Tennessee River (EPA, 1991).

In addition to several potential sources of pollution to the creek, 42 known or suspected hazardous waste sites surround the creek. Of the 42, 12 are state Superfund sites. There are 15 known industrial and sewage discharges. An overwhelmed city wastewater treatment plant discharges raw sewage during heavy rain. Local residents dump garbage and old tires in and along the creek. Finally, large coal-tar waste pits line about two miles of the creek's banks. Some of the pits may be up to six feet deep. The surfaces are unstable and do not support the full weight of an adult (ATSDR, 1993a).

The South Chattanooga communities of Alton Park and Piney Wood surround the creek. A mix of residential and undeveloped areas are at the south end, and industrial complexes are to the north. Access to the creek is unrestricted. Signs are posted that read: "Water is contaminated. Do not swim or fish. Water contains toxic chemicals and waste that can cause cancer, birth defects and disease." Many of the signs are faded and in disrepair, and some are grown over the kudzu. A junior high and high school border the creek, and four other schools are within a mile. Evidence of contact with the creek by schoolchildren included potato chip bags and soda cans littering the banks near one of the schools (ATSDR, 1993b).

Environmental Contamination

SURFACE WATER.   Extensive sampling had been conducted by USEPA, the Tennessee Valley Authority (TVA), and the Tennessee Department of Environment and Conservation (TDEC) in the 1980s and early 1990s. Results showed fecal coliform counts up to 94 times the safe recreational water standards (ATSDR, 1993b).

SEDIMENTS.   Soils surrounding the creek were sampled by USEPA in 1990. Polychlorinated biphenyls (PCBs) were found at levels as high as 12,000 mg/kg soil. The maximum level of carcinogenic polycyclic aromatic hydrocarbons (PAHs) detected was about 3400 mg/kg soil (ATSDR, 1993b).

FISH.   Fish from Chattanooga Creek were monitored for heavy metals and pesticides in 1991 and 1992. PCBs were found at 3.29 mg/kg fish tissue, about 1.5 times the Food and Drug Administration standard (ATSDR, 1993b).

■ANALYSIS
Exposure Pathways
Once an assessment of all available information had been completed, the information was analyzed by using exposure pathway and toxicological analyses (Neufer & Narkunas, 1994). The exposure pathway is the process by which an individual is exposed to contaminants that originate from some source of contamination (ATSDR, 1992). Put simply, the exposure pathway describes how people contact and absorb hazardous wastes from their environment. An exposure pathway consists of five elements: a

source of contamination (the facility responsible for the hazardous substance release); an environmental medium (air, soil, surface water, groundwater, or food chain); a point of exposure (a location of human contact with the contaminated medium); a route of exposure (inhalation, ingestion, and/or dermal exposure); and a receptor population (people who are exposed or potentially exposed to the contaminants of concern at a point of exposure) (ATSDR, 1992).

For the Chattanooga Creek site, there was documented and observed evidence of area residents swimming, playing, and consuming fish. A survey of fourth, fifth, and sixth graders found that the fifth graders reported having the most contact: 9% swim in the creek, 20% play in the creek, 23% fish in the creek, and 8% have eaten fish from the creek. Also, the health clinic serving the homeless population reported that two men had recently been treated for gastroenteritis after drinking water from the creek. Evidence of human activities at the creek was also noted during the site visit, including soda cans and trash around the creek banks (ATSDR, 1993b). (See Table 13-1).

Toxicological Analysis

After the exposure pathways were identified, a toxicological analysis was conducted. The results of the analysis indicated that a public health hazard existed, particularly for frequent and long-term exposure via ingestion of contaminated soils, sediments, and fish. For example, fish concentrations of PCBs were as high as 3.29 mg/kg, exceeding the present FDA guideline of 2 mg/kg for the average person consuming store-brought fish. Frequent meals of fish caught from Chattanooga Creek could expose individuals to unacceptable levels of PCBs. There is no reliable epidemiological evidence that PCBs cause cancer in humans. However, because

TABLE 13-1   Exposure Pathways for Chattanooga Creek

PATHWAY NAME	SEDIMENT	SURFACE WATER	FISH
Source	Local industries	Local industries	Local industries
Environmental Media	Sediment	Surface water	Food chain/fish
Exposure Point	Chattanooga Creek	Chattanooga Creek	Chattanooga Creek
Exposure Route	Ingestion, dermal absorption	Ingestion, dermal absorption	Ingestion
Receptor Population	Children, fisher-, men homeless people	Children, fisher-, men homeless people	Fish consumers
Contaminants	PCBs[1], c-PAHs[2]	Bacteria	PCBs, chromium

[1]Polychlorinated biphenyls.
[2]Carcinogenic-polycyclic aromatic hydrocarbons.

there is some evidence of hepatocarcinogenicity in rodents, PCBs are classified as probable human carcinogens (ATSDR, 1993c).

Frequent skin contact with substances high in PAHs, such as soot and coal tar, has been associated with adverse dermal effects. Patients and volunteers receiving a 1% benzo(a)pyrene solution topically for four days to four months experienced aggravation of existing verrucae and pemphis vulgaris, nucleolar enlargement, pigmentary changes, and slight verrucous effects (ATSDR, 1990c). Frequent dermal exposure for many years, in conjunction with poor hygiene, may also increase risks for skin cancer.

▰NURSING DIAGNOSES

Based on the environmental assessment, and the exposure and toxicological analyses, the following nursing diagnosis was developed (Neufer, 1994):

> *Potential for injury: Residents who play in or consume fish or water from Chattanooga Creek are at risk for adverse dermal effects and gastroenteritis. Long-term, frequent ingestion of fish and contact with sediments may increase risks for skin or liver cancer.*

In addition, the large coal-tar deposits lining the creek banks posed a concern for safety, since they did not support individuals walking or standing on the banks. Another nursing diagnosis was the following:

> *Potential for injury: Residents who play in or near the coal-tar deposit areas may be at risk for physical injury because of the instability and size of the coal-tar deposits.*

▰GOALS/INTERVENTIONS

Preventing exposure was the key to protecting the health of residents from contaminants in Chattanooga Creek. In extreme situations, preventing exposure means relocating entire neighborhoods; however, relocation is very expensive and a logistical nightmare. Practically speaking, exposure is prevented in two ways: removing contamination and educating residents on minimizing exposure. As health professionals, public health nurses play a pivotal role in accomplishing the latter, but we may also influence the former as well. The public health actions for protecting the health of residents from contaminants in Chattanooga Creek required preventing exposure of residents to contaminants in Chattanooga Creek's surface water, sediments, and fish. Preventing these exposures transcended both education and removal activities.

Education

1. Local Health care providers were targeted for raising awareness about potential health hazards at Chattanooga Creek. The goal was as follows:

Local health care providers will be aware of potential health hazards at Chattanooga Creek, and possible signs and symptoms of exposure (i.e., gastroenteritis, skin rashes, and infections). Specific target audiences included:

- *school nurses who serve South Chattanooga*
- *area health center*
- *staff of clinic serving homeless population*
- *county health department*

The initial health education program will be completed by the first day of summer, 1993.

To accomplish this goal, an information package was developed and presented to the above audiences in the first two weeks in June 1993. Included in the package were ATSDR's Case Studies in Environmental Medicine for PCBs and PAHs. These publications provided information on signs and symptoms of exposure to PCBs and PAHs and recommended treatments (ATSDR, 1990a; ATSDR, 1990b). The package also included a fact sheet that highlighted the basic issues at the site, and literature on taking exposure histories (ATSDR, 1993b).

2. Elementary school-age children had been identified as a receptor population by the exposure survey described in the exposure pathways analysis section. Schools in the immediate area surrounding the creek were targeted. The goal was as follows:

Children, teachers, and school nurses at schools near Chattanooga Creek will be aware of potential health hazards at Chattanooga Creek, and possible signs and symptoms of exposure. The initial education program will be completed by the first day of summer, 1993.

Age-appropriate lessons were developed for children in kindergarten through eighth grade by ATSDR staff and school nurses. The slogan for the lessons was, "Don't be a creek geek." Lessons included a poster drawing contest, a "fish dance," and a simple experiment for the older children.

The "fish dance" taught younger children about the food chain pathway by having them dance a "happy dance" like fish in a clean creek, and a "sad dance" for ill fish swimming in a dirty creek. The lesson taught children about the effect polluted water may have on fish and encouraged children not to eat an "unhealthy" fish.

For the science experiment, the children passed around a jar of "clean water" to see. The jar was actually full of vinegar, as children discovered when they opened the jar and sniffed. The lesson taught children that although the creek water may look clean, there may be pollution that cannot be seen, and it may still be unsafe.

The take-home message of all these lessons was to avoid playing or fishing in the creek. Fact sheets were distributed for the children to take home to their parents. School nurses collaborated with ATSDR staff in development of the lessons and facilitated their approval by the school superintendent. The lessons lasted about a half hour and were given on a classroom-by-classroom basis. Teachers, especially science teachers, community volunteers, school nurses, and ATSDR staff all helped implement the program. Teachers and school nurses were provided with copies of lesson packets for use in the curriculum for years to come (ATSDR, 1993b).

3. Parents and residents who fish in Chattanooga Creek may have been unaware of potential health hazards at Chattanooga Creek. The following was the goal for general community health education:

> *Residents in South Chattanooga will be aware of potential health hazards at Chattanooga Creek, and possible signs and symptoms of exposure. Specific target audiences include the following:*
>
> - *activist groups*
> - *media*
> - *community leaders*
> - *local health care providers.*
>
> *The initial community health education will begin by the first day of summer, 1993, and continue until the creek is no longer a health hazard.*

The activist group that contacted ATSDR initially, STOP, was contacted first. This group had monthly meetings, which offered opportunities for planning and implementing community health education activities, such as developing and distributing fact sheets and meeting fliers, planning open community meetings, and contacting health care providers and other community leaders. A proactive approach was taken with local media. Efforts were made to contact newspapers, which were the primary media contacted, ahead of scheduled meetings or events. One newspaper had been running "environmental health" articles and was very receptive to printing items that raised awareness about potential health and safety hazards at Chattanooga Creek. Supplying fact sheets promoted accuracy in these articles, and often the fact sheets were printed verbatim on the front page of the major paper (Chattanooga Times, 1993). Television reporters and camera crews appeared at some of the community meetings, and "on camera" interviews were provided as requested.

Meetings were also scheduled with the mayor of Chattanooga, city council members, the director of the local health center, and staff members of the TDEC, the County Health Department staff, and the Tennessee Department of Health (TDH). Having media participation helped in making these contacts; in fact, on several occasions, community leaders became aware of activities through the newspapers and made the initial contacts. Providing thorough information and a scientific basis for the public health activities was required to gain support from leaders for these activities. Open lines of communication were also established.

Clean-Up Activities

4. Coordination with other agencies—including USEPA, TDEC, the Tennessee Valley Authority (TVA), and the City of Chattanooga—was needed to begin working toward reducing the potential for exposure. Of particular concern were the coal-tar deposits, since they presented both a physical and a chemical hazard. A goal for this immediate problem was set:

> *Appropriate federal, state, and local agencies will be aware of the health and safety hazards of the coal-tar deposits in Chattanooga Creek, and will be provided with health-based recommendations. These agencies will be contacted as soon as possible.*

Through community health education activities, open lines of communication were already established with these agencies. To address the coal-tar deposit issue, ATSDR issued a Public Health Advisory to EPA, which stated that the coal-tar deposit areas around Chattanooga Creek were an imminent health and safety hazard. The Public Health Advisory also included recommendations to fence these areas as soon as possible; repost the entire 7.5 miles of the creek; and propose the deposits for the National Priorities List (ATSDR, 1993a). Sound scientific and public health information supported these recommendations. USEPA and TDEC erected several miles of fences and new warning signs during the summer. The city stepped up efforts to upgrade the sewage treatment facility. The coal-tar deposit areas were proposed for the National Priorities List in February 1994 (ATSDR, 1993b). Placing these coal-tar deposits on the National Priorities List opens the door to Superfund money needed to plan and implement clean-up and remedial strategies.

■CONCLUSION

In a recent editorial in *Public Health Nursing,* Marla Salmon proposed that public health nurses have two key roles in the field of environmental health: hazard assessment and communication (Salmon, 1993). New methods for implementing these roles effectively are evolving, as more public health nurses gain experience in environmental health. The importance of succeeding in these roles is demonstrated by the public health nursing activities for the Chattanooga Creek community. First, the importance of including environmental issues in a community assessment cannot be stressed enough. As in the case of Chattanooga Creek, assessing environmental health meant more than a "windshield survey." It meant networking with other agencies and local community groups, requesting and analyzing environmental monitoring data, and researching possible exposure pathways and toxicological characteristics of the environmental contaminants. In Chattanooga, this assessment led to the identification of a health and safety hazard at a site that is now proposed for the National Priorities List.

Second, whether as educator or facilitator, performing the role of communicator was also key to developing and implementing public health activities. Education programs for community members and leaders, health care professionals, children, and the media can be a primary environmental health activity for public health nurses, as demonstrated in Chattanooga. Education is one way to protect your community from environmental hazards. Another is removing the environment hazards. Public health nurses may participate by facilitating communication. In Chattanooga, open lines of communication between federal and state agencies led to making public health recommendations, and ultimately to this site's being proposed for the EPA National Priorities List.

Acknowledgments

This project could not have been a success without the help of ATSDR staff from the Division of Health Education and Regional Operations. Thank you to Drs. Cynthia Lewis-Younger and Fredrick Rosenburg, and Saju Isaac for their time, energy, and creativity. Special thanks go to Dr. Alan Susten for his technical assistance with the Toxicological Analysis Section.

▬ REFERENCES

Agency for Toxic Substances and Disease Registry (ATSDR). (1990a) *Case studies in environmental medicine: Polynuclear aromatic hydrocarbon (PAH) toxicity.* Atlanta: U.S. Department of Health and Human Services, Public Health Service.

Agency for Toxic Substances and Disease Registry (ATSDR). (1990b) *Case studies in environmental medicine: Polychlorinated biphenyl (PCB) toxicity.* Atlanta: U.S. Department of Health and Human Services, Public Health Service.

Agency for Toxic Substances and Disease Registry (ATSDR). (1990c). *Toxicological profile for polycyclic aromatic hydrocarbons (PAHs).* Atlanta: U.S. Department of Health and Human Services, Public Health Service.

Agency for Toxic Substances and Disease Registry (ATSDR). (1992). *Public health assessment guidance manual.* Chelsea, Mich.: Lewis Publishers.

Agency for Toxic Substances and Disease Registry (ATSDR). (1993a). *Public health advisory for the Tennessee Products Site.* Atlanta: U.S. Department of Health and Human Services, Public Health Service.

Agency for Toxic Substances and Disease Registry (ATSDR). (1993b). *Public health assessment for the Tennessee Products Site (a/k/a Chattanooga Creek).* Public Comment Release: Atlanta: U.S. Department of Health and Human Services, Public Health Service.

Agency for Toxic Substances and Disease Registry (ATSDR). (1993c). *Toxicological profile for selected polychlorinated biphenyls (PCBs).* Atlanta: U.S. Department of Health and Human Services, Public Health Service.

The Chattanooga Times. (May 14, 1993). *Health officials issue early warning on creek.*

Environmental Protection Agency. (1991). *The environmental quality of Chattanooga Creek.*

Neufer, L.M. (1994). The role of the community health nurse in environmental health. *Public Health Nursing, 11*(3), 155–162.

Neufer, L.M., Narkunas, D.M. (1994). Analyzing potential health threats of hazardous substance releases at the community level: A practical approach. *AAOHN, 42*(7), 329–335.

Salmon, M.E. (1993). Editorial: An open letter to public health nurses. *Public Health Nursing, 10*(4), 211–212.

Chapter 14

Occupational Health Nursing:
A Public Health Perspective

RUTH ANN JACOBSON   ELAINE RICHARD

The health of people in the workplace is another important focus for community health nursing practice. It is in the work setting that many individuals spend a quarter to almost a third of their working lives. From janitor to corporation executive, each working person faces certain conditions and develops certain patterns on the job that affect her or his health. The occupational health nurse is in a prime position to assess the health needs of this population group and design healthful interventions. The authors of this chapter describe occupational health nursing and discuss integration of public health theory and principles with this role to increase its effectiveness in serving the working population.

Occupational health nursing is the practice of nursing utilizing public health principles and theories for the promotion and maintenance of healthy workers. As occupational health nurses representing both education and service, we present our views of the framework and practice for this expanding speciality field in nursing. It is our belief that occupational health nursing practice has become more comprehensive in scope and therefore will require baccalaureate and advanced preparation to fulfill the needs and expectations of both labor and industry.

This chapter will address four major areas: 1) public health, the origin and basis for occupational health practice; 2) the application of public health principles in occupational practice settings; 3) roles and preparations for occupational health nursing; and 4) trends in occupational health.

▬PUBLIC HEALTH—BASIS FOR OCCUPATIONAL HEALTH PRACTICE

The practice of occupational health nursing began in 1895 when the Vermont Marble Company employed a public health nurse to visit ill employees and the families of workers.[1] Public health agencies also became

This chapter was written especially for the second edition of this book.

providers of occupational health services through contractual agreements: The Boston Visiting Nurses Association in 1908 provided such services to the Lowrey Chocolate Factory.[2] At the turn of the century, factories, department stores, and hotels began employing "industrial nurses" to provide on-site health care to employees. By 1930, over 3,000 nurses were employed by industry.[3,4]

As nurses began to practice in occupational settings, there was a professional concern that nurses who were isolated from other health professionals would be in danger of servicing the employer only and that they would not uphold professional standards of practice.[5] Thus, to meet the needs of industrial nurses, the National Organization of Public Health Nursing began to represent nurses in commerce and industry. The scope of occupational health nursing also was in danger of being limited to the acute care of individuals. In her 1933 book, *Public Health Nursing in Industry*, Hodgson made the following statements:

> *Public health nursing in industry may be defined as the application of nursing skills and procedures to the sick or injured workers, and the sharing of information in the fundamental principles of healthful living as applied to the needs of the worker in his daily environment. All too often the nurse's function is limited to the care of the sick and injured, but it is the second service which determines the true preventive value of her contributions to the health of the employee. It is the second service which should receive increasing emphasis as a means of enriching the contribution of the nursing service to the plant and community health program.[6]*

Industry and business provide an economic base for a community, jobs for its workers, and products or services for its people. The type and size of the industry or business will determine the kinds and numbers of workers, their skills and education, and the potential health and safety hazards to both the community and its work force. For example, an insulation manufacturing company, the major employer in a hypothetical community, hires a primarily blue-collar work force with high school and/or vocational technical preparation. Its use of asbestos creates a health hazard for the community. Citizens of this community look to the company for civic leadership, source of income, health and welfare benefits, and job satisfaction. The population is composed of various ethnic groups with limited education, diverse value systems, and differing attitudes toward health that do not include prevention. Thus the population lacks the values and knowledge necessary to control the transmission of hazardous asbestos material into their homes, thereby exposing other family members.

■APPLICATION OF PUBLIC HEALTH PRINCIPLES TO OCCUPATIONAL HEALTH NURSING

The practice of occupational health nursing requires an integration of public health principles. This is so because of the interrelatedness of the community, the workplace, and workers. The goals and objectives of an occupational health program, therefore, will require utilization of public health skills to plan and manage appropriate health programs for the working adult population that take into account their impact on workers' families and the community.

The public health skills that will assist the nurse in performing this leadership role will include the following:

1. Knowledge of the community's demographic data, including morbidity and mortality statistics
2. An assessment of the work force to determine populations at risk for occupationally related injury or illness
3. Application of epidemiology in determining the relationship of work and injury or illness
4. Interdisciplinary planning with a safety specialist, an industrial hygienist, a toxicologist, and an occupational health physician
5. Intervention at the aggregate level, where maximum benefits can occur
6. Networking with appropriate community resources
7. Evaluation of programs that address cost-benefits and cost-effectiveness

These public health skills provide the framework for development of an occupational health program. Each of these skills will be utilized by the occupational health nurse. Examples of the application of each skill are given in the following paragraphs.

Community Assessment

Data on disease trends, birth and death rates, and social environmental conditions provide pertinent information for the establishment of priorities in planning and implementing occupational health programs. Therefore, the occupational health nurse seeks information about the community's demographic characteristics, including mortality and morbidity statistics. In addition, data on economic, cultural, and psychological factors that determine the community's health attitudes and behavior become essential.

Consider a hypothetical community. It has few structured social organizations, and statistics reveal a high incidence of accidental deaths and injuries, including those related to suicide. Community officials relate many of these accidents to drug and alcohol usage. Hospital admissions for treatment of alcohol- and drug-related problems support this contention. The only community-based industry, a manufacturing plant employing mostly younger people, experiences considerable loss of productivity directly related to this community problem. Based on a community assessment, the company occupational health nurse may choose to develop a chemical-dependency program. The program includes education to prevent chemical abuse, to promote early detection and treatment of abusers, and to successfully employ recovering chemical abusers.

Worker Assessment

The characteristics of the work force will determine populations at risk for occupationally related injury or illness. Classification of groups of employees by age, sex, race, type of work, and presence or absence of disability provides the occupational health nurse with the data necessary for analysis of health risks. For instance, female assembly-line workers of childbearing age must be protected from exposure to substances having teratogenic properties. Workers of Scandinavian descent exposed to direct sunlight for long periods should be taught proper techniques to prevent skin cancer, such as the use of barrier creams.

Application of Epidemiology Principles

To determine the relationship of work and illness or injury, occupational health nurses apply the epidemiological method. Investigation of causation of illness or injury begins with a thorough description of its occurrence. This pattern of occurrence permits identification of the population at greatest risk. Application of such sciences as toxicology, pathology, and ergonomics provides the basis for developing theories of causation. Approaches to prevention can then be tested to confirm or disprove these theories. The experience of a group of polyvinylchloride workers illustrates the value of an epidemiological approach:

> In the early 1970s, three residents of a Kentucky community died of angiosarcoma. A relationship of these cases was not evident, as each individual was treated by a different physician. However, after the third death from angiosarcoma, interest and concern about this rare disease developed. Subsequent investigation led to the discovery that all three individuals were employed by the same plant that manufactured polyvinylchloride resins.[7]

The occurrence of angiosarcoma in these three cases led to an exploration of this occupational exposure as a potential hazard for the entire worker population in that plant.

Team Approach

Occupational health efforts, to be most effective, require team work. A team of occupational health professionals assesses, plans, implements, and evaluates programs. A multiplicity of data collected from a variety of disciplines enhances the development of a comprehensive occupational health program. Ideally, collaboration among specialists such as safety engineers, industrial hygienists, toxicologists, physicians, and nurses produces appropriate, effective, and efficient occupational health services. For example, an occupational health nurse in a hypothetical utility company notes an unusually high number of workers visiting the health service complaining of "pain in the wrist." An investigation establishes that these workers experiencing tendonitis all have similar jobs involving the splicing of cable. Further study reveals that 6 weeks previous to the onset of symptoms, productivity engineers developed and implemented a new splicing technique. The ergonomist is consulted. This specialist is concerned with fitting a job to man's biological and psychological characteristics in order to enhance human efficiency and well-being. The ergonomist studying the procedure finds that it involves considerable repetitive motion of the wrist. Problem-solving by the nurse, safety engineer, ergonomist, and productivity engineer results in a revision of the procedure to minimize repetitive motion without loss of production time or violation of safety principles. Ultimately, protection of both worker health and safety is provided without placing productivity in jeopardy.

Program Planning and Implementation

Program planning and implementation, a major focus of occupational health nursing, must take place at the aggregate level, where maximum benefits occur. Carolyn Williams emphasizes the distinction between the focus of programs designed for personal care of individuals and of programs designed to affect groups. Aggregates, she maintains, are individuals who have in common one or more personal or environmental characteristic. These characteristics may identify groups at high risk of developing certain personal health problems. Health needs of populations, therefore, can be anticipated, and programs, including health promotional activities and personal health services, can be designed.[8]

The primary goal of the occupational health program is the promotion of wellness and the prevention of illness and injury among workers. However, illness and injury do occur, necessitating occupational health programs aimed at all levels of prevention: primary, secondary, and tertiary. Since these programs are the major activities of occupational health nursing, an in-depth description is appropriate.

PRIMARY PREVENTION. Access to well adults creates the opportunity for the application of primary prevention principles in occupational health. A program to ensure the health of prospective employees includes a history and physical examination to assess level of wellness. Maintenance of that level is provided through appropriate job placement. For example, a potential stockroom worker, a healthy young female of extremely small stature, is screened for ability to lift and push heavy objects. She is able to safely manipulate boxes weighing up to 40 pounds. Assignment to a stockroom storing supplies under 40 pounds may prevent potential musculoskeletal injuries.

The workplace is surveyed periodically to protect employees from potential health hazards. Environmental conditions may be changed to prevent illness or injury. For example, the occupational health nurse touring a plant may notice a wet surface on a walkway. Correction will eliminate many falls and injuries. Subtle hazards, such as color schemes and lighting techniques, when identified, can be modified to diminish eye fatigue among clerical work groups.

The dissemination of health and safety information and instruction are also common prevention techniques directed toward employee groups. One-to-one health counseling remains an effective motivator of safe and healthy behavior, but the impracticality of individual instruction forces the occupational health nurse to develop innovative and cost-effective methods for instructing aggregates of workers. The prevention of occupational illness and injury depends on employee knowledge and understanding of many safety procedures, including use of protective equipment and clothing and of proper body cleansing techniques.

Efforts to prevent nonoccupational injuries and illnesses are also underway in increasing numbers of organizations, both large and small. Morbidity and mortality statistics specific to people of employable age reveal a need for preventive services focused on motor vehicle, home, and recreational safety, and the importance of maintaining a healthy life-style. Involvement in these efforts ranges from the distribution of printed material to elaborate in-house health and fitness facilities. Campaigns designed to promote off-job activities, such as safe driving and the use of seat belts, smoke detectors, and proper sports equipment, are occurring in the workplace. Many such programs are currently flourishing, and they include teaching principles of nutrition, exercise, and stress management. They also aim to modify health habits, such as alcohol consumption and cigarette smoking, and to promote consumer involvement in health care. Activities during working hours as well as those carried out in the employee's free time include support groups to facilitate behavioral change and incentive programs to reward such change. The motivation of employees to adopt healthy life-styles is becoming a common goal of organizations.

SECONDARY PREVENTION. Despite primary prevention efforts in occupational health, disease and disability continue to exist, necessitating the development of secondary preventive services. Early detection and treatment of both work- and nonwork-related health problems constitutes a major portion of health services available to workers.

Screening and monitoring of workers exposed to potential hazards are carefully performed to comply with company policy and government regulations. For example, exposure to lead, a frequently used element in industry, constitutes a threat to workers and must be closely evaluated. A surveillance program may consist of serum lead levels performed on all workers exposed. These results are carefully scrutinized and recorded, and tests are repeated periodically to ensure early detection of overexposure. Health screening for nonwork-related illnesses, such as diabetes, may be provided by companies. For example, mass screening in conjunction with community agencies, such as the American Diabetes Association and the American Cancer Society, can be performed with minimum expense to the employer.

Workers may be unable to meet productivity standards because of undetected illness. Encouraging supervisors to refer these employees to the occupational health department for evaluation will frequently result in the identification of an emotional, chemical, or physical health problem. Improvement of health status will enhance the potential of the employee to function at a high level of productivity.

Accident reporting and monitoring systems are developed to ensure that injured employees are treated promptly and appropriately and that all possible disability is prevented. The nature of injuries experienced in the work place will determine the type of emergency care facilities provided by the organization. The occupational health nurse, notified when an injury occurs, will assess the need for treatment. A worker with a muscle strain, for instance, may be assessed and treated within the company medical department, while an employee with a large laceration may be transported to a hospital for emergency care. Investigation of accidents is undertaken to determine causation, thereby making possible prevention of similar incidents.

TERTIARY PREVENTION. Primary and secondary prevention programs in occupational health decrease the number of workers permanently disabled but do not eliminate the need for tertiary prevention. Rehabilitation efforts are directed toward workers disabled by occupational and nonoccupational problems. These efforts include evaluation of current status, enhancement of employability, and appropriate job placement of disabled employees. Whether performed within company facilities or within a variety of community agencies, evaluation will focus on increasing the capabilities of the worker. The services of such disciplines as physical, occupational, and speech therapy; vocational training; chronic pain clinics; and remedial reading and mathematics programs may be enlisted. Placement in a job involves careful analysis of the work, tools, and work place to ascertain necessary modifications. Communication with and preparation of the employee's supervisor will promote successful placement.

A hypothetical situation illustrates the point. Following an automobile accident that took place while driving a company vehicle, a male worker is unable to use his right arm because of nerve damage and permanent paralysis. It is no longer possible for him to perform his job, which consisted of driving a delivery van and loading and unloading large boxes. Positions not requiring use of both arms are highly technical in this organization, requiring advanced mathematics and electronic and computer skills. Assessment of the individual's interests and capabilities reveal that he is not a candidate for advanced education. Therefore, the nurse and personnel staff review the driver delivery jobs in the company to ascertain modification methods possible to accommodate this worker. Job functions within the department are realigned, and a position of shipping clerk is created. After an orientation period, this handicapped worker is successfully returned to work.

The occupational health department spearheads the creation of a positive company atmosphere within which rehabilitation may take place. All levels of management and employee groups must be involved and committed to the process of returning handicapped employees to fulfilling positions within the organization.

Referral to Community Resources

Occupational health nurses enhance their practice through the development of a network of appropriate community resources. Appropriate referral and follow-up provide more comprehensive, cost-effective service to workers. Utilization of community health agencies and professionals as well as institutions, such as education, finance, law, and recreation, supplements and enhances the effectiveness of occupational health programs. For instance, occupational health nurses frequently deal with workers experiencing situational stress. In cases when more intense intervention is needed, a referral to community inpatient mental health treatment centers becomes appropriate. Counseling on financial and legal matters may be needed by some employees. Referral to a community support group for divorced persons or single parents may be appropriate for others. Additional sources may include services for career counseling, vocational training, day care of children, emergency medical care, and protection from an abusive spouse.

Program Evaluation

Assessment of programs to determine benefits in terms of decreasing loss of productivity related to employee health problems is carried out. Cost-effectiveness is established, for example, when an occupational health program demonstrates an increase in worker productivity. Occupational health professionals are increasingly expected to justify their program goals and costs. One occupational health nurse studied a company employee counseling program using several parameters.[9] These included tabulation of days away from the job because of illness, injuries, or visits to the doctor; days in the hospital; personal leave; and disciplinary action (suspension) for employees prior to and after receiving counseling. These workers and their supervisors were asked to evaluate the workers' job performance and attitudes toward the job and co-workers. The results demonstrated that, in the majority of employees counseled, there was a decrease in days spent away from work and an improvement in performance and attitude. Dollar values can be assigned to these changes so that cost-effectiveness can be assessed. Other areas that have been used to measure cost-effectiveness are programs and/or activities aimed at reducing worker compensation costs.

The public health skills, although described separately, operate simultaneously in practice. Each one is interrelated and, therefore, interdependent. The omission of one component will diminish the effectiveness of the collective whole.

■ ROLES AND PREPARATION

The planning and managing of occupational health programs will require the skills of a master's-prepared occupational health nurse. However, the implementation of occupational health programs will be carried out by staff occupational health nurses, who provide direct care to workers. The practice of occupational health nursing has become more comprehensive and more preventive in orientation, requiring knowledge and skills in public health science, interviewing and counseling, research process, and most important, oral and written communication. In order to meet these increasing demands, baccalaureate education in nursing will become the basis for nursing practice in the field of occupational health.

   The role and responsibilities of the staff occupational health nurse may vary depending on the goals of the organization (industry or business) and the skills of the registered nurse. Definitions and standards of practice have been developed by both the American Association of Occupational Health Nurses and the American Nurses' Association. Certification in occupational health nursing is also available to nurses who have 5 years experience in the field and who demonstrate competencies in occupational health nursing through a written examination.

▬TRENDS IN OCCUPATIONAL HEALTH

In 1978 the National Institute of Occupational Safety and Health (NIOSH) conducted a nationwide survey to examine the supply and demand of occupational safety and health personnel. The report revealed that the supply of nurses prepared in occupational health would not meet the projected demands for the 1980–1990 period.[10] This increased demand for occupational health nurses is the result of a growing change in focus and approach to health in our society. A shift in attitude toward health is witnessed by recent legislation targeted to occupational and environmental concerns, a government commitment to prevention in health delivery, and society's interest and involvement in personal life-style changes. Concomitantly, nursing education has responded to these changes by better preparing nurses in public health sciences and for work with the well adult population.

   A growing concern for the high incidence of occupationally related illness and injuries in the 1960s led to the passage of the Occupational Safety and Health Act of 1970. This act assured every American worker a healthy and safe work environment. It also mandated NIOSH the responsibility for conducting educational programs to provide qualified occupational safety and health personnel. By 1980, ten educational resource centers had been established in universities throughout the nation, most of which offered a master's degree program in occupational health nursing.

   Another significant law that concerned the worker and his health was the Toxic Substance Control Act of 1976. In an effort to protect the environment and human health, this law requires the testing and restricting of chemical substances.

   A major shift in health policy came in 1979, when the Surgeon General's *Report on Health Promotion and Disease Prevention* clearly emphasized prevention as the focus for the 1980s.[11] The chronic diseases, namely, cardiovascular conditions, cancer, and stroke, currently lead the list of mortality and morbidity statistics in the United States. Therefore, efforts to develop ways of preventing their occurrence and/or reduce their effects are a priority of government's involvement in health care.

   Occupational health is a targeted program in public health because the work force is a high-risk group for chronic diseases resulting from exposure to carcinogens and other toxic substances.

   Personal life-style intervention programs have become very popular among well adults. These "wellness" programs are aimed at population groups identified as at high risk for cardiovascular and other chronic diseases. Many of these programs are offered as a benefit to employees at the work place. Company participation is high because employers are interested in cutting costs for illness care, improving workers' health, and increasing productivity. The work place becomes an ideal setting to reach this well population and to coordinate a wellness program with existing occupational health and safety activities.

The 1980s, therefore, became the decade for occupational health. There was interest and concern in society, government, labor, and industry to assume responsibility and allocate monies for preventive health intervention. This prevailing atmosphere provides the nursing profession an opportunity to demonstrate its unique abilities to plan and implement health programs and to improve and maintain the health of the working adult population.

▬REFERENCES

1. The National Organization for Public Health Nursing. *Manual of Public Health Nursing* (3rd ed.). New York: Macmillan, 1939, p. 311.
2. Public Health Service, National Institute of Occupational Safety and Health. *Community Health Nursing for Working People*. Public Health Service Publication No. 1296, 1971. P. 1.
3. Hodgson, V. *Public Health Nursing in Industry*. New York: Macmillan, 1933. P. xi.
4. Gardner, M. S. *Public Health Nursing*. New York: Macmillan, 1916. P. 301.
5. Hodgson, V. *Public Health Nursing in Industry*. New York: Macmillan, 1977. P. xii.
6. Hodgson, V. *Public Health Nursing in Industry*. New York: Macmillan, 1933. P. 49.
7. Creech, J. L., Jr., and Johnson, M. N. Special Communication—Angiosarcoma of Liver in the Manufacture of Polyvinyl Chloride. *J. Occup. Health Med.* 16(3): 150, 1974.
8. Williams, C. Community Health Nursing—What Is It? *Nurs. Outlook* 25(4): 250, 1977.
9. Scrivner, R. A. Handling Stress Makes Dollars and Sense. *Occup. Health Nurs.* 29:3, 1981.
10. Public Health Service Center for Disease Control, National Institute of Occupational Safety and Health. *A Nationwide Survey of the Occupational Safety and Health Workforce.* Cincinnati, Ohio, 1978.
11. Public Health Service, Office of the Assistant Secretary for Health, and Surgeon General. *Health of People: The Surgeon General's Report on Health Promotion and Disease Prevention.* PHS Publication No. 79-55071, 1979.

Chapter 15

Innovative Practice Models in Community Health Nursing

CHERIE RECTOR

> Since its inception, the field of public health nursing has demonstrated its ability to develop innovative responses to meet community health needs. Today that tradition continues as community health nurses practice in countless settings, adapting to changing circumstances and designing creative programs to address the needs of aggregates and populations at risk. In this chapter, Dr. Rector describes some of these programs and shows how community health nurses exercise creativity and resourcefulness to meet the needs of the communities they serve.

Since the days of Lillian Wald, visiting families in their homes has been at the core of public health nursing. Certainly, what distinguishes this speciality practice of nursing is the ability of its practitioners to know the community best by seeing firsthand the difficulties experienced by individuals and families in their homes and neighborhoods. The effectiveness of home-based interventions on health and social outcomes for mothers and infants, for example, has been demonstrated in several studies (Barnard, Magyary, Sumner, Booth, Mitchell, & Spieker, 1988; Olds, Henderson, Tatelbaum, & Chamberlin, 1988; Olds & Kitzman, 1990; Kristjanson & Chalmers, 1991; Brooten et al., 1986). In low-density, rural areas, home visiting may be the only method of contact for public health nurses (PHNs) and their clients (Davis & Droes, 1993). However, even Lillian Wald and her Henry Street Settlement House nurses sought less labor-intensive methods of delivering care to aggregates by organizing mothers' clubs, a convalescent center, and first aid stations (Buhler-Wilkerson, 1993). And, today, Zerwekh (1992) proposes that community health nurses work simultaneously with individuals, families, and aggregates to improve the health of our society.

With changing structures of health care delivery, shrinking budgets, and a move to more population-based care, public health departments will undoubtedly have to examine many alternative methods of delivering care to the public. While health departments have generally offered clinics for

This chapter was especially written for this edition of this book.

various groups (eg, perinatal services, immunization and Early and Periodic Screening Diagnosis and Treatment [EPSDT] services, sexually transmitted disease and tuberculosis screening), most have been fixed services provided at a central location, or, perhaps, a few satellite centers. However, are the greatest number of clients being served using this approach? Also, the method of delivery of care at these clinics may need to be examined (Corcoran et al., 1988). Is it more effective to have clients come on specific days to receive one specialized service at a block clinic with no scheduled appointment time (taking up a good deal of the client's day), or is a more integrated approach (eg, several programs available on the same day using scheduled appointments) better?

■ COMMUNITY-BASED SERVICES

Lillian Wald and her nurses moved into the neighborhoods they served. This provided them with easier access to clients and a greater knowledge of the barriers to care and the health and social needs of the public (Buhler-Wilkerson, 1993). Nursing services which are geographically defined (eg, block nursing, district nursing, neighborhood nursing) have been shown to promote greater access, be more cost-effective, and provide greater continuity and outcome satisfaction. Dreher (1984) described the benefits of district nursing (then a dying specialty) in a small, rural New England community. Contrary to the misconception of being "behind the times," district nurses were viewed by their clients as more readily available and accessible, more accountable and acceptable to the public, and able to provide more comprehensive, coordinated services than the newer, more widely available home health nursing services. The district nurse handled preventive and health maintenance duties as well as care of the chronically ill. The home health care agency only dealt with the latter.

Block nursing was described by Jamieson (1990, p. 250) as a "cost-effective and ... innovative solution to the delivery of health and long-term care services." In block nursing, nurses who live within the neighborhood boundaries act as case managers for elderly clients in need of housekeeping, help with activities of daily living, or aid in accessing other local agency services. Volunteers supplement the duties of paid staff, and families of elderly clients work with nurses in developing care plans that meet clients' needs. As a result of this innovative program, less elderly in the study were forced to enter nursing homes, more families were involved with their elderly relatives, and the community demonstrated increased sensitivity to the needs of the elderly. This program decreased hospitalizations, increased the time the elderly could remain in their homes, and was found to be generally cost-effective and innovative in its approach.

In a similar approach, parish nursing was described by Miskelly (1995) as a means of providing screening, counseling, advocacy, and education to a church community as the service population. This approach was developed by a "Lutheran chaplain" in 1983 (p. 1). Parish nurses use a community health nursing model to assess the needs of their clients and design appropriate interventions. Miskelly did a needs assessment and identified at-risk aggregates within her church population (eg, nonexercising and overweight adults, adults under age 50 without regular blood pressure and cholesterol screening, adults who lacked access to primary care services and health insurance coverage). A population-specific program plan was designed which included support group facilitation, educational classes (eg, stress management, exercise, nutrition, health promotion), community resource referrals, and health counseling/screening. In communities without parish nurses, community health nurses could join with local churches in health promotion and needs assessment, as well as for provision of health services at the church site.

Joining with churches and other community entities can extend the role of the PHN. Universities can be interested partners in providing care for communities. Community nursing centers, established by university schools of nursing, often provide care for the public and educational opportunities for students, as well as offer sites for faculty practice and research. Barger and Kline (1993) and Walker (1994) describe center services provided to individuals and families and the derived benefits for students and faculty. One center, operated by the Rochester School of Nursing, extended their services to local community businesses and organizations (Walker, 1994). They offered expert consultation in grantwriting and research, educational programs for management and employees in first aid and cardiopulmonary resuscitation and employee wellness programs, along with other services, in an effort to broaden their financial base. They relied heavily on marketing principles and diversification of revenue streams to ensure financial success.

The University of Pennsylvania School of Nursing organized a community-based nursing center to improve access to primary care for an impoverished neighborhood in West Philadelphia (Whelan, 1995). They joined with the local community and the public health department in assessing barriers to care and designing a nursing center tailored to community needs. They started small, in a well-accepted and highly frequented local community center, offering well child care services to daycare clients, calling their clinic the Health Corner. Gradually, under the direction of the neighborhood advisory council and the public health department, other services were added (eg, a teen-specific family planning clinic, and walk-in pregnancy testing and counseling for women of all ages). The times and dates of these services were adjusted to meet the needs of the population they served (eg, well child clinic hours were set during dropoff and pickup times for daycare, teen clinics were during school hours). Linkages were established with local agencies and referral mechanisms were designed. The clinic used the services of nurse practitioners, a social worker, a community health aide, and a health educator, with funding from a federal Healthy Start grant.

In an effort to meet the needs of another unique underserved population, Visiting Nurses and Hospice of San Francisco designed the Hotel Project to provide care for residents of a tenement hotel in the Tenderloin district who were substance users infected with HIV (Robb, 1994). A team approach was used with this aggregate, as nurses, social workers, and home health care aides visited patients at the hotel. Basic needs were addressed first and volunteers assisted in providing necessary items (eg, dishes, linens, clothes). These clients, who had virtually no social support networks, were hesitant to use hospital and residential hospice services because of feelings of alienation and stigmatization. Also, access to illicit drugs is denied in these settings. Gradually, clients began to consider placement in residential hospices. Benefits derived from the project included improved nutrition and personal hygiene, better symptom management and pain control, fewer emergency room visits, and a greater number of clients accepting primary medical care.

Another frequently underserved population, the homeless, are receiving services at nurse-managed clinics designed for their specific needs (Bowlder & Barrell, 1987; Turner, Bauer, McNair, McNutt, & Walker, 1989; Reilly, Grier, & Blomquist; 1992). Reilly (1994), using an ecological approach, determined environmental, natural, and personal/social/cultural hazards for the homeless population in an urban area of the southeastern United States. Homeless shelters and soup kitchens which provide meals for the homeless often operate on schedules which do not take these risk factors into account. They are frequently closed at periods of high risk, forcing the homeless into hazardous situations. This is a key factor in providing appropriate services to this vulnerable population. In planning for targeted services, Bowdler and Barrell (1987) assessed the homeless population of Richmond, Virginia, using a systems approach. They found that most of the homeless were single, had family problems, and were under- or unemployed. Common problems included substance abuse, mental illness, and circulatory or respiratory disease, as well as infectious disease. Suggestions for a new nurse-run clinic were made, including regular availability of services, development of outreach programs to link clients to appropriate community services and better coordinated health care, and development of specific health education programs for this population.

▬OTHER METHODS OF REACHING THE PUBLIC

Telephone services were used in a model program offering public health nursing consultation and services to family daycare homes and daycare centers. Phone consultation, home visits, and group training sessions for daycare workers were provided by PHNs in Minneapolis, and expansion of services was requested (Lie, 1992). Health promotion for children that use daycare centers and daycare homes was an expected outcome of this project, although no formal evaluation of health outcomes was cited by the author. However, telephone follow-up has been shown to be effective in improving use of services to a targeted population. Oda and Boyd (1988) used a telephone call or a single home visit to increase use of EPSDT services for children of low-income families. Oda, Fine, and Heilbron (1986) used telephone follow-up to increase numbers of dental visits following screening. These approaches were deemed a cost-effective method for reaching this client group.

EPSDT services are available for Medicaid-eligible children under age 21; however, many families may not qualify for this service because of income eligibility guidelines, even though they may not have access to other preventive primary health care due to their under- and uninsured status. To address this health care gap, Wisconsin initiated a pilot project to provide services to this population through a program called KidsCare (Clarridge, Larson, & Newman, 1993). Health benefits counselors worked with these families to determine their coverage, and to assist them in filing appeals and engaging legal counsel (if needed). These counselors worked closely with PHNs who provided EPSDT-equivalent services to children in the KidsCare group. They found children within this group (non-EPSDT eligible, but under- or uninsured) had noticeably worse health status than children who were EPSDT eligible. Also, KidsCare children were significantly more likely to have been off-schedule for dental visits than EPSDT-eligible children. Providing preventive health care services for the burgeoning numbers of under- and uninsured is a formidable challenge, and one that public health departments may need to examine.

However, achieving full use of EPSDT by eligible clients can be a challenge. Only 25% to 30% of eligible clients nationwide use this service (Selby, Riportella-Muller, Sorenson, & Walters, 1989). Using a health promotion model (PRECEDE) and components of other models related to health promotion and disease prevention, as well as concepts derived from learning and crisis theory, PHNs in a rural area of North Carolina designed a model for intervention with poor, nonwhite single mothers and their children (Selby, Riportella-Muller, Sorenson, & Walters, 1989). Targeted pamphlets, telephone calls, and home visits were selected as the most potentially effective methods to increase the use of EPSDT services. These methods were used in a later pilot study, and found to be helpful in improving use of EPSDT services by this aggregate (Selby et al., 1990). Mailed pamphlets followed up with a PHN phone call were found to be effective, and less labor-intensive than home visits, although home visits were found to be most effective in motivating clients without telephones.

Another health promotion model, the Health Belief Model, was used to develop a health education intervention, using commercial television (Braun & Conybeare, 1995). Ten one-half hour programs were developed on various topics (eg, breast cancer, diabetes, asthma, skin cancer) and each program was followed by a physician-staffed phone bank, available to answer viewer questions for 90 minutes. Also, a fact sheet for each of the 10 topics was available at a local drug store chain and physician offices. Viewers were enticed into answering quizzes on the back of each fact sheet by offering a Healthy Weekend Sweepstakes at the end of the series. Authors cited numbers of phone calls to the phone bank, Nielsen ratings, and the number of contest entries as evidence of a significant audience size for the programs. The series was considered such a success that sponsors agreed to finance program repeats at a different day and time. This relatively low-cost approach to health education was felt to be an impetus for some viewers to learn more about their health and to take action on health concerns.

The use of paraprofessionals and lay volunteers can extend PHN services in underserved communities. *De Madres a Madres* is a program in Texas which uses lay community volunteers to reach mothers who demonstrate risk factors for obtaining late or no prenatal care (Mahon, McFarlane, & Golden, 1991). The intent of the program was to increase community awareness regarding the problem of not seeking early prenatal care, and to engender community support and activism. Community leaders were informed about the program, and 14 volunteer mothers subsequently completed an 8-hour training program on the importance of prenatal care, community resources for pregnant women, and how to be an advocate and effective communicator. Over 2,000 contacts with at-risk women were made in the first year, and further evaluation was to be done during the second year of the program (eg, comparing use of prenatal services and referrals for social services pre- and post-intervention, as well as structured interviews with at-risk mothers).

Paraprofessionals (community health aides) from the Fresno County Health Department have been instrumental in initiating Walking Clubs in outlying rural communities in California. Because of the high numbers of Type II (adult-onset) diabetics in these largely Hispanic areas, health educators and PHNs designed this innovative method of increasing exercise and participant numbers have grown. Other outreach programs target senior aggregates (Silver Screen, available to neighborhood senior nutrition centers) or children (immunization vans which operate on weekends in local fast food, grocery store, or shopping center parking lots).

■SCHOOL-BASED OR SCHOOL-LINKED INTERVENTIONS

Public health nurses have long participated in school health, either as consultants to school districts or as actual providers of services (Wold, 1984; Woodfill & Beyrer, 1991; Hawkins, Hayes, & Corliss, 1994). School nurses plan, deliver, and manage school health services, including health education and maintaining a healthy environment (Igoe, 1994). School-based clinics have employed nurse practitioners to provide primary care for some time (Igoe, 1975). However, the numbers of these clinics are increasing (currently there are over 500 across the country), and linkage with other community agencies has been found to be beneficial (Igoe, 1994). Public health nurses, working in conjunction with nurse practitioners and school nurses, can perform community assessments and epidemiologic studies, assist in policy development, and design appropriate interventions. Health education is a vital component of this new model, as is case management for medically fragile or chronically ill students. Also, provision of ready access to immunizations and EPSDT services for all school children is vital and can be facilitated by public health agencies (Kirby, 1990).

In settings where PHNs are not currently located in schools, there are several current models which can include public health services to school children and their families. School-linked services are also coming of age, as schools are becoming neighborhood service centers for children and families (DeFriese, Crossland, MacPhail-Wilcox, & Sowers, 1990; Igoe, 1994). Public health clinics can be periodically housed at school sites to provide immunizations, tuberculosis (TB) screening, family planning services, well-baby care, and health education. Other agencies and "helping professionals" can also be brought onto school campuses (eg, social service or welfare workers, employment development specialists, literacy program volunteers, mental health counselors). Federal and state government agencies have encouraged this movement of health and social services into the schools (Cohen, 1992). Educators and health and social service providers have recognized the advantages of coming together to better meet the needs of clients by offering a more easily accessible setting and coordinated services (Dryfoos, 1994; Wang, Haertel, & Walberg, 1995). In fact, comprehensive service models, coalition building, and collaborative models of practice are necessary to meet the needs of an increasingly vulnerable population of students (Igoe, 1994). No longer can schools ignore the social and emotional problems of children and families, as they are now recognized as having a significant impact on learning outcomes. In California, Healthy Start grants to local school districts have promoted the development of school-based clinics, school-linked services, and school–agency partnerships. In one such program, which did not get funded under Healthy Start, the Visalia Unified School District is working with the local hospital, which donated the services of a school nurse/nurse practitioner to work as a case manager for children and families at two at-risk school sites. In the Tulare County Office of Education's Early Intervention Program for at-risk infants and children (ages 0 to 3), an expert panel (including a PHN) screens cases for referral to special education teachers who work with parents and infants in their homes to improve outcomes. Another innovative program at Clovis Unified School District combines a school-based clinic and services provided by local community agencies. A school nurse/pediatric nurse practitioner provides EPSDT screenings, TB skin testing, well-baby care and immunizations, as well as Women, Infants, and Children nutrition program referrals. The nurse also provides school nursing services such as health and developmental assessments for special education; vision, hearing, and dental screenings and referral; and health counseling for students and families. Because the local health department services are not easily accessible (over one hour and several bus transfers away), the school district supported this effort until reimbursement for services could be made by accessing various public funding streams. A school social worker helps to coordinate services that link with the school and provides counseling and referrals to outside agencies, as well as organizing local events (eg, yearly parades, a Safe Halloween Festival). A local church provides volunteers who staff a food and clothing distribution center, the Boys and Girls Clubs provide assistance with homework and after-school activities, and the Fresno Parks and Recreation Department operates various programs at a nearby community center (eg, AA meetings, seniors activities, and blood pressure and glucose testing provided by a local hospital). The local police and fire departments also are involved with the Pinedale C.A.R.E.S. (Community Agencies Resources & Expanded Services) Safety Team in violence and crime prevention. Mental health services are provided through a county agency, and even the local library, located nearby in the community center, provides expanded services for children and their families. This is truly a concerted effort to improve the health and well-being of this community.

Hospitals and health maintenance organizations may find it beneficial to join with public health departments and schools to promote healthy lifestyles and community safety. Unintentional injuries could be addressed by programs which promote infant car safety seat and bicycle helmet safety, for example. Programs also could be designed to impact dental health and nutrition, smoking prevention and cessation, healthy lifestyles, and common disease risk factors. The upcoming cohort of citizens could be reached early in the schools and society as a whole could benefit.

■SUMMARY

Public health nurses need to look for innovative and unique ways to better serve the public. With many gaps in service and changing funding sources, along with the rise again in communicable diseases, public and community health agencies will be strained to meet the needs of the communities they serve. Once again, like Lillian Wald and her Henry Street Settlement House nurses, PHNs can be in the forefront—on the cutting edge. Only this time, our very existence as a profession may depend on the depth of our creativity and resourcefulness.

■REFERENCES

Barnard, K.E., Magyary, D., Sumner, G., Booth, C.L., Mitchell, S.K., & Spieker, S. (1988). Prevention of parenting alterations for women with low social support. *Psychiatry, 51,* 248–253.

Barger, S.E. & Kline, P.M. (1993). Community health service programs in academe: Unique learning opportunities for students. *Nurse Educator, 18*(6), 22–26.

Bowlder, J.E. & Barrell, L.M. (1987). Health needs of homeless persons. *Public Health Nursing, 4,* 135–140.

Braun, K.L. & Conybeare, C.R. (1995). HealthScope: A model for a low cost health education program using commercial television. *Public Health Reports, 110*(4), 483–491.

Brooten, D., Kumar, S., Brown, L.P., Butts, P., Finkler, S.A., Bakewell-Sachs, S., Gibbons, A., & Delivoria-Papadopoulos, M. (1986). A randomized clinical trial of early hospital discharge and home follow-up of very low birth weight infants. *New England Journal of Medicine, 315,* 934–939.

Buhler-Wilkerson, K. (1993). Bringing care to the people: Lillian Wald's legacy to public health nursing. *American Journal of Public Health, 83*(12), 1778–1786.

Clarridge, B.R., Larson, B.J., & Newman, K.M. (1993). Reaching children of the uninsured and underinsured in two rural Wisconsin counties: Findings from a pilot project. *The Journal of Rural Health, 9*(1), 40–49.

Cohen, W. (1992). The role of the federal government in promoting health through the schools. *Journal of School Health, 62*(4), 126–127.

Corcoran, J., Hill, N., Credle, J., Lowe, P.H., Dever, G.E., Lofton, T.C., & Anderson, S.L. (1988). Improving the delivery of services in a local health department: Integration versus block. *Public Health Nursing, 5*(2), 76–80.

Davis, D.J. & Droes, N.S. (1993). Community health nursing in rural and frontier counties. *Nursing Clinics of North America, 28*(1), 159–169.

De Friese, G.H., Crossland, C.L., MacPhail-Wilcox, B., & Sowers, J.G. (1990). Implementing comprehensive school health programs: Prospects for change in American schools. *Journal of School Health, 60*(4), 182–187.

Dreher, M. (1984). District nursing: The cost benefits of a population-based practice. *American Journal of Public Health, 74*(1), 1107–1111.

Dryfoos, J.G. (1994). *Full-service schools: A revolution in health and social services for children, youth, and families.* San Francisco, CA: Jossey-Bass Publishers.

Hawkins, J., Hayes, E., & Corliss, C. (1994). School nursing in America—1902 to 1994: A return to public health nursing. *Public Health Nursing, 11*(6), 416–425.

Igoe, J.B. (1975). The school nurse practitioner. *Nursing Outlook, 23*(6), 381–384.

Igoe, J.B. (1990). School Nursing. *Nursing Clinics of North America, 29*(3), 443–458.

Jamieson, M.K. (1990). Block nursing: Practicing autonomous professional nursing in the community. *Nursing and Allied Health Care, 11*(5), 250–253.

Kirby, D. (1990). Comprehensive school health and the larger community: Issues and a possible scenario. *Journal of School Health, 60*(4), 170–177.

Kristjanson, L.J. & Chalmers, K.I. (1991). Preventive work with families: Issues facing public health nurses. *Journal of Advanced Nursing, 16,* 147–153.

Lie, L. (1992). Health consultation services to family daycare homes in Minneapolis, Minnesota. *Journal of School Health, 62,* 29–31.

Mahon, J., McFarlane, J., & Golden, K. (1991). De Madres a Madres: A community partnership for health. *Public Health Nursing, 8*(1), 15–19.

Miskelly, S. (1995). A parish nursing model: Applying the community health nursing process in a church community. *Journal of Community Health Nursing, 12*(1), 1–14.

Oda, D.S., Fine, J.I., & Heilbron, D.H. (1986). Impact and cost of public health nurses' telephone follow-up of school dental referrals. *American Journal of Public Health, 76,* 1348–1349.

Oda, D.S. & Boyd, P. (1988). The outcome of public health nursing service in a preventive child health program: Phase I, health assessment. *Public Health Nursing, 5,* 209–213.

Olds, D.L., Henderson, C.R., Tatelbaum, R., & Chamberlin, R. (1986). Improving the delivery of prenatal care and outcomes of pregnancy: A randomized trial of nurse home visitation. *Pediatrics, 77,* 16–28.

Olds, D.L. & Kitzman, H. (1990). Can home visitation improve the health of women and children at environmental risk? *Pediatrics, 86,* 108–116.

Reilly, F.E., Grier, M.R., & Blomquist, K. (1992). Living arrangements, visit patterns, and health problems in a nurse-managed clinic for the homeless. *Journal of Community Health Nursing, 9,* 111–121.

Reilly, F.E. (1994). An ecological approach to health risk: A case study of urban elderly homeless people. *Public Health Nursing, 11*(5), 305–314.

Robb, V. (1994). The hotel project: A community approach to persons with AIDS. *Nursing Clinics of North America, 29*(3), 521–531.

Selby, M.L., Riportella-Muller, R., Sorenson, J.R., & Walters, C.R. (1989). Improving EPSDT use: Development and application of a practice-based model for public health nursing research. *Public Health Nursing, 6*(4), 174–181.

Selby, M.L., Riportella-Muller, R., Sorenson, J.R., Quade, D,, Sappenfield, M.M., Potter, H.B., & Farel, A.M. (1990). Public health nursing interventions to improve the use of a health service: Using a pilot study to guide research. *Public Health Nursing, 7*(1), 3–12.

Turner, S.L., Bauer, G., McNair, E., McNutt, B., & Walker, W. (1989). The homeless experience: Clinic building in a community health discovery-learning project. *Public Health Nursing, 6,* 97–101.

Walker, P.H. (1994). A comprehensive community nursing center model: Maximizing practice income—a challenge to educators. *Journal of Professional Nursing, 10*(3), 131–139.

Wang, M.C., Haertel, G.D., & Walberg, H.J. (1995). The effectiveness of collaborative school-linked services. In L.C. Rigsby, M.C. Reynolds, & M.C. Wang (Eds.). *School/community con-*

nections: Exploring issues for research and practice (pp. 283–310). San Francisco, CA: Jossey-Bass Publishers.

Whelan, E. (1995). The Health Corner: A community-based nursing model to maximize access to primary care. *Public Health Reports, 110*(2), 184–188.

Wold, S. (Ed.) (1984). *School nursing: A framework for practice.* North Branch, MN: Sunrise River Press.

Woodfill, M.M. & Beyrer, M.K. (1991). *The role of the nurse in the school setting: A historical perspective.* Kent, OH: American School Health Association.

Zerwekh, J.V. (1993). Commentary: Going to the people—public health nursing today and tomorrow. *American Journal of Public Health, 83*(12), 1676–1678.

Zerwekh, J.V. (1992). Community health nurses: A population at risk. *Public Health Nursing, 9*(1), 1.

Unit 3
Assessing and Building Healthy Communities

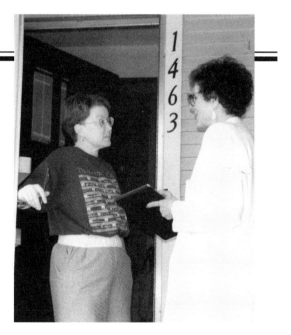

Community health nursing has as its primary focus the health of aggregates. That is, this field of nursing is concerned with the health status of populations and communities of people. In clinical nursing, one learns to assess an individual client's health status and plan nursing interventions. But how does one assess needs and plan health services for an entire community? Before that question can be answered, the nurse must first understand what a community is. What does that concept mean and are there different kinds of communities? What is the nature of a community and what are its characteristics? Let us examine this concept briefly.

The concept of community may be defined and interpreted in various ways. For many people, the term "community" suggests a place. One can speak of the community in which one lives, meaning a certain neighborhood or section of a city. Some think of community as that geographic area surrounding and external to a hospital or other institution. Others think of community in ethnic or sociological terms—the African American community, the Scandinavian community, the feminist community, or the gay community. Yet another use of community refers to people living together or in close proximity to one another, such as a religious community. This variety of definitions can be confusing unless we realize that each is valid, because each serves a specific purpose. A definition has a particular meaning in a particular context. For community health nurses, then, it is important to clarify the meaning of community as it applies to nursing practice.

The concept of community, for community health nursing, includes two important variables. One is people. The other is having something in common. Simply stated, a community is a collection of people who share some important feature(s) of their lives; that is, they have personal and/or environmental characteristics in common. For community health nursing, a community may be a collection of people who have a common location. It may include the residents of a town, the employees of a factory, or the students in a school. A community may be a group of people who share a common interest. Couples interested in parent education, church members concerned about ethical issues in health care, or senior citizens wanting an exercise program are examples. Such groups may share the same location or be widely scattered geographically. Moreover, a community may be a collection of people who share common problems, such as postmastectomy women, diabetics, and the homeless. Again, the group of people involved may or may not live near one another. Community assessment, then, first requires a clear definition of the community to be studied. The nurse needs to define the precise group of people and the boundaries of the community.

How does the nurse assess community health needs? Community assessment means studying the interacting variables that influence a community's health. Every community is a system made up of parts, each influencing the others. A community defined by common location may require study of many features. The political structure determines numerous decisions affecting the people of a community. A conservative faction may keep the community from developing an innovative health program. Schools, churches, and clubs influence the thinking and behavior of people. Geography can influence the local economy. Location on a river may encourage certain types of industry and may provide jobs for many area residents. A town situated in the center of a farming area may bring in migrant farm workers with their special needs and concerns. The health care system of a community is not isolated from these other features of community life. It must be seen as one part of a complex system. Only then will assessment be complete and service to the community be effective.

A community defined by a common interest or a common problem requires assessment of other variables. To assess the needs of teenage alcoholics, for instance, one must study physical, social, and psychological influences on their health, such as peer influence or pressure to succeed. These teenagers must be viewed in the context of the community in which they live. What characteristics of the community have influenced these teenagers? Assessment also includes analyzing the community's resources to determine what is available and what is lacking.

Community health nurses are compelled to understand the community to plan and carry out services effectively. Nurses must know what resources are available and how to put people in touch with these resources. They need to understand the influence of various community characteristics on the families and populations they are serving. This is only one aspect of community health nursing, however. Its broader goals also must be considered. Community health nurses are members of an extensive team of public health professionals; they are also members of the community. Therefore, they have a dual responsibility to know about and be involved in larger community concerns. Their charge is to help build a healthier community.

One needs to keep in mind that community health nursing is future oriented, because it seeks to increase the level of health in communities. This requires an emphasis on distributive justice and preventive services which, in turn, require effective long-range planning. Planning for health services to aggregates, now more than ever, demands a business orientation and the development of business skills. An important business application that encompasses assessment and planning is the concept of marketing. Marketing asks basic questions, such as, "What are we in business to do?" "Who are we aiming to serve?" "What are our revenue sources?" "What resources do we have and need to conduct our programs?" Although not a part of our basic preparation as nurses, skills in marketing and strategic planning must be acquired to meet community health needs judiciously. The chapters in Unit III present essential information concerning how to define and assess a community's health needs, how to plan for and implement primary health care programs, the need to incorporate a broader ethical paradigm of social justice into nursing practice, how to partner with communities, and how to apply marketing concepts to build healthier communities.

Chapter 16

The Next Step: Creating Healthier Communities

LEANNE KAISER CARLSON

> As a central focus and mission of community health nursing, creating healthier communities poses a considerable challenge. Health system structure and incentives, as well as limited resources available for prevention and health promotion programs, all make the task more difficult. Yet there is much that can be done and that is being done to create healthier communities. Leanne Carlson describes some of the problems in health system design and demonstrates ways in which innovative health providers have overcome these and are collaborating to promote healthy communities.

Late one afternoon, high in the San Juan Range of the Rocky Mountains, our small group arrived at the edge of a crevasse. We stared into the yawning gap that separated two rocky shelves midway up the mountain. Each of us had to decide: Am I willing to make the leap to the other side leading to the summit?

A different group of expeditionists—leaders creating healthier communities—are poised at a similar testing point today. The challenge in this case is not a gap of empty space, but a system in dire need of redesign. And like our group on that afternoon in the Rockies, each one must decide whether to put everything at risk and take the next step.

In many communities, the first step in a journey of transformation has been made. Organizations have formed new relationships, redefined problems, and sought systems solutions. Literally hundreds of communities have created coalitions, formed action plans—even bridged competitive histories. A new direction has been set, and a new future made possible.

The journey began with the birth of a new vision. A vision of health as the ability to achieve one's potential, rediscovered connectedness, and community. A vision of well-being, partnership, healthy children, safe streets, and supportive environments. Enfolded in this vision is the potential for complete regeneration of health and healthcare.

For this to become a reality, however, we must take another giant step, and in many ways, it will be more difficult than the first. This next step re-

From *Healthcare Forum Journal* May/June 1995, 14–18. Reprinted by permission of Kaiser and Associates.

quires us to move into the hard work of system redesign. We must tackle the nuts and bolts of real change: 1) redesigning the way healthcare is financed and delivered, 2) providing incentives for healthy individual choices, and 3) measuring and defining outcomes. These and other challenges stand between us and the summit—the creation of healthier communities.

■AN OVERHAUL, NOT JUST A TUNE-UP

Healthcare leaders are working within a structure that was never designed to accomplish the objectives central to healthy communities. Prevention, primary care (other than as a feeder for speciality and hospital services), care for the poor where a disproportionate share of health problems cluster, and community (rather than institutional) objectives are not rewarded by mainstream medicine.

Ultimately, we must face the challenge of total health systems redesign if community health improvement is to become more than an ancillary "outreach" effort.

Most healthy communities initiatives exist on the periphery of the healthcare system, funded either from the profits made by the "real" business of the healthcare system—illness—or dependent upon voluntary initiatives.

In the coming environment of narrow institutional margins, funding activities that do not contribute directly and immediately to institutional survival will become increasingly difficult. As long as community health must be funded from healthcare's primary business, the two will be in competition. It is a testament to the commitment of providers that so many have committed so much in today's environment.

Organizing and staffing community initiatives solely through volunteer effort solves the problem of fiscal competition. In many communities, much has been done solely through volunteer effort. Yet such initiatives will never have the power or stability of the established systems where the vast amount of resources, talent, and attention are deployed.

Capitation offers new possibilities.* Health systems will have the ability to redeploy resources and find freedom from the volume-driven systems of the present. For this reason, some providers—Mid-Columbia Medical Center in The Dalles, Oregon is one example—are accelerating the development of capitation in markets where it would normally take many more years to evolve.

Even capitation may not be a real solution, however. In intensely competitive markets, employers and individuals scrutinize health plans, search-

*Editor's note—Capitation is a reimbursement strategy for care delivery that focuses on number of covered lives and cost per life. It reverses financial incentives in health care. High capitation and universal coverage are most favorable to public health. See Williams, C. (1995). Beyond the Institute of Medicine Report: A Critical Analysis and Public Health Forecast. *Family & Community Health* 18(1);12–23.

ing for the lowest monthly costs. Returns from prevention accrue over the long term, which presents two fundamental problems.

First, if prevention requires an up-front financial investment, the provider or health plan risks losing enrollees because of higher short-term costs.

Second, even if a provider or payer were to take this risk, there is no guarantee the enrollees will still be members of the plan five or ten years into the future.

In some communities, providers have agreed to broad-based collaboration in prevention and community health, so no one loses in the short term and everyone wins in the long term as costs decline community-wide. In Michigan, for example, the four hospitals in Macomb County have come together to create a $1 million cash fund (in addition to in-kind contributions) to launch a community health improvement initiative. Competitors in Portland, Oregon are working together on immunizations, and in Orlando, Florida the two dominant health systems have joined forces in a broad-based healthy communities effort.

This kind of collaboration enables true community initiatives, the benefits of which cannot be confined to any one enrolled population.

▬SIGNS OF TRANSFORMATION

Despite the challenges, there are signs of a healthcare system transforming itself. A large number of providers have recrafted their mission statements to embrace improved community health status as their reason for being. For many this is not just a formality, but a commitment to a new direction supported by action. There are also many more vice presidents for community development, and community health status objectives have become the core elements of strategic planning for some health systems.

A growing number of organizations and health systems have even begun to link senior executive compensation to community health status objectives.

At Winchester Hospital in Winchester, Massachusetts, for example, senior executives receive compensation according to the accomplishment of six planned achievements—three corporate goals and three identified by the individuals themselves. No cost-of-living increases or other compensation are given outside this program.

Last year, one of the three corporate planned achievements related to community health and half of the senior managers also had a personal planned achievement focused on community health.

Similarly, 100 percent of the incentive compensation at Crozer-Keystone Health System in Delaware County, Pennsylvania is tied to performance goals. This fiscal year, three of the eight goals relate directly to community health improvement.

Major HMOs, insurers, and providers are setting health status objectives for populations. Health Partners, a managed care organization in Minnesota representing nearly 600,000 members, set the following four-year goals in 1994:

1. Reduce the number of heart disease events (such as heart attacks) among our members by 25 percent.
2. Increase from 75 to 95 percent the number of children in our system who are fully immunized for childhood diseases by age 2.
3. Improve the early detection of breast cancer among our members, reducing by 50 percent the cases that reach an advanced stage before being detected.
4. Increase the early detection of adult-onset diabetes by screening 90 percent of high-risk members. Reduce by 25 percent the progression from a high-risk state to active diabetes. Reduce by 30 percent the onset and progression of eye, kidney, and nerve damage resulting from diabetes.
5. Reduce by 30 percent the infant and maternal complications among our membership.
6. Reduce new dental cavities by 50 percent for all age groups in our dental membership.

Lastly, and perhaps most importantly, a number of state and local experiments are underway that attempt, in one way or another, to redesign the structure of healthcare. These range all the way from small and relatively unknown communities like Muskegon, Michigan, where a comprehensive health systems redesign is in progress, to the growing number of states actively reforming both the delivery and financing of health services.

■ WHY MAKE HEALTHY CHOICES?
Optimizing health requires a balance of community and individual responsibility. The creation of a healthier community means supportive environments and the opportunity for personal growth and potentiation. That does not describe the many places in America that are ridden with decay and deterioration. A neighborhood on the west side of Chicago is representative of many such communities: Approximately one-third of births are to teen mothers. More than 60 percent of the area's residents live in poverty. Nearly as many never graduate from high school. Infant mortality rates loom at 22 per 1,000. Substance abuse, domestic violence, crime, and gangs are part of the fabric of life.

The messages that environments like these send are grim: "The future is tenuous, live only for today." "No one cares about me, why should I care for myself?" It is hardly surprising that a teenager in circumstances like these becomes pregnant when that infant may be the only means to give and receive love. Likewise, alcohol abuse may seem an inevitable choice for the person who perceives no other way out of hopelessness.

But no matter how earnest our organizational endeavors to create healthier communities, we can't supplant the power of individual responsibility for healthy choices.

According to the Centers for Disease Control (*Morbidity and Mortality Weekly Report* 43, 1994), for example, the roughly 20 billion packs of cigarettes smoked each year lead to an estimated $2.06 each in healthcare costs, $0.89 of which is paid through public sources. Colorado recently calculated (as noted in "Tobacco and Health" in *Hospitals for Healthy Communities* published by the Colorado Hospital Association, 1994) that if the $260 million in public funds spent each year on tobacco-related medical care in that state were instead divided among the state's 176 school districts, each one would receive $1.4 million. Aside from the financial costs, there are the human costs. Roughly 435,000 Americans will die from tobacco use in 1995—more than the number who succumb to AIDS, auto accidents, cocaine, alcohol, heroin, gang violence, drunk driving, fires, suicide, and homicide combined.

Health is shaped not by the single element of tobacco use, though. It emerges from a confluence of factors ranging from diet and exercise to attitude and genetics. Some communities and health plans are beginning to seriously consider the legal and other implications of rewarding people for "good" behavior. What if, for example, the benefits of a recommended lifestyle change such as exercise or weight loss are offset by other risks? Clearly, the reforming of healthcare in America will require much greater individual responsibility, and fostering this responsibility without moving into legal, ethical, or other quagmires will be one of the defining challenges of the healthy communities movement.

Evidence exists that success can be achieved, and, surprisingly, the motivators and leverage points aren't always obvious. Some healthcare/school partnerships, for example, have found that mentoring is effective in reducing teen pregnancy rates. Jobs and recreation for teenagers, rather than traditional styles of law enforcement, have been the primary factors in lowering youth crime rates in some cities. Many other leverage points exist for those willing to search for them and seek to understand the psychology of human motivation.

■ AVOID THE PITFALLS OF MEASUREMENT

To succeed in the long run, the healthier communities strategists must demonstrate tangible outcomes. Measuring the impact of the initiatives now underway, without falling prey to the pitfalls of such measurement, will be a challenge.

Outcomes measurement for population health is still in its early stages. However, from the array of tools and methodologies developed so far, important insights are emerging. These include the need to:

1. *Find measures that truly reflect health.* The challenge is the same whether the system is a person, a community, or a whole ecosystem: Single measurements within systems give us hints about possible problems and progress, but cannot fully reflect the overall health of the system. Furthermore, some elements are easier to measure than others, and those that are most measurable may not necessarily be

those that are most important. A blood pressure reading may register in the normal range, but it provides no hint of cancer developing at the cellular level. Graduation rates may improve or decline, but they do not tell us anything about the quality of education.

The science of outcomes and health status measurement is becoming more sophisticated, enabling us to better understand and measure health. Also, new measures are emerging that are not limited to the old standards, which really evolved around "dishealth"—morbidity, mortality, complications. These newer measures—which include such factors as function enhancement, social and emotional wellness, vitality, lifestyle, and preventive measures—more fully reflect the expanding concept of health.

2. *Develop information systems that encompass the whole community.* Such information systems should support community-wide assessments of health status and integrate the resulting information, as appropriate, into the various community sectors.

In most communities, health information may be found in bits and pieces in an array of places, including hospitals, clinics, public health departments, ambulatory and other health service providers, insurers, state agencies, city and county offices, business and industry groups who commission private surveys, school systems, and numerous other coalitions, councils, and local organizations—in addition to federal bureaus and national institutes. The scope, quality, timeliness, methods of calculation, and reporting procedures vary widely, making it difficult to obtain a clear and consistent picture of health over time for specific populations.

Of course, the way we design our information systems reflects our mindset. If we think public health is different from primary care or the concerns of hospitals and insurers, we develop separate, distinctly different information systems for each. If, however, the intent is to manage health across lines, such distinctions no longer make sense, and the focus moves toward integrating (if not actually physically consolidating) aspects of such information.

Currently, many of the old lines are being redrawn with the consolidation of clinical and financial information across a continuum of care—a necessity fueled by the system integration taking place in healthcare. CHINs (community health information networks) are emerging in places as diverse as Chicago, Milwaukee, San Antonio, and Sierra Vista, Arizona. CHINs begin to move the interconnectedness beyond individual health systems to include other providers, pharmacy, laboratories, managed care, employers, purchasers, public health, government, and even patients. Statewide information linkages and standards are also being developed in places such as Minnesota.

The financial investment is significant, but such information is necessary to truly manage health seamlessly. Although the primary focus today is centered on institutional information needs, the integration now underway must expand beyond individual health systems and sectors if we are to truly manage the health of the community.

Once community health indicators are determined and the necessary information and other support systems created, outcomes management will take a quantum leap. This will contribute toward a new accountability throughout all community systems.

Even with sophisticated systems, however, some of the most important benefits of healthy communities initiatives will never fully be measured. The intangibles that accrue as a result of the participation experience—new relationships and ideas, the building of community capacity, problem-solving across disciplines, adverse events such as crimes and diseases that do not happen, lives redirected, and contributions to the community made possible—may never be fully understood, let alone quantified.

■ ARE WE MAKING A DIFFERENCE?

Even before systems redesign can take place, efforts to enhance community health can and do make a measurable difference. Stories of success are arising from nearly every region of the country on a wide array of health issues. These successes with focused initiatives and programs offer a hint of what could be achieved through comprehensive system redesign. Here is a sampling of early successes:

- In Aiken, South Carolina, infant mortality fell 40 percent, from 12.1 per 1,000 births in 1989 to 7.2 in 1993. The multi-faceted approach created to lower this rate includes case management, widespread education, improved clinic conditions, a pregnancy hotline—even collaboration with community-oriented police (COPS) and the Health Department to identify women in need of prenatal care. The Growing Into Life Taskforce, at the forefront of organizing the community around this issue, has set a goal of 5.01 per 1,000 births for the future.
- In Detroit, Michigan, teen pregnancies at Hutchins Middle School dropped from 14 in 1991 to zero in 1993–94—a decrease attributable primarily to a comprehensive partnership among the Henry Ford Health System, Hutchins Middle School, the Kellogg Foundation, and the community. In 1995, the model will be taken to 12 new schools.
- In Dallas, Texas, Community Oriented Primary Care clinics are transforming the face of health services. Among the many impacts is an increase in immunizations from 30 to 70 percent and earlier detection of health problems among clinic patients, according to R. Blankenau, writing in the October 1994 issue of *Trustee*. When the clinics first opened, for example, providers were finding breast tumors 2.5 times larger among the clinic population than among the insured population. Today, breast tumors identified among COPC patients are no larger than those of the insured women in Dallas.

■ In Stockton, California, burglaries, robberies, assaults with deadly weapons, and homicides in targeted areas declined 24.8 percent in 1994, the third year in a row of crime reduction since implementation of the Safe Stockton Plan. During the same period, crime rates outside the target areas have increased. Community initiatives range from neighborhood betterment committees (made up of residents, business owners, and property owners) reclaiming their neighborhoods to problem-oriented policing teams, neighborhood cleanup and graffiti removal, employment development, recreation in parks and schools, housing, substance-abuse prevention and treatment, and the participation of 61 different nonprofit organizations that provide services in the target areas.**

We need to hear stories and see evidence of success like this. Particularly for those just beginning down the road to a healthier community, such stories send an important message. They are like signposts on the road from those who have been there before, saying: "We have been where you are, and we are accomplishing what we set out to do. You can too."

■FOCUS ON THE LONG TERM

Most of the results of healthy communities initiatives are likely to occur over the long term. This is true because healthy communities efforts change systems rather than ameliorate symptoms. If too much emphasis is placed on short-term outcomes, it may shift the focus from systemic change to short-term, easily reportable gains. In the rush to demonstrate success, we must not become captive to the quick fix or be satisfied with symptomatic improvements while underlying structures remain unchanged.

Until the foundation of healthcare is redesigned, even the most successful initiatives will be fragile. Far too many successes exist today, only to fall victim to economic pressures, political forces, or leadership changes tomorrow. Even the future of such nationally recognized, community-based healthcare systems as that of Parkland Memorial Hospital in Dallas, is not assured. Parkland's Community Oriented Primary Care clinics budget is assessed annually by local officials and is subject to cutbacks or even elimination.

We are not yet at the summit. Early successes provide evidence that the vision of healthier communities is not just a dream. Dramatic achievements in health and quality of life are being made across the country. But ahead lies a chasm of financial incentives, accountability measures, and structures—all of which must be fundamentally reshaped for us to move forward.

**1994 California Healthy Cities Project Special Achievement Award Nomination, Stockton, CA, 1994, and personal communication with Sergeant Ed Wunsch, Special Services Unit, City of Stockton Police Department.

Many of us in healthcare have taken the first step toward achieving a healthier community by supporting the creation of a collective vision. What is not yet clear is which of us will take the next step—the more difficult step of restructuring systems to support that vision. That will determine whether we will see the vision from the perspective of the next century as a reality—or as a possibility that once existed.

Chapter 17

An Epidemiological Approach to Community Assessment

LORNA FINNEGAN   NAOMI E. ERVIN

To achieve the goal of creating a healthy community, community health nurses must first assess that community to determine its health status and needs as a basis for program development. Using epidemiological principles, Lorna Finnegan and Naomi Ervin in this chapter provide a conceptual model to facilitate the community health assessment process. They describe community assessment as consisting of three elements: data collection, data analysis, and community diagnosis. After explaining the process for completing each step within the context of the community assessment model, they illustrate the model's use with a helpful case study.

Community assessment has long been considered an important component in the practice of community health nursing. Moreover, it has recently been reconfirmed as an appropriate aspect of nursing practice at the specialty level. Thus it should constitute a strand throughout undergraduate and graduate education programs in community health nursing (Division of Nursing, 1985).

One of the difficulties in teaching and learning the community assessment process is the small number of models or conceptual frameworks. Although theories about community exist and offer raw material for the nurse–researcher, community health nursing has been slow both in testing and developing relevant theories and conceptual frameworks. Notable exceptions are the work by Goeppinger and colleagues (Goeppinger & Baglioni, 1985; Goeppinger, Lassiter & Wilcox, 1982).

An additional need for community assessment models arises from the ranks of practicing community health nurses. Today the need for this type of assessment skill is even greater because of rapid changes experienced by society in almost all areas of life—economic, social, moral, political, and cultural. A model would provide nurses with an organized approach for capturing data about and making sense of these changes. We developed

From *Public Health Nursing* 6(3):147–151. Reprinted by permission of Blackwell Scientific Publications, Inc.

an approach to allow students and practicing nurses to apply the principles of epidemiology to community assessment. It provides a possible structure for agencies faced with the need to justify funding, or a basis for program planning.

COMMUNITY ASSESSMENT

Community assessment consists of three components: data collection, data analysis, and community diagnosis. The collection of data is the gathering of information, facts and opinions about demographic, health, environmental, and other characteristics of the community. Some of the methods used to collect data are reviews of written materials, interviews of key informants, and surveys. The data are then carefully examined, synthesized, and evaluated. Community diagnosis is currently defined as the identification of health problems in communities or populations (Watson, 1984). An additional key aspect is based on the purpose of preventing problems in a community. Viewed as a concept in prevention of disease, injury, or other problems, the definition of community diagnosis must be expanded to include the identification of trends and potential problems.

DEFINITION OF COMMUNITY

A logical approach to community assessment requires the determination of a definition of community that is related to the framework to be used. For an epidemiological approach, community may be viewed as "people and the relationships that emerge among them as they develop and use in common some agencies and institutions and a physical environment" (Moe, 1977, p. 128). An operationalization of this definition is offered by Shamansky and Pesznecker (1981) who proposed four dimensions of community: who; what; where and when; and why and how. They view the community itself as the "what." The "who" dimension consists of the people factors and includes social, economic, demographic, cultural, and attitudinal features. "Where and when" refer to the time-space framework in which the people factors coexist. Characteristics of the population change with time and with the physical environment. Frequently, geographic or political boundaries are used to define the space framework for a community assessment. The "why and how" dimension includes the functions of the community; it accounts for the "interplay of such forces as communications, power, and authority" (Shamansky & Pesznecker, 1981, p. 183). Functions of the community are seen in Moe's (1977) definition as the development and use of agencies and institutions.

EPIDEMIOLOGICAL PRINCIPLES

MacMahon and Pugh (1970) defined epidemiology as "the study of the distribution and determinants of disease frequency in man" (p. 1). Clemen-Stone, Eigsti, and McGuire (1987) adapted this definition to include the "determinants of health and disease frequencies in populations, for the purpose of promoting wellness and preventing disease" (p. 322).

One goal of epidemiology is to identify populations at risk so that measures can be used through programs and services to prevent or halt the progression of disease (Clemen-Stone et al., 1987). This is consistent with the goal of the community assessment process, which is to establish a community diagnosis that addresses a population at risk. By determining significant host–agent–environment relationships (through data collection and analysis), such populations can be identified and a community diagnosis can be formulated. The community diagnosis is then used as the basis for planning and implementing programs and services.

Identification of host–agent–environment relationships takes into consideration the concept of multiple causation; that is, more than one factor must be present in order for a disease to develop. An example of this is myocardial infarction, which is due to the interplay of several factors such as atherosclerosis, hypertension, obesity, and lack of exercise (Friedman, 1974). This concept of multiple causation is also evident in community assessment. A community diagnosis is not supported by one factor alone but based on the presence of several factors. For example, a high infant mortality rate in a specific community is usually related to a combination of low family income, low education level, smoking, drug use, insufficient prenatal care, teenage births, and a high rate of low-birth-weight infants.

To determine the relationships that exist among the host, agent, and environment, it is necessary to identify measurable variables that can facilitate data collection. The variables commonly used in epidemiological studies are person (who is affected), place (where affected), and time (when affected) (Clemen-Stone et al., 1987). They also may be used by public health nurses to facilitate and organize data collection.

▬COMMUNITY ASSESSMENT FRAMEWORK

Shamansky and Pesznecker's (1981) definition of community is consistent with epidemiological principles and can be compared to the dimensions of the classic epidemiological triangle of host, environment, and agent (Fig. 17-1). An agent can be defined as "an animate or inanimate factor which must be present or lacking for a disease or condition to occur"; host is a "living species (humans or other animals) capable of being infected or affected by an agent"; and the environment is "everything external to a specific agent and host, including humans and animals" (Clemen-Stone et al., 1987 p. 331). Interaction among the host, the environment, and the agent determines health or disease within a community. When these variables are in a state of equilibrium, health is maintained; when equilibrium is disturbed due to a change in any one of these variables, disease occurs. The "who" dimension of Shamansky and Pesznecker's definition encompasses the host factors in the epidemiological triangle, and the "where and when" dimension describes the environment. The relationship between the agent of the epidemiological triangle and the "why and how" dimension deserves further explanation.

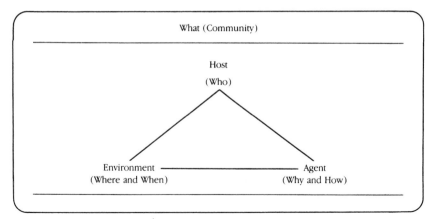

FIGURE 17-1   Community assessment framework.

When the focus of epidemiology was on infectious disease, the infecting organism was separated out of the environment and given a separate status as an agent. Now that this focus has shifted to other diseases and conditions, many epidemiologists consider the agent as an integral part of the environment (Mausner & Kramer, 1985). The "why and how" can be analyzed in this same manner. This "interplay of such forces as communication, power, and authority" (Shamansky & Pesznecker, 1981, p. 183) can be viewed separately (as an agent) or as an integral part of the community environment.

■ USE OF COMMUNITY ASSESSMENT FRAMEWORK

The community assessment framework provides an organizing scheme for the collection of data about any community. Person variables include age, sex, ethnic group or race, income, occupation, education, health status, cultural norms, and values. Place factors are those of the physical, biologic, and social environment, as well as resources and services within or provided to the community. Time takes into consideration time of year, time of day (e.g., for automobile accidents), and trends of an event over time.

Because the categories of data that could be collected are numerous, the nurse or instructor may designate, based on experience and knowledge, those that are most pertinent to a specific community. Without experience to choose more pertinent categories, a nurse may collect data in a wide variety of areas, as time allows. The ability to use a community assessment framework successfully is based on the fact that the nurse or student has knowledge (or is gaining knowledge) about such areas as the concept of community, risk factors, epidemiology, and disease processes. Thus data collection becomes a thoughtful process rather than an exercise in trying to amass information about every possible aspect of a community. The process also contains an element of detective work, with the collectors delving deeper into areas that appear to hold promise for the identification of existing and potential problems. For example, initial data about population distribution show that community A has two times the proportion of elderly than the county. This statistic alerts the data collector to gather more information related to the elderly.

Various methods of data collection may be used within a framework for community assessment. A windshield survey, in which information is noted on a map while one drives through a community, provides a good deal of information, such as the locations of businesses, parks, schools, hospitals, physicians' offices, and other agencies. This method also provides information about the locations, conditions, and types of housing. Characteristics about the community as place can be noted on a map, such as physical barriers to access to health care and the proximity of hazards to neighborhoods.

Interviewing key informants, such as the mayor, school administrator, health center director, and school nurse, provides information about person, place, and time factors. Given their experience, profession, or elected office, such individuals can contribute valuable insight into community issues that may provide a more thorough understanding of problems through different perceptions of them (Dignan & Carr, 1981).

Available statistics can provide much needed person and time data. Vital statistics, census figures, and morbidity data should be collected for specified time periods to allow for the analysis of trends. A single statistic or statistics from one year give a static view of an event, which is inadequate for formulating a community diagnosis.

A community diagnosis that fits within an epidemiological framework contains person, place, and time references. For example, it may be stated as follows:

> *An infant mortality rate in the city of Middletown for 1984 of 14.7 deaths per 1000 live births has decreased 10 percent since 1980, is 20 percent higher than the national rate, and is composed of 9.1 for whites and 16.3 for blacks. Related risk factors are (1) 40 percent of minority women begin prenatal care after the first trimester of pregnancy; (2) 15 percent of all births are to females 10 to 19 years of age; (3) 40.5 percent of the population have incomes below the poverty level.*

This diagnosis gives us an idea of who (infants) and where and when (in Middletown in 1984). The related risk factors address the why and how.

Case Illustration

The following example is presented to illustrate the use of the community assessment framework. Although the data are about an actual community, the name of the community has been changed to retain anonymity. Not all the available data are presented. The community diagnosis that was formulated after data collection and analysis is: risk of pregnancy among females age 15 to 19 years.

ENVIRONMENT: WHERE AND WHEN. Chester is a community of 10,110 people as of 1980, with a racial composition of 76 percent white, 16 percent black, and 8 percent other. The total population has decreased 0.9 percent since 1970. The majority of the population (61 percent) is between 18 and 64 years of age, with 28 percent under 18 and 11 percent over 65 years of age. These statistics are similar to those of New County in which Chester is located, except for the racial composition of New County, which is 67 percent white, 26 percent black, and 7 percent other (Census of population and housing, 1980).

The unemployment rate in Chester increased from 4.3 percent in 1970 to 10.4 percent in 1980. The differences in unemployment rates by population subgroups are large: for example, 8.3 percent for whites, 16.2 percent for blacks, and 15.8 percent for Hispanics in 1980. Forty-two percent of the town's residents are employed in manufacturing and industry, whereas in New County only 26 percent of residents work in those occupations. Among the black population in Chester, 13.8 percent of children under 18 years are living with both parents; in New County 39 percent live with both parents.

HOST: WHO. From 1982 to 1985, 13.2 percent of the 560 live births in Chester were to females age 10 to 19 years. In New County 6.8 percent of the 6587 live births during that time were to the same age group. In both Chester and New County most of these births occurred in females age 15 to 19 years: 100 percent and 98.6 percent, respectively. The estimated pregnancy rate for the same three years was 58.9 per 1000 families age 10 to 19 years in Chester and 21.7 per 1000 for New County. A group for teenage parents that is based at the local high school has a membership of approximately 15 pregnant students per year. In addition, some students become pregnant and choose not to join the group or to terminate the pregnancy.

AGENT: WHY AND HOW. Most of Chester's black population is concentrated in an area on the south side of the community. Of these individuals, 37.2 percent have incomes below the poverty level.

According to a key informant, no formal sex education is provided in the elementary schools. The seventh-grade science class discusses reproduction on the technical level. The elementary school nurse uses a question box in a class given to fifth-grade girls on menstruation. Questions asked reflect concerns about timing of intercourse and pregnancy.

Contraceptives are available through a local health center for females age 13 and older, without parental consent. The health center is in a conspicuous location in the main business district, however, which may prevent teenagers from using its family planning services. The health center director stated that most of the teenagers use the center for pregnancy testing.

Factors Related to the Risk
Flick (1986) reviewed current research on adolescent parenthood and concluded that it may be a result of four decisions. Two of those decisions relate to the risk of pregnancy, and two concern having and raising the

child. These data from Chester can be examined in light of the two factors that relate to the risk of pregnancy in females 15 to 19 years old: (1) increased likelihood of engaging in sexual activity and (2) ineffective or lack of contraceptive use. This examination is aimed at identifying the interaction among the host, environment, and agent to give depth to understanding the community diagnosis and the many factors that contribute to it:

1. Race (black), low socioeconomic status (SES), residence in a segregated poverty area, single-parent households, and lack of sex education are significantly associated with an increased likelihood of engaging in sexual activity (Flick, 1986).
2. Race (black and Hispanic), low SES, single-parent households, lack of contraceptive information, and lack of family planning without parental consent all decrease the likelihood of effective contraceptive use (Flick, 1986).

Viewed as environment, host, and agent, Chester contains these factors. The combination of minority groups with high unemployment and incomes below the poverty level living in a segregated area presents an environmental profile of factors related to the risk of pregnancy for females 15 to 19 years of age. Additional risk factors are related to the agent or functions of the community, such as lack of sex education and underused family planning services. Factors related to the host are likelihood of being sexually active, ineffective or lack of contraceptive use, and probability of being raised in a one-parent home.

This approach to community assessment using epidemiological principles is appropriate for nursing students in undergraduate and graduate programs and for practicing community health nurses. The skill and depth to which the framework is applied will vary with the knowledge and background of the student or nurse. In addition, the framework would be useful to community health nursing supervisors, directors of community health nursing services, and multidisciplinary teams that contribute to or conduct community assessments as a basis for program planning. To develop programs specifically related to the amelioration of problems identified within community diagnosis, further analyses are required. This type of assessment and diagnosis provides a basis for meaningful and effective program planning.

▀REFERENCES

Census of population and housing. (1980). Washington DC: U.S. Government Printing Office.
Clemen-Stone, S., Eigsti, D. G., & McGuire, S. L. (1987). *Comprehensive family and community health nursing* (2nd ed.). New York: McGraw-Hill.
Dignan, A. S., & Carr, P. A. (1981). *Introduction to program planning: A basic text for community health education.* Philadelphia: Lea & Febiger.
Division of Nursing. (1985). *Consensus conference on the essentials of public health nursing practice and education.* Report of the conference, September 1984. (NTIS Publication No. HRP.0906582). Springfield, VA: National Technical Information Service.
Flick, L. H. (1986). Paths to adolescent parenthood: Implications for prevention. *Public Health Reports, 101,* 132–147.

Friedman, G. E. (1974). *Primer of epidemiology.* New York: McGraw-Hill.

Goeppinger, J., & Baglioni, A. J., Jr. (1985). Community competence: A positive approach to needs assessment. *American Journal of Community Psychology, 13*(5), 507–523.

Goeppinger, J., Lassiter, P. G., & Wilcox, B. (1982). Community health is community competence. *Nursing Outlook, 30*(8), 464–467.

MacMahon, B., & Pugh, T. F. (1970). *Epidemiology—Principles and methods.* Boston: Little, Brown.

Mausner, J. S., & Kramer, S. (1985). *Mausner & Bahn epidemiology—An introductory text.* Philadelphia: W.B. Saunders.

Moe, E. O. (1977). Nature of today's community. In A. M. Reinhardt & M. L. Quinn (Eds.), *Current practice in family-centered community nursing* (Vol. 1) (pp. 117–137). St. Louis: C. V. Mosby.

Shamansky, S. L., & Pesznecker, B. (1981). A community is.... *Nursing Outlook, 29*(3), 182–185.

Watson, N. M. (1984). Community as client. In J. A. Sullivan (Ed.), *Directions in community health nursing* (pp. 69–90). Boston: Blackwell.

Chapter 18

Primary Health Care and Primary Care: A Confusion of Philosophies

DONELLE BARNES　　CARMEN ERIBES　　TERESA JUARBE

MARTHA NELSON　　SUSAN PROCTOR　　LINDA SAWYER

MURIEL SHAUL　　AFAF IBRAHIM MELEIS

The distinctions between primary health care and primary care are important for community health nurses to understand to create healthy communities. The authors of this chapter show how the two concepts are often confused and that such confusion limits the achievement of health for all both nationally and internationally. They compare the two concepts and then analyze principles basic to the practice of primary health care as proposed by the World Health Organization. These principles include a focus on essential services, community participation, access to health care, and community empowerment. The practice of these principles is already promoting healthier communities in many countries.

In 1978 the term *primary health care* (PHC) was coined by the World Health Organization (WHO) and the United Nations International Children's Emergency Fund (UNICEF) in the World Health Assembly, which included 24 member countries and organizations.[1] At that time, member countries expressed outrage at the low life-expectancy averages and the high mortality rates among children of a majority of the world's population, whose living conditions were substandard and improverished.[2] It was acknowledged that advances in science had helped eradicate many of the major communicable diseases, but it was noted that the most dramatic decreases in morbidity and mortality rates were achieved by simple, local, inexpensive solutions to health problems, such as rehydration programs. Health indicators pointed toward the need to combine economic and social development with health.

As a result of these discussions and deep concern over health care for a majority of the world's population, the World Health Assembly prompted the formation of a global health strategy called primary health care, and all members of the WHO were invited to act toward attaining health for all by the year 2000. That declaration is commonly known as the Alma-Ata

From *Nursing Outlook* 43(1):7–16, 1995. Reprinted by permission of Mosby-Year Book, Inc.

declaration, referring to the geographic location within the Soviet Union where the conference took place.[1,3]

The adoption of PHC as the means to achieve health for all implied the concurrent acceptance of a new world view of health and a new strategy for the delivery of health care. Health was now viewed as an integral constituent of social and economic relationships, and the responsibility for health was transferred from the physician, as a healer, to a primary health care worker, as a partner.

Internationally nurses have participated in numerous meetings for planning and implementing health care based on the Alma-Ata declaration. Similar collaborative activities have occurred in the United States. However, we believe that the way PHC is currently conceptualized and implemented in the United States is frequently confused with the concept of primary care (PC), as delivered by nurse practitioners, and that PC qualitatively differs from what was proposed at Alma-Ata in 1978. The clarification of the PHC and PC concepts is critical in the light of the current dialogue related to health care reform.

The purpose of this article is to challenge nurses to discuss some fundamental issues related to health care reform. More specifically we describe PHC from an international perspective and compare and contrast the most prevalent conceptualization of PC used by nurses in the United States. We argue that PC as commonly expressed in the United States violates the principles and intent of PHC as proposed internationally. We further argue that the current use of PHC in the United States reflects PC, or institutionally driven and controlled medical care, rather than community-driven comprehensive health care. We demonstrate that the current prevailing definition of PC in the United States may constrain nurses from joining in a vigorous international dialogue about PHC, and may limit the potential sharing of models designed to implement PHC as a strategy. The clash of definitions could further limit the potential of joining the rest of the WHO/UNICEF member countries in realizing health for all by the year 2000. To support these arguments, we compare the definitions and origins of PHC and PC, and present and analyze principles of essentiality, community participation, intersectoral collaboration, access, and empowerment, as proposed at Alma-Ata. Finally, we suggest how PC can fit within the broader philosophy of PHC as a component, rather than as a replacement.

▬PRIMARY HEALTH CARE AND PRIMARY CARE
Definitions
The Alma-Ata declaration sought to emphasize health, or well-being, as a fundamental right and a world-wide social goal, to address inequality in the health status of persons in all countries, and to target government responsibility for policy that would promote economic, social, and health development. These goals could be achieved through PHC, defined as:

> . . . *essential health care based on practical, scientifically sound and socially acceptable methods and technology made universally accessible to individuals and*

families in the community through their full participation and at a cost that the community and country can afford to maintain at every stage of their development in the spirit of self-reliance and self-determination. It forms an integral part both of the country's health system, of which it is the central function and main focus, and of the overall social and economic development of the community. It is the first level of contact of individuals, the family and community with the national health system bringing health care as close as possible to where people live and work, and constitutes the first element of a continuing health care process.[2]

Progress toward PHC implementation worldwide was analyzed in 1988 at Riga, Latvia, U.S.S.R.[3] At that time, five subject areas were identified for critical attention and emphasis: 1) strengthening political and social interventions, 2) strengthening the organization and management of health systems, 3) supporting community-based and home-based health activities; 4) facilitating applications of science and technology to PHC, and 5) developing leadership for "Health for All" (Box 18-1).[3]

The WHO Executive Board studied the future effect of nurses within PHC.[4] They concluded that the role of nurses would move from the hospital to everyday life in the community, that nurses would become resources to people, rather than to physicians, and that nurses would become leaders and managers of PHC teams, including supervising nonprofessional community health workers.

PC, on the other hand, was born in 1965, when Silver and Ford originated the role of the pediatric nurse practitioner as a physician extender on the health care team.[5,6] The nurse practitioner literature chronicles the health care crisis in the United States from 1965 to the present, outlining the shortage of primary physicians, the unequal distribution of health care personnel, the reduced services available to impoverished and rural populations, and the rising cost of all health care.[6]

The American Nurses Association and the National League for Nursing defined PC as advanced practice based on generalist (BSN) preparation,

---

BOX 18-1   Definitions of Primary Health Care and Primary Care

PRIMARY HEALTH CARE	Essential health care based on practical, scientifically sound and socially acceptable methods and technology made universally accessible through their full participation and at a cost that the community and country can afford.[2]
PRIMARY CARE	Delivery of a complex set of services, which include the first contact and the maintenance care. It assumes responsibility for referral to distinct services in response to the client needs and cultural values.[8]

predicated on the construct of PHC, with concepts of direct contact, comprehensive care, case management, prevention, health, and wellness.[5] Nurse practitioners provide direct client (individual or family) care, but also assume indirect roles, including those of educator, administrator, clinical supervisor, consultant, and researcher.[5]

Current issues for nurse practitioners within PC revolve around the autonomy debate for independent professional practice and labor market competition involving reimbursement practices.[6,7] Some authors argue that, in the future, the term *nurse practitioner* would describe only a master's prepared nurse and encompass critical elements of advanced practice.[8] Reifsnider[9] encouraged nurse practitioners in the United States to support Nursing's Agenda for Health Care Reform, since it is the only plan that addresses the role of the nurse practitioners in the provision of health care.

Both PHC, as defined by WHO, and PC, as manifested in the U.S. health care system, evolved in response to the recognition of health disparities among socioeconomic, ethnic, age, and gender groups. The poorer health of the disadvantaged—whether viewed as individuals, aggregates, or nations—is the basic problem addressed by both approaches. They differ fundamentally, however, in the conceptualization of the underlying sources of the problem and, consequently, in the strategies adopted to bring about a solution. They also differ in their definition of health. The PHC model targets social, political, and economic environments as the key determinants of health for populations, as well as for individuals. Thus intervention at the community level or above, to bring about health-promoting environmental changes for individuals and groups, is integral to the PHC approach. In contrast, PC models identify unequal access to health services as the principal cause of health disparities. Efforts are focused on removing some of the health care access barriers affecting individuals and families, but not communities. Essentially, differences in the conceptualization of the problem of health inequities are evidenced as differences in the level at which disparities in health are addressed, and differences in importance assigned to the provision of medical services in improving health.

Practice

PHC refers to an array of essential services, those without which a healthy life is not possible. These services are to be provided to every citizen, regardless of degree of health risk, and at a reasonable cost. PHC does not necessarily go beyond a guarantee of essential services, but does commit to access, equity, and affordability with particular emphasis on vulnerable populations.[10] PHC services are both curative and restorative, as well as preventive and promotive.[11] PHC involves not only access, availability, and service delivery, but community participation, remediation of the causes of health inequities (e.g., poverty, unemployment), and a subscription to the right of all citizens to health care. Universal distribution of essential services with emphasis on vulnerable (high risk) groups is a principle of PHC that differentiates it from PC. PHC embodies not only principles of PC but also principles of public health and is currently practiced in the United States by public health nurses, school nurses, and other health professionals.

The practice of PC can be contrasted with the practice of PHC. PC refers to first-line medical and health care, controlled by the providers, but often community-based and frequently rendered in community clinics, physician's offices, or health department facilities. Access may be a hallmark of PC services; however, PC providers do not guarantee essential services to everyone; nor do they necessarily offer services at affordable costs to those without health insurance. They do frequently provide services beyond what is an "essential" level of care through referral and a systematic use of third-party insurers to cover cost. PC services do not focus as much on prevention and promotion as they do on curing and restoring, including the use of advanced technologies.

While discussing each of the five principles of PHC covered below, we will demonstrate the similarities, differences, or absence of the principle in PC practice in the United States (Table 18-1).

▬ PRINCIPLES
Essentiality
A hallmark of PHC is the concept of essentialness, or essentiality. PHC is considered to be "essential care."[1] A dictionary definition of *essential* is "necessary or indispensable." The Alma-Ata declaration specifies which services are considered essential:

> *Primary health care includes, at least, education (about prevailing health problems), promotion of food supply and proper nutrition, adequate supply of safe water, basic sanitation, maternal and child health care. . . . immunization. . . . prevention and control of locally endemic diseases, appropriate treatment of common diseases and injuries, promotion of mental health and provision of essential drugs.[1]*

Further, *essential* assumes economic and social development as basic to the attainment of health for all.[1]

In the United States, what is considered essential in one setting or one community may not be considered so in another. Essential services, in the spirit of Alma-Ata, are considered to be those that the populace cannot do without for a healthy life. They extend beyond traditional health care services and involve issues of housing, the environment, and economic, political, and social opportunity. Further, essentiality requires that services be based on practical, scientifically sound, and socially acceptable methods and technology.[12]

PC, while usually scientifically sound, may be neither practical nor socially acceptable. Within the context of PC, *essential* refers to clinically delivered physical or mental health services. Several professional organizations have identified a common scope of health care essentiality as comprehensiveness, prevention, diagnosis, a therapeutic focus, health maintenance, and rehabilitation.[13–15] Specific services identified as consti-

TABLE 18-1   Differences and Similarities Between Primary Care and Primary Health Care

	PRIMARY CARE	PRIMARY HEALTH CARE
Essentiality	■ Tends to be driven by private, for-profit sector ■ Primary focus on treatment and restoration ■ Limited preventive care ■ Provides entry to secondary and tertiary care, dependent on eligibility ■ Focus on resource allocation or tertiary/high-tech care	■ Tends to be publically driven ■ Minimum level of care is defined by the community ■ Universally available regardless of payment source ■ Focus of resources on health care services for the majority/preventive health care
Community participation	■ Provider directed ■ *Community* defined as *power brokers* ■ *Professional role: experts, providers, authority, team leader*	■ Client directed ■ As grassroots effort, client participates as partner. ■ Professional role: facilitator, consultant, catalyst, resource
Intersectoral collaboration	■ Occurs among health care professionals, members of health care team ■ Individual/family focus ■ Competition for resources	■ Goes beyond the health care sector ■ Includes collaboration among health, employment, education clients, and other sectors ■ Community/aggregate focus ■ Collaboration on resource appropriation
Access	■ Limited availability to medically oriented health care services ■ Access to health care limited by eligibility for third-party reimbursement	■ Universal availability and eligibility to health care services and resources
Empowerment	■ Focus on individual being able to obtain resources for self-care ■ Paternalistic patterns of interaction ■ Provider-assisted process	■ Collective decision making and action ■ Redistribution of power ■ Collaborative, enabling; a process and outcome

tuting a "package" or a "core" of essential services include "primary health care services" (undefined), "hospital care, emergency treatment, inpatient and outpatient professional services, home care services, prevention services including prenatal, perinatal, infant and well-child care, school-based disease-prevention programs, screening tests, prescription drugs, medical supplies and equipment, laboratory and radiology services, mental health services, substance-abuse treatment and rehabilitation, hospice care, long-term care services of relatively short duration, and restorative services determined to prevent long-term institutionalization."[13,15] A presidential campaign paper on health care reform identified health education as an essential component of health care services.[16] Further, there is some concurrence that certain groups should be targeted for services initially: women and children[13,15]; the elderly[14,15]; and the poor.[13] The recognition of these populations as deserving of special attention is compatible with the PHC principle of emphasis on the most vulnerable.

However, while there is considerable agreement among professional organizations with regard to what constitutes a package of essential health care services, they nonetheless remain within the purview of traditionally delivered health services. There appears to be little consideration given to the larger sociopolitical context within which the health care is delivered and in which health evolves, that is, to the inextricable relationships between health status and levels of poverty, employment, education, quality of life, and general community development. In this sense, the treatises cited must be judiciously considered as to whether or not they meet the spirit of essentiality within PHC.

In sum, the scope of PC and of PHC differs in what is involved in minimum essential care that should be accessible to *all* populations. In PC there is more focus on privatization, on treatment and restoration of physical health and functioning, on providing referral to secondary and tertiary care, and on limited preventive care. The driving force for PC is ascertaining eligibility for services. On the other hand, PHC is driven by public institutions and by providing services that are initiated by the consumer communities. These services are expected to be available universally to all, with eligibility also defined by the community. The primary focus of PHC is on providing health care services for the majority, with a particular emphasis on preventive health care.

Community Participation

The Declaration of Alma-Ata asserted that people, both individually and collectively, had the right and duty to participate in their health care.[1] This assertion is radical for the health professional to consider, since most professionals are socialized as, and expected to be, experts advising individuals and communities on what is best for their health. PC lacks community participation as defined and proposed by proponents of PHC. The difficulty in planning and implementing community participation in PC is manifested in the definition, the components, and the roles of PHC providers.

Rifkin et al.[17] defined community participation as "a social process whereby specific groups with shared needs living in a defined geographic area actively pursue identification of their needs." Community participation implies that there is equity in relationships between health care workers, administrators, and the people, and equity in the provision and accessibility of services and programs.

Meleis[18] identified several components that need to exist for community participation to occur. First, a framework for defining communities should be developed and utilized. Definitions of *community* include geography, common interests, and vulnerability to a health concern. A second necessary component is the level of members' awareness that they belong to a community. Other necessary components include mechanisms to mobilize the community, awareness of community needs, community recognition by the political system, willingness of health professionals to work in partnership with the community, a clear definition of participation, and the development of a "culture of participation."

Participation can be categorized in several ways: as contribution, as organization, and as empowerment.[19] Participation as contribution includes voluntary or other contributions made by people to already existing or planned programs. Participation as organization focuses on the process by which people participate. Finally, participation as empowerment includes the development of skills that enable people to make decisions and take action which they believe is essential for their health.

Rifkin[20] described three approaches to participation: 1) the medical approach, which is aimed at curing disease and is controlled by medical professionals; 2) the health services approach, which mobilizes people to take an active part in the delivery of services; and 3) the community development approach, which requires active involvement of people in decisions to improve health. The first two approaches imply a "top down" approach that is expert driven and typical of PC, and the last is a "bottom up" approach that is community driven and more consistent with PHC.

Even when communities have been defined and identified, the question of Who participates needs to be addressed. Communities are not homogeneous entities, and leaders may only represent a segment of the community. Some groups, particularly women, children, and minorities, may be prevented from participating because of oppression. Rifkin[20] described five levels of participation: People may participate as recipients in the program, actively participate in activities of the program, participate in the implementation of the program, monitor and evaluate the program, or participate in the planning of the program. True participation, according to Arnstein,[21] includes partnership, delegated power, and citizen control.

The role of the professional varies from manipulator to team leader to resource.[22] The role of the professional as a resource for the community is most consistent with the principles of PHC. Professionals may be threatened by community involvement because it requires the sharing of knowledge and skills, the professional's source of power. Some authors assert that there must be de- or re-professionalization for true community participation to occur.[23] Community participation cannot simply be viewed as an intervention to improve health care. It is a dynamic process and is supported by the belief system inherent in PHC. If participation is to be sustained, it requires time, energy, and constant dialogue among all involved. Nurses as community resources are expected to continue to strive toward the development of respect, trust, and common goals with the community. The PC model, with a focus on reimbursement for services, does not provide the conditions necessary for community participation.

Intersectoral Collaboration

Intersectoral collaboration is the cooperative effort of different community and organizational sectors (e.g., health, social welfare, housing, education, sanitation, among others) toward mutually agreed on goals. It can occur at different levels of society, from international efforts to local efforts. In the context of PHC, the goals of intersectoral collaboration center on health and wellness but do not exclude economic, environmental, and social well-being, or political empowerment, since these components are interwoven and interdependent with health.[24] Social and economic development must be integrated with PHC to successfully improve the quality of life in a population.[12] It is precisely this broad context—the integration and interaction of community sectors toward mutually defined economic, social, health, and political goals—that differentiates PHC from PC.

Intersectoral collaboration provides the framework within which individuals in the community can work. It is the means by which international, national, regional, and local policies can be translated into local concerns and by which resources can be allocated and programs developed. The community establishes the goals for collaborative effort. These goals direct the process of interpreting policy into a plan of action that addresses the needs of the people in a manner that is congruent with the cultural beliefs of, and is sustainable by, the community.

The essential elements for successful intersectoral collaboration, as listed in Box 18-2, include national policy that supports PHC through the allocation of resources, decentralized control, local goal-setting, planning and provision of services, mutual accountability, responsibility, coopera-

---

BOX 18-2   *Essential Elements of Intersectoral Collaboration in PHC*

- National policy supports PHC
- Allocation of human and monetary resources
- Decentralized control
- Formal and informal linkages
- Local interpretation of goals
- Local development of plans
- Local accountability and responsibility
- Cooperation and mutual respect

tion, and respect. Goals for health must be made in the context of the social, political, and economic realities of the community,[25] while being supported by national policy and decentralized control. The community's goals must be translated into local plans that are supported by an equitable allocation of human and monetary resources.[26]

The constellation of sectors involved in a particular community will depend on the community's needs, culture, and level or stage of development, among other factors. Sectors include both private and public health care sectors, governmental and nongovernmental entities, social and economic sectors, politicians, and representatives of the consumers of health care services. Formal and informal linkages between sectors must be developed such that mutual goal setting and program planning, development, and evaluation may occur. These linkages must be able to sustain collaborative efforts through the facilitation of communication, work flow, development of new programs, evaluation of program effectiveness, and monitoring of program congruence with outcomes and community needs.[27]

Another component of intersectoral collaboration is the mutual and ongoing accountability and responsibility for the services provided, and for the ongoing support and direction of those services. Community needs may change and essential health care services must be responsive to those changing needs. In the case of a rural community, the priority need may be for basic medical services, transportation, and nutrition services. Other needs may revolve around the economic development of the community to sustain the population. With development may come a different array of problems or needs that the existing health care services are not equipped to address. Thus intersectoral collaboration is a dynamic process that evolves with the growth and development of the particular community.

Finally, there must be a spirit of mutual cooperation and respect. The competitiveness that is familiar to business and industry must become secondary to cooperative participation in achieving goals that support the common good. The notion of social justice must supersede individual gain so that those people in a community that are least advantaged receive equal care and service.

Barriers to intersectoral collaboration include historical, political, technical, cultural, linguistic, environmental, or geographic constraints. These vary with each community and can interfere with the successful implementation of the collaborative process. Furthermore, resource inadequacy or the inequitable distribution of resources can impede collaboration, as can the effects of complex bureaucracy, which impede well-intended plans and programs. It is essential that barriers be identified and minimized by the community. Dean et al.[28] noted that in the United States the National Health Planning and Resources Development Act of 1974 designated local health agencies to plan for the health care of the residents of specific geographic areas. Studies were conducted and plans made, but the barriers to health care persisted. The effects of bureaucracy, inadequate resources, and resource distribution, social inequities, and overreliance on technology are among the many reasons for the failure of this Development Act to improve health care outcomes.

When the social, economic, and health care problems of a society are treated independently of one another, the programs and plans have a lesser chance of success. In the United States, the collaborative efforts of health care professionals providing primary care are largely confined to the health care sector, and thus are intrasectoral, rather than intersectoral. It is only through intersectoral collaboration that the necessary links to support health within the community are formed. Intersectoral collaboration is enhanced when communities participate in identifying problems, needs, resource requirements, and implementation strategies. The process of collaboration is itself empowering to those who participate. Fundamental to this process is the belief that individuals within their own communities can and will direct their own development, whether economic, health related, or educational, and that national and regional policies must support that process.

Access

Access to health care is a core element of Nursing's Agenda for Health Care Reform,[13] a central component of nursing practice, and an arena for nursing action.[29] However, one of the most conflictive issues regarding access to health care is the current meaning, definition, and focus of access to health care. The confusion between the definitions of PHC and PC, as shown in Box 18-1, is partly responsible for the difficulties in defining and directing access.

Defining access to health care from a PHC perspective implies a focus on the communities to be served, and suggests continual community participation and involvement of individuals and families in defining 1) what are essential health care services and resources, 2) what are culturally and sociably accessible health care services, and 3) what are affordable health care services.

A PHC perspective also requires that health care be available where people live and work. Community settings, therefore, are ideally suited to enhance health protection and promotion. From a PHC perspective, accessible, affordable, and essential health care services, as well as resources, must be defined by the communities served according to their own priorities and needs. This implies a commitment to community participation and involvement in the definition.

On the other hand, from a PC perspective, access to health care suggests entry into a complex arrangement of health care services. The emphasis of access is on the individual's need for disease prevention and curative services. The PC perspective also includes access to the delivery of services by nurse practitioners. This implies access to nursing services in which nurses are accountable for complex medical services within a given health care institution. From this perspective, health care priorities and needs are determined by health care providers. Furthermore, issues of accessibility, affordability, and appropriateness of health services are defined by providers from a profit perspective, which is essential to compete in the market-driven U.S. health care economy. As stated by Levine,[30] these entities have "failed to provide either universal access or cost control."

To provide access in the United States within a PHC perspective, a reassessment of access is necessary. Stevens[29] provided a reconceptualization of access congruent with nursing practice and the principles of PHC. Stevens acknowledged that social justice and social equity are essential conditions for health care to be accessible and affordable. Consistent with the philosophy and principles of PHC, the following conditions for access were identified:

1. Cost experiences are to be equal across all groups.
2. The availability of services and resources must be based on the needs and geographical distribution of the population.
3. Health care encounters must be of equal quality and comprehensiveness for all groups.
4. Positively perceived interactions with the system must be experienced by all clients.

This reconceptualization of access is congruent with the principles of access as identified by the Nursing's Agenda for Health Care Reform and by PHC.[13] Essential health care services ought to be affordable and "as close as possible to where people live and work, and constitute the first element of a continuing health care process."[1] The clarification of these concepts and their philosophic approaches will enhance the efforts to improve the issues of access to health care in congruence with nursing and PHC.

Empowerment

The acceptance of the Alma-Ata declaration resulted in the emergence of empowerment as a means to achieve world health. Although first identified as a community approach to guide mental health policy, the philosophic base for empowerment has extended into nursing. Empowerment implied people would be helped to control their own lives. It also conveyed the ideology of persons helping themselves and other people, without the assistance of structured helping systems.[31,32] The definition of empowerment varies and depends on the characteristics of the people, community, and context where it is used. In comparing PHC and PC perspectives on empowerment, consideration needs to be given to the assumptions and values framing the concept and the activities that will provide empowerment.[33]

The application of empowerment in the health care system begins with a fundamental belief in the capability of people to create healthy environments. Through social, political, and economic advocacy, nurses can acknowledge their partnership with people in a movement for better health.[34] *Social advocacy* implies cultural sensitivity, respect, and loyalty to the community. *Political advocacy* includes familiarity with the health care system and understanding the processes that govern resource allocation. It also means a working knowledge of the mechanisms for developing health policies. *Professional advocacy* implies that nurses work as a group through their nursing associations and conferences.

The implementation of empowerment as a process to achieve the goals of PHC depends on the community's ability to overcome the challenges posed by social, political, and economic constraints. These challenges include: 1) a lack of congruency between the health care delivery philosophy and PHC, 2) the need to gain acceptance of PHC principles by the dominant political establishment, 3) availability of resources, and 4) the community's acceptance of PHC principles.

There are barriers to using empowerment as a goal and a strategy which need to be understood in relationship to the basic PHC concepts of accessibility, equity, community participation, and intersectoral cooperation.[35] The first barrier to be overcome in the implementation of empowerment as a process is the values of nursing professionals. Currently, the philosophic underpinnings of nursing come from both medicine and nursing, and some have argued that these are grounded in the values of inequality, competition, and individualism[36]—values contrary to those of PHC. Nurses will need political skills and cultural competency to assist people in identifying their health issues and concerns and the most appropriate strategies to deal with them. Nurses may also need to address their own empowerment as individual professionals before assisting in the empowerment of the client.

A second barrier, and perhaps the most formidable to be overcome in implementing any community strategy, may be the local governing body. The political establishment within the community is a determining factor in the decision to allow for the definition of PHC concepts to prevail.[37] It may be to the advantage of the dominant society or ruling party to keep people in a powerless, dependent position. As a result, a collective consciousness may be threatening to the political establishment.[37] A third barrier to the success of PHC program implementation is the accessibility and equitable distribution of resources.[38] The political system of the community will ultimately facilitate or constrain accessibility and equity of means necessary to achieve productive goal outcomes.

Empowerment, unlike community participation and intersectoral collaboration, is a PHC principle that is discussed in PC models in the United States. The meaning and expression of empowerment in PC, however, is very different from that described in the PHC literature. Empowerment from a PC perspective is grounded in the ideology of individual responsibility. It is viewed as the process through which individuals become aware of and able to make meaningful choices affecting their health. It is assumed that once empowered, individuals will make appropriate choices that are consistent with the values and beliefs of health care professionals. However, empowered individuals may also make choices that are contrary to medical recommendations; thus so-called noncompliance could be viewed as a manifestation of empowerment and reasoned decision making.[39] This is a problem from a PC perspective.

When personal empowerment is the focus, attention is drawn away from the social, economic, and political structures that constrain individual choices. In contrast to the PC emphasis on personal empowerment, PHC emphasizes collective empowerment, which is the process through which communities become activated toward health issues. It is through the empowerment of groups and communities that health-promoting changes in the environment may be accomplished.

Empowerment can be the catalyst to achieving health for all by the year 2000. In working with the community in a spirit of cooperation, in having the community identify their own problems, objectives, and strategies, barriers may be reconciled or overcome.

▄ IMPLICATIONS

PC and PHC share ideals of equity and justice, and acknowledge the prevention and promotion aspects of health and well-being; however, there are differences in the goals and the emphasis, as demonstrated in Table 18-1. Primary care advocates decided that extending the services of physicians with specially trained nurses would significantly reduce inequalities in the system. Primary health care advocates designed an approach to health and health care that would radically change the system itself. The role of the nurse practitioner fits well within PHC; however, PHC also covers the larger issues of government involvement to change policy, the community as the basis of care, and collaboration between health professionals and community groups.

Empirical evidence exists to show that in the past 20 years health changes have occurred in under-developed countries as a result of changes in political, economic, and social structures; and these have occurred independent of changes in the health sector.[37] If health is dependent on social, economic, and political structures within a community, the implementation of essentiality, community participation, intersectoral collaboration, access, and empowerment will also be determined by these structures. Primary health care advocates implementing these principles at the structural, as well as individual, level of intervention.

Nursing practice within a PHC framework takes place in hospitals, clinics, and diverse community settings. Hospital nursing is not abandoned in any way, but its emphasis is reduced in favor of simpler services and health-promotion efforts where people live and work. The location of nursing practice will be altered as more nurses respond to community needs for local services. The style of nursing practice will change as nurses work in professional teams with physicians, social workers, and others, at levels of intervention that increasingly target prevention, education, and social change, as well as treatment of disease.[40] Nursing for the future will deliver cost-effective care to an aging and diverse population, emphasizing management of care with a community orientation.[41] Additionally, nurses will find new ways of working with the public and being a public resource.[42,43]

Implications for nursing education from a PHC perspective include preparing nurses for multiple levels of practice, contingent on the needs of the community. In some regions, nonnurse community health workers have been very successful at basic health education and intervention. Nurses often serve in a supervisory role in this case, and act collaboratively, rather than adversarially, with community and other health workers. At another level, community health/public health nurses need increased clinical preparation in and with communities, rather than in classrooms or hospitals. Some argue that baccalaureate nurses' preparation should include epidemiology, biostatistics, health services administration, and clinical experiences in and with the community.[42] Nurse practitioners' preparation should also include experience with elderly and vulnerable populations, in settings closer to the community than to the hospital.

Nurses at all levels need education in public health policy and the use of both personal and group influence to bring about change.[44,45] For too long nurses have complained about a lack of equity for their patients, while remaining ignorant of ways to change the system. Nurses must be able to analyze the influence of health care policy and the strategies for implementing change at the organizational, community, state, and national levels.[5]

Nursing research should also be directed by principles of PHC. Research questions should be proposed around concepts of PHC, such as participation, access, and empowerment. Research should target vulnerable populations, such as women, children, the chronically ill, immigrants, and minorities. Nurses should be asking questions that address not only individuals as clients, but also larger groups at the local community, city, state, and national levels.[40] Those questions must take into account the social, political, and economic environment of the client, as well as client behavior.

Finally, research questions need to consider different health outcomes. It is no longer useful to study whether or not nurse practitioners can do a pap test as effectively as a physician. Proving clinical competency must give way to showing healthy outcomes in response to nursing interventions. If health is a result of economic, social, and political resources and limitations, then changes in these variables can be considered as outcomes of nursing interventions. Health outcomes cannot be measured by disease indicators alone. Nurses, along with medicine, social work, and other health disciplines, can and should measure indicators of quality of life, well-being, and social equity, to name a few.

▬ CONCLUSION

Primary care and primary health care need not be mutually exclusive concepts. There are, undoubtedly, nurses who deliver PC within a PHC philosophy. They strive for universal access and affordability, espouse empowerment of the client, and target those at risk for health problems, particularly preventable health problems. In addition, PHC subscribes to a philosophy that aims to alter major sociopolitical barriers to achieving and maintaining health, such as poverty, unemployment, and racial, ethnic, gender, and religious discrimination.

A key feature of PHC is that public institutions and governments (i.e., schools, public health departments, city councils, state governments) are involved with and committed to the health of the population. *Further, the system which delivers PHC is integral to the entire health care system of the country.* Consumers must be involved in the planning and delivery of care. These issues are key to the current debate on health care reform. As nurses, we must decide if it is enough to alter current insurance-driven health care services, or if we must engage in reworking the entire system with PHC principles in mind.

Finally, the intent of this article is to initiate a forum for discussion and to promote debate about some of the fundamental differences and similarities between PC and PHC, as we have outlined. We believe that without such discussion and debate, nurses' participation in health care reform may perpetuate the definitions and framework that reflect institutional needs, rather than the needs of the people who are to be served.

Supported, in part, by an institutional research grant (T32) from the National Institute of Nursing #NR 07055.

■REFERENCES

1. World Health Organization. Primary health care: report of the International Conference on Primary Health Care, Alma Ata, USSR, 6–12 September. Geneva: World Health Organization Health for All Ser No 1, 1978.
2. World Health Organization. Global strategy for health for all by the year 2000. Geneva: World Health Organization Health for All Ser No 3, 1981:32.
3. World Health Organization. From Alma-Ata to the year 2000. Geneva: World Health Organization, 1988.
4. World Health Organization. WHO executive board emphasizes key role of nurses in primary health care. Geneva: World Health Organization Press, 1985 Jan 14.
5. Price MJ, Martin AC, Newberry YG, Zimmer PA, Brykezynski KA, Warren B. Developing national guidelines for nurse practitioner education: an overview of the product and the process. J Nurs Educ 1992;31(1):10–15.
6. Koch LW, Pazaki SH, Campbell JD. The first 20 years of nurse practitioner literature: an evolution of joint practice issues. Nurse Pract 1992;17(2):62–71.
7. McGivern DO, Mezey MD, Glynn PM. Evolution of primary care roles. Nurse Pract Forum 1990;1(3):163–8.
8. McGivern DO. The evolution of primary care nursing. In: Mezey MD, McGivern DO, eds. Nurses, nurse practitioners. Boston: Little, Brown, 1986:3–14.
9. Reifsnider E. Restructuring the American health care system: an analysis of nursing's agenda for health care reform. Nurse Pract 1992;17(5):65–75.
10. Sebastian JG. Vulnerable populations in the community. In: Stanhope M, Lancaster J, eds. Community health nursing: promoting the health of aggregates. Philadelphia: WB Saunders, 1992:365–90.
11. World Health Organization and United Nations International Children's Emergency Fund. Primary health care: report of the international conference on primary health care, Alma Ata, USSR. Geneva: World Health Organization, 1978.
12. Collado CB. Primary health care: a continuing challenge. Nurs Health Care 1992, 13:408–13.
13. American Nurses Association. Nursing's agenda for health care reform. Kansas City: American Nurses Association, 1991.
14. American Public Health Association. A national health program for all of us: the American Health Association's guide to the health care reform debate. Washington: American Public Health Association, 1992.
15. California League for Nursing. National League for Nursing's proposed health care plan. Newsletter: California League for Nursing 1990;3(3):4–5.
16. [Anonymous.] Bill Clinton's American health care plan: national health insurance reform to cut costs and cover everybody. Little Rock, Arkansas: The Clinton Campaign, 1992.

17. Rifkin SB, Muller F, Bichmann W. Primary health care: on measuring participation. Soc Sci Med 1988;26:931–40.
18. Meleis AI. Community participation and involvement: theoretical and empirical issues. Health Serv Manage Res 1992;5(1):5–6.
19. World Health Organization. Community involvement in health development: challenging health services. Geneva: World Health Organization Tech Rep Ser No 808, 1991.
20. Rifkin SB. Lessons from community participation in health programs. Health Policy Plan 1986;1:240–9.
21. Arnestein S. A ladder of citizen participation. Am Inst Planners J 1969;35:216–24.
22. Rifkin SB. The role of the public in the planning, management and evaluation of health activities and programs, including self-care. Soc Serv Med 1981;15A:377–86.
23. Woelk GB. Cultural and structural influences in the creation of and participation in community health programs. Soc Sci Med 1992;35:419–24.
24. Flynn BC. Healthy cities: a model of community change. Fam Community Health 1992;15(1):13–23.
25. Butterfield PG. Thinking upstream: nurturing a conceptual understanding of the societal context of health behavior. Adv Nurs Sci 1990;12(2):1–8.
26. Holzemer WL. Linking primary health care and self care through case management. Int Nurs Rev 1992;39:83–9.
27. Ulin PR. Global collaboration in primary health care. Nurs Outlook 1989;37:134–7.
28. Dean D, Jorgensen KT, Loose DS, Duffy ME. Local health planning: a report of a collaborative process between a university and a church. Fam Community Health 1988; 10(4):13–22.
29. Stevens PE. Who gets care? Access to health care as an arena for nursing action. In: Kos-Munson BA, ed. Who gets health care? An arena for nursing action. New York: Springer, 1992:11–26.
30. Levine JS. A political perspective on health care access. In: Kos-Munson BA, ed. Who gets health care? An area for nursing action. New York: Springer, 1992:51–4.
31. Rappaport J. Studies in empowerment: introduction to the issue. Prevention in Human Services 1984;3(2–3):1–7.
32. Rappaport J. Terms of empowerment/exemplars of prevention: toward a theory of community psychology. Am J Community Psychol 1987;15:121–48.
33. Swift C, Levin G. Empowerment: an emerging mental health technology. Journal of Primary Prevention 1987;8(1–2):71–94.
34. McMurray A. Advocacy for community self-empowerment. Int Nurs Rev 1991; 38(1):19–21.
35. Maglacas A. Health for all: nursing's role. Nurs Outlook 1988;36:66–71.
36. McPherson KI. Health care policy, values, and nursing. Adv Nurs Sci 1987;9(3):1–11.
37. Navarro V. A critique of the ideological and political position of the Brandt report and the Alma Ata declaration. Int J Health Serv 1984;14:159–72.
38. Higgenhougen HK. Will primary health care efforts be allowed to succeed? Soc Sci Med 1984;19:217–24.
39. Donovan J, Blake D. Patient non-compliance: deviance or reasoned decision-making? Soc Sci Med 1992;34:507–13.
40. Berland A. Primary health care: what does it mean for nurses? Int Nurs Rev 1992; 39(2):47–8, 52.
41. de Tornyay R. Reconsidering nursing education: the report of the Pew Health Professions Commission. J Nurs Educ 1992;31:296–302.
42. Beddome G, Clarke HF, White NB. Vision for the future of public health nursing: a case for primary health care. Public Health Nurs 1993;10(1):13–18.
43. ACHNE. Essentials of baccalaureate education for community health nursing. Lexington, Kentucky: Association of Community Health Nurse Educators, 1991.
44. Clay T. Education and empowerment: securing nursing's future. Int Nurs Rev 1992;39(1):15–18.
45. Williams A. Community health learning experiences and political activism: a model for baccalaureate curriculum revolution content. J Nurs Educ 1993;32(8):352–5.

Chapter 19

Caring is Not Enough: Ethical Paradigms for Community-Based Care

KATHLEEN CHAFEY

As community health nurses seek to build healthy communities they must examine the ethical basis for their practice. Is it enough to operate on the basis of "caring" about people or is more needed? In this chapter Dr. Kathleen Chafey forcefully argues for a broader ethical paradigm that incorporates a social justice orientation. As in the days of Lillian Wald, she states, we must not only care but we must put social justice to work in community-based practice. She proposes that nurses promote the health of communities by caring enough to ensure that the principles of justice are universally applied and gives examples of how this can be done.

In the waning years of the 20th century, just as in its beginning, there is once again a need for a community-based practice ethic that can address the just allocation of scarce resources, universal access to health care, and benevolent public policy governing the distribution of social goods. At the end of the 19th century, government assumed limited responsibility for, and had little apparent interest in, such matters as health care, public assistance, child labor, and working conditions and wages. It was in this environment that nurse and feminist Lillian Wald began her career as a social reformer. Wald led major social reform movements aimed at improving health care, housing, and labor conditions suffered by immigrants and others who made up the laboring classes of adults and children in a rapidly urbanizing, industrializing America. Wald worked continuously and successfully on progressive causes until after the decline of liberalism in the post-World War I era. Even then, her biographer notes, "She kept her objectives alive and helped train a new generation which came into its own during the New Deal" (Daniels, 1989, p. 1). It is the central thesis of this paper that in the waning years of the 20th century, just as in its beginning, there is once again a need for a community-based practice ethic that can address the just allocation of scarce resources, universal access to health care, and benevolent public policy governing the distribution of social goods.

From *N&HC: Perspectives on Community* 17(1):10–15. Reprinted with permission. Copyright 1995 National League for Nursing.

In the late 20th century, the government has again turned away from a liberal social agenda and aims to trim government spending for social and health programs, seemingly without regard for long-term outcomes. Gains in the public's health, education, working, and aging conditions realized during the years of the New Deal and the Great Society of the 1960s have gradually eroded with the emergence of a growing underclass that includes increasingly larger numbers of women and children, just as in Wald's day.

▄WALD CONVINCED THAT THE PUBLIC WOULD SEE THE NEED FOR JUST AND HUMANE SOCIAL POLICIES

"Caring" was certainly an important part of what motivated Wald's work. She admitted long after the fact that, although she and co-founder Mary Brewster wanted to help people better their lives, they really did not know how to do so when they moved to Henry Street and the settlement house: "[We] were both quite ignorant, but this we did know, . . . we cared for these neighbors" (Wald, cited in Daniels, 1989, p. 34). But if Wald cared for those she came to know as "neighbors," it was also a deep and enduring sense of the principles of justice and equality that brought her to the neighborhood in the beginning. It was a sustained belief that she could, by her own efforts, create and shape public opinion for "progressive, reasonable, and right projects" that kept her moving forward (Wald, cited in Daniels, p. 4). Wald told of her "baptism of fire" that culminated in the founding of the Henry Street Settlement and the Visiting Nurse Service. She was taken by a child to visit his sick mother in the filthy, crowded tenements of lower Manhattan. There, she felt "embarrassed . . . and ashamed of being part of a society that permitted such conditions to exist" (Daniels, 1989, p. 33). She naively thought that, just as she had been ignorant of such appalling conditions, so too was the general public. She was convinced that if informed and inspired, they too would surely see the need for more just and humane social policies.

▄THE MORE THINGS CHANGE, THE MORE THEY STAY THE SAME

In many ways, the hard won battles for social and health care justice waged by Wald and the early reformers in public health have been lost to the marketplace. The current environment for the care of aggregates bears strong resemblance to the Wald era. The composition of the populace is changing, immigration (both legal and illegal) is increasing rapidly, and job security for all but the wealthiest and best educated is increasingly illusory. Until about 50 years ago, health care in America was largely an individual and family responsibility. There were few company pensions or insurance plans, no worker's compensation, and until 1935, no social security. The quest for national health insurance was begun 77 years ago, prompted by the Progressive movement, in which Lillian Wald was a leader. Yet, approximately 40 million Americans were without *any* health insurance whatsoever in 1993. An estimated 13.7 percent or 10 million of these are children. Another estimated 50 million are underinsured, and only 48 percent of those living in poverty in 1993 were eligible for Medicaid (Bureau of the Census, 1995).

Health care programs and policies as we know them were yet to be created when Wald began her work. Public health programs, save those few established by reformers like Wald, focused largely on the control of infectious diseases and sanitation. Recently, health care goods and services accounted for an estimated 15 percent of a five-trillion-dollar economy (Fein, 1992). In fact, the U.S. spends more of its gross domestic product on health care than any of the 23 members of the Organization of Economic Cooperation and Development (Fein, 1992), including Canada with its single-payer, universal access system. Clearly, some progress has been realized since Wald's time. Life expectancy has increased. For the population as a whole, both maternal and infant mortality have decreased. The aged and the poorest of the poor are insured through social programs, if only partially, for the most basic services.

Yet, millions of our citizens continue to do without the minimum assurances of almost every other democratic society (Beauchamp, 1988). The health care "system" is out of control in terms of cost and expenditures per capita, and the U.S. is still among the worst of industrialized nations in terms of health care access. Furthermore, the nation's health indicators are beginning to show the stresses of an uncoordinated and chronically underfunded health infrastructure and a gradual decline in living standards. In the past, surveillance and education were employed to alert the nation to new health threats and to prevention and control measures coordinated by state and local health agencies. However, the AIDS epidemic epitomizes the deterioration in the U.S. health care infrastructure during the last two decades. Without surveillance and control programs, we are again vulnerable to emergent diseases and the recurrence of lingering public health menaces that refuse to go away. As in Wald's era, a shameful number of citizens live in poverty. The best health care is reserved for the rich or well insured (a rapidly shrinking pool of Americans); for the rest, health care is rationed. Significant segments of the population suffer from disease of poverty and chronic conditions that, untreated, lead to premature death and disability. Disproportionately large numbers of women and children are uninsured, poorly nourished, jobless, homeless, and increasingly, victims of domestic and community violence (Institute of Medicine, 1993).

▬ THE U.S. HEALTH CARE SYSTEM HAS FAILED TO MAKE HEALTH CARE PROGRAMS ACCESSIBLE TO ALL

The most urgent health problems that threaten the health of the population reflect the injustice of health care policies during the past two decades that have downsized public health programs. Health problems are both "untreated" and unprevented," as the federal government has gradually left the distribution of health goods and services to marketplace forces. In so doing, the system has failed to make health care programs, including minimum protections, accessible to all, or even to most of those who should be its beneficiaries. The following represent the most pressing aggregate health problems related to inequities in the distribution of and access to health and illness care:

- *Women go without preventive care.* The *overall* rate of infant mortality is worse than that of 22 other countries in the world (Singh & Yu, 1995). The infant mortality rate for people of color—African-Americans, Hispanics, Native Americans—is still twice that of European Americans (Beauchamp, 1988) and the disparity is likely to continue (Singh & Yu, 1995). Only one half of African-American women are estimated to receive adequate prenatal care, and a significant percentage of women, particularly African American and Hispanic, are not receiving Pap smears and mammograms (Institute of Medicine, 1993).

- *Immunization rates have fallen to dangerously low levels.* Immunization levels have fallen to below that of 25 other countries in the Americas (Beauchamp, 1988). In 1985, for example, only 63.6 percent of European-American children and 48.8 percent of all other children between ages 1–4 were immunized for measles (Institute of Medicine, 1993).

- *The uninsured are likely to go without physician care.* Differences in access to expensive discretionary procedures emerge according to patient health insurance status, race, and other sociodemographic factors. The poor are only two thirds as likely to obtain the needed services.

- *Evidence of excess mortality rates by race continues.* Even controlling for behavioral risk factors, the gap between mortality rates of middle-aged African and European Americans persists, and in some cases, such as low birth weight and late stage cancer diagnoses, the gap is widening (Rice & Winn, 1991; Institute of Medicine, 1993, p. 3).

- *Social Security, without supplements, limits access.* Previously one of the most secure cohorts in the population, the elderly now find themselves paying higher out-of-pocket costs and higher insurance premiums, often with less choice. Prescription and drug coverage and provisions for long-term care are simply not available for most, and basic entitlements may soon be reduced.

- *Environmental hazards threaten global health.* Global trade, travel, and changing social and cultural patters make the population vulnerable to diseases endemic to other parts of the world and even to those previously unknown. Degradation of air, water, and soil to support industry and technological advances contributes to pathogen mutations and threatens public health.

▬MORAL PROBLEMS COMMONLY CONSTRUED FROM EITHER A CARING OR A JUSTICE ORIENTATION

The history of health care in this country reflects fundamental differences of opinion as to whether health is a right or a privilege, a public or private good, market driven or government provided, the responsibility of the individual or the community, a concern of social justice or free enterprise. The conflicting paradigms about the direction and control of health care are likely to continue, since most health policy issues cannot be resolved independent of political and social values (Batistella, Begun & Buchanan, 1991).

The debate over appropriate paradigms continues in the nursing literature as well. "Care" or "caring" has recently been promoted as the ethical basis, or sometimes as *the ethic,* for nursing practice wherein the nurse-patient relationship is morally fundamental (Fry, 1989). Following the formulations of writers outside the profession of nursing (Gilligan, 1982, 1987; Noddings, 1984), theorists such as Fry (1989), Leininger (1981), and Watson (1985) have adopted the viewpoint shared by many feminists that moral problems are commonly construed from *either* a caring *or* a justice orientation. The "justice orientation" comes from the liberal tradition of Locke, Kant, and in this century, the American philosopher John Rawls (1971). The justice perspective emphasizes autonomy, impartial reason, and moral judgment based on universal rules and principles and has been the predominant paradigm in the literature on morality (e.g., Kohlberg, 1984) and biomedical ethics (e.g., Beauchamp & Childress, 1989). The nursing literature, however, often describes the "justice perspective" as excessively individualistic, detached, impersonal, abstract, and more likely to be preferred as a mode of thinking by men (Chinn, 1985; Cooper, 1989; Fry, 1989; Watson, 1985). The caring orientation, on the other hand, focuses on relationship, connection, context and responsibility, and sensitive, empathic concern for others. While either gender may view moral problems from this perspective, it is often presented as preferred by women.

Some feminist writers have argued that, by itself, either ethical position is incomplete (Card, 1988). Noddings (1984), on the other hand, has taken a position that an ethic of justice, based on principles and rules, should be supplanted by an ethic of caring. According to this view, "One's responsibility to care for those close to one takes priority over or entirely replaces . . . obligations to a broader range of people, or even humanity at large" (Okin, 1989, p. 247). To the extent that nursing models of caring parallel Nodding's (1984) theory, they are likely to "reject principles and rules as the major guide to ethical behavior, . . . and also reject the notion of universalizability" (p.5). Thus, the ethic of caring is ultimately grounded in the subjective experience of those who care. Its action guidelines are not based on ethical principles but on affective self-searching and "development of an ideal self . . ." (Noddings, 1984, p. 94). However, such an ethic of caring ignores principles that should apply to all. Ethical obligations apparently extend only to those in one's "own circle," those for whom one *chooses* to care. Thus, the ethic is inadequate in and of itself to address important issues of social justice, including those affecting the health of populations.

Unlike Noddings, for whom there is no rapprochement between the "voice" of caring and the "voice" of reason, others such as Gilligan (1987) are more optimistic that the two voices come together in the morally mature individual. Some critics have argued that, in fact, the claims for two distinct ethics are unjustified. Nunner-Winkler (1984) has pointed out that concern and responsibility, even caring, are already accounted for in the justice ethic, though these features have not received enough emphasis in theory development. For example, in defense of Rawls's theory of justice (1971), Okin (1989) states that the theory:

> . . . *is most coherently interpreted as a moral structure founded on the equal concern of persons for each other as for themselves, a theory in which* emphathy with and care for others *[emphasis added], as well as awareness of their differences, are crucial components (p. 248).*

The same accommodation for justice has not been made within the caring paradigm, however, although Cooper (1989), for example, has acknowledged that the ethic of caring "must be understood as a necessary but not sufficient framework for moral activity" (p.14).

Wholesale alignment with the ideal of care and rejection of the justice ethic can invite perpetuation of the stereotype nurses have struggled to change. To suggest that nurses are more inclined to reject principled thinking and impartiality itself hints at gender stereotyping. Suggestions about "inclination" or "preference" for certain modes of thinking can slide all too easily into time-worn discussions about women's innate *capacity* to be moral, or to conceptualize and reason about moral problems. Adoption of caring as *the* ethic for nursing may also invite disenfranchisement from nursing's rightful participation in the arena in which justice issues in health care are being debated.

Problems in today's health care system cry out for models of ethical thinking that reflect a synthesis. It must be recognized that current complex health issues can be best understood within the context of multiple orientations. In situations involving individual nurse-patient actions, there is indisputably a need for caring responses. However, issues of autonomy, conflicting claims, truth telling, the distribution of scarce resources, and access to those resources may be better understood through the lens of justice.

▬IN A JUST DISTRIBUTION OF PRIMARY GOODS, THERE MUST BE A PLACE FOR HEALTH PROMOTION

At the end of the 20th century and beyond, health and social policies must take into account that humans (including the unborn) are organisms, internally related to their surrounding ecosystem (Callicott, 1992), including their physical, social, and psychological environments. An ethical paradigm for community-based nursing practice must promote healthy communities. According to World Health Organization guidelines, such communities have a clean and safe physical environment and a sustainable ecosystem, satisfy basic human needs, provide an optimal level of high-quality and accessible public health and illness care, offer life-long educational opportunities, and enjoy a diversified, vital economy. However, health care today and in the foreseeable future is as dependent on policy makers and insurers, on economic policy, and on political philosophy as it is on service providers, including, of course, nurses. Ethical problems are increasingly related to problems of distribution and access, cost and financing, and the exploitation of resources for private convenience at the expense of the common good. Nursing practice in community-based delivery systems is constrained by policies designed to limit rather than increase access. And, without significant health care reform, access will continue to be controlled by marketplace forces, largely under insurer control and drive by the profit motive. A perspective of justice in health care (following Rawls, 1971) should be based on benevolence and fairness with regard to the allocation of the primary goods of society. In community-based care, a Rawlsian approach might very well be used to advance the agenda of equality of health opportunities for all. After all, in a just distribution of primary goods, there is a special place for health promotion and protection (Daniels, cited in Beauchamp, 1988). The "special place" is based on the assumption that health and safety are essential to the completion of one's plan of life, regardless of what the plan might be. Furthermore, "Ill health constitutes a serious impediment to exploiting the existing range of opportunities for each individual" (Beauchamp, 1988, p. 39). At the end of this century, the central ethical issue in the health of the communities relates to remediation of past and present market and social inequities in the distribution of resources and to uncaring practices that impede access to resources that *are* available.

Unfortunately, a broad cross-section of Americans are curiously intransigent on the issue of equal access to health care, and universal health insurance is widely regarded as utopian (Beauchamp, 1988). However, there is a growing consciousness about health care reform and the shift back to community-based care. Nurses in both education and practice may wish to consider adopting an ethical paradigm that is both socially just and benevolent. By so doing, nurses in community-based practice would be well positioned to move the agenda of promoting healthy communities.

▬PUTTING JUSTICE TO WORK
IN COMMUNITY-BASED PRACTICE

Nurses can work on problems of distribution of health and related services such as housing, protection from violence, nutrition, and public assistance programs. Nurses can be spokespersons and advocates. They can bring to the attention of local-, county-, and state-level policy makers the need for essential services by those either locked out of, or invisible to, the system. Nurses can help both elected officials and the electorate understand and value the public health agenda. Working through community organizations and more directly with local government and voluntary agencies, nurses can help empower communities to address distribution problems. They can identify aggregates in the community (elderly, youth, minority groups) and involve them in planning and problem solving to increase the distribution of resources where the resources are most needed. Nurses can collect and analyze data and advocate or negotiate with policy makers for needed resources on behalf of groups that are unable to negotiate for themselves. There is need, for instance, for nurses to talk with policy makers about the necessity in their community for services to address protective and mental health needs of children, or clinics to serve minority women in neighborhoods where they have support systems, or immunization clinics to target children at highest risk.

Nurses can activate communities to be concerned about problems that affect the community as a whole. They can work for better health care, broadly defined, as Wald did. They can form partnerships with special interest groups and coalitions in the community to ensure clean air, water, soil, and food; improve emergency services; reduce occupational hazards; provide shelter for the homeless; assist the elderly; improve nutritional services; reduce violence; and increase awareness of the effects of racism and xenophobia. In almost every community, there are groups, or coalitions of groups, concerned about these and a myriad of health-related issues; if there are not, nurses can help form coalitions. Nurses can lend these groups the benefits of their knowledge of community assessment and health interventions and their experience working with high-risk groups. In short, nurses can work in partnership with the community to empower and teach communities to be healthy.

Nurses can work not only to improve the just distribution of common resources, but to reduce barriers to access as well. Often, clients are unable to access services because of isolation, lack of transportation, and lack of awareness of what is available. Sadly, many clients have also had experience with uncaring providers who were insensitive to client needs related to religious and cultural beliefs or language or particular health problems. Many members of these groups may believe the health care system has stereotyped and discriminated against them and therefore, existing services *cannot* meet their needs. Nurses can improve access to care within existing programs and program budgets by using and teaching others to use caring interventions. Attention to the special needs of individuals, families, and communities in ways that reduce barriers to access is an important ethical component of community-based practice.

■CARING IS NOT ENOUGH

Nurses must, of course, "care" in community-based practice, but the focus and nature of that care cannot be limited to those one knows personally or those "with whom one has established some 'close' or intimate relationship," as Noddings suggested (Matthew, 1993, p. 56). The "ideal of care" as an ethical paradigm seems most relevant and powerful in nursing's one-to-one interaction: In caring as a moral ideal, there still remains a focus and commitment to the particular experience of specific persons in concrete circumstances within a living context wherein intersubjective sensitivities are evoked and engaged (Watson, 1992, p. 170).

However, the focus of community-based nursing is building and developing the health of *communities*. As such, nurses must care about what happens to groups of citizens, as well as particular clients. A more suitable ethical paradigm for practice in this setting is one that is not solely dependent on particular relationships or "engrossment" in the life and circumstances of particular others. Although proponents of "caring" seem to have drawn a distinction between an ethic of justice and an ethic of care that is bipolar, even antithetical, building the health of communities requires universal application of the principles of justice. It further requires that nurses care enough about their communities and the individuals in them to do battle in the political, social, and economic arenas. It requires a moral ideal perhaps best described by Brabeck (1989) as reflecting:

> . . . *reasoned, deliberate judgments that ensure justice be accorded each individual while maintaining a deep concern for the well-being of all people. This moral ideal is directed toward transcendence of masculine and feminine aims and virtues and calls upon all to care (p. xvii).*

The legacy of Lillian Wald is that caring alone is not enough. Nurses today, as Wald did throughout here career, must reason well, make deliberative judgments, and speak forcefully about the conditions that diminish the quantity and quality of people's lives. In short, nurses must care enough to work for justice in building healthy communities.

■ REFERENCES

Batistella, R.M., Begun, J.W., & Buchanan, R.J. (1991). The political economy of health services: A review of major ideological influences. In T.J. Litman & L.S. Robins (eds.) *Health politics and policy* (2nd ed.). Delmar Publishers, Inc.

Beauchamp, D.E. (1988). *The health of the republic: Epidemics, medicine and moralism as challenges to democracy.* Philadelphia, PA: Temple University Press.

Beauchamp, T. & Childress, J.F. (1989). *Principles of biomedical ethics.* New York, NY: Oxford University Press.

Brabeck, M. (ed.) (1989). *Who cares? Theory, research, and educational implications of the ethic of care.* New York, NY: Praeger.

Callicott, J.B. (1992). La nature est morte, vive la nature! *Hastings Center Report, 22*(5), 17–23.

Card, C. (1988). Women's voices and ethical ideals: Must we mean what we say? *Ethics, 99*(1), 125–135.

Chinn, P. (1985). Debunking myths in nursing theory and research. *Image, 17*(2), 45–49.

Cooper, M.C. (1989). Gilligan's different voice: A perspective for nursing. *Journal of Professional Nursing, 5*(1), 10–16.

Daniels, D.G. (1989). *Always a sister.* New York, NY: The Feminist Press.

Fein, R. (1992). Health care reform. *Scientific American,* November, 46–53.

Fry, S.T. (1989). Toward a theory of nursing ethics. *Advances in Nursing Science, 11*(4), 9–22.

Gilligan, C. (1982). *In a different voice.* Cambridge, MA: Harvard University Press.

Gilligan, C. (1987). Moral orientation and moral development. In E.V. Kittay & D.T. Meyers (eds.) *Women and moral theory.* Totowa, NJ: Rowman & Littlefield.

Institute of Medicine. (1993), *Access to health care in America.* Washington, DC: National Academy Press.

Kohlberg, L. (1984). *Essays on moral development: Vol. II. The psychology of moral development.* New York, NY: Harper & Row.

Leininger, M. (ed.) (1981). *Caring: An essential human need. Proceedings of three national caring conferences.* Thorofare, NJ: Slack.

Matthews, M.W. (1993). *An ethic of care: A methodological critique.* Unpublished doctoral dissertation, University of Minnesota.

Noddings, N. (1984). *Caring: A feminine approach to ethics and moral education.* Berkeley, CA: University of California Press.

Nunner-Winkler, G. (1984). Two moralities? A critical discussion of an ethic of care and re-sponsibility versus an ethic of rights and justice. In W.M. Kurtines & J.L. Gewirtz (eds.), *Morality, moral behavior, and moral development.* New York, NY: John Wiley & Sons.

Okin, S.M. (1989). Reason and feeling in thinking about justice. *Ethics, 99*(2), 229–249.

Rawls, J. (1971). *A theory of justice.* Cambridge, MA: Harvard University Press.

Rice, M.F. & Winn, M. (1991). Black health care and the American health system: A political perspective. In T.J. Litman & L.S. Robins (eds.), *Health politics and policy.* Delmar Publish-ers Inc.

Singh, G.K. & Yu, S.M. (1995). Infant mortality in the United States: Trends, differentials and projections, 1950 through 2010. *American Journal of Public Health, 85*(10), 957–964.

U.S. Bureau of the Census. (1995). *Statistical abstract of the United States.* Washington, DC: U.S. Government Printing Office.

Watson, J. (1985). *Nursing: Human science and human care.* New York, NY: Appleton-Century-Crofts.

Watson, J. (1992). Response to "Caring, virtue theory, and a foundation for nursing ethics." *Inquiry for Nursing Practice. 6*(2), 169–170.

Chapter 20

Building Community Capacity for Health Promotion: A Challenge for Public Health Nurses

REBECCA KANG

Essential to the creation of healthy communities is community-wide participation in the process. Nurses must work in partnership with the communities they serve to promote people's ability to solve community health problems and to develop health protection, illness prevention, and health promotion initiatives. In this chapter, Rebecca Kang discusses the issues involved in accomplishing these goals. She further describes the ways in which public health nurses can partner with communities to achieve the three core public health functions of assessment, policy development, and assurance. Through these partnerships, nurses can enhance the competencies of communities and successfully build community capacity for health promotion.

▬ INTRODUCTION

Public health nurses have a challenging opportunity to work with communities on prevention initiatives in the context of health care reform. The overall endeavor of health care reform is to control health system costs, ensure universal access to health services, regulate insurers, and exercise equity in the distribution of health care resources and costs (Washington State Department of Health, 1994). Inextricable from a cost-efficient health system is the prevention of illness conditions to improve the collective state of health. Concomitant reform in public health focuses on improved population-based and community-based prevention of disease, injury, disability, and premature death. Public health nurses are vital for building the capacity of communities to create a responsive public health system for health promotion and disease prevention. They are essential in facilitating community capacity by encouraging public participation, strengthening community health services, and coordinating public policy (Epp, 1986). Their strength in developing community capacity is their fa-

From *Public Health Nursing* 12(5):312–318, 1995. Reprinted by permission of Blackwell Scientific Publications, Inc.

miliarity with the internal working of communities and the lives of people in them.

▰A TRADITION OF BUILDING COMMUNITY CAPACITY FOR HEALTH

One hundred years ago, Lillian Wald began public health nursing in response to debilitating health and deplorable living conditions of immigrant families living in New York tenements (Buhler-Wilkerson, 1993). Public health nurses brought care to individuals and families where they lived. They taught mothers to care for children, visited the sick in their homes, developed communicable disease programs, and initiated social welfare programs for families. They respected the ability of families to participate in developing strategies to alleviate their own problems. Ms. Wald organized agencies to draw resources into the community and advocated for policies to increase appropriation of funds for expanded public health programs. She believed that public health nurses were vital in orchestrating the link between economic, social, and health needs of families and the services required to promote their health. Public health nursing embraced the ideals of respect for individuals, families, and communities; distributive justice; and beneficence in deeds.

The centennial celebration of Lillian Wald's work is a strong reminder of the tradition and practice of public health nursing. Reinvestment in community care by public health nurses is being summoned today by costly health conditions such as heart disease, cancer, teenage parents, and AIDS. Combining public health and professional nursing practice, public health nursing is concerned with all levels of prevention in individuals, families, populations, and total communities.

Primary prevention of disease and health promotion are central to public health nursing practice. Public health nurses teach mothers about caring for children, including feeding, immunization schedules, and accident prevention. In schools, public health nurses have classes on dental hygiene, nutrition, and sexual health. They conduct stress management and back injury prevention in workplaces. They work with older adults in making changes in the home environment to prevent falls.

In secondary prevention, public health nurses focus on case-finding, early detection, and screening for prompt diagnosis and treatment. Public health nurses monitor the health of pregnant women to detect early signs of toxemia, and conduct hearing, vision, and scoliosis screening of children in day care and schools.

For tertiary prevention, public health nurses provide care to limit disability and rehabilitate those with chronic conditions. Public health nurses are active in providing care to children with disabilities and to those with acquired immunodeficiency syndrome along with their families, loved ones, and friends. At all levels of prevention, public health nurses coordinate resources, advocate for clients, and work toward creating services to fulfill health needs. A practice focused on prevention is grounded in the eyewitness of life-styles and living conditions related to illness and disease.

Intimate knowledge of communities and prevention-oriented nursing practice make public health nurses essential contributors to public health initiatives (Swanson & Albrecht, 1993).

CONTEMPORARY CHALLENGE

Recommendations for revitalization of public health were proposed by the 1988 Institute of Medicine (IOM) report *The Future of Public Health.* The report calls for concerted effort by public health agencies to improve their capacity to assure conditions to protect, promote, and restore the health of people. Three core functions of public health agencies were identified: assessment, policy, and assurance. Regular assessments of communities are needed to describe and monitor current and emerging health problems, risks, and resources. Patterns of health conditions shape policies and appropriation of resources. Services and programs established by policy must be assured and monitored for quality by public health or other, private health agencies.

Achievement of core functions is dependent on the capacity of public health infrastructure in several areas. Agencies need technical competence in establishing data sets, analyzing health problems, and disseminating findings for policy and program development. Public health agencies have a responsibility to cultivate citizen participation, develop closer community ties, and build relationships with other private and public institutions. Organizational, fiscal and personnel responsibilities require qualified managerial staff. Effective community-wide interventions are needed to foster healthy living conditions, to control and reduce environmental hazards, and to implement quality assurance programs. An adequate financial structure is critical to fund services and personnel resources to fulfill public health missions and goals (Institute of Medicine, 1988).

The IOM recommendations lean heavily on physicians and public health officials to lead the way in public health revitalization. Public health nurses, however, receive little recognition as major assets in capacity building. According to the Association of State and Territorial Health Officials Foundation (1985), 20% of state public health agency staff in 1982 were nurses, a 2.4% increase from 1977. This statistic merely hints at the immensity of the proportionate contribution of public health nurses to public health. The number and dispersion of public health nurses throughout the nation positions them well for building capacity in communities for health promotion and health protection.

HEALTH AND COMMUNITY: ESSENTIAL CONCEPTS

Building community capacity for prevention rests on ideas about health. In 1946 The World Health Organization (WHO) defined health as "a state of complete physical, mental and social well-being and not merely the absence of disease or infirmity." Health is holistic in nature with multiple determinants. Health evolves from daily experiences of individuals in social contexts involving the family, community, social-cultural structures, and the physical environment (Green & Raeburn, 1990). Promotion of health, therefore, is best practiced where people live. The practice of health care within the context of living is primary health care. Primary health care requires maximum community and individual self-reliance and participation in planning, organizing, and implementing health care initiatives (World Health Organization, 1978). Facilitating participation has been a hallmark of public health nurses while working with individuals, families, and communities.

Understanding the concept of community as different from population is essential to define the focus for capacity-building effort. Population refers to a collective of individuals with common properties, such as sex, gender, age and health- or illness-related characteristics. Populations may be circumscribed by geopolitical boundaries (e.g., city limits or county or state boundaries) and by time, such as a cohort of individuals born after World War II, colloquially known as the baby boomers. A community exists when individuals share a locale and engage in patterned social interaction, share common identity, participate in interdependent activity, and work toward shared goals and collective action (Hillery, 1955; Poplin, 1979; Schultz, 1987). Thus, a population of Ethiopian refugees may reside in a public health nursing district. The cultural group assumes characteristics of a community when members interact on a regular basis for mutual aid, emotional support, and material resources to achieve common goals of adaptation and survival. The Ethiopian community is a likely focus for encouraging participation in community-based prevention because of its existing social order.

Theoretical perspectives about communities are fundamental for organizing knowledge about community structures and processes that influence health. The ecological approach organizes communities by typography, residential patterns, and the physical dispersion of neighborhoods, institutions, resources, and services (Poplin, 1979). The functional perspective specifies responsibilities of communities that involve: production, distribution, and consumption of goods and services; socialization of members; social control; opportunities for social participation by members; and provision of mutual support (Warren, 1972). The social system approach focuses on the availability and interaction of structures and organizations involving status, roles, social groups, and institutions. Social subsystems have responsibility for important functions concerned with government and economic, education, religious, and family activities (Poplin, 1979). These theoretical perspectives provide a framework to organize relationships between health conditions and ecological, functional, and social facets of communities. Such relationships pinpoint areas for public health intervention.

▬MEDIATING STRUCTURES: PARTNERS FOR BUILDING COMMUNITY CAPACITY

A critical feature of building community capacity is facilitating the participation of communities in prevention initiatives. Participation in planning, organizing, and implementing health programs, however, is foreign to many individuals and communities. Yet, social groups in which people congregate for a variety of reasons offer a starting place to encourage participation for health. Social groups usually found in communities are families, clans, churches or other spiritual units, associations, and neighborhoods. These social entities function as mediating structures by enhancing the interaction of members with each other and with the larger community (Berger & Neuhaus, 1977). Group members form social networks though which they exchange elements of social support: material aid, affirmation, and information. Social support is vital for helping people to cope with sudden life events, such as illness and injury, and long-term challenges and stresses from poverty, discrimination, and other health-damaging social conditions (Israel & Rounds, 1987; Levin & Idler, 1981). Furthermore, the breadth and quantity of resources multiply when social networks overlap. Interconnections unite people into intricate webs to form communities (Berger & Neuhaus, 1977; Poplin, 1979).

Schools, churches, associations, and other mediating structures also stand between members as private persons and large public institutions, such as government and the health care system (Berger & Neuhaus, 1977). These organizations coalesce identities of members and represent them as a collective to the outside world. They are able to secure resources for the group that each member could not get alone. They also may wield considerable social and political power to influence policies to benefit their members. Power can be formidable when many organizations in the community unite through personal networks and common values and beliefs. These organizations have deep roots into communities for tapping the voices of people, in particular those who are traditionally marginal and disenfranchised as single entities. Trusting relationships facilitate efficiency and fidelity in communication, and diffusion of information. Forming partnerships with these community groups is basic for community capacity-building to influence policies and programs for health promotion.

Partnership with communities has been a long tradition of public health nursing and is fundamental to primary health care. Lillian Wald was adamant that public health nurses work in partnership with families and communities to share the responsibility for alleviating health problems and debilitating living conditions (Buhler-Wilkerson, 1993). Partnership is the informed, flexible, and negotiated distribution (and redistribution) of power among participants involved in the process for improved community health (Goeppinger, 1984). A basic condition of partnership is trust, in which there is confidence in the integrity of parties to uphold informal or formal agreements. Underlying elements of partnership are mutual respect for and contribution of capabilities by involved parties, and their willingness to work together to achieve shared goals. Influence over the course of events is negotiated continuously as situations change and demand contribution of different resources from partners (Goeppinger, 1984). There is observable and perceived equality in levels of status, control, and responsibility in the relationship to others (Stewart, 1990). Mutuality in contribution secures investment in alleviating problems and engenders commitment to measures for successful change.

Partnerships are vital for building community capacity. Through contact with multiple social groups and agencies, public health nurses have the perfect opportunity to solicit the concerns of key members of these groups and organize them into coalitions to respond to common concerns in the community. Their devotion to the community can unify them into another mediating structure to work on behalf of the community by creating more responsive and effective strategies for health promotion. Partnerships between these social organizations and public health nurses provide the foundation for achieving core public health functions.

▬BUILDNG COMMUNITY CAPACITY FOR ASSESSMENT

Public health nurses are in a prime position to conduct community health needs assessments. They have knowledge of current and emerging health concerns through contact with people and the communities they serve. These established relationships allow public health nurses to establish alliances with key members of community groups to form advisory committees to plan community needs assessments. Advisory members have insight into community concerns and can evaluate social indicator and epidemiological data in relation to their communities with public health nurses. Public health nurses can collaborate with key community members to organize focus groups, identify primary informants, and develop descriptive methods that are culturally sensitive to individual, family, and community needs, values, language, and cultural differences.

Using a holistic approach to health, public health nurses may stimulate community members to think about the political, social, and cultural context of health to shape needs assessments that include different sectors, such as food distribution practices, housing, or the community's economic base.

Appreciation of the intricacies of community social networks gives public health nurses insight into ways to reach the silent or uninvolved, such as people of color, the elderly, and the homeless. Honest expression of values, beliefs, and intimate concerns is more likely divulged to trusted individuals. Members of the community can interpret findings from assessments to identify strengths and problems that have priority and relevance to community residents by considering the context of community life. Identifying relevant concerns is an initial step to successful public health campaigns (Minkler, 1990).

▬BUILDING COMMUNITY CAPACITY FOR POLICY

Public health policy is crucial in shaping the environment and the options available for living. Creating health promotion initiatives through public policy requires active participation by communities. Toward this endeavor, public health nurses may serve as consultants and advocates for communities. Public health nurses can gather findings from needs assessments and summary reports for critical analysis by the community. They may work with community groups to propose new programs, changes in policies, and allocation of resources to public health officials and other agency administrators. Public health nurses and organized communities can collaborate to stimulate changes in local policies of various sectors, such as education, commerce, food industry, and transportation. Public health nurses can encourage communities to participate in developing research to examine the effect of health policies on a variety of issues, such as access to services, efficacy of programs, adequacy of fiscal allocation, community participation, organizational linkages, and changes in collective behavior and health status of community residents.

Through knowledge of community concerns from research and informal sources, communities and public health nurses can lobby for changes in health policy at public forums, legislative hearings and city council meetings. Public health nurses can be instrumental in building support for health policies by assuring that the needs of communities are visible in policy documents and by disseminating these policies throughout the community for review. By encouraging community involvement in health policy, public health nurses narrow the gap between communities and decision-making bodies for improved accountability in community health.

■ BUILDING COMMUNITY CAPACITY
FOR ASSURANCE

Community contribution to health needs assessments and public policy activities creates ownership in determining public health programs. Participation encourages investment of communities in planning health initiatives to benefit residents. Public health nurses can work with communities to sift through identified health issues and to select those to work on, such as adolescent violence or infant mortality. Community health services that are culturally appropriate may be developed through collaboration between communities and public health nurses. Careful listening and respectful research of values and health beliefs are essential for sculpting user-friendly education, media, and behavior-change programs for cancer screening, sexual health, tuberculosis, and other sensitive topics. Health promotion programs may be disseminated by public health nurses through mediating structures, such as churches, schools, workplaces, adult centers, and other organized social groups.

One-to-one assistance between network members facilitates adoption of new ideas and novel competencies, such as breast self-examination, new dietary practices, and conflict resolution skills. Informed lay helpers are especially effective in disseminating health information to communities of color in which language and culture are barriers to health care. Public health nurses can assist community groups to broaden their goals to include delivery of health promotion services to members. They can identify health services and strengthen linkages of these services to community groups to support disease prevention goals. Public health nurses are effective in coordinating health services for organized delivery to increase access of preventive health services to the community.

Through partnership with communities, public health nurses can assure implementation of primary, secondary, and tertiary prevention programs. For primary prevention, community groups are excellent places for health education about a variety of issues. Work sites, churches, and other organizations congregate people for health promotion programs applicable across the life span, such as home accident prevention, fire prevention, nutrition education, and environmental home safety. Workplace education can target parent programs on immunizations, child development, adolescent health, and parent–teenager communication. Neighborhood women's groups and women's ethnic organizations can be engaged to disseminate education about mammography, Pap screening, and breast self-examination in culturally sensitive and language-appropriate ways. Neighborhood sites also serve as centers for immunizations and blood pressure readings. School-based health promotion programs can emphasize health hygiene, conflict resolution, and interpersonal skills, relationship issues, sexual health, stress management, and drug-use prevention. Organizations that attract older persons are appropriate for providing meals and teaching about fall prevention.

Public health nurses will continue to have active involvement in delivering primary preventive services to at-risk families with young children. Home visit intervention is effective in reaching families in communities with high rates of poor child health outcomes and infant mortality, and in working with disenfranchised families at risk for child abuse. The broad scope of intervention services involves parenting education, child care, behavioral management, and preventive child health care. These families also benefit from coordinated community support services involving counseling, respite services, crisis care, job training, and educational programs. Public health nurses can work with neighborhoods to develop creative solutions to reconnect these families into community life to bond them into a social network for social support.

Practice in the community allows public health nurses to plan secondary prevention involving case finding and early diagnosis and treatment of health conditions. Public health nurses can organize community groups to serve as sites for blood pressure and cholesterol screening. They can make visits to homeless shelters, nursing homes, substance abuse treatment centers, and ethnic associations for tuberculin testing. They can conduct hearing and scoliosis screening in schools, and receive referrals from teaching staff about children with observed developmental delay or conduct disorders that need further assessment and treatment. Public health nurses can hold educational meetings involving HIV-infected persons to support health-promoting lifestyles and increase access to community services.

With health care reform, primary providers and their clients will bear the responsibility to manage disabling and chronic conditions. Public health will provide tertiary prevention activities for health conditions that threaten the health of public, such as tuberculosis, AIDS and other infectious diseases. Public health nurses have been involved in one-to-one follow-up of those with active tuberculosis or untreated infectious conditions to assure treatment compliance. In addition, public health nurses can work with various communities in which there is a prevalence of certain health conditions to support educational campaigns to encourage follow-up tests and completion of treatment regimens by those with positive tests or active infectious diseases. Public health nurses may conduct educational programs on heart disease, diabetes, and other chronic conditions to improve public recognition of these problems and to educate them on self-care management to reduce complications. Increasing access to health services through coordination of agencies is an essential contribution of public health nurses for improved health among those with chronic and disabling conditions, such as children with special needs and the elderly.

▬OUTCOMES OF COMMUNITY CAPACITY BUILDING

Public health nurses have a major role in building community capacity through fostering public participation, strengthening community health services, and coordinating public policy. Their contribution to community capacity building is documented in improved competencies at individual, family, organization, and community levels in response to a variety of health conditions. Kuehnert (1991) describes the outcome of a community-wide AIDS program developed through the collaborative effort of a public health nurse who served as an AIDS coordinator, other public health nurses, and community agencies. The program involved implementing an HIV-education public campaign aimed at health providers, the general public, and those with high-risk behaviors, creating a consortium of local and health service providers to coordinate support services for those with HIV and AIDS, providing in-home nursing visits, and developing a continuum of residential services for HIV/AIDS-affected persons. The AIDS coordinator was instrumental in getting the approval of a municipality to adopt personnel policies to protect government employees from HIV-related discriminations and mandate their attendance at HIV/AIDS-prevention education. In addition, an intergovernmental AIDS Task force secured a formal standing AIDS committee on the community's board of health to monitor the effect of AIDS on the community and to advocate for policies and needed services.

Effective public health nursing involvement in building capacity in a community of color is illustrated by the De Madres a Madres, a program designed by Hispanic women in a Texas community to reduce barriers to prenatal care (Mahon, McFarlane, & Golden, 1991). The program involved community partnerships among business, the general public, and volunteer women. The program's goal was to disseminate information about prenatal care, community resources, low birthweight, and family life through a network of volunteer mothers who had positions in the community that brought them into daily contact with other women. Culturally relevant social support, coupled with community resource information, was viewed as an effective method to reduce barriers to prenatal care for Hispanic women. The public health nurse, employed as the project director, trained the volunteer mothers and mingled in the community to build trust, network, and gain support for the program. After the first year of implementing De Madres a Madres, more than 2,000 at-risk women for late prenatal care had received information from volunteer mothers. Contact with volunteer mothers improved access to prenatal care, social services, and food supplements.

Public health nurses have demonstrated effective community capacity-building effort through work in various organizations and centers. The network of day care centers provides an opportunity for systemic organizational effect on health promotion and disease-prevention activities for very young children. In one situation, public health nurses worked with 38 centers providing full day care to 1,500 children from ages 1 to 5. They collaborated with day care providers and parents to develop a systematic and comprehensive network of public health services involving vision, hearing, and dental screening, health education programs, and early referral of at-risk children and families to appropriate providers and services. The success of the program stimulated the health department to appropriate tax dollars to expand the program from three public health nurses to 13 field-based public health nurses to serve day care centers in the community (Schmelzer, Reeves, & Zahner, 1986).

Home visiting for family-centered care has always been the hallmark of health care provided by public health nurses to the vulnerable, especially the very young and old. Home visiting has been a primary program delivery method for improving pregnancy outcomes, preventing child abuse, improving child health outcome, and limiting disability among children with special needs. Outcomes of public health nursing intervention with high-risk pregnant women include increased use of health services, enhanced social support, and improved self care, including better nutrition and less tobacco smoking, and high rates of full-term infants (Barnard, Magyary, Sumner, Booth, Mitchell, & Spieker, 1988; Olds, Henderson, Tatelbaum, & Chamberlin, 1986). Home visits that extend through the first years of life produce improved maternal psychological health, greater social support, enhanced capacity in appropriate child care, improved parent-infant interaction skills, and positive child development outcome (Barnard et al., 1988; Olds et al., 1986; Olds, Henderson, Chamberlin, & Tatelbaum, 1986). These findings indicate that home visits by public health nurses for at-risk families improve parent competencies necessary for supporting the health of children.

■ SUMMARY

The climate of health care reform heralds tremendous opportunity for revitalization of public health for health promotion through population-based and community-based initiatives. Public health nurses are positioned in the community to enhance the competencies of communities to shape a responsive public health system for health promotion. Through facilitating community participation, enhancing community health services, and coordinating public policy, public health nurses contribute to the overall capacity of communities to respond to a wide variety of health concerns. Some overall effects of enhanced community capacity are increased service utilization, greater health knowledge, and improved self-care practices by individuals and families. Enhanced connections among residents and stable residential patterns may flourish. Residents may report increased social support, resources for coping with personal concerns, and willingness to work on problems together. More resources and services may be available in community groups through service linkages and coordination among social and health agencies. Communities may be more involved in advocating for their residents for policies and programs that promote health.

Public health nurses have been steadfast in their commitment to communities. They travel rural roads and walk urban streets to bring care to people. They are needed more than ever as modern life has made old diseases more virulent and burdened society with costly preventable diseases and chronic health conditions. Guiding principles of respect, distributive justice, and beneficence undergird partnerships between public health nurses and communities. Public health nurses therefore have fiduciary responsibility to be actively involved in public health initiatives. Public health nurses and communities together can create responsive prevention programs to complement the needs, values, and cultural diversity of American people. Public health nurses are vital to improving health for all.

▄ REFERENCES

Association of State and Territorial Health Officials Foundation. (1985). *Staffs of state health agencies.* Washington, D.C.: Association of State and Territorial Health Officials Foundation.

Barnard K.E., Magyary, D., Sumner, G., Booth, C.L., Mitchell, S.K., & Spieker, S. (1988). Prevention of parenting alterations for women with low social support, *Psychiatry, 51* (248–253).

Berger, P.L., & Neuhaus, R.J. (1977). *To empower people: The role of mediating structures in public policy.* Washington, D.C.: American Enterprise Institute for Public Policy Research.

Buhler-Wilkerson, K. (1993). Bringing care to the people: Lillian Wald's legacy to public health nursing. *American Journal of Public Health, 83*(12), 1778–1786.

Committee for the Study of the Future of Public Health. Institute of Medicine. (1988). *The future of public health.* Washington, D.C.: National Academy Press.

Epp, J. (1986). Achieving health for all. *Canadian Journal of Public Health, 77* (November/December), 393–407.

Goeppinger, J. (1984). Community as client: Using the nursing process to promote health. In M. Stanhope & J. Lancaster (Eds.). *Community health nursing: Process and practice for promoting health* (pp. 379–387). St. Louis, Mo.: C.V. Mosby.

Green, L.W., & Raeburn, J. (1990). Contemporary developments in health promotion. In N. Bracht (Eds.). *Health promotion at the community level* (pp. 29– 44). Newbury Park, Calif.: Sage Publications.

Hillery, G.A. (1955). Definitions of community: Areas of agreement. *Rural Sociology, 20,* 111–123.

Israel, B.A., & Rounds., K.A. (1987). Social networks and social support: A synthesis for health educators. *Advances in Health Education and Promotion, 2,* 311–351.

Kuehnert, P.L. (1991). Community health nursing and the AIDS pandemic: Case report of one community's response. *Journal of Community Health Nursing, 8*(3), 137–146.

Levin, L.S., & Idler, E.L. (1981). *The hidden health care system: Mediating structures and medicine.* Cambridge, Mass.: Ballinger Publishing Company.

Mahon, J., McFarlane, J., & Golden, K. (1991). De Madres a Madres: A community partnership for health. *Public Health Nursing, 8*(1), 15–19.

Minkler, M. (1990). Improving health through community organization. In K. Glanz, F.M. Lewis & B.K. Rimer (Eds.). *Health behavior and health education* (pp.257–287). San Francisco: Jossey-Bass.

Olds, D.L., Henderson, C.R., Tatelbaum, R., & Chamberlin, R. (1986). Improving the delivery of prenatal care and outcomes of pregnancy: A randomized trial of nurse home visitation. *Pediatrics, 77*(1), 16–28.

Olds, D.L., Henderson, C.R., Chamberlin, R., & Tatelbaum, R. (1986). Preventing child abuse and neglect: A randomized trial of nurse home visitation. *Pediatrics, 78*(1) 65–78.

Poplin, D.E. (1979). *Communities: A survey of theories and methods of research* (2nd ed.). New York: Macmillan Publishing Co.

Schmelzer, M., Reeves, S.R., & Zahner, S.J. (1986). Health services in day-care centers: A public health nursing design. *Public Health Nursing, 3*(2), 120–125.

Schultz, P.R. (1987). When client means more than one: Extending the foundational concept of person. *Advances in Nursing Science, 10*(1), 71–86.

Stewart, M. (1990). From provider to partner: A conceptual framework for nursing education based on primary health care premises. *Advances in Nursing Science, 12*(2), 9–27.

Swanson, J.M., & Albrecht, M. (1993). *Community health nursing: Promoting the health of aggregates.* Philadelphia: W.B. Saunders Company.

Warren, R.L. (1972). *The community in America.* Chicago: Rand McNally & Company.

Washington State Department of Health. (1994). *Public health improvement plan* (Progress Report). Olympia, Wash.: Washington State Department of Health.

World Health Organization. (1978). *Alma-Ata 1978: Primary Health Care* (Report of the International Conference on Primary Health Care, No. 1). Geneva: World Health Organization.

Chapter 21

Planning for Success: The First Steps in New Program Development

CASSY D. POLLACK

In the process of building healthy communities, nurses collaboratively develop many new initiatives, projects, and programs. A systematic approach to program development ensures greater effectiveness and efficiency and promotes successful program outcomes. In this chapter Cassy Pollack outlines a four-step planning process to be used prior to implementing a program. The process is called the "pre-start up plan" and includes mission statement clarification, stakeholder analysis, problem identification, and a SWOT (strengths, weaknesses, opportunities, and threats) analysis. Applying this to a school health program, she illustrates how the nurse carries out the four-step planning process.

Suzanne Jones had noticed an increased number of students in the middle school who appeared to be overweight. Previous efforts to teach weight control had failed. As the school nurse, she was concerned about the obesity-related risks for the student population. She wasn't sure how to address the problem.

■ INTRODUCTION

Most of us can look around and recognize many problems waiting to be "solved." How can the school nurse transform a problem into a successful program? Even when ideas for new services come easily, it can be unclear how to go about launching a new program. Program development can be an exciting process when supported by careful, deliberate planning. Early identification of issues that will "make" or "break" a new endeavor increases the odds of success. An approach that helps the nurse organize and clarify early planning efforts can result in a reduction of wasted time, energy, and dollars.

Management literature (Bryson, 1988; Garner, Smith & Piland, 1990; Van Slyke & Stevenson, 1985; Vogel & Doleysh, 1988) clearly stresses careful planning as the beginning point in starting any new program or service. The founder of a successful program strives to launch an effort that

From *Journal of School Nursing* 10(3):11–15, 1994. Reprinted with permission of National Association of School Nurses.

is: 1) effective in addressing the identified problem; 2) appropriate for the parent organization; 3) viable; and 4) sustainable. To accomplish these goals, a clear planning process must be in place.

As plans develop, it is common to have changes in definition, scope, and audience. Examples of potential changes include the manner in which the service is delivered, how it is priced or funded, the necessary personnel to manage the project, or the location of the service. For instance, consider the start-up of an obesity prevention program. Many choices exist in how the program could be constructed.

- Students could learn to cook and assist in meal planning for the cafeteria;
- A contest for consistency of the quality of bag lunches could be held;
- A promotion in collaboration with a local supermarket could focus on quality school lunches, with coupons and prizes;
- A series of public service spots on risks of obesity could be delivered by the school nurse on local radio and television;
- A weight loss program focused on only those children identified as overweight could be developed in conjunction with the physical education teachers;
- Programs could focus solely on the children or include their parents and family;
- Programs could take place only at the school, or instead could include other locations, such as a local mall, YMCA—or might even be in a mobile van visiting individual neighborhoods.

Once the list begins, many choices begin to emerge, some less logical than others. Only with initial careful information gathering and subsequent planning can decisions be made as to the more viable or appropriate options. (Budgen, 1987; Singleton & Nail, 1985). Therefore, it can be beneficial to begin with a series of preliminary steps that clarify the project at hand. These have been called "planning to plan" or "pre-start up planning" (Aaker, 1984; Benz, 1984). The pre-start up plan sets the direction of a new endeavor, enabling subsequent planning efforts to occur with fewer roadblocks.

For discussion purposes, the scope or complexity of the project under consideration is irrelevant. This planning framework can be applied to projects of any size, be it a health promotion newsletter or the construction of a school-based clinic. Given the variety of programs nurses start, the terms *service, program venture, project* and *enterprise* are used interchangeably.

▬THE PRE-START UP PLAN

There are four major components in the pre-start up plan. Each component requires a specific set of tasks. As the planning process evolves, additional issues may be uncovered that need to be included in each phase; go ahead and add them to the list. The framework described is intended as a starting point and, if employed, should create a flexible planning environment. The steps or phases in the pre-start up plan are:

1. Mission Clarification
2. Stakeholder Analysis
3. Problem Identification
4. Strengths, Weaknesses, Opportunities, and Threats (SWOT) Analysis

MISSION CLARIFICATION.   To be effective, organizations should have a clear sense of their mission. The mission statement drives the activities of the organization and sets the expectations for all functions within that organization (Andrews, 1990). There should be no activities incongruent with the mission. A problem common to many organizations is attempting to undertake programs that really are a result of multiple missions or a very broad, unclear mission (Bryson, 1988).

A well-written mission statement will clearly state:

- whom the organization serves
- what the organization is going to accomplish
- why the organization provides the service; and
- how the organization will know it has provided the service

The mission drives the goals and objectives of the institution. Goals serve as the language to set overall direction; they are neither concrete nor quantifiable. On the other hand, objectives are measurable, quantifiable targets the organization uses to reach the goals and to assess progress. In this context, any new program or service must match with the institution by furthering its mission. A program that causes the organization to stray from its explicit mission can over-extend the institution and deplete resources, rather than accomplish the goal of expanding and augmenting the current organization.

At Suzanne's school, the mission statement includes language about "creating an environment conducive to the learning process, supporting and protecting the individuality of all members of the school community, fostering the physical and psychological well-being of all students, and increasing their ability to learn." Any program designed to address the issues of obesity needs to support and further the stated mission. It would be congruent to develop a program that reduced the number of overweight children in the school, for that would foster their physical and psychological well-being. To expand beyond the school community, for example, to the entire city population, could over-extend the resources of the school and confuse the purpose of a program, reducing its effectiveness.

It is well worthwhile to take the time to write a mission statement, or to seek clarification of the mission. This effort assures that everyone involved in the planning effort is in agreement and helps to keep the message of the organization clearly stated in everyone's mind. For example, in developing a program to decrease the number of school-aged obese children, one member of the committee might urge creation of a nutrition counseling service for parents as part of the town's adult education program while others think efforts should be limited to the children. As valuable as nutrition counseling for adults may be, the question is, "Does the new service further the work of the organization as defined by the school's mission statement?"

Even in organizations with current well-written statements, time should be given to revisiting the mission prior to general program planning. Questions that assist in identifying mission issues are:

- What purpose do we serve/why do we exist?
- What problems are we attempting to solve?
- What about us is different/unique?
- What can we offer that no one else can/how can we service clients differently than others?
- Do we have the ability to maintain our uniqueness?
- What are our values and beliefs? (Bryson, 1988; Van Slyke & Stevenson, 1985.)

STAKEHOLDER ANALYSIS.   The second phase in pre-start up planning is a stakeholder analysis. Stakeholders are those individuals or groups of individuals who have a vested interest in the organization, or in whose participation the organization has a vested interest (Bryson, 1988; Coddington & Moore, 1987). In effect, they are the people who either can assure the success or the failure of the venture. Anyone who can influence the program, demand results from the program, or hold the program accountable to regulations or standards is a stakeholder. Students, parents, teachers, student teachers, staff, administration, school board members, legislators, grant-makers, townspeople, and licensing agencies are all examples of stakeholders.

Taking the time to identify who the stakeholders are, what they expect from the organization, and how well the organization performs in meeting their needs is an important step in the planning process. This is called a *stakeholder analysis.*

Successful programs balance the needs and expectations of the critical stakeholders. Not all stakeholders have equal importance in each situation. For instance, included on Suzanne Jones' complete list of stakeholders would be the students, the teachers, and the town political leaders. In determining the significance of each stakeholder, Ms. Jones would probably put the students and the teachers above the political leaders for a weight loss program. If she were developing a venture that would be considered politically "hot", such as condom distribution, the political leaders take on a different level of importance; without their support the project could be forbidden.

Problems arise when powerful stakeholders have conflicting expectations of the organization. Prior to beginning a new program, careful consideration should be given to potential differences in the stakeholders' assumptions regarding the project. If the needs of critical stakeholders are not addressed, the program will be up against serious survival issues, if not guaranteed failure. With a school-based obesity program the students would be considered critical stakeholders. If the students felt embarrassed or degraded by the program's efforts, it is unlikely they will participate willingly, eliminating any chance for success.

There are four steps in conducting a stakeholder analysis. First, identify those people or groups who constitute stakeholders. Second, determine the criteria you think the stakeholders would use to assess the performance of the program. Note that these are not the criteria you would use, rather, the ones you believe a stakeholder would identify. There may be many for the more important stakeholders.

Third, evaluate the capability of the venture to meet the stakeholder criteria. It is difficult to meet successfully all of the criteria. For this process to be effective, an honest appraisal is necessary. Here, redefinition of the project may occur. As stakeholder criteria are identified, adaptation in the program may become necessary to ensure support from critical individuals. For example, if a program were one that required licensure, the licensing agency would be a stakeholder. All aspects of the regulations would have to be met, or the project would need to be completely redefined.

Ranking the importance of each of the criteria along with the necessary timing for meeting the criteria is the fourth step. There will be some tasks that must be completed prior to others. The school administration is a stakeholder expecting to grant approval prior to the start of significant school projects. If the criteria for approval are not met, planning for the venture will not be able to continue.

The ranking of stakeholders and their perceptions of success serve as a guide to recognizing people of potential support and those of possible disapproval. This is important information in establishing a successful program and may lead to changes in overall program scope and design.

A method for handling the steps of this analysis is to make a chart (Table 21-1). Down the left side list all the stakeholders. Across the top list the stakeholders' assessment criteria, the rating of the organization's abil-

TABLE 21-1 Example of a Stakeholder Analysis

STAKEHOLDER	STAKEHOLDER ASSESSMENT CRITERIA	MEET CRITERIA	IMPORTANCE	EARLY PLANNING
Students	Provide emergency care Provide health education "Be there for me"	excellent very well inconsistent	very	yes
Teachers	Assist in health education Supportive resource Provide emergency care Provide health screening	inconsistent inconsistent excellent very well	very	yes
Townspeople	Provide emergency care Provide health screening	very well very well	not very	not necessary

ity to meet the criteria, and the ranking of each by its critical nature, noting those who must be incorporated into initial planning. Then, fill in the chart as appropriate for the project. This information is valuable throughout the development of a program, not just in the pre-start up process. It also provides a beginning for later project evaluation.

PROBLEM IDENTIFICATION.   Usually the motivation for a new program or service is the identification of a problem not suitably addressed by the organization's current offerings. A gap between what is available and what is perceived as needed becomes apparent (Kearns, 1992; Stanhope & Lee, 1991). Even though problem definition may seem simple and easily stated, data that support the overall problem definition must be collected (Triebsch & Frank, 1991). As simple as this may sound, most problems can be viewed from different perspectives, altering the approach to a solution.

The following questions will assist in further clarification of the problem:

- What is the problem you are attempting to solve?
- How or why do you know this is a problem?
- Is the problem simply stated, or is it complex and therefore difficult to articulate?
- What is an acceptable/successful outcome if the problem is solved?
- What are the implications of not solving the problem, or what will happen if the problem is not solved?
- Is there a critical time frame in which the problem must be solved or a "price will be paid?" If so, what are the ramifications if the problem is not solved at all, or not in the critical time frame?
- Is the problem readily acknowledged by others encountering the situation? If so, is it defined similarly? If not, how is it perceived?
- How big is the problem? Define "big" by the units of the problem (e.g., dollars, attendance, vacancies in positions, birth weights, deaths, incidence of new cases).
- Is there information that needs to be gathered in order to answer any of these questions? If so, what would it take to gather the data?

By answering these questions, new issues will come forward that assist in clarifying the problem and in shaping the way in which the service is offered. Identifying problems is less difficult than formulating the best solution. There can be many ways of approaching the same problem, some more successful than others. In this lies the challenge.

Suzanne decided to investigate what others in the middle school thought about the numbers of overweight students. She spoke with classroom teachers, physical education teachers, the administration, food service personnel, some of the students, and parents. At the completion of her interviews she was confused. Everyone agreed it was becoming a problem. But the classroom teachers thought the children sat in front of the television as soon as they went home and wanted to eat only what was advertised. The physical education teachers thought the amount of time spent in physical activity during the day was too little. The ad-

ministrators thought parents were responsible for general health of the students. And the food service personnel complained that the children didn't eat any of the "good food"—just threw it away.

Each of Suzanne Jones' findings could become the basis for a different new program at the school. In response to the teachers' comments, a module could be integrated into classroom activities, thereby teaching the students to interpret advertising on television coupled with a nutritional analysis of commonly advertised foods. If the physical education teachers were the only source of information, then methods for increasing physical activity would be considered. If the administrators had the only voice, all efforts would either be aimed at changing parental behaviors or ignored as a school concern. The food service personnel clearly see what is eaten in the cafeteria and may or may not have insight on what may be done. Each of these is potentially a different approach and a different program. Not until the definition of the problem is clarified and the stakeholder analysis completed will the school nurse have the necessary information to shape the program.

SWOT ANALYSIS. A Strengths, Weaknesses, Opportunities, and Threats (SWOT) analysis becomes valuable at this point in the pre-start up planning process (Bryson, 1988; Coddington & Moore, 1987). As with each of the previous steps, insight gained in this part of the plan might cause a revision of the overall venture.

Strengths and weaknesses generally have an internal focus. The strengths of an organization are those elements that contribute to its success (Bryant, Dobal & Johnson, 1990; Kearns, 1992). Examples might include exemplary teaching capabilities, a strong and supportive administration, a community commitment to the school, or a strong financial position. New programs should be positioned to take advantage of the organization's strengths.

The Weaknesses of an institution are those attributes that may impede success. Weaknesses are considered in program planning, for they could offer barriers to the well-being of the new enterprise. Examples could be a deteriorating physical plant, large budgetary cuts that could jeopardize a program, or an ineffective management team. Weaknesses can be handled in two ways: work to solve them or work to minimized them. It appears obvious that one would not emphasize a weakness, but it *is* frequently done. An overworked principal who has very little extra time could be a weakness. To put him in charge of a new program would probably mean that something important would not be done—possibly, the program. Or to have a very poor public speaker become the community spokesperson for a new project might create more harm than good.

Strengths and Weaknesses often are linked together. For example, a strength might be the presence of a strong dynamic leader. A weakness might be singular dependence upon that one person to make things happen. In considering strengths and weaknesses, be sure to give thought to the "other side" of the identified attribute.

Opportunities and Threats tend to be more external to an organization. They are the *p*olitical, *e*conomic, *s*ocial, and *t*echnological occurrences (sometimes called P.E.S.T.s) that influence the operation of an organization (Kearns, 1992; Triebsch & Frank, 1991). Recognizing environmental opportunities and threats allows the positioning of new programs to take advantage of potential opportunities while preparing for future threats.

Creative thinking often can turn threats into opportunities. With health care reform posing as a threat to many of the current practices in health care, opportunities may well exist for the school nurse. School-based clinics may well expand: immunization programs and pediatric primary care may have an increased place within the school setting; programs addressing primary prevention may have an increased role in formal classroom curriculum. In addition, there will be a need to establish comprehensive data bases, coordinating the acute care setting with community-based care. One starting point might be with information tracking school-age children.

Suzanne finally decided that the only way to initiate a successful weight loss program was to involve representatives from all of the stakeholder groups in the planning process. The physical education teachers were very excited about starting something new. The regular classroom teachers readily agreed that a program could and should be launched, but they felt their workload was already too heavy. The food service people said they were willing to plan new menus, but the food purchasing agreements and the budget could not be changed. They asked for help in knowing what to do. The assistant principal thought she had heard of the possibility of obtaining some governmental funding for supporting the increased physical fitness of school-aged children. A new town administration had just been elected and they were supporting child-focused programs. Suzanne realized that her new program would need to balance the needs and interests of all of the stakeholders to have a chance of success.

SUMMARY

Designing, implementing, and managing a new program is a time-consuming endeavor. Successful projects must fit within the parent organization and assist in carrying out its goals and objectives. Taking the time to clarify the mission, analyze the expectations of the stakeholders, and conduct a SWOT analysis will increase the viability of the new program. These processes become valuable planning tools as they assist in the clarification of the problem and determination of the program options. All necessary modifications can occur prior to the development of the final plan. These steps also signal the administration that care is being given to the planning process and so the outcome is worthy of attention.

REFERENCES

Aaker, D.A. (1984). The process of developing business strategies. In *Developing business strategies* (pp. 23–39). New York: John Wiley & Sons.

Andrews, M.M. (1990). Strategic planning: Preparing for the twenty-first century. *Journal of Professional Nursing, 6*(2). 103–112.

Benz, P.D. (1984). Strategic planning. In M. Penberth-Valentine (Eds.), *Health planning for nurse managers* (pp. 71–112). Rockville, MD: Aspen Publishers.

Bryant, L., Dobal, M., & Johnson, E. (1990). Strategic planning: Collaboration and empowerment. *Nursing Connections, 3*(3), 31–36.

Bryson, J.M. (1988). An effective strategic planning approach for public and nonprofit organizations. In *Strategic planning for public and nonprofit organizations* (pp. 46–70). San Francisco: Jossey-Bass Publishers.

Budgen, C.M. (1987). Modeling: A method for program development. *Journal of Nursing Administration, 17*(12), 19–25.

Coddington, D., & Moore, K. (1987). Strategic planning. In *Market-driven strategies in health care* (pp. 232–247). San Francisco: Jossey-Bass Publishers.

Garner, J.F., Smith, H.L., & Piland, N.F. (1990). Planning for strategic visions. In *Strategic nursing management* (pp 63–94). Rockville, Md.: Aspen Publishers.

Kearns, K.P. (1992). From comparative advantage to damage control: Clarifying strategic issues using SWOT analysis. *Nonprofit management & leadership, 3*(1), 3–22.

Singleton, E.K., & Nail, F.C. (1985). Guidelines for establishing a new service. *Journal of Nursing Administration, 15*(10), 22–26.

Stanhope, M., & Lee, G. (1991). Program management. In M. Stanhope & J. Lancaster (Eds.), *Community health nursing: Process and practice for promoting health* (pp. 201–214). St. Louis: Mosby - Year Book, Inc.

Triebsch, H.C., & Frank, R.A. (1991). Program planning and costing: A blueprint for success. *Caring Magazine, 10*(1), 10–12, 14–17, 61–63.

Van Slyke, J., & Stevenson, H. (1985). Prestart analysis: A framework for thinking about business ventures. (Case study). Cambridge, Mass.: Harvard Business School.

Vogel, G., & Doleysh, N. (1988). Entrepreneurship: A nurse's guide to starting a business. (NLN Report #41-2201). New York: National League for Nursing.

Chapter 22

Applying Marketing Concepts to Promote Health in Vulnerable Groups

SUSAN A. FONTANA

In order to build healthier communities, nurses need to determine what the community needs and wants and incorporate this information into health interventions. This is known as marketing—a useful strategy for community health nursing. Marketing is an exchange relationship, Dr. Susan Fontana states. She goes on in this chapter to explain exchange relationships and a second marketing concept, channels of distribution, and shows their application to nursing practice. When marketing concepts are incorporated into the planning and delivery of community health nursing services, they hold the potential for greatly increasing the relevance and impact of those services on the community's health.

Marketing strategies have increasingly been applied to health promotion activities since the mid-1980s when competitive health care financing and delivery systems emerged. During this time, investor-owned health systems gained over 15% of the market, which is expected to double in the next five years (Editors, 1986). However, the acceptance and adoption of marketing strategies by public health nurses and other health professionals has been very limited, and is perhaps due to the scarcity of resources available to guide these professionals as well as the distinctive problems of marketing professional services.

Since health promotion and primary prevention are major activities in their practice, public health nurses must think strategically and analytically about marketing their services in a marketplace confronted by a concern with cost and a multitude of trends. Some of these trends are 1) a revised legal and ethical climate that has lifted restrictions against the use of advertising, soliciting, and competitive bidding for professional services; 2) increased consumer dissatisfaction with the quality of the health care product; 3) growth in the medical profession, and 4) rapidly changing technologies that make some services obsolete while creating opportunities for other services (Andrews, 1986; Kotler & Bloom, 1984).

From *Public Health Nursing* 8(2):140–143, 1991. Reprinted by permission of Blackwell Scientific Publications, Inc.

Given these trends, together with the widespread application of marketing by health care organizations with regard to health promotion and prevention services, a marketing orientation that is meaningful for public health nurses is necessary. A sound marketing orientation can assist public health nurses better to understand and satisfy the health needs of their clients.

Broadly defined, marketing is a way for any type of organization to learn about its customer/client wants and to use this information internally to satisfy these consumers. To date, some controversy still exists over the use of marketing concepts and techniques in nonprofit and public sector organizations. This stems from the belief that such concepts and techniques should be confined to the "sale" of goods and services. It is important to understand, however, that the goal of government and social service agencies to satisfy customer/client groups is exactly the same one pursued by private sector organizations. The social and economic justification of both types of organizations depends on their abilities to satisfy consumer wants (Crompton & Lamb, 1986). This view demonstrates the relevance of marketing for use by public health nurses whether they practice in public, private, or for-profit organizations.

Marketing as a field developed over several economic and social eras beginning in the early decades of the twentieth century. By the 1950s, the orientation changed, as some business organizations began to realize that their success was dependent on customers' perceived value of their goods and services and not on aggressive selling or production efforts. This is useful to keep in mind as one considers the several types of marketing strategies that exist today in the health care marketplace (Table 22-1).

The four types of marketing orientations are production, products, sales, and societal. Organizations that focus on products, production, or sales are likely to become preoccupied with programs, services, or internal needs. Moreover, the services or programs they provide are dominated by

TABLE 22-1 Comparison of Marketing Orientations

ORIENTATION	MAJOR TASK(S)
Production	Pursue efficiency in production and distribution of goods/services. Example: Immunize as many persons as possible.
Product	Offer as many goods/services as are thought to be good for the clients. Example: A variety of prenatal classes for first-time mothers.
Sales	Stimulate interest of potential clients in existing goods/services. Example: Hire a public relations firm to recruit more clients to attend a smoking cessation program.
Societal	Systematically study clients' needs, wants, perceptions, and preferences, and satisfy them efficiently. Example: Use of focus group and state family planning clinics in planning, implementing, and evaluating a campaign to market state family planning services.

their own needs rather than by those of the clients. The goal is to have maximum numbers of persons enrolled or seen, rather than client satisfaction. In contrast, in a societal marketing orientation an organization determines the needs, wants, and interests of target markets, and adopts its methods to deliver satisfaction that preserves and enhances the consumer's and society's well-being (Kotler & Clark, 1987).

A societal marketing orientation has a number of advantages for public health nursing organizations engaged in health promotion and illness prevention. Some of these are 1) promoting innovation and creativity of programs and services by suggesting many ways to deliver to similar client groups; 2) keeping services relevant by stimulating an awareness of changes in client group wants as they occur; and 3) defining the public health nursing agency's role more broadly, resulting in remaining abreast of clients' and society's wants (Crompton & Lamb, 1986).

With a societal marketing orientation, a strategic marketing plan for public health nursing agencies or organizations can be conceptualized as a continuous process involving the following six steps congruent with the nursing process:

Step 1. Analyze environment: demographic, economic, technical, political, social, cultural changes through time.

Step 2. Identify the desires, preferences, and priorities of actual and potential clients (opportunities, resources, threats).

Step 3. Establish goals, objectives, and outcomes (set by priority, specified, benefit-oriented).

Step 4. Formulate long-term strategies and action programs (how do we get there?).

Step 5. Implement incrementally.

Step 6. Evaluate program- and agencywide activities.

These steps can provide a frame of reference from which to view service delivery decisions as well as generate ideas for problem solving. In addition, they can assist public health nursing agencies to avoid the two critical mistakes in marketing professional services: defining and limiting efforts to getting new clients, and misunderstanding or refusing to examine the organizational implications for effective marketing (Kotler & Bloom, 1984). Thus, an important distinction between the strategic marketing plan and the structure of a public health nursing agency must be highlighted. That is, the agency's structure should not dictate the strategic marketing plan but rather the plan should shape the agency's structure.

In delivering public health nursing services, exchange relationships and channels of distribution are marketing concepts that are especially relevant. By being aware of such concepts, public health nurses can better organize and deliver services, particularly in the area of health promotion, that are effective in reaching larger numbers of vulnerable groups.

An exchange relationship centers around the act of offering something of value to someone who voluntarily accepts the offer in exchange for something else of value (Cooper, 1985). Values can be characterized as tangible or intangible, similar or dissimilar, and related or not related to a desired health behavior (DeMusis & Misoulis, 1988). The something of value may be either a product or a service.

Distinctive problems exist if the exchange relationship involves a professional services as opposed to a product. Some of these relate to issues involving third-party accountability, allocation of a professional's time to marketing, maintenance of quality control, and the constant demand to provide services on short notice (Kotler & Clark, 1987; Gould, 1988).

Channels of distribution center around how services are made available as well as accessible to targeted groups or populations. Decision making related to creating a channel of distribution focuses on three major types of access: physical, time, and information/promotional. Examples of decisions involving physical access include where to locate facilities, and those involving time access include what hours services are to be provided. Information and promotional access decisions have to consider which intermediaries, if any, are necessary to inform and promote the service to the consumer/client.

The concept of exchange relationships and channels of distribution applied to health promotion from a public nursing perspective can be illustrated by a well-baby clinic. Consider a single, unemployed woman who takes her toddler to the clinic advertised through the local newspaper. The mother wishes to have the child immunized so that the child will be eligible for day care and she can obtain work. She arrives at 8:30 A.M. in the basement of a local church where the clinic is set up. The child's immunization status is reviewed by a nurse. By 10:00 A.M. the child has received the appropriate immunizations as well as hearing and vision tests. In addition, hemoglobin has been measured and noted to be slightly below the normal value for the child's age. The mother receives information on nutrition (i.e., dietary sources of iron; Women, Infants, and Children program) and is advised to have the child's hemoglobin and hematocrit rechecked within the month. She returns the next month as scheduled because she feels the information and counseling she has received have been valuable.

This example outlines a marketing exchange process from beginning to completion. That is, there are at least two parties, each offers something the other perceives as valuable, each is capable of communication and delivery, and each is free to accept or reject the offer (Kotler & Clark, 1987). It is likely that many organizations and individuals have participated in the well-baby clinic (e.g., dietitian, volunteer group, local media, local church, state health department, etc.). Moreover, the public health nursing agency probably secured the services of many organizations that usually do not work together in providing services, and many values, mainly intangible, have been exchanged among them. Thus the clinic has served as a medium for transforming the varied services into a cohesive unit of values desired by consumers/attenders.

The well-baby clinic also illustrates a channel of distribution and how it provides for forward movement of products or services to consumers (DeMusis & Misoulis, 1988; Kotler & Clark, 1987). A channel follows the flow of a product or service. The goal is to deliver the products or services in a more effective and cost-efficient manner than in a nonchannel process. Typically, it involves one or several intermediaries who are selected based on their ability to make products and services readily available to targeted populations. The result is that more consumers/clients are reached.

A number of key determinants must be kept in mind if public health nurses are to be successful in creating a channel of distribution that can be successful in reaching a targeted population. Foremost, the exchange of values between the health care providers, especially primary values or values sought more than others, has a direct impact on channel efficiency (Demusis & Misoulis, 1988). In addition, some values can be achieved only by channel membership. Knowledge of these is especially important in systems in which several levels of values must be exchanged by health organizations.

Figure 22-1 illustrates the channel of distribution created by the well-baby clinic and depicts the intermediaries selected to facilitate forward movement of its services. In this example the values associated with health education and positive health behaviors were exchanged between the nurse providers and the targeted group. The double arrows between the nurse providers and selected intermediaries indicate the values that have been exchanged between these groups. These probably include public image, visibility, local recognition, and mission fulfillment.

In summary, a number of marketing concepts and issues are relevant to public health nursing practice. This knowledge can be useful in designing health promotion programs targeted at reaching the largest proportion of

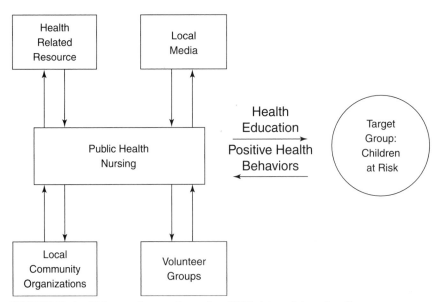

FIGURE 22-1   Value exchange through a PHN channel (one-level).

a vulnerable group. A production, product, or sales orientation to health promotion can be compared to looking through the wrong ends of the telescope; that is, starting with what one has and trying to make people buy it (Altenburg, 1988). Conversely, societal or sound marketing applied to health promotion can assist public health nurses to find out what their clients want and to gauge the impact of their services in a proactive manner.

■ REFERENCES

Altenburg, T. (1988). Developing a marketing strategy for health care services. *Strategic Management Concepts, 1*(4), 1–3.

Andrews, L.B. (1986, Jan-Feb). Health care providers: The future marketplace and regulations. *Journal of Professional Nursing, 1,* 51–63.

Cooper, P.D. (1985). *Health care marketing issues and trends* (2nd ed.). Rockville, MD: Aspen.

Crompton, J.L., & Lamb, C.W. (1986). *Marketing government and social services.* New York: Wiley.

DeMusis, E.A., & Misoulis, G. (1988). Channels of distribution and exchange concepts in health promotion. *Journal of Health Care Marketing, 8*(1), 60–68.

Editors. (1986). Ten trends to watch. *Nursing and Health Care, 7,* 17–19.

Gould, S.J. (1988). Macrodynamic trends in health care: A distribution and retailing perspective. *Health Care Management Review, 13*(2), 15–22.

Kotler, P., & Bloom, P.N. (1984). *Marketing professional services.* Englewood Cliffs, NJ: Prentice-Hall.

Kotler, P., & Clark, R. (1987). *Marketing for health care organizations.* Englewood Cliffs, NJ: Prentice-Hall.

Unit 4
Tools for Community Health Nursing Practice

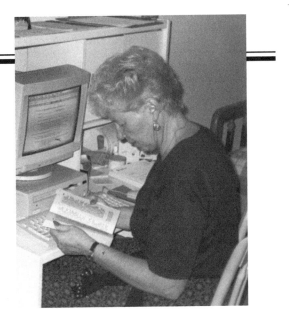

M any skills are required to effectively practice community health nursing, and to employ these skills, the nurse must have the appropriate tools ready for use. The nursing process, a primary tool, provides the framework for all community health nursing activity. It involves a series of steps that, when taken, lead toward the goal of raising the level of health for targeted communities. This field of practice emphasizes health and normality and the prevention of problems in groups at risk, and dealing with problems is only one part of the community health nurse's endeavors.

The community health nurse uses the nursing process in all aspects of her or his practice. For example, to help a community meet the needs of its homeless population, the nurse will use each step of the nursing process. First, data must be gathered and analyzed. Who are the homeless in this city? Where can they be found? What are their needs and which ones are most urgent? Next, a diagnosis must be made. What exactly is the problem that needs to be addressed? Perhaps the data show that food and shelter must take priority as the first programs of service to be developed; thus planning, the next step, can begin. The nurse and other professionals involved will establish goals and objectives, determine what resources are available and/or needed, and develop a plan for implementing the program. Finally, they will evaluate the program's effectiveness in meeting the food and shelter needs of the homeless persons in their community and determine what other needs should be addressed. The steps of the nursing process—assessment, diagnosis, planning, implementation, and evaluation—require the use of more specific tools for the nurse to carry them out effectively. What are these tools and how does the nurse become proficient in their use?

Tools used in community health nursing come primarily from the two fields that make up this specialty; nursing is one, the other is public health science. From nursing the community health nurse draws on many basic tools for applying the nursing process. Clearly the knowledge of health and illness, including normal growth and development and crisis prevention and intervention, is essential for assessing aggregate health needs and planning nursing interventions. Equally important, communication skills make up a core set of tools that include the ability to listen attentively and without bias, to engage in expert questioning, to encourage feedback and increase understanding between clients and nurse, and to promote healthy interpersonal relationships. A related tool, health teaching, also serves the community health nurse because much of health promotion and illness prevention depends on proper education and knowledge assimilation. Research is a critical tool for gathering descriptive data, generating and testing hypotheses, sharing new information, and developing concepts and theories for community health nursing practice. From research come models of care and advanced technology that frame health care delivery in the community.

Today, terms such as critical or clinical pathways, client outcomes, case management, and clinical or community partnerships are a part of health care language. Critical or clinical pathways and client outcomes denote a process used to deliver cost-effective quality care to individuals which incorporate time frames to achieve measurable criteria and goals. Case management and clinical or community partnerships are broader systems of caregiving that involve a specific management structure of programs or whole agencies. These processes are in place and influence the nurse–client relationship in the community. Advances in technology, especially the computer, have also dramatically affected how nurses collect, record, and use data. The effective community health nurse has always needed the skills of flexibility, open-mindedness, and adaptability to manage her or his role in the community. However, these new tools provide new challenges. Each of these and many more are important pieces in the nurse's repertoire to be kept ready for constant use.

The community health nurse draws on additional tools from public health science. Knowledge of aggregates—how to identify, assess, relate to, and intervene with population groups—is a particularly significant set of tools. So too is the use of epidemiologic processes. Epidemiology, the study of the distribution and determinants of health, health conditions, and disease in population groups, forms the core of public health. It is by means of epidemiologic processes that nurses can accurately assess such things as accident rates, disease occurrences, environmental hazards, and what groups are at risk for certain illnesses. Nurses are dependent on this set of tools for certain kinds of critical data collection in public health planning. Similarly, public health science offers the tool of biostatistics as another essential data-gathering device that enables nurses to analyze the community's health, draw inferences, and plan health services. Social policy and public health philosophy and values also strongly influence the nature of community health nursing and provide additional tools for practice. For example, concern for the greatest good for the greatest number and other social justice issues guide the nurse's decision making in community health planning. Understanding the structure and function of the health care delivery system, how healthcare policies are formulated, how to use the principles of management and organization for public health, and how to engage in health care planning at the aggregate level are among still other essential tools derived from the public health sciences.

Some of the preceding tools mentioned are discussed in other sections of this book. More are covered in depth in other nursing texts and will not be repeaed here. Unit IV presents selected tools to emphasize certain important traditional, changing, and/or new aspects of community health nursing practice.

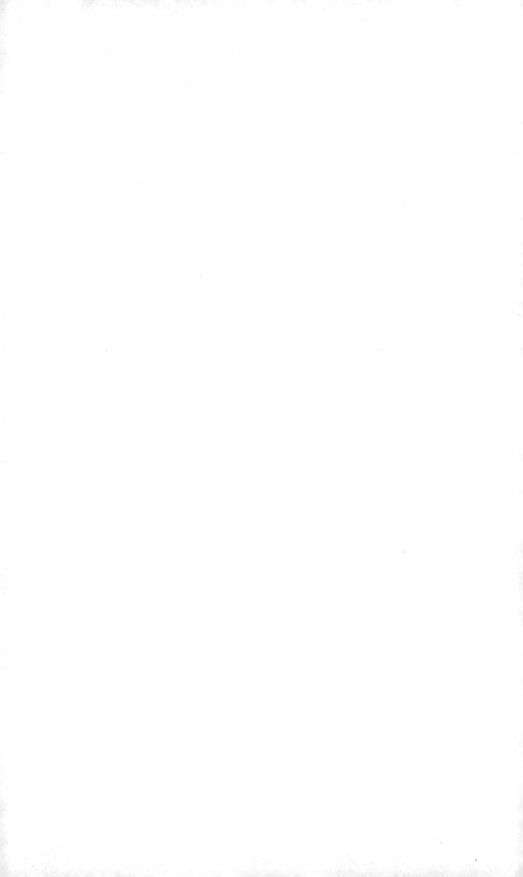

Chapter 23

Epidemiological Approach to Health Promotion

RICHARD LAUZON

A critical theory base for community health nursing practice is derived from the public health science of epidemiology. Epidemiology studies the distribution and causes of health and illness states in population groups. For many years epidemiologists have used the host–agent–environment model as a basis for studying disease and designing interventions. In any given situation, there is always a susceptible host (the person or persons at risk), causative agent(s), and environmental factors that either inhibit or foster the conditions for illness or accident to occur. Today this model is used as the basis for newer multiple-causation models. However, this classic approach to health promotion is presented by Richard Lauzon with specific and useful interventions for promoting client health. This chapter is an introduction to epidemiology for some and is a review for others; nevertheless, it offers a foundational tool on which community health nurses can build their practice.

Health promotion is a concept that has received a good deal of recent attention from health professionals.[1-3] Although most health workers appear relatively comfortable with the substance and implications of health promotion, few new insights have resulted from the now extensive discussion of the concept. Unfortunately, there are indications that the rhetoric surrounding health promotion is nothing more than a semantic game, a form of word wizardry in which the health education activities of yesterday are transformed into the health promotion programs of tomorrow.

The working document *A New Perspective on the Health of Canadians* outlines a health promotion strategy "aimed at informing, influencing and assisting both individuals and organizations so that they will accept more responsibility and be more active in matters affecting mental and physical health."[1] Undoubtedly, health promotion means much more than health education. Health promotion should be concerned with both positive and negative influences on the health consumer recognizing the reinforcing, competing, and contradictory impact of education messages, media advertising, availability of products and services, regulations and laws, and the environment in which they interact.

From *Canadian Journal of Public Health* 68:311–317, 1977. Reprinted with permission.

The purpose of this article is to propose a health promotion paradigm. This model attempts to consolidate past and present health-related influence strategies into a taxonomy of health-promotion activities. I hope such a model will stimulate further meaningful discussion on health promotion. The necessity for proposing such a model has been explained most forcefully by Thomas S. Kuhn:

> *In the absence of a paradigm or some candidate for a paradigm all the facts that could possibly pertain to the development of a given science are likely to seem equally relevant.[4]*

▬ EPIDEMIOLOGY AND HEALTH PROMOTION

The point of departure used in drafting this health-promotion model was Leavell and Clark's description of health promotion as the first phase of primary prevention (Figure 23-1). Furthermore, the authors suggest that health promotion activities can be identified through a study of the interrelations of host, agent, and environment, insofar as they may influence the natural history of disease.[5] As can be seen in Table 23-1, host, agent, and environmental factors form the basis of the proposed health promotion model.

The general strategy in the employment of the traditional epidemiological model is threefold: 1) to make the *host* more resistant; 2) to decrease the virulence of the *agent;* and 3) to create a barrier in the *environment* which will prevent the agent from reaching the host.[6] The discussion about each component will be oriented to describing the author's conception of the tripartite strategy indicated above.

The epidemiological model enables health professionals to acquire an ecological or systems perspective for various health problems. Such a perspective facilitates the identification of potential courses of action which may be useful in moderating or eliminating health risks.[7] The dynamic in-

Prepathogenesis Period		Period of Pathogenesis		
Health Promotion	Specific Protection	Early Diagnosis and Prompt Treatment	Disability Limitation	Rehabilitation
Primary Prevention		Secondary Prevention		Tertiary Prevention
Levels of Application of Preventive Measures				

FIGURE 23-1   Diagram showing the application of preventive medicine. (Adapted from Leavell and Clark.[5])

TABLE 23-1 A Health Promotion Model

EPIDEMIOLOGICAL COMPONENT	TARGETS	SELECTED HEALTH PROMOTION ACTIVITIES
Host	Low-risk individuals Average-risk individuals Excess-risk individuals	Instruction Education Persuasion Behaviour modification Proselytizing Screening Advertising
Agent	Alcohol Automation Automobiles Food Health services Illicit drugs Licit drugs* Tobacco	Marketing Product modification Engineering Substitutes Regulation Legislation
Environment	Physical Social–cultural Economic Mass media	Physical influence Social–cultural influence Economic influence Media influence

*Licit drugs: excluding alcohol and tobacco.

terrelationship among the three components must be recognized in order to conduct risk-reduction programs in an effective and efficient manner and to evaluate them appropriately. Unlike the model's application in the infectious or communicable disease sector, its application in the chronic or non-communicable disease sector is less exclusive regarding intervention among epidemiological components, a situation which makes it difficult to categorize the various influence activities presented at Table 23-1.

Figure 23-2 describes the problem inherent in applying the epidemiological model in a non-infectious disease setting. The reader will no doubt consider some examples mentioned later in the article which might better have been discussed under another component. Nevertheless the various classifications presented express the author's opinion at the time.

There are a number of precedents for employing the epidemiological model to describe the dynamics of preventive health for non-communicable or non-infectious disease states. Leonard and Arnold[6] reviewed its application in studies of mental health, nutrition, and accident prevention in their description of the epidemiological model in a general educational approach. In an accident prevention program, Suchman[8] applied the epidemiological model to analyze the acceptance or rejection of a protective glove for sugar-cane workers. This interesting article translates each of the epidemiological components—host, agent and environment—into social-

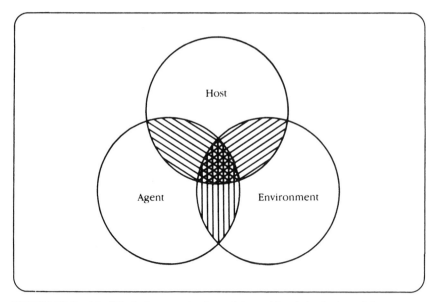

FIGURE 23-2   Modified characterization of the epidemiological model.

psychological factors relevant for health-related behaviour change. This approach is perhaps one of the most detailed and sophisticated modifications of the model in a noninfectious or non-communicable disease program.

The present application of the model adopts a grosser, methodological purview. The following section in the article will be devoted to explaining the substance of the proposed health promotion paradigm. Each component of the epidemiological model has been analyzed according to Targets and according to Health Promotion Activities perceived to be most applicable to influencing health. Each of the Health Promotion Activities may be employed to influence one or more items listed in the Target section of Table 23-1.

In viewing the proposed health promotion model, one of the most important contributions it makes is the recognition of the non-health professional and situation as having a major influence in health promotion.[9] There is little doubt that major health-related breakthroughs were oftentimes stimulated not by specific health efforts in the health care delivery system or in health education but through changes in legislation, modification of the environment, or the appearance of new products and commodities in the marketplace.

▬HOST-ORIENTED VARIABLES

The "at-risk concept" is used to specify more precisely the target populations in a health promotion program. It takes into consideration the fact that some individuals may be at low risk, for some factors, e.g., not smoking, and yet may be at excess risk for other factors, e.g., sedentary lifestyle.

It is a general rule of thumb in programs to change health behaviour that individuals who feel that they are more susceptible to a given health risk respond differently from individuals who do not feel highly susceptible.[10, 11] A well-conceived health promotion program would attempt to identify the target populations of excess-risk individuals in order to direct more appropriate messages to them; in addition, it may be very worthwhile to employ some form of reinforcing message to low and average risk individuals for practicing a particularly good health habit.

A significant body of research has indicated that individuals who recognize that they are at excess risk for some particular health threat become more attentive and receptive to information related to the diminution of this threat to health.[10] However, certain additional variables must also be present. The health threat must be perceived as important and immediately relevant; moreover, the health message should provide one or more realistic behavioural alternatives capable of reducing personal susceptibility or at least reducing the severity of the threat once it occurs.[10]

Recent encouraging results have been reported by Meyer and Henderson regarding multiple risk-factor reduction in a cardiovascular disease prevention program.[12] It may be that significant behavioural gains could be made by emphasizing to individuals the need to maintain an average or lower than average composite health-risk profile. Such a strategy would be consistent with popular psychological models of behaviour.[13, 14] A popular tool in the field of family practice, Health Hazard Appraisal, is based fundamentally on this concept.[15, 16]

■MAKING THE HOST MORE RESISTANT

Many personal health programs of the past have been host-oriented. The basic premise was the assumption that as people became more knowledgeable about some health risk, they would subsequently alter their behaviour to minimize the risk. However, our experience with cigarette smoking and alcohol abuse support the notion that "man is a rationalizing, rather than a rational, creature."[17] The inability of a mastery learning program to improve compliance with a hypertensive therapeutic regimen confirms the accepted notion that information alone is not sufficient to stimulate health behaviour.[18]

A selection of host-oriented, health-promotion activities is described in Table 23-2. In extending the infectious disease analogy, one could consider the methods in Table 23-2 as the various means of "immunizing" the individual with effective information or behavioural responses to resist the potential threat of disease.[19]

Under certain conditions, the methods would be employed prior to exposure to the health threat, i.e., drug education programs for elementary school children. In other cases, the methods would be applied following exposure, i.e., behaviour modification program on smoking withdrawal. In either case, the purpose would be to make the host more resistant to messages advocating maladaptive lifestyles.

TABLE 23-2   Host-Oriented Health Promotion Activities

Instruction	Teaching of very specific information or skills. Emphasis on factual material
Education	A logical and rational approach to information in which cognitive and affective objectives predominate
Persuasion	Intensive messages intended to stimulate compliance to some target behaviour. Often rely on fear-arousing appeals
Behaviour modification	Altering of behaviour by modelling and selective reinforcement
Proselytizing	Process of recruiting others to one's own beliefs
Screening	Evaluation used to identify health risk factors. Such evaluation may stimulate awareness and personal relevance for some particular health threat
Advertising	Any paid form of non-personal presentation and promotion of products, services, or ideas by an identified sponsor
Counseling	Personal guidance of an individual using various techniques of the personal interview

AGENT-ORIENTED VARIABLES

One approach in viewing the agent component within a health promotion context would be to characterize agents as facilitative mechanisms (such as more facilities and equipment with regard to encouraging physical activity). However, this article will retain the original analogical perspective and thus characterize agents along causal-association factors having bearing upon the disease state.

The agents identified here are those lifestyle-related agents which have been associated with high rates of mortality and morbidity.[1, 15] A study of disease precursors implicates the consumption of alcohol with mortality from cirrhosis of the liver, motor vehicle accidents, and pneumonia. Our increasingly sedentary lifestyle has evolved from increasing automation, a trend which manifests itself in the individual's cardiovascular health and emotional stability.[20] The major cause of death for males aged 15–44 is motor vehicle accidents. Factors contributing to automobile accidents are the driver's ability behind the steering wheel, the design of the car, and the driver's state of mind. The choice of food and the amount consumed may be reflected in certain deficiency states or accelerate the natural history of some diseases such as diabetes, obesity, or atherosclerosis. The immoderate use of licit or illicit drugs has demonstrated their debilitating qualities through habituation, dependence, and addiction, as well as factors related to motor vehicle accidents and suicide.

Automation has been added as an agent to account for the probable health effects due to sedentary behaviour. Health services have been included as an agent to reflect the prevalence of iatrogenic conditions which Illich[21] claims is the result of the "medicalization" of life.

▬DECREASING THE VIRULENCE OF THE AGENT

In this context the agents described are those substances or factors which have been related directly or indirectly to some particular disease state. The major concern here is to control the potential for harm inherent in the agent. In part this may relate to a "dose-response" effect and efforts to minimize the toxicity of the particular agent, or in a social influence sense; to recognize the detrimental health effect from the promotion of various maladaptive lifestyles.

Each of the selected health promotion activities in Table 23-3 may be employed to minimize the threat of harm for the human host. For example, in considering the adverse health effects of alcohol, considerable attention has been devoted to minimizing lifestyle-oriented advertisements used by the various breweries in marketing their product.[21] The effect of producing low-alcohol beer has not been studied sufficiently at this time to determine whether reduced alcohol content will have a measurable health effect. The most potent influential activities in moderating the effect of an agent such as alcohol are regulation and legislation whereby factors such as the price and availability of alcohol could be controlled.[22]

▬ENVIRONMENT-ORIENTED VARIABLES

The environmental component has been subdivided into four areas (Table 23-4). In addition to the usual environmental breakdown—physical, socio-cultural, and economic—mass media have been added as a separate component because of their pervasive influence in modern society.

▬CREATING A BARRIER IN THE ENVIRONMENT

There seems to be universal consensus that the most significant gains in preventive health have come from influences on the environmental factors associated with disease.[1, 23] One modification is suggested to the basic epi-

---

TABLE 23-3   Agent-Oriented Health Promotion Activities

Marketing	Discovering the wants of target audiences and then creating goods and services to satisfy them
Product modification	Changes in existing products having a positive or negative effect on health behaviour
Engineering	Improvements in the design of structures, machines, products, systems, and processes
Substitutes	Alternative choice of some product or behaviour
Regulatory controls	Authoritative rules governing certain details or procedures associated with availability of goods or services
Legislative controls	Establishment of laws to control certain details or procedures associated with the availability of goods or services

TABLE 23-4   Environment-Oriented Health Promotion Activities

Physical influence	Effect or change in the physical space; equipment or facilities inhabited or employed during work or leisure
Sociocultural influence	Effect or change in current or traditional social customs or mores
Economic influence	Effect or change in the economic factors which may facilitate or hinder the availability of some particular opportunity, product, service, or standard of living
Media influence	Effect or change in the mass media

demiological strategy. As much if not more attention should be devoted to strategies for increasing the environmental opportunities as to strategies for creating barriers designed to prevent hazardous agents for adversely affecting the host. Some splendid examples have occurred in Canada. The decision by the National Capital Commission in Ottawa to remove the snow and flood the Rideau Canal has increased physical recreation opportunities for Ottawa inhabitants during the winter. Many civil servants now skate to work and experience the physiological and psychological health benefits incidental to their main reason for skating, namely, as a means of traveling to work.

The recent activism on the part of non-smokers has undoubtedly exerted a definite social influence on smoking behaviour. A burgeoning number of companies and businesses have adopted restricted smoking policies for their employees and clients as a result of an increasingly vociferous demand on the part of the non-smoking majority. Non-smoking areas on commercial airlines are extremely popular.

Leventhal[11] stated that under certain situations, people are far more obedient and conforming than one might anticipate. Consider the case in a general hospital or health clinic where visitors are asked by doctors, nurses, and other health workers to respect the institution's non-smoking policy. Moreover, consider the reinforcing impact upon other community smoking and health efforts. Perhaps Leventhal's point helps to explain why liminal peer pressure has such a socially reinforcing impact on smoking among teenage girls.

Whereas the host characteristics could be considered as internal factors, the environment characteristics can be considered as external factors. Lalonde's development of the Health Field Concept[1] recognizes the environment as a unique area comprised of those influences on health over which the individual has no control. I do not view environment in such an exclusive sense. Although the individual may have little control over macro-environmental health problems, micro-environmental issues are certainly within the individual's control.

With regard to economic influence, there are significant reports which advocate the potential health influence of responsive social welfare programs.[24, 25] Comprehensive and universal health insurance has removed the financial barrier to medical care in Canada. In another sphere, some life insurance companies reduce premiums for non-smokers or alcohol abstainers while levying higher premiums for clients who are overweight, have a history of excessive drinking or otherwise have been judged to have an excessive mortality risk.[26] This financial incentive has likely reinforced healthy habits.

We should comment on the potential efficacy of reinforcing healthy lifestyle. Much of the work in modifying lifestyles has been host-oriented, and more particularly oriented toward excess-risk individuals. Few programs have attempted to reinforce individuals in the practice of healthy lifestyles. Notable exceptions would be certain occupational safety programs providing employee incentives for accident-free work periods. Imagine the potential savings of reinforcing the 85–90 percentage of nonsmoking grade 9 students for their current behavioural preference as opposed to encouraging smoking cessation by the 45–50 percent who are smokers by the time they reach the twelfth grade.

Media influence activities have recently been shown to be quite effective in stimulating community health behavioural changes. Alexander[27] reported that mass media had a powerful influence on knowledge and dietary behaviour, and a less significant effect on smoking behaviour in a mass media program to stimulate reductions in coronary heart disease risk factors. Jackson's study of the Participation Saskatoon project[28] noted that a comprehensive local mass media campaign was able appreciably to increase the amount of physical activity among Saskatoon inhabitants.

MEDIA-MIX CONCEPT

The epidemiological approach is in essence a systems approach to deal with a problem. A similar tactical effort can be observed daily in our mass media. Advertising agents have long ago recognized the value of employing a range of media to present their message. Their objective was to determine the optimal "media mix," that is, what percentage of resources should be allocated to the broadcast media versus special events. The proponents of the media-mix strategy suggest that there are a number of reasons to justify a multipronged approach: 1) a particular medium may have more appeal for certain groups than others;[29] 2) the reinforcement of complementary messages appearing in different media; and 3) the possible synergistic potential of complementary messages, i.e., the effect of two media working together is greater than either alone.[30]

An epidemiological approach to health promotion would provide a sound point-of-departure in mobilizing a media-mix strategy. From this perspective health promotion programs would not be organized in a vacuum and deliberate efforts would be made to determine the most effective medium (i.e., influence activities) complemented by secondary and tertiary thrusts among other epidemiological component activities.

A casual review of many personal health campaigns of the past would reveal that most have relied entirely on the use of one medium. And in the majority of these cases the medium of choice was education. It is especially disheartening to be subsequently confronted with the opinion that education has failed, for example, in smoking and health programs, sex education, or alcohol abuse. Perhaps closer to the point is that certain aspects of society have failed. What is the impact on cigarette smoking of five 30-minute periods on smoking during the child's high-school career compared to the mass of print and broadcast media advertising as well as the social reinforcement of parents and peers? Is it not remarkable that *only* 45–50 percent of our grade 12 graduates are smokers?

Chisholm has suggested that we should consider a spectrum of health promotion effects within the community.[31] It would be theoretically possible to divide independent or cumulative health-influencing events into three categories: 1) those having a positive effect; 2) those having a negative effect; and 3) those with a neutral or no perceived effect.

This point of view recognizes the mutually reinforcing nature of health messages and is consonant with the multiplicative nature of disease causation. In a general sense it conforms to a McLuhanistic analysis of health influences in that the "medium is the message."[39] Table 23-5 describes a personal assessment of this health promotion spectrum using smoking behaviour within the community as a dependent variable. This is akin to Suchman's thinking when he suggested that the resolution of all factors in his use of the epidemiological model represented "a balance between positive 'pulls' towards the action and negative 'pushes' away from it."[8]

TABLE 23-5   Spectrum of Health Promotion Influences Using Smoking Behaviour as an Example

HEALTH PROMOTION EFFECT		
Positive	*Neutral*	*Negative*
Regulation of *all* cigarette advertising[32]	Health warning on cigarette packages[36]	Smoking tolerated in health institutions
Smoking cessation clinics	Moderate cigarette tax increase[35]	Exemplar who smokes[38]
Non-smoking areas[33]		Tobacco company sponsored sporting events
Low-tar and nicotine cigarette[34]	Anti-smoking education[37]	
High cigarette tax increase[35]		

▬HEALTH PROMOTION AND SOCIAL MARKETING

Recent trends in personal health campaigns have signalled a change in the planning and operation of health promotion efforts. Perhaps the greatest influence on the Canadian scene comes from the implications of the concept of social marketing. Social marketing is concerned with "the design, implementation and control of programs calculated to influence the acceptability of social ideas."[40] In general, it is a multiprogram, multimedia strategy which is highly coordinated to achieve very specific objectives under selected conditions. Perhaps the only documented program in health promotion based upon social marketing techniques is the Stanford University Three Communities Project currently in progress.[27]

The gains assumed for effective health promotion will only be possible when program planners accept an ecological and epidemiological perspective of health behaviour. Although the element of time has not been discussed, the comprehensive strategies will of necessity be effective over the long term. The constraints of short-term, fiscal year oriented objectives must be replaced by more responsible, longitudinal efforts.

▬CONCLUSIONS

Effective health promotion programs for the future must be founded upon sound principles which recognize the multiplicative dynamics of health behaviour. In addition, health workers must be prepared to commit themselves to very specific objectives over definite time-periods. As Bass has said in a very recent article, "Without defining goals which we can fail to achieve, we also eliminate our chance to win real success. Furthermore, once we define population-wide targets, alternative means of accomplishing them can be explored."[41] Health promotion needs a model. The success of the epidemiological method warrants its consideration as a candidate paradigm for health promotion.

Acknowledgments
The author wishes to recognize the valuable suggestions of Dr. H. N. Colburn and Mr. Neil E. Collishaw in the preparation of this paper.

▬REFERENCES

1. Lalonde, M. *A New Perspective on the Health of Canadians—A Working Document.* Ottawa: Government of Canada, 1974.
2. CPHA Policy Statement—Health Promotion. *Can. J. Public Health* 65:140, 1974.
3. Niblett, D. Health Promotion—A Rediscovered Social Imperative. *Ibid.* 66:357, 1975.
4. Kuhn, T. S. *The Structure of Scientific Revolutions.* Chicago: University of Chicago Press, 1962.
5. Leavell, H. R., and Clark, E. G. (Eds.). *Preventive Medicine for the Doctor in his Community* (3rd ed.). Toronto: McGraw-Hill, 1965.
6. Leonard, A. R., and Arnold, M. F. An Epidemiologic Approach to Health Education. *Am. J. Public Health* 51:1555, 1961.

7. Colburn, H. N., and Baker, P. M. The Use of Mortality Data in Setting Priorities for Disease Prevention. *Can. Med. Assoc. J.* 10:679, 1974.
8. Suchman, E. A. Preventive Health Behavior: A Model for Research on Community Health Campaigns. *J. Health Soc. Beh.* 8:197, 1967.
9. Science Council of Canada. Report No. 22. Science for Health Services. Ottawa, Information Canada, 1974.
10. Becker, M. H. (Ed.). The Health Belief Model and Personal Health Behaviour. *Health Educ. Mono.* 2(4):324, 1974.
11. Leventhal, H. Changing Attitudes and Habits to Reduce Risk Factors in Chronic Disease. *Am J. Cardiol.* 31:571, 1973.
12. Meyer, A. J., and Henderson, J. B. Multiple Risk Factor Reduction in the Prevention of Cardiovascular Disease. *Prev. Med.* 3:225, 1974.
13. Festinger, L. *A theory of Cognitive Dissonance.* Stanford: Stanford University Press, 1957.
14. Insko, C. A. Rosenberg and Abelson's Affective-Cognitive Consistency Theory. In *Theories of Attitude Change.* New York: Appleton-Century-Crofts, 1967. Pp. 177–197.
15. Robbins, L., and Hall, J. *How to Practice Prospective Medicine.* Indianapolis: Methodist Hospital of Indiana, 1970.
16. Colburn, H. N., and Baker, P. M. Health Hazard Appraisal—A Possible Tool in Health Protection and Promotion. *Can J. Public Health* 64:490, 1973.
17. Le Riche, W. H., and Milner, J. *Epidemiology as Medical Ecology.* London: Churchill Livingstone, 1971.
18. Sackett, D. L., et al. Randomized Clinical Trial of Strategies for Improving Medication in Primary Hypertension. *Lancet* 1:1205, 1975.
19. Insko, C. A. McGuire's Inoculation Theory. In *Theories of Attitude Change.* New York: Appleton-Century-Crofts, 1967. Pp. 296–329.
20. Sharkey, B. J. *Physiological Fitness and Weight Control.* Missoula, Mt.: Mountain Press, 1974.
21. Illich, I. *The Medical Nemesis—The Expropriation of Health.* London: Marion Boyars, 1975.
22. Clifford, E. Lifestyle Ad Guidelines Could Affect All Media. *Globe and Mail,* Wednesday, August 25, 1976, p. B4.
23. Terris, M. A Social Policy on Health. *Am J. Public Health* 58:5, 1968.
24. Task Force Reports on the Cost of Health Services in Canada. Ottawa: Queen's Printer for Canada, 1970.
25. *Health,* Report of the Commission of Inquiry on Health and Social Welfare. Quebec: Government of Quebec, 1970.
26. Sterba, J. P. Nonsmoker is Winning Right to Clean Indoor Air. *New York Times,* Sunday, September 30, 1973, p. 1.
27. Alexander, J. Mass Media: The New Health Provider? Paper presented at the 26th Annual Meeting of the International Communication Association, Portland, Oregon, April 1976.
28. Jackson, J. J. Diffusion of an Innovation: An Exploratory Study of the Consequences of Sport Participation Canada's Campaign at Saskatoon. Doctoral dissertation, University of alberta, 1975.
29. Cox, D. F. Clues for Advertising Strategists. In L. A. Dexter and D. M. White (Eds.), *People, Society and Mass Communications.* New York: Free Press, 1964.
30. Bogart, L. *Strategy in Advertising.* New York: Harcourt, Brace and World, 1967.
31. Chisholm, D. Personal communication, September 1975.
32. Hamilton, J. L. The Demand for Cigarettes: Advertising, the Health Scare and the Cigarette Advertising Ban. *Rev. Econ. Stat.* 54:401, 1972.
33. Katz, S. Non-smokers Fight Back—They Start to Organize. *Toronto Star,* Wednesday, October 9, 1974.
34. Wynder, E. Quoted in *Smoking Health Newletter* 8:2, 1972.
35. Russell, M. A. H. Changes in Cigarette Price and Consumption By Men in Britain, 1946–71. A Preliminary Analysis. *Br. J. Prev. Soc. Med.* 27:1, 1973.
36. Cotter, N. Cigaret Firms' Marketing Strategy More Refined. *Globe and Mail,* Wednesday, May 1, 1974, p. B4.
37. Bradshaw, P. Q. The Problem of Cigarette Smoking and Its Control. *Int. J. Addict.* 8:353, 1973.

38. Levitt, E. E. A Multivariate Study of Correlative Factors in Youthful Cogarette Smoking. *Dev. Psychol.* 2:5, 1970.
39. McLuhan, M. *Understanding Media: The Extensions of Man.* New York: Signet Books (New American Library), 1964.
40. Kotler, P., and Zaltman, G. Social Marketing: An Approach to Planned Social Change. *J. Marketing* 35:3, 1971.
41. Bass, F. A Public-Health Approach to Illness-Producing Behavior, the Example of Tuberculosis Control Applied to Cigarette Smoking. In *Preventive Medicine.* New York: Prodist 1976. Pp. 148–162.

Chapter 24

Florence Nightingale as Statistician

EDWIN W. KOPF

Health statistics comprise an important tool for community health practice. From statistics we learn about a community's morbidity and mortality rates, accident patterns, demographics, and use of systems and resources. Statistics provide the data from which positive changes in health care can be launched. They form the basis for designing community health nursing interventions, for planning and evaluating community health programs, and for analyzing and developing health policy and legislation. Florence Nightingale long ago recognized the value of statistics and used them, described in this classic chapter by Edwin Kopf, as a basis for major reforms in the health care of her day.

The somewhat legendary accounts of this remarkable woman contain but few references to that part of her life and work which should appeal to the students of the history of modern social statistics. More or less is understood of her radical innovations in the nursing care of the sick in institutions and especially in military hospitals; a definite idea exists of her capacities as reformer, administrator, and nurse. Comparatively little is known of her, however, as a constructive compiler and interpreter of descriptive social statistics. One biographer alone, Sir Edward T. Cook, speaks with sympathy and understanding of her as a statistician. He calls her a "passionate statistician."

The activities of Miss Nightingale in statistics may be classed under several broad categories. We may think of her in terms of her forty years of thought and achievement in the Indian question; in safeguarding the health of the British soldier; in reorganizing civil and military hospital administration at home and abroad; and, in this latter regard, of her pioneer services to the profession of nursing. Her keen intellect, applied to these major projects of her career, comprehended the utility of the statistical method as a means of developing a basis of established fact for social reform.

In early life, Miss Nightingale showed peculiar aptitude for collecting and methodically recording current historical facts. Her observations during the travels of the Nightingales in Europe over the period 1837–1839 are a curious mixture of comment and criticism on the then existing laws,

From *Journal of the American Statistical Association* 15(116):338–404. Reprinted by permission of American Statistical Association.

land systems, social conditions, and benevolent institutions. Throughout her life she collected an immense number of pamphlets, reports, and returns which she skillfully analyzed with telling effect in her campaigns for hospital and sanitary reform. Following her nursing apprenticeship with the Fliedners at Kaiserswerth, she undertook further training at the *Maison de la Providence* in Paris; here she proceeded to collect hospital reports, returns, statistical forms, and general information on hospital construction and sanitation. Among her papers then were elaborately tabulated analyses of hospital organizations and nursing systems and their end results. These inquiries extended to both France and Germany. She seems also to have addressed circulars of inquiry on the same subjects to representative hospitals in the United Kingdom.

Miss Nightingale was profoundly influenced by the works of Adolphe Quetelet, the Belgian astronomer, meteorologist, and statistician. Perhaps her practice of methodically recording the facts of her botanical researches led her to one of Quetelet's laws of flowering plants. The common lilac flowers, he averred, when the sum of the squares of the mean daily temperatures, counted from the end of the frosts, equals 4264° centigrade. While this "law" delighted her, she regarded it as a lesser example of Quetelet's researches and statistical conclusions. She was fascinated most by Quetelet's "*Sur l'Homme et le Développement de ses Facultés*," published in 1835, in which he outlined his conception of statistical method as applied to the life of man. From Quetelet, Miss Nightingale learned much of the science and art which describes human society in terms of numbers. From him she learned the methods, general aims, and results of qualified inquiry into social facts and forces.

MILITARY AND SANITARY STATISTICS OF THE CRIMEAN WAR

The discipline of Quetelet's new science of social inquiry was to have its first influence upon the military and sanitary statistics of the Crimean War. Miss Nightingale found the medical records of the Scutari hospitals in lamentable condition. Even the number of deaths was not accurately recorded. The three separate registers then maintained gave each a totally different account of the deaths among the military forces. None of the statistical records was kept in uniform manner. She was able to introduce an orderly plan of recording the principal sickness and mortality data of the military hospital establishments which came within the sphere of her influence.

Miss Nightingale's experience in the Crimea filled her with an ardent desire to remedy the scandalous neglect of sanitary precautions in the Army; her study of the available data convinced her that the greater number of deaths in hospitals need not have occurred at all. During the first seven months of the Crimean campaign, a mortality of 60 percent per annum from disease alone occurred, a rate of mortality which exceeded even that of the Great Plague in London, and a higher ratio than the case mortality of cholera. Miss Nightingale's vigorous use of these facts resulted in a series of reforms, which in turn reduced this terrible rate of mortality. She observed, also, that if sanitary neglect prevailed in the Army afield, it probably affected the Army at home in considerable degree likewise. She compared the mortality in civil life with the mortality in army barracks. Between the ages of 25 and 35 she found that the mortality among soldiers was nearly double that in civil life. In writing to Sir John McNeill she said: "it is as criminal to have a mortality of 17, 19, and 20 per thousand in the Line, Artillery and Guards, when that in civil life is only 11 per 1,000, as it would be to take 1,100 men out upon Salisbury Plain and shoot them."

Her further observations on the Chatham military hospitals were: "This disgraceful state of our Chatham Hospitals is only one more symptom of a system, which, in the Crimea, put to death 16,000 men—the finest experiment modern history has seen upon a large scale, viz., as to what given number may be put to death at will by the sole agency of bad food and bad air." Among her private notes of 1856 her biographer found this: "I stand at the altar of the murdered men, and while I live, I fight their cause." The one weapon upon which she placed most dependence was her collection of sanitary statistics.

■ HEALTH, EFFICIENCY, AND HOSPITAL ADMINISTRATION OF THE BRITISH ARMY

The results of her personal studies of army medical statistics were embodied in a report, from the first intended as a confidential communication to the War Office and the Army Medical Department. There had been considerable delay in the formation of the Royal Commission on the health of the Army which she had requested in her November, 1856, interview with Lord Panmure. The Royal Warrant establishing the Commission was not issued until May 5, 1857. During this exasperating period of delay Miss Nightingale held in reserve her array of statistics, until, having begun her agitation with the sovereign and continuing through the politicians, she was almost ready to plead her cause with the people. In three months from the day the Royal Warrant was issued, the Commission presented its report. In the meantime, Lord Panmure had asked Miss Nightingale for her "Notes Affecting the Health, Efficiency and Hospital Administration of the British Army." These notes are the least known of her works, because they were never officially published. It has never become know how much of the final Report of the Royal Commission was actually the work of Miss Nightingale. Printed at her private expense and circulated among influential people, her "Notes" made a profound impression. They have been termed "a treasury of authentic fact . . . affording a complete elucidation of the causes which had brought about failure, and showing the means by which the country could best hope to safeguard the truly sacred task of providing for the health of its troops in future wars." Another of her friends who read the proof said: "It has so much the character of good, sincere, enlightened conversation on a subject which is thoroughly understood and appreciated, and so little the appearance of having been 'got up' or of pretension of any kind, literary or artistic." Another reader said: "I regard it as a gift to the Army, and to the country altogether priceless."

The preface to the Notes gave the keynote. Hospitals were shown to be but part of wider programs involving the general health and efficiency of the Army. This was emphasized by the fact that those who fell before Sebastopol by disease were above seven times the number who fell by the enemy. The introductory chapter gave the history of the health of the British Armies in previous campaigns. Six of the twenty sections of the Notes dealt with the medical history of the Crimean War. Two other sections discussed the mortality of armies in peace and war and the necessity for a statistical department of the army. There were also numerous appendices, supplementary notes, and graphic illustrations and diagrams.

▬PIONEER IN GRAPHIC ILLUSTRATION OF STATISTICS

It must be remembered that these Notes were written by Miss Nightingale in the short space of six months, and while in delicate health. In the preparation of her report she had but little assistance; the gathering of the data was facilitated, however, by the friendly cooperation of many broadminded men in the public service. Dr. Farr, for instance, aided materially in the preparation of the comparisons between the mortality of civil and army life and in editing the graphical illustrations which he especially commended. These graphical diagrams were at that time somewhat of an innovation in statistics, and had no significant precedent save in the statistical works of A. M. Guerry, a contemporary of Quetelet. The Report of the Commission, containing some thirty-three written answers by Miss Nightingale to leading questions by the Commission, together with her original tabulation of the appalling morbidity and mortality statistics of the British Army, was issued to the public in January, 1858. The graphical illustrations in her own Notes portrayed, by means of shaded or colored squares, circles and wedges, 1) the deaths due to preventable causes in the hospitals during the Crimean War and 2) the rate of mortality in the British Army at home. "Our soldiers enlist," as she put it, "to death in the barracks." She reprinted this graphic section and distributed it, with a brief memorandum, to leading members of Parliament and to medical and commanding officers throughout the country, in India, and in the Colonies. "It is our flank march upon the enemy," she said.

▬STATISTICAL DEPARTMENT OF BRITISH ARMY FOUNDED

The chief product of the Commission's work of interest from the statistical standpoint was the report of the subcommittee on Army Medical Statistics. This committee, consisting of Mr. Sidney Herbert, Sir A. Tulloch, and Dr. Farr, reported in June, 1858, and published its "First Annual Statistical Report on the Health of the Army" in March, 1861. The compilations were directed by Dr. Thomas Graham Balfour, under whose leadership British army statistics became the best and most useful obtainable in Europe.

The facts published in the "Notes" did not go unchallenged. A pamphlet appeared anonymously calling them in question. Miss Nightingale immediately prepared a reply. This second note was entitled "A Contribution to the Sanitary History of the British Army during the late War with Russia," and constituted a scathing and eloquent account of the preventable mortality which she had witnessed in the East. The graphic charts of the "Notes" were reproduced.

CONSTRUCTION, ORGANIZATION, AND MANAGEMENT OF CIVIL HOSPITALS

The opposition to the recommendations of the subcommission on Army Barracks stimulated Miss Nightingale to prepare a more extended discussion of hospital construction, organization, and management. From her extensive experience in and study of hospital systems in Germany, France, and Ireland and in the Crimea, she prepared two addresses on hospital construction and sanitation for the Liverpool meeting of the National Association for the Promotion of Social Science. These papers were reprinted as "Notes on Hospitals." These "Notes" in three editions, the last in 1863, revolutionized ideas of hospital construction.

It was pointed out that the hospital statistics then available gave little information of real value on the proportion of recoveries, of deaths, and the average duration of hospital treatment for different diseases, duly qualified by sex and age. A common agreement on the number and nature of statistical data to be tabulated was recommended. A unique feature of this Liverpool address was a mortality table for hospital nurses and attendants showing the greatly increased prevalence of communicable diseases among this class of hospital employees, as compared with the mortality from the same causes in civil life. The deplorable existence of "hospital gangrene" and "hospital septicemia" in that day of defective hospital sanitation and construction was effectively portrayed by these mortality statistics.

A brief inquiry into the precedent circumstances will be of interest. When Miss Nightingale returned from the Crimea she directed much thought and attention to hospital statistics as an adjunct to administration of institutions for the care of the sick. She found a complete lack of scientific coordination. The statistics were not kept along uniform lines. Each hospital followed its own nomenclature and classification of diseases. The available data had never been tabulated upon forms which would render the statistics of one hospital comparable with those of another. The data had little value for advancing medical knowledge or as an adjunct to hospital management. With the assistance of Dr. Farr, and of other friendly physicians, she drew up a standard list of diseases (largely a selection from the d'Espine-Farr System) and a set of model hospital statistical forms. She had her model forms printed in 1859 and persuaded some of the London hospitals to adopt them experimentally. She and Dr. Farr studied the tabulated results, which had sufficient value to show how large a field of qualified statistical inquiry had been opened by the introduction of her forms.

Miss Nightingale's skill in so effectively employing the statistical method in army sanitary reform had led to her election, in 1858, to fellowship in the Royal Statistical Society. On October 16, 1874, the American Statistical Association elected her an honorary member.

INTERNATIONAL STATISTICAL CONGRESS OF 1860

This growing association with the leaders of thought in the statistical world of her time enabled her to take an active part in drawing up the program of the second section of the International Statistical Congress, held at London in 1860. This Section dealt with sanitary statistics. Miss Nightingale and Dr. Farr incorporated the forms for uniform hospital statistics, which had been experimentally introduced into a group of London hospitals in 1859, in a paper read for her before the Section by Dr. McMillian. Additions and recommendations, chiefly by Dr. Berg of Sweden and Dr. Neumann of Berlin, were concurred in by the author in a letter to the Earl of Shaftesbury, President of the Section.

This paper on uniform classifications and forms for hospital statistics was afterward widely circulated among physicians and hospital officials. Large quantities of the forms were supplied to hospitals in various parts of the country. The Paris hospitals took up the plan. Guy's Hospital, London, prepared a statistical analysis of its experience for the years 1854 to 1861; St. Thomas' for the years 1857 to 1860; and St. Bartholomew's, for 1860. At a meeting held at Guy's Hospital on June 21, 1861, it was unanimously agreed to adopt a uniform plan of registration, that each hospital should publish its own statistics annually, and that the forms devised by Miss Nightingale should be used so far as practicable.

ELEMENTS OF HOSPITAL MEDICAL STATISTICS

Miss Nightingale then prepared the detailed paper on "Hospital Statistics and Hospital Plans" for the Dublin meeting of the National Association for the Promotion of Social Science in 1861. In this paper she emphasized the seven primary tabulation elements of hospital sickness statistics, which were:

1. Number of patients remaining in hospital on first day of year.
2. Patients admitted during year.
3. Patients recovered or relieved during the year.
4. Patients discharged as incurable, unrelieved, for irregularities or at own request.
5. Patients died during year.
6. Patients remaining at end of year.
7. Mean duration of cases in days and fractions of a day.

These tabulation "elements" were to be compiled as seven separate tables, each showing diseases classified thereunder by sex and age (by single years under five and by five year periods thereafter). The additional consideration of diseases contracted in hospital while under treatment was also provided for. These extensions of the original paper were suggested by Drs. Berg and Neumann. Miss Nightingale held that these supplementary tables would bring out the fact of the then scandalous prevalence of "hospital diseases" such as gangrene and septicemia.

The statistics of the various hospitals adopting her forms were published in the *Journal* of the Royal Statistical Society for September, 1862. Miss Nightingale's system of uniform hospital statistics was never generally successful over any considerable period of time. The plan, but partly realized in the requirements of the King's Hospital Fund, demands for its complete and effective operation a more intelligent appreciation of and a finer enthusiasm for statistical facts than is afforded even by present day voluntary and competitive hospital systems in metropolitan districts.

A further example of Miss Nightingale's use of the statistical method in hospital economy was her study of the questions relating to the possible removal of St. Thomas' Hospital at the instance of the Southeastern Railway. The railway company proposed the removal of the hospital to provide for an extension of the right-of-way from London Bridge to Charing Cross. She analysed the origins of cases served by the hospital, tabulated the proportions of cases within certain radial distances, and showed the probable effect upon patients of the removal of the hospital to the several possible sites suggested. This method of fitting hospital accommodation to the needs of populations has only recently been revived. It represents a legitimate application of demographic principles of the study of the relief of dire human needs.

The statistics of surgical operations from the standpoint of hospital cost and practical end results were next considered by Miss Nightingale. In a commentary of St. Bartholomew's statistical report, Miss Nightingale outlined the minimum requirements of a report form for the nature and result of surgical operations. The subject was further developed in a paper read for her before the Berlin meeting of the International Statistical Congress in 1863.

Before the close of the London meeting of the International Statistical Congress, 1860, Miss Nightingale addressed a letter to Lord Shaftesbury. The letter was read to the whole Congress and adopted by it as a resolution. The resolution impressed upon governments the prime necessity for publishing more extensive and numerous abstracts of the statistical information in their possession.

▄MISS NIGHTINGALE AND THE CENSUS OF ENGLAND, 1861

Miss Nightingale made a determined effort to extend the scope and application of the Census of 1861, largely in the direction of collecting statistics which would serve as a foundation for sanitary reform. Her aim was twofold: one was to enumerate the sick and infirm on Census Day. To those who denied that it could be accomplished, she pointed out that it had been done elsewhere, notably in Ireland. Her second ambition was to obtain complete data on the housing of the population; this, too, had been practicable in Ireland, she urged. In pressing her point with the Census officials she said: "The connection between the *health* and the *dwellings* of the population is one of the most important that exists. The 'diseases' can be approximated also. In all the more important—such as smallpox, fevers, measles, heart disease, etc.—all those which affect the *national* health, there will be very little error. Where there *is* error in these things, the error is uniform . . . and corrects itself . . ." These few remarks still serve as prolegomena to any future census plans for England or any other country.

The Census Bill came up late in the session and not much comment can be found on the foregoing suggestion for a development of Census inquiry. The only critical comment made in the debate proceeded from Lord Ellenborough, who, far from considering the innovations of sickness and housing statistics, proposed to exclude most of the inquiries already suggested. Miss Nightingale, in her conception of census methods and results, was far ahead of her day and generation. Subsequent censuses, chiefly in the United States, in Tasmania, and in one or two other countries, have included sickness and housing inquiries.

▬SCOPE AND USE OF STATISTICS

Miss Nightingale's activities in furthering statistical progress were the outgrowth of her deep conviction, variously expressed in her several papers, that the social and moral sciences are in method and substance statistical sciences. In her several papers on metaphysical topics, she asserts that statistics were to her almost a religious exercise. Her conception of theology was that its true function was to ascertain the "character of God." Statistics, she mused, discovered and codified law in the social sphere and thereby revealed certain aspects of "the character of God." Doubtless, in these speculations she was profoundly influenced by the studies of Quetelet in moral statistics, as typified in his "*Recherches statistiques sur le Royaume de Pays-Bas.*"

Statistics as an element in political education also appealed with peculiar force to Miss Nightingale. In a letter to Benjamin Jowett she said: "The Cabinet Ministers, the army of their subordinates . . . have for the most part received a university education, but no education in statistical method. We legislate without knowing what we are doing. The War Office has some of the finest statistics in the world. What comes of them? Little or nothing. Why? Because the Heads do not know how to make anything of them. Our Indian statistics are really better than those of England. Of these no use is made in administration. What we want is not so much (or at least not at present) an accumulation of facts, as to teach men who are to govern the country the use of statistical facts."

She proposed a number of leading questions which she desired to see investigated by the statistical method: What had been the result of twenty years of compulsory education? What is the effect of town life on offspring in number and in health? What are the contributions of the several social classes to the population of the next generation? In proposing these inquiries she anticipated by more than a generation the work of the eugenists and biometricians of the Galton-Pearson school. Her friend, Adolphe Quetelet, had inaugurated studies of this character. Both he and Dr. Farr had hoped that she would pursue her inquiries more extensively. In conversation with Benjamin Jowett she proposed to found at Oxford a Professorship or Lectureship in Applied Statistics. Mr. Jowett seems to have discussed the matter with Mr. Arthur Balfour and Professor Alfred Marshall. Miss Nightingale, on her part, consulted Mr. Francis Galton, who responded earnestly and worked out a detailed plan. There was more or less discussion over the matter, but in the press of other affairs, the proposition was discarded. It is certainly of very great interest in this connection to observe that many years afterward such an enterprise was undertaken by the University College in London; probably, however, not directly issuing from Miss Nightingale's suggestion.

▬ VITALITY OF ABORIGINAL RACES

Following her disquisitions on army, medical, and civil hospital statistics, came her statistical investigations into colonial questions: the first into the vitality of native or aboriginal races in the Colonies; the second into the sanitary condition and material welfare of the population and military establishment of India. In a paper before the National Association for the Promotion of Social Science, meeting at Edinburgh in 1863, she discussed the gradual disappearance of the native races when brought into contact with the influences of civilization. The paper was suggested by Sir George Grey, who, at that time, was deeply engaged with questions of Colonial policy. The preliminary inquiry related to the probable effect of European school usages and school education generally, upon the health of children, of parents, and of races which had not heretofore been brought under any system of education. With the assistance of the Duke of Newcastle, she prepared a form which was sent by the Colonial office to the governors of the various colonies. From the returns of 143 schools she deduced the mortality of school children by age period and by sex, and further classified the statistics by causes of death. A second inquiry into the statistics of colonial hospitals gave important information on the causes of high institutional mortality among the native races. The numbers involved were small, and the results were necessarily considerably in error; but, in the main, the conclusions as to the neglect of sanitary precautions and the change in the living habits of native races were sound.

A further paper on the aboriginal races in Australia was read before the same Association at York, England, in 1864. This essay contained copious quotations from correspondence with colonial governors over points raised by the first paper. The Colonial Office circulated the reprint of the Edinburgh paper widely. Miss Nightingale has been considered a pioneer in work for arresting the decline of native races, so far as such work has been possible.

BRITISH ARMY IN INDIA

After the death of Sidney Herbert, Miss Nightingale devoted the larger portion of her time and attention to the Indian question. Her earlier years of service to the British Army at home were not more significant than her later years of endeavor for the army and people in India. The greater proportion of the lives of soldiers lost in India was not chargeable to battle, but to disease caused by insanitation and general ignorance of military tropical hygiene. In 1859, it was found that the average annual death rate of the British armies in India had been 69 per 1,000 since the year 1817.* In recent times the figure has been 5 per 1,000. The changes in living and working accommodations which brought about this reduction in army mortality are directly traceable to the recommendations of the Royal Commission, appointed in 1859, which reported in 1863. An unrecorded fact, however, is that Miss Nightingale's suggestion led directly to the appointment of the commission and that the greater part of the Report was her handiwork. The suggestions upon which permanent reforms in army sanitation in India were based were also her work.**

For eight months, during the latter part of 1858 and the earlier part of 1859, Miss Nightingale importuned Lord Stanley for the appointment of a Royal Sanitary Commission which would do for the armies in India what had been done for the armies at home. She had contemplated for two years before, the appointment of a Commission to investigate the entire question of the armies in British India. The mutiny of almost the whole of the Bengal native army and the contingents in northern India in 1857, which had filled the minds of the British population with thoughts of vengeance and repression against the native army, had only served to fix her attention upon sanitary and other administrative reform on behalf of the soldiers. Her analysis of the statistics of army mortality in India con-

---

*While this figure included battle casualties of the campaigns of the forty years ending with 1856, the mortality figure was still excessive. It was stated that the registered mortality among British troops in India was six times that of Englishmen of the same ages at home. Again, in an earlier investigation into mortality from disease among troops in the East Indies (including for the most part British India) death rates varying from 40 to 98 per 1,000 of mean strength over the period 1840–1848 were found.

**British soldiers in India today live in barracks which surpass in comfort and sanitation any that can be found in other countries. Every regiment, battery, and depot has its regimental institute, a sort of soldier's club, library, reading and recreation room, a temperance association, and a theatre. The use of alcoholic beverages is discouraged and every encouragement is given to useful employment for the men.

vinced her that there was murder committed not by the Sepoys alone. To her mind, it was murder to doom British soldiers to death by neglect of the most elementary sanitary precautions.

Anticipating the appointment of the Commission, she began collecting, tabulating, and interpreting data she derived from circulars of inquiry which she had drafted and sent to all the stations in India. The inquiry form lacked little in requisite completeness and precision of detail. In the meantime, Miss Nightingale and Dr. Farr searched the sickness and mortality records of the India Office.

The report of the Indian Sanitary Commission when issued in 1863 comprised in all 2,028 pages, mostly in small print. The greater part of the statistical work in the Report bore clear evidence of Miss Nightingale's influence. Her inquiry blank, in the first instance, provided the vehicle for the transmission of much of the evidence. The replies to her questions occupy the whole of the second volume of the Report. In October, 1861, the Commission requested her to submit her interpretation of these Stational Reports. Her observations upon these reports occupied 23 pages and are the most remarkable of her published works. Her unusual treatment of the subject by the addition of illustrative wood-cuts describing Indian hospitals and barracks, made the Treasury demur, however, at the cost, but Miss Nightingale was permitted to pay for the printing out of her private purse. Copies of these observations were sent to the queen and to influential members of the government. Sir John McNeill wrote: "The picture is terrible, but it is all true. There is no one statement from beginning to end that I feel disposed to question and there are many which my own observation and experience enable me to confirm." In detail, her notes related to the camp diseases which follow the selection of poor sites, defective disposal of human wastes, overcrowding in barracks, lack of suitable occupation and exercise, dietaries and defective hospital arrangements. The sources of statistical data for the armies in India were also criticised. In addition to her observations, Miss Nightingale prepared with Dr. Sutherland an abstract of the returns upon which her "Observations" were founded.

Moreover, when the Report was published she moved with her characteristic decision to secure for it the newspaper and periodical publicity which it deserved. She contributed a popular résumé of the Royal Commission's Report to the National Association for the Promotion of Social Science, meeting at Edinburgh in 1863, entitled "How People may Live and not Die in India." The paper was republished in 1864, with a preface and an account of what the Commission had actually achieved in sanitary works and measures. In 1868, the Secretary of State printed her résumé of the Indian Sanitary Question from 1859 to 1867 and her memorandum of advice and suggestions on the entire situation as it then stood. The dispatch from Sir Stafford Northcote under date of April 23, 1863 (drafted by Miss Nightingale), was printed at the same time. This dispatch resulted in the first of the annual series of Indian Sanitary Reports. In the reports for 1868 and 1869 appear two of Miss Nightingale's contributions; in the first an Introduction of eight pages and in the second her paper on "Sanitary Progress in India."

Her statistical enterprises of this period are well summarized in a few phrases which are here quoted from one of her letters: "I am all in the arithmetical line now . . . I find that every year . . . there are in the Home Army, 729 men alive every year who would have been dead but for Sidney Herbert's measures, and 5,184 men always on active duty who would have been 'constantly sick in bed.' In India the difference is still more striking. Taken on the last two years, the death rate of Bombay is lower than that of London,* the healthiest city in Europe. And the death rate of Calcutta is lower than that of Liverpool and Manchester. But this is not the greatest victory. The Municipal Commissioner of Bombay writes that the 'huddled native masses clamourously invoke the aid of the Health Department if but one death from cholera occurs; whereas formerly half of them might be swept away and the other half think it all right."

In 1873, the National Association for the Promotion of Social Science invited her to contribute a paper on the ten years of progress in India since her "How People may Live and not Die in India" paper appeared. Her title for this later paper was "How some People have Lived and Not Died in India." The India Office reprinted the paper in its 1874 bluebook. The salient fact developed in this report was that the death rate in the Indian Army had been reduced from 69 per 1,000 to 18 per 1,000. This summary of ten years of sanitary progress in India she was qualified to prepare in consequence of her editorial work on the annuals issued by the sanitary department of the India Office.

In 1877, Miss Nightingale published two letters on famine in India and followed these by an article in the *Nineteenth Century* magazine. This article, "The People in India," gave the principal facts about the Indian famines and proceeded further to describe in considerable detail the evils of usury in the Bombay Deccan. Beginning with 1874, Miss Nightingale collected statistics of irrigation in India, and of the effect of irrigation on the life and health of the people. These data, the appendix of the second part of an unpublished work on the Indian Land Question and Irrigation Systems, were afterward partially used in several isolated papers. She thought much on education in India. There had been a neglect of elementary education. The exception was found in the system of village schools established by Lieutenant-Governor James Thomason, of what is now the Agra Province. The report of the Indian Education Commission of 1883 directed attention to the essential difficulties residing in the language, credal, race, and traditional differences of the populations of the several provinces. The two chief difficulties in the way of a diffusion of education among the masses in India are the large agricultural population, among whom it is in all countries difficult to advance any system of education, and the existence of a hereditary class, whose object has been to maintain their monopoly of learning as the chief buttress of their social

*These figures related only to conditions prevailing at the time this letter was written.

supremacy. Questions such as these occupied Miss Nightingale's attention in the years 1881 and 1882.

The succeeding years were taken up in turn by Army Hospital Service reform, district nursing organization, nursing education and Indian finance problems.

In 1891 Miss Nightingale finally laid aside her ambition to found at Oxford a Professorship in Applied Statistics. This relinquishment of active interest in the progress of statistics was indicative only of her failing physical powers. The gradual failure of sight, memory, and mental apprehension proceeded during the last fifteen years of her life. Her death occurred on August 13, 1910.

▬FLORENCE NIGHTINGALE AS STATISTICIAN

Florence Nightingale may well be assigned a position in the history of social statistics next to those occupied by Quetelet and Farr. Her ardent, genuine sympathy for the sick and distressed was greatly augmented by a positive genius for marshalling definite knowledge of the forces which make for disease and suffering. The same intellect which sharply separated the formulae, procedures, and practical methods of nursing from its abiding principles as one of the humanities, also discerned the statistical facts of sickness and other forms of disharmony between the individual and his environment. In hospital care of the sick, as an instance, Miss Nightingale replaced the astigmatic case viewpoint with one embodying a grasp of total situations. This is one function of statistics.

Her earnest perception of this truth—an essential in the equipment of the statistician—was firmly supported by her control over laborious detail and by her scrupulous care in testing the statistical foundations of her premises. The interpretations she placed upon the facts developed in her researches show a careful regard for the competent counsel which she so often consulted. In all these respects Miss Nightingale exhibited the prime qualities of one thoroughly versed in the art of preparing and reflectively analyzing social data.

Chapter 25

Outcomes: The Mainstay
of a Framework for Quality Care

DONNA AMBLER PETERS

Quality assurance, quality management, and quality improvement are
terms used to describe what nurses have always thought they were delivering—a system of quality nursing care. However, this may not always be the
case. Another factor, cost of care, is an issue more recently of concern to
community health nurses and their agencies. When these two issues are
reckoned with, how nursing care is planned, delivered, documented, and
evaluated must change. By using a conceptual framework for organizing all
the relevant practice components, such as professional standards, protocols, critical paths, and care plans, the delivery of quality care can be measured more effectively. Donna Peters presents such a framework in this
chapter that focuses on client outcomes and defines and incorporates all
the other essential elements that are used to reflect quality nursing care.

Paradigm, a word once used only by the educational elite, is becoming
more of a household term as society becomes increasingly aware of fundamental shifts that are occurring. A shift in paradigm means that people are
changing the way they view the world, that they are altering their fundamental assumptions about reality. For example, it used to be that patients
sought health care for an illness, a problem, to be fixed by a health care
practitioner, an expert. Now, clients or persons seek health care for an illness, a challenge, to be approached by a health care practitioner, a partner.[1]

This paradigm shift is further reflected in health care as the industry
moves from quality assurance to quality improvement and from fee for service to managed care. The philosophical differences are evident. For example, in home health care under current Medicare reimbursement, an
agency benefits most by maximizing the number of visits; under managed
care the benefit is in providing the service in as few visits as possible while
maintaining the same or better outcomes. Thus new ways of planning and
implementing care are appearing on the scene, including the concepts of
outcomes, guidelines, critical paths, and flowcharts. These concepts are
mingling with existing ideas, such as protocols, standards, and policies.

From *Journal of Nursing Care Quality* 10(1):61–69, 1995. Reprinted by permission of
Aspen Publisher, Inc.

The result is confusion, misinterpretation, inconsistent use, and questionable relevance. The real questions are: What do these concepts mean, and when and how do they all fit together in rendering quality care?

This article sorts out these concepts, defines them, and places them into a relevant picture or conceptual framework for quality care. The resulting configuration (Figure 25-1) is useful and appropriate for all client care, although the focus in this article is community care. The structure was inspired by a previous conceptual framework developed to enhance the quality assurance program at Johns Hopkins Hospital.[2, 3,]

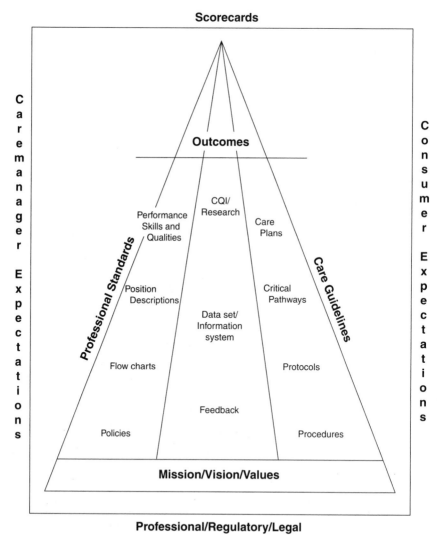

FIGURE 25-1   Organizing framework for quality care.

▬ELEMENTS IN A FRAMEWORK FOR QUALITY

A conceptual framework enhances the definition and understanding of client care. Using a common framework allows for the universal understanding and sharing of terminology and concepts, organizes the components of practice, facilitates the investigation and evaluation of the elements of care through quality management, assists in understanding the process of change, encourages participation, and promotes the effectiveness of quality management tools. It can be valuable in educating staff during times of change.

Multiple elements influence care and must be accounted for in a framework for quality care, although the most important element is the outcomes that are used to reflect quality. Other crucial elements are:

- the external environment that influences client care
- the mission/vision/values of the organization
- professional standards that define care manager behaviors
- care guidelines that define care management
- unifying tools that provide the opportunity to bring together professional and client/consumer viewpoints

The framework presented here encompasses excellence in both professional practice and management of care and delineates the unifying tools that bring these two sides into alignment. Thus it promotes the attainment of negotiated client/professional outcomes that are a true measure of professional accomplishment and quality care. Following is a more detailed examination of the key elements in the framework and how they contribute to the whole.

▬OUTCOMES

Outcomes are the conditions to be achieved and provide the backbone for organizing and managing care and quality in the age of paradigm shifts and health care reform. Specific outcomes provide for feedback during the process of rendering care. They indicate whether interventions are effective, how well standards are being met, and whether changes need to be made. The example of a guided missile can be used to illustrate the importance of outcomes. Guided missiles are programmed with their destination and then given constant feedback about whether they are on course. If they are on course, fine; if they are off course, they are given course corrections. If the destination is unknown or not programmed into the missile, however, there is no way to know whether the missile is off course, so there is no way to offer course corrections. So it is with outcomes. They are the picture of the destination of the client so that the effectiveness of the interventions can be monitored. If there is no agreed-upon picture of where the care is to take the client, there is no clear way to evaluate what is being done. If there are agreed-upon outcomes and the care being given is not bringing clients closer to their destinations, then changes can be made.[4]

Quality care can be evaluated in terms of professional outcomes, consumer outcomes, or shared outcomes. Professional outcomes are measured through the use of professional standards, and client outcomes are measured through the use of client care guidelines (see Figure 25-1). Quality outcomes, described in terms of the performance of the professional and the status of the client, are the result of the integration of professional standards and client care guidelines using identified unifying tools. It is these negotiated and agreed-upon outcomes that should be used to determine the caliber of performance of individuals and institutions and for which they should be held responsible.

▬EXTERNAL ENVIRONMENT

The external environment provides the context in which outcomes are met and activities such as client care occur. Under the old paradigm, cause and effect were used to explain relationships, and environment was not considered important because cause itself was seen as sufficient to explain an event. Under systems thinking in the new paradigm, however, the environment is crucial in explaining what is occurring (i.e., what outcomes are being measured and to what degree they are being met).

For care in the community, some of the critical factors in the environment are care manager expectations; consumer expectations; professional, regulatory, and legal directives; and score cards (see Figure 25-1). Each of these factors is discussed in more detail below.

Care managers include the professionals and any other formal health care providers involved in the care of the client. Professionals enter the health care system with their own expectations. Nurses, for example, have predetermined ideas about the provision of care, compensation, professional mobility, role autonomy, continuing education, and opportunities for recognition and advancement.[3] Physicians have expectations about the role of the nurse and other team members. Physical therapists expect certain equipment to be readily available. How closely compatible these care manager expectations are with each other and with the organization influences the quality of care.

Concurrently, the media blitz on health care reform and rising interest on the part of the consumer have produced more and more expectations of the system from the clients. Those expectations are influenced by media opinions on rising costs, diminishing resources, technological complexity, and ethical dilemmas and by previous exposure of self or friends to the system.[3] The closer these expectations are to the care provided, the higher the perception of quality.

Inherent in the environment are the regulatory and professional directives and legal mandates by which all within the health care system must abide. Examples include Medicare regulations, state licensing laws, nurse practice acts, accreditation standards, and reimbursement policies. Standards set by these regulatory groups usually focus on secondary or tangential aspects of quality (e.g., mortality and readmissions) not because they constitute quality but because they are measurable.[5] Even when they indicate that there is a problem, they fail to provide direction regarding the origination of the problem.[6]

Score cards or report cards are new to the environment and are about to become a powerful force in the health care system. Score cards are simply a set of measures that allow for a fast but comprehensive view of a business focusing on key concepts of quality.[7] In health care, agency score cards are envisioned to be available to consumers to facilitate the consumer's ability to make an informed choice for quality care. There is still much discussion about what items will be on the score cards, but more intrinsic, creative, and relevant measures of quality are what the consumer is seeking.

▬ MISSION/VISION/VALUES

To get people to work together, there must be a clear and well-defined shared vision or common identity, something agreed upon toward which the institution is striving. It is a description of what the future will look like if the institution meets the dreams of its collective leadership. It can be viewed as a projected composite outcome. For example, the vision of a managed care organization may be to have a healthy population in the geographical community it serves. When there is genuine vision, people excel and learn because they want to.[8] Without a predetermined shared vision, it is impossible to render care with any degree of organization because no one is clear about what he or she is seeking to create. Therefore, everyone goes ahead and creates what is important for him or her, never knowing whether this agrees with what everyone else is doing.

A shared vision is actually one part of the three governing ideas that provide the structure under which care is rendered within an enterprise. The other two governing ideas are mission and values.[8]

The mission of an organization is the unique contribution that the agency strives to make, or in other words why that organization exists. For example, the mission of a pediatric high-technology agency may be to improve the health of children. The mission provides the why that inspires the how. The missions of successful organizations encompass more than just providing for the needs of their owners and employees (e.g., a mission of financial viability is not enough); their sense of purpose includes a service to a defined population.[8, 9]

Values answer the question of how the persons in the organization want to act, consistent with the mission and along the path to achieve the vision. Values are the guiding stars that are used to navigate the path to the vision and to make the necessary decisions along the way.[8, 10] For example, behaviors will be different if an agency values seniority instead of equal opportunity for team members. One of the difficulties with a paradigm shift is a changing of values and the resulting confusion when differing values coexist in an agency at the same time. Therefore, it is important that agency values are clarified for all staff.

▰ PROFESSIONAL STANDARDS

Professional standards are authoritative statements by which the profession describes the responsibilities for which its practitioners are accountable. The effectiveness of these behaviors is measured through the achievement of professional outcomes. Standards may pertain to general or speciality practice.[11] In essence, they describe the expected care manager behavior in ways that allow for the evaluation of performance. Rather than defining a maximum (standards of excellence) or minimum level of performance, the American Nurses Association (ANA) is now defining standards in terms of competency.[11]

Although professional standards exist as discrete entities, such as the ANA standards of professional performance, they can be operationalized through policies, flow charts, position descriptions, and performance skills and qualities.

Policies represent the nonnegotiable aspects of practice and allow for no professional judgment or interpretation in their implementation. Because they are ironclad statements, there are usually few policies within an agency. Furthermore, because there is seldom an unalterable aspect of practice, policies tend to focus on the resources or conditions that are required to facilitate practice.[3] An example of a policy statement is: "All patients admitted to service will have a home visit within 12 hours of referral."

Flow charts depict the predetermined steps for key agency processes. Philosophically, both quality improvement and reengineering concepts assert that there are a limited number of key processes that are crucial to the organization of the agency. Diagramming the steps of these processes ensures that everyone knows the steps and also enables unnecessary steps to be eliminated. An example of an agency process that could be represented in a flow chart is scheduling.

Position descriptions reflect the qualifications and responsibilities for all persons within a position or job category. They reflect the competence, education, and experience of the professional role.[3] An example of a job category is public health nurse. The position description for a public health nurse within an agency would be the same regardless of individual professional differences or differences in practice settings (home or clinic).

Performance skills and qualities identify individual attributes that determine a specific level of performance based on knowledge and personal and professional development. These attributes are the capabilities and characteristics of staff that set each person apart from all others. In the emerging paradigm, they will become an agency's most important asset.

Examples of performance skills include any type of certifications or special knowledge, such as a second language. Performance qualities can include personal characteristics that may affect the relationship with the client. For example, whether a home health aide smokes may be important in placement in a client's home. Personal growth experiences can also be important; whether the care provider has experienced the death of someone close may be instrumental in assigning him or her to a dying client.

CARE GUIDELINES

Care guidelines are systematically developed statements to assist in determining how diseases, disorders, and other health conditions can be most effectively and appropriately prevented, diagnosed, treated, and clinically managed.[12] They are thought to promote the appropriate management of potential or defined health problems. The degree of appropriateness is measured through the attainment of client/consumer outcomes.

Because guidelines are recommendations rather than authoritative statements, they allow for more flexibility than standards. This flexibility is important for two reasons. First, there is little information regarding the enigma of client care and what interventions yield the best outcomes under what circumstances. Therefore, the ability to adjust care in accord with the amount of progress toward the client's expected outcome is significant. Second, the individuality of client/family response to care is great and has many intervening variables, so that it is impossible to predict all the potential events during an episode of care. Therefore, the ability to respond in various ways to these unique events is critical.

Like professional standards, care guidelines are operationalized at a more discrete level in the form of procedures, protocols, care plans, and critical pathways (see Figure 25-1).

Procedures are step-by-step outlines of how to perform a particular psychomotor skill. They are primarily task oriented and require both cognitive abilities and manual dexterity.[3] An example of a procedure is how to perform the task of removing sutures.

Protocols outline the steps to be taken in treating a certain condition. They establish a course of action to be taken in specific terms under specific conditions. There are three types of protocols defined by the need to involve the physician: dependent, interdependent, and independent.[3] An example of an independent protocol is the management of decubitus ulcers.

Critical paths comprise the predetermined care activities involved in a specific project (client care) from start to finish and the time to complete each of the activities. They are interdisciplinary guides to the usual treatment patterns for a group of clients with similar needs.[13] In health care, the expected outcome and intervening milestones to be attained by what date have been added to the activities (interventions) to provide a visual picture of the care to be rendered. These paths reflect the most appropriate path to take, not the perfect path. Within the critical path there is room for variance, mistakes, and corrections. In fact, it is impossible to eliminate all variation in care from the path. The intent is to reduce major course corrections (or changes in care) to more subtle and gentle ones.[9]

A critical pathway for a population with similar needs will consist of client problems, expected outcomes, and intermediate outcomes or milestones specified by visit or client day for an entire episode of care. Pathways incorporate generic guidelines and protocols into the care of a specific group of clients. Their value lies in agreement by the caregiving team on the critical steps involved in the care of a given group of clients and in their potential for decreasing the number of visits or length of time on service. In addition, by monitoring variance and what interventions are used to accomplish what milestones, or outcomes, changes can be made in the pathways to incorporate those interventions that work best, thus constantly improving care.

Care plans are critical pathways that have been individualized to meet the needs of a specific client. They are customized by deleting, modifying, or adding problems, outcomes, milestones, interventions, or time frames in the critical path for a generic client with the kinds of needs specified by that path. If there is no critical pathway available for a client, the care plan is developed for the client by adopting guidelines and protocols into that client's care. Such a care plan would include identified problems, expected outcomes with a time frame, possibly intermediate outcomes or milestones with time frames, and specific interventions to meet those outcomes.

▬UNIFYING TOOLS

The professional side of care (professional standards) and the client's side of care (care guidelines) are integrated by using certain identified tools. These critical tools include feedback, an information system that incorporates and builds a data set, and a system for continuous quality improvement and/or research. The purpose of these tools is to unify and improve on the professional standards and care guidelines to optimize the attainment of the agreed-upon client outcomes.

Feedback is essential to determine the expectations and needs of the internal (staff) and external customers and the strengths and weaknesses of the caregiving process. Client feedback measures how well client communication is occurring. Traditional client satisfaction is not sufficient; what is needed is a continuous system for gathering information through complaint solicitation, market service surveys, focus groups, and employee surveys.[14] The goal is to listen continually to what the customer says, to make clients a partner in their own care, and to make staff collaborators in how to provide quality services.

Making clients a partner in their own care requires proficiency in the following areas within the nursing process:

■ for assessment, the nurse must observe, explore the areas of need, and above all listen to what the client is really saying
■ for planning, the nurse must negotiate outcomes, interventions, and time frames with the client and explore resources that play a role in the circumstances
■ for interventions, the nurse must assign tasks and responsibilities with the caregiving team, including the client; confirm a commitment from

the client and others to fulfill those tasks and responsibilities; and teach, when necessary, how to accomplish those tasks

- for evaluation, the nurse tracks the variation from the established plan (critical path); renegotiates outcomes, interventions, and time frames with the client as necessary; establishes commitment to new or modified interventions; and terminates the care when outcomes are met

An information system with a consistent data set allows for the tracking and synthesis of care planned, care rendered, and variations that occurred during the process. It also allows for costs to be attached to each of the elements of care and tracked.

It is the foundation of a client classification system that measures intensity of need and classifies clients accordingly. Ultimately, it provides the capacity to understand which care alternative using what procedures and protocols achieves the best outcome at what cost using what care manager.

The information system is the data repository for information about the performance skills and qualities of the care manager and the care requirements of the client so that the two partners in care can be better matched. Ultimately, the abilities and experiences of the staff member need to match the unique requirements in the client care plan. The better the match, the more conducive the environment for meeting the agreed-upon outcomes in the shortest period of time.

Furthermore, the more comprehensive and detailed the data set and the information system, the more factual information the care manager will have to make knowledgeable decisions rather than blind selections or best guesses. The better the information system is understood and continually updated, the more quality client care will be defined by the actual caregiving process rather by the demands or regulations of the external environment. For example, if a managed care organization authorizes only three visits for a particular client, but the agency has information that shows historically that only three visits on this type of client results in a readmission, whereas six visits provides for optimal outcomes, the agency can strongly negotiate for the additional three visits.

The information system also is the infrastructure for quality improvement or research. The difference between these two concepts is often obscure, the most prevailing distinction being that research has a broader applicability, usually spanning more than one area or institution. Regardless, the tracking of variations provides information about which variations on standards, guidelines, or their integration are significant and require investigation for possible change and improvement. Organizing the data available, gathering additional data, and describing what the data say become the basis for solutions (or hypotheses), further learning, or demonstration of improved integrated processes of care and resulting outcomes.

Generating standards and guidelines that are constantly monitored and improved is the determinant for improving quality. The key to improving these standards and guidelines is outcomes. Outcomes provide the benchmarks for measurement that ascertain how well standards and guidelines are working. To do that, standards and guidelines must be used consistently. Therefore, policies, flow charts, job responsibilities, care plans, critical paths, and procedures must be well defined and integrated into agency operations. Measurements of outcome achievement using these components must take place internally by institution and also collectively among institutions to elicidate the strengths and weaknesses of the health care system. It is these outcome measurements that will move health care to its next level of quality.

In this time of rapid change and shifting of beliefs, it is important to have a picture or conceptual framework to assist in our understanding of the world. This article has presented such a picture in the shape of a framework for quality care. The mainstay of this framework is outcomes. Other components include the external environment, shared visions, professional standards, care guidelines, and tools for unifying the patient and care manager perspectives and for improving care. Understanding the components of client care and the tools required to integrate care with professional standards provides care managers the best opportunity for maintaining quality.

▬REFERENCES

1. Cassidy, C.M. "Social Science Theory and Methods in the Study of Alternate and Complementary Medicine." *Journal of Alternative and Complementary Medicine* 1 (1995): 19–40.
2. Peters, D.A. "An Example of an Existing Quality Assurance Program: A Hospital-Based Agency." In *Assurance in Home Care,* edited by C. Meisenheimer. Gaithersburg, Md.: Aspen, 1988.
3. Poe, S.S., and Will, J.C. "Quality Nursing-Patient Outcomes: A Framework for Nursing Practice." *Journal of Nursing Quality Assurance* 2 (1987): 29–37.
4. Peters, D.A. "Strategic Directions for Using Outcomes." *Remington Report* 11, (1994): 9–11.
5. Vladek, B.C. "Quality Assurance through External Controls." *Inquiry* 25 (1988): 100–107.
6. Berwick, D.M., Godfrey, A.R., and Roessner, J. *Curing Health Care—New Strategies for Quality Improvement.* San Francisco, Calif.: Jossey-Bass, 1990.
7. Kaplan, R.S., and Norton, D.P. "The Balanced Scorecard—Measures That Drive Performance." *Harvard Business Review* 70 (1992): 71–79.
8. Senge, P.M. *The Fifth Discipline: The Art and Practice of the Learning Organization.* New York, N.Y.: Doubleday, 1990.
9. Garfield, C.A. Peak Performers. New York, N.Y.: Avon, 1986.
10. Covey, S. *The Seven Habits of Highly Effective People.* New York, N.Y.: Simon & Schuster, 1989.
11. American Nurses Association. *Standards of Clinical Nursing Practice.* Washington, D.C.: American Nurses Association, 1991.
12. American Nurses Association. "Task Force on Nursing Practice Standards and Guidelines: Working Paper." *Journal of Nursing Quality Assurance* 5 (1991): 1–17.
13. Hofmann, P.A. "Critical Path Method: An Important Tool for Coordinating Clinical Care." *Journal on Quality Improvement* 19 (1993): 235–246.
14. Berry, L. L., Parasuraman. A., and Zeithaml, V.A. "Improving Services Quality in America: Lessons Learned." *Academy of Management Executive* 8 (1994): 32–44.

Chapter 26

Case Management and Nursing Practice

ANN RHEAUME   SARA FRISCH

ANNE SMITH   CAROLINE KENNEDY

Case management, a system of assessing clients and families, planning and establishing outcomes of care delivered by other health care providers, delivering care or by delegating, coordinating, and collaborating with an interdisciplinary team, and monitoring care and outcomes, is a current model being used in the managed care arena of health care delivery systems in North America. Many agencies are adopting this model as a framework for nursing care delivery and it is becoming an accepted framework of practice. Does adopting a case management model alter nursing practice? The authors of this chapter examine the effect case management has on nurse–client relationships and nurse–colleague relationships. Relationships may not always be trouble free if the case manager's role is not understood clearly by client and colleague. Based on a literature review of case management and interviews with community-based nurses, the authors explore case management as a vehicle to achieve professionalism.

Case management is becoming an accepted framework of practice within the nursing community, as evidenced by its endorsement by prominent groups, such as the American Nurses Association.[1] Although there are various case management models, the core elements usually include an individual who coordinates and monitors care given to clients by multiple services. The use of case management is based partly on the assumption that people with complex health problems need assistance in using the healthcare system effectively. Nurses are adopting case management across community and hospital settings in an attempt to decrease service fragmentation and improve the quality of care for people who require numerous or long-term health services.

The proliferation of nursing articles on case management in the past few years reflects nurses' interest in this approach. However, many authors present case management as a panacea and do not ask how using this model affects nurse care giver roles and relationships. We examine the effects case management can have on nurse–client and nurse–colleague re-

From *Journal of Nursing Administration* 24(3):30–36, 1994. Reprinted by permission of Lippincott-Raven Publishers.

lationships within community settings. The link between case management and the pursuit of professionalism in nursing practice is also explored.

METHODS

The purpose of the project was to examine case management and its usefulness to Canadian community health service agencies. We sought information from several sources. Literature was identified by searching computerized databases and following up on references in the retrieved articles. Unpublished information, primarily internal documents or reports from existing programs, was also sought, although not much was obtained. Finally, interviews were conducted with 17 nurses who were practicing case management in publicly supported community-based agencies across Canada. Our working definition of case management for this project was a model in which the case manager assesses clients and families, plans and establishes the outcomes of care with other healthcare providers, provides the care directly or by delegation, coordinates and collaborates with an interdisciplinary team, and monitors care and outcomes.[2] More than half of the nurses interviewed were not officially designated case managers; however, all of the nurses viewed themselves as case managers and met our definition of case management practices. In addition, many of the home care programs were in the process of developing case management frameworks with their healthcare workers.

Project resources allowed us to record telephone interviews with nurses from at least one program in each Canadian province and the Yukon. Seven interviews were conducted with nurses working in Montreal-area community health and social service centers (local community service center [CLSC]). Interviews lasted from 30 to 90 minutes. Data were summarized from the tape recordings and integrated with the findings from the published and unpublished material.

CASE MANAGEMENT
AND THE NURSE–CLIENT RELATIONSHIP

Nurse–client relationships usually are discussed within the framework of primary care giver roles in community and hospital settings. Case management, however, assumes that some primary care giving will be exchanged for care coordination roles. Although certain care coordination responsibilities always have been a part of community-based nursing, service provision rather than service coordination usually has been the central component of nurses' practice.[3, 4]

SERVICE COORDINATION AND PROVISION

The case manager has many care coordination responsibilities, including service coordination and monitoring.[1, 5] Service coordination is defined as the linkage of clients to service providers in the community, and involves the processing of referral forms, delegation of tasks to other healthcare workers, and coordination of interventions with the client. The delegation of tasks may include delegating many or all primary care giver roles to other nurses while maintaining case manager responsibilities; "the nurse case manager ... may carry out the remaining aspects of case management while arranging for other nurses to provide the necessary nursing care.[1(p1)]

Whether delegation occurs in practice varies according to situational factors, such as type of case management model, accompanying role responsibilities, service provision, and the client organization relationship. For example, in the brokerage model, case managers do not provide any direct services to clients other than case management services.[3] Direct services are provided to clients by other agencies, associations, or groups. The case manager acts as a broker, linking clients to other service providers (e.g., medicine, social work, nursing), but does not provide care. In contrast, the casework model is characterized by case managers who provide the most care to clients. Delegation occurs to others within the same agency instead of to outside organizations.

In essence, case management has the potential to shift the usual nursing roles of community nurses; service coordination roles may expand and primary care giver roles may decrease. Some of the more well-known nurse case manager models reflect these dimensions.[6, 7] Nurse case managers in the Nursing Network have multiple coordinating responsibilities that enable them to move with their clients from the hospital to the community setting.[7] Nursing care can be given by the nurse case manager or delegated to associate nurses or nurse practitioners.

Several of the nurse case managers interviewed delegated all or some nursing care to other nurses. Caseloads from our study ranged from 5 to 450 clients. Nurse case managers who had large caseloads did not provide direct hands-on care to their clients. They usually assigned physical care to other nursing colleagues involved in the community, such as public health nurses. These nurse case managers appeared to operate under the brokerage model described previously. On the other hand, nurse case managers with small caseloads usually gave some primary care to their clients. Routine nursing care was often delegated to public health nurses; more complex tasks were maintained by the nurse case managers.

▬SERVICE MONITORING

Another care coordination responsibility within case management is service monitoring.[1] Service monitoring involves ensuring that the client receives the agreed on services. At times, this entails supervising other healthcare workers. Furthermore, many case managers are part of a multidisplinary team that they coordinate or manage.

A respondent from the present study described this aspect of her role. The nurse case manager indicated that she spent a great deal of time contacting agencies involved with her client to instigate or monitor care given by other service providers. She worked in a home care program in which the healthcare workers were given clients according to their own skills and expertise. As a result of this system, this nurse case manager spent more time in her office accessing other service providers and less time giving nursing care to her clients.

■NURSE–CLIENT RELATIONSHIPS

Ultimately, the case manager's coordination roles may influence the nature of nurse–client relationships. Although there presently are no studies examining this issue, a review of the nursing literature enables us to draw some conclusions. First, the abundance of articles on nurse–client relationships within the nursing literature demonstrates the high value placed on these relationships by both nurse theorists and researchers. Peplau's conceptualization of nursing in the 1950s laid the groundwork for further research regarding the interactive relationship between these care givers and their clients.[8] Other interactive theorists, such as Travelbee and Orlando, have also made interpersonal relationships between nurses and clients a central part of their theories.[9, 10] This continuing interest in nurse–client relationships reflects the belief that a special type of relationship must be established for nurses to become successful in healing and promoting their clients' health. Bonding is the term often used to describe this particular relationship.

Second, recent studies examining the development of nurse–client relationships have identified several variables that affect the nature of these relationships.[11, 12] Morse[12] used the grounded theory approach to analyze 86 interviews with nurses from different specialty areas ranging from hospital to community settings to learn more about the nature of the nurse–client relationship. Morse concluded that the relationship between nurses and their clients is initially superficial and develops to one that is agreed on covertly by both parties. It develops according to situational circumstances, such as the needs or desires of the nurse and patient, or the length of time the nurse and patient are together. Four mutual relationships were identified, ranging from clinical relationships (where interactions between the nurse and client are superficial) to over-involved relationships (where the attachment between nurse and client is at a very intense level). Outside variables that made relationship formation more difficult and increased fragmentation of care included the number of care givers treating the client, the specialization within the nursing profession that can interrupt therapeutic bonding, and the amount of time that the nurse, as a primary care giver, can spend with the client.

The following two themes are emerging from the nursing literature on nurse-client relationships: 1) many nurses view the therapeutic interaction between nurse and client as the essence of nursing; and 2) the development of this relationship is dynamic and influenced by outside variables. Although part of the nurse case manager's mandate is to decrease service duplication and service fragmentation, the presence of one creates another healthcare worker with whom the client must deal. The delegation of some nursing care roles to other nurses while maintaining other nursing responsibilities also may contribute to fragmentation of care. Given the nature of case managers' coordination responsibilities, the development of a therapeutic relationship with clients may be more difficult to achieve.

Although the nurse case manager may have a positive impact on client health outcomes, it may be unrealistic to expect all nurse case managers to achieve the kind of relationship that primary care giver nurses have with their clients. In fact, nurses who gave primary care to clients while working alongside nurse case managers may be in better positions to develop therapeutic relationships with their clients. The caring relationship described in the literature that bonds nurse and client may be replaced under case management by a more formal relationship that may also benefit the client, but in a different way.

▬COLLEGIAL RELATIONSHIPS AND CASE MANAGEMENT

Case managers deal regularly with other healthcare providers as part of their mandate; the most frequent contact is with physicians, social workers, and other nurses. Effective case management occurs when healthcare workers share power with others and do not dominate or allow themselves to be dominated by other disciplines. This, of course, represents an idealistic way of practicing that may be difficult for all healthcare workers to achieve.

Healthcare Workers

Case management has the potential to alter fundamentally the usual lines of authority between nurses and physicians. This occurs because the nurse case manager may have the mandate to plan total client care, coordinate and monitor other service providers, and evaluate care given without physician supervision or consent. In essence, this mandate provides nurses with an expanded power base. The relationship between nurse case managers and physicians appears to evolve over many years. Several respondents in the present study described difficulties with physician relationships at the beginning of their case management practice. During the beginning phases, physicians were often skeptical about the nurse case managers' mandate. The nurse case managers had to work hard to establish their credibility with physicians and counteract this skepticism. Eventually, collaborative, supportive relationships were established between both healthcare workers, although older physicians often had more difficulty accommodating to the nurse's new role as case manager.

Although the literature describes most professional relationships under case management as collaborative, there are occasional difficulties encountered. Problems between hospital discharge planners and case managers in community settings were cited in some studies.[13, 14] Discharge planners felt that case management was job duplication, and were concerned that case managers would supplant them. Bremer's study on the Block Nurse Program in Oregon suggests that nurses credibility with physicians depended on the nurses' knowledge of healthcare, the formal social service system, program eligibility criteria, client health problems, and the nurses' communication skills.[6]

Team Settings

Our interviews with nurses in Quebec enabled us to examine more closely the relationship changes occurring within the context of nurses practicing case management in the local community service centers. There are currently 159 centers located in different regions of Quebec providing primary care, such as healthcare and social services. The centers develop programs to meet the needs of the community that they serve. As a result of changing population demographics, many of the centers' programs are geared to meeting the needs of the aging population. Local community service centers are funded by the provincial government and services are free of charge to the client. These services are part of the broader Quebec healthcare system.

The nurse case managers in these centers practice within a multidisciplinary team setting usually consisting of a social worker, physician, physiotherapist, and other nurses. Client plans of care are discussed between the nurse case manager and other team members during regularly held meetings at the center. The nurse case manager provides some nursing services to the client at home and coordinates the care of other service providers involved with the client. All nurse case managers regarded their relationship with other team members positively, indicating that they were open, informal, collaborative, and supportive. These centers were established in 1972, and the relationships among healthcare workers have developed over the past 20 years.

In the mid 1980s, Grau expressed concern with the growing use of case management teams, fearing that nurses may not be treated as equal team members and not emerge as frequently as primary case managers because of other team members' struggle for power.[4] There is no documented evidence of this power struggle between nurses and other healthcare workers in the nursing literature. Also, there was no sense that this situation occurred for the nurses and other team members in the CLSC setting. In fact, one respondent indicated that she recently asked a social worker to become her client's primary case manager because the client had multiple social problems that matched the social worker's expertise. The nurse case manager in this clinic indicated that it is not uncommon for clients to be shared by a team of nurse and social worker if their problems are both physical and psychosocial.

Relationships with other healthcare workers can be troublesome if the case manager's role is not understood clearly. This is even a potential problem in relationships with other nurses. For example, conflict might occur because of perceived duplication of services between nurse case managers and other nurses. A respondent from our study who worked in a small home care program described how she worked with the public health nurses to resolve difficulties that arose in the overlap of their work and her position as case manager. Boundaries of expertise were delineated between the nurse case manager and public health nurses to avoid duplication of services.

The delineation of boundaries resulted in public health nurses focusing on the younger population in the community and the case managers focusing on the elderly population. Short-term interventions were handed over to the public health nurses, whereas long-term care and follow-up were done by nurse case managers. Eventually, a system that enabled both groups of nurses to communicate with each other on a regular basis regarding client needs and care was developed. In this situation, the nurse case managers and public health nurses had overlapping roles. Although the extent of overlap is difficult to assess, it was significant enough for both parties to define clear boundaries. The choice was to divide the client population into two groups, rather than a task-based division of labor.

Overall, case management appears to improve the quality of working relationships with other healthcare workers. The literature on case management and the interviews with our respondents indicate that egalitarian collegial relationships are possible under case management. The pursuit of a collaborative practice with other healthcare workers has always been an issue with nurses. Case management appears to be the most current way of making this collaborative practice happen.

CASE MANAGEMENT AND THE PURSUIT OF PROFESSIONALISM

The endorsement of case management by nurses is reminiscent of the widespread support given to primary nursing in the 1980s. Although this study looked at community-based management and much of the primary nursing literature is hospital-based, parallels can be drawn between both approaches. Both models are intended to enhance personal and professional autonomy within nursing practice. For the leaders of nursing, these models facilitate the redefinition of nursing from a semiprofessional occupation to a full-fledged profession. For nurses, practicing according to these models promises more autonomy over working conditions. This section explores the adoption of primary nursing and case management as strategies to achieve professionalism.

The distinction between professions and occupations has been proposed by several social scientists. Goode[15] identified two key characteristics of a profession—prolonged training in a body of specialized knowledge and a collectivity or service orientation. Freidson[16] took these concepts further and concluded that autonomy in defining and organizing work were essential to professionalism. This last criterion, professional autonomy, has been difficult for nursing to achieve.

Nurses have also examined autonomy. Schutzenhofer[17] states that autonomy has been difficult for nurses to achieve because of a combination of female and nursing socialization experiences. She argues that changes are necessary in the academic and clinical setting to foster professional autonomy. Singleton and Nail[18] state that nurses often do not exercise the autonomy they have within clinical settings. Furthermore, complete autonomy within the hospital is difficult to attain, given the nature of the hospital organization and interdependence of healthcare workers.

Although Manthey[19] introduced primary nursing as a work modality to improve quality of nursing care, primary nursing soon became viewed as a vehicle to achieve both personal and professional autonomy. Autonomy in the work place was achieved through nurses gaining control over nursing decisions regarding their primary patients, ". . . autonomy and authority for patient care decisions are best delegated to the (primary) nurse who knows the most about the individual patient provided that the nurse is a professional nurse with expertise in assessment, care planning, care giving, and care evaluation."[20(p1)] Primary nursing was considered a professional model of practice because it encompassed the concepts of accountability, collaboration, and autonomy. It also supported a more advanced educational background and knowledge-based practice. Although primary nursing encouraged the move toward professional status, nurses still do not possess the mandate to define and organize all of their work, as stated by Freidson, within the hospital setting. Physicians and hospital administrators play a large role in nurses' day-to-day practice.

Nurses view primary nursing as a panacea—it is described as a way of reaching all of nursing's long-term goals. It is beyond the scope of this article to examine critically all the alleged merits of primary nursing; nonetheless, it has been cited as a way of dealing with problematic issues, such as costs of healthcare, patient satisfaction levels, quality of care outcomes, job satisfaction among nurses, and the attainment of professional status. Primary nursing is not only identified as a solution to nursing problems, but as the solution to the ailments of the healthcare system. Given this perspective, it is not surprising that few studies have examined primary nursing more critically.

Case management is viewed as another way of enhancing nurses' professionalism by encouraging the acquisition of specialized knowledge and autonomy within practice. Qualification for nurses practicing case management are fairly high. The American Nurses Association recommends the baccalaureate degree with several years of clinical experience as the minimum requirement for nurse case managers.[1] There is also unanimous support for the acquisition of special knowledge for nurses related to case management, community services, and the target population. In fact, the University of Kansas School of Nursing has developed an educational program to assist nurses to become case managers.[5] Autonomy in the practice setting is encouraged through the nurse case manager's mandate to plan and coordinate all aspects of client care (without this practice being restricted to nursing care alone). The structure in which the case manager works enables this autonomous type of practice. Thus, case management also appears to encourage professionalism.

The respondents in our study were asked about the skills and qualifications needed for case management. Reflecting the characteristics of professionalism, the most frequently mentioned qualifications were initiative, autonomy, managerial and organizational skills, dynamism, and communication skills. Several of the respondents also felt that a baccalaureate degree in nursing should be a minimum requirement for a case manager and that special knowledge of the target population were extremely important.

Case management has been cited as a way to improve quality care, enhance client quality of life, improve nurses' satisfaction levels, and contain healthcare costs.[1] These long-term goals are identical to those expressed for primary nursing. Although much of the recent nursing literature claims that use of case management enables nursing to accomplish these goals, there was no consistent evidence in the literature reviewed for its cost-effectiveness or connection to improved client outcomes.[21] Could nursing be trying, once again, to accomplish the difficult task of reconciling issues of healthcare costs, quality healthcare, and professionalism this time through case management?

■ CONCLUSION

This article explored the ramifications case management can have on nursing practice. On one hand, case management has the potential to make more nurses become administrators of care rather than care givers themselves. This may change the central position that therapeutic relationships have had within nursing practice. On the positive side, case management may actually make collaborative practice with other healthcare workers feasible. Nurses are given the structural support necessary to overcome the subordinate role usually allocated to them in the healthcare system.

Case management, whether practiced in the community setting or hospital setting, is not an extension of primary nursing. But, the development of case management is not unlike that of primary nursing a decade ago. Regardless of whether case management alters quality of care, nurses should evaluate more carefully how it effects nursing practice and whether it truly forwards nurses' quest for professional status.

■ REFERENCES

1. American Nurses Association Task Force on Case Management in Nursing. *Nursing Case Management.* Kansas City, MO: American Nurses Association: 1988. Publication No. NS–32.
2. Frisch S, Smith A, Kennedy C, et al. *Nursing Case Management: A Model of Community-Based Health Services Delivery for the Elderly* (unpublished manuscript). Montreal; 1991.
3. Stanhope M. Lancaster J. *Community Health Nursing.* 3rd ed. St. Louis: Mosby Yearbook; 1992.
4. Grau L. Case management and the nurse. *Geriatr Nurs.* 1984; 5(8):372–375.
5. Wahlstedt P, Balser W. Nurse case management for the frail elderly: a curriculum to prepare nurses for that role. *Home Health Care Nurse.* 1986; 4(2):30–35.
6. Bremer A. A description of community health nursing practice with the community-based elderly. *J Community Health Nurs.* 1989; 6(3):173–184.
7. Ethridge P, Lamb GS. Professional nursing case management improves quality, access and costs. *Nurs Manage.* 1989; 20(3):30–35.
8. Peplau H. *Interpersonal Relations in Nursing.* New York: GP Putnam's Sons; 1952.

9. Travelbee J. *Interpersonal Aspects of Nursing.* 2nd ed. Philadelphia: FA Davis Co; 1971.
10. Orlando IJ: *The Dynamic Nurse-Patient Relationship.* New York: GP Putman's Sons; 1961.
11. Ramos MC. The nurse-patient relationship: theme and variations. *J Adv Nurs.* 1992; 17:496–506.
12. Morse JM. Negotiating commitment and involvement in the nurse-patient relationship. *J Adv Nurs.* 1991; 16:455–468.
13. MacAdam M. Capitman J, Yee D, et al. Case management for frail elders: the Robert Wood Johnson Foundation's program for hospital initiatives in long-term care. *Gerontologist.* 1989; 29(6):737–744.
14. Quinn J, Segal J, Raisz H, Johnson C. *Coordinating Community Services for the Elderly.* New York: Springer Pub Co; 1982.
15. Goode WJ. The profession: reports and opinion. *Am Sociol Rev.* 1961; 25:902–914.
16. Freidson E. *Profession of Medicine.* New York: Dodd, Mead; 1970.
17. Schutzenhofer KK. The problem of professional autonomy in nursing. *Health Care for Women International.* 1988; 9:93–106.
18. Singleton EK, Nail FC. Autonomy in nursing. *Nurs Forum.* 1984; 21(3):123–130.
19. Manthey M. *The Practice of Primary Nursing.* 1st ed. Boston: Blackwell Scientific Publications; 1980.
20. Marram G, Barrett MW, Bevis EO. *Primary Nursing—A Model for Individualized Care.* St. Louis: CV Mosby Co; 1979.
21. Weissert WG, Cready CM, Pawelak JE. The past and future of home-and community-based long-term care. *Milbank Q.* 1988; 66(2):309–388.

Chapter 27

Nurse Practitioners and Community Health Nurses: Clinical Partnerships and Future Visions

MELINDA L. JENKINS   EILEEN M. SULLIVAN-MARX

In restructuring our health care system, innovative practice models are emerging. What they look like is varied and several are described elsewhere in this text. One model of care, the clinical partnership between community health nurses and nurse practitioners, is a unique model that promotes a partnership between one of the oldest nursing disciplines with one of the newest, enhancing client access to primary care nursing in community-based settings. A primary care delivery pyramid is presented, with principles of public health science at its foundation. At a second level are community nursing centers for traditional population-based care for the healthy and ill. Home care and nursing home care is at a third level with medical management and acute and critical care at the top of the pyramid. A future vision of these authors is a system of care in the community where the necessity for physician approval for payment is removed and nurses coordinate and refer between nursing systems for care—a system from which clients and society would benefit.

Nurse practitioners (NPs) are advanced practice nurses who provide personal health care with a community health focus. They are autonomous expert community health nurses who promote health and prevent disease in the population while diagnosing and managing individual patient problems. NPs and community health nurses need to work together to define care settings and services that will ensure continuity of care for individuals and population groups in the new American health system.

Community health nurses have traditionally specialized in providing preventive services to an aggregate population. Such services include case management, teaching, and counseling aimed at health promotion and disease prevention. Principles of health promotion are integral to primary care. It is not surprising, therefore, to find the historical roots of primary care NPs grounded in public and community health nursing.[26]

In today's system of health care, however, there is a strain between primary care NPs and community health nurses. The strain is caused by a

From *Nursing Clinics of North America* 29(3):459–470, 1994. Reprinted by permission of W. B. Saunders Company.

disease-oriented "health" delivery system that emphasizes disease cure rather than disease prevention and health. This disease emphasis focuses on episodes of illness and shifts power and authority toward the medical discipline. As a result, control of practice and financial payments for integrated preventive and curative services provided by NPs or community health nurses often hinge on a physician's signature.

Direct payment for nursing case management and direct payment to primary care NPs is needed to ensure access to care. Why are nurses not paid directly for case management? How did preventive and curative care become divided? What must be done to create direct consumer access to community health nurses? An explanation is found in history.

▬PREVENTION VERSUS CURE:
LESSONS FROM HISTORY

Starr[21] details the social development of the American medical system. According to Starr, a split between public and private health care occurred in the 1920s with the "artificial separation of diagnosis from treatment, and more generally, of preventive from curative medicine . . . [resulting in] the 'fragmentation' of the medical system" (p 196). Physicians sanctioned public payment for the identification of problems but fought to reserve private physician payment for treatment of problems. Thus, well-baby, school health, and geriatric screening sites were maintained and administered by public health nurses. Only a few treatments, notably for sexually transmitted diseases and tuberculosis, were funded as public services because of perceived risks to the public at large.

At the same time, disease-oriented scientific medicine was raised as the standard in the United States. Physicians set up a system of professional authority in health care, regulating professional education and licensure and consumer purchase of patent medicines.[21]

From 1900 to 1930, public health nurses were involved in the disintegration of prevention and cure as these functions were segregated by public and private payers.[7] At the turn of the century, most preventive programs were privately funded and initiated by voluntary visiting nurse societies caring for both the sick and the well in the community. A case management process was undoubtedly used to integrate prevention and cure for complex physical, psychosocial, and environmental needs of low-income patients and families.

Even though most preventive programs were initiated by nurses, the authority for these endeavors was taken over by public health departments or boards of education that were careful not to treat illness in order to avoid antagonizing local physicians. Visiting nurses were left with the care of the sick at home. Payment sources were also split. Public monies and charities paid for preventive education and screening. Funds for visits to the sick were provided first by urban lady philanthropists and later by insurance companies and Medicare.[6,7]

Private health insurance flourished after 1930. In 1934, the American Medical Association (AMA) stipulated that "all features of medical service in any method of medical practice should be under the control of the medical profession"[21] (p 299). Efforts to provide prepaid comprehensive and preventive health care, similar to "primary health care" or "managed care" today, were repeatedly sabotaged by the medical profession and eventually outlawed in most states.[21]

In the 1960s, public programs such as Medicare, Medicaid, and community health centers were begun as strategies to increase access to health care. NPs were created in an effort to boost the supply of primary care providers, especially for underserved groups. In 1965, when the first pediatric nurse practitioner program was initiated, nurses gained "the opportunity to reclaim ground they had lost in the 1930s when the American Academy of Pediatrics claimed all of well child care for pediatricians"[11] (p 288). Unfortunately, most insurers at the time, including Medicaid, did not pay for well-child or well-adult care. Moreover, beneficiaries of Medicaid and Medicare were limited in their access to the services of NPs, because NPs were not reimbursable providers in these or other third-party-payer systems. This is still largely true today.

PAYMENT FOR HEALTH CARE

In 1966, AMA developed the current procedural terminology (CPT) codes that have become the framework for all billing claims in the United States.[1] The AMA, in contractual agreement with the Health Care Financing Administration (HCFA), classifies and assigns values for specific CPT codes used by physician and "nonphysician" providers. Consequently, the AMA controls classification of services for *all* provider services billed under Medicare and other insurers.

In December 1992, the AMA, under direction from the HCFA, created the Health Care Professional Advisory Committee (HCPAC). Providers other than physicians who used the CPT codes for billing are represented in the HCPAC (nursing is included) and have input into the review of CPT codes and the relative value scale for services provided by their respective disciplines. This is a unique opportunity for nursing to review and possibly add codes that reflect the work of nurses.

Currently, the CPT code for case management, a common service provided by both community health nurses and NPs, is under review by the HCFA and the AMA.[14] Organized nursing is responding by defining the nature of case management as nurses' work and emphasizing the need for direct payment to nurses for this work. Autonomy of nursing practice will be ensured through defining case management practice and being directly paid for the service.

CURRENT CHALLENGES TO PAYMENT REFORM

Health care costs rapidly escalated after Medicare and Medicaid were enacted in 1965. Because physician specialists, billing with CPT codes, received more money from Medicare for services provided, there was an incentive for physicians to become specialists, continuing the rise of costs. In an attempt to control costs, the Physician Payment Review Commission (PPRC) was established by Congress in 1986. A nurse has had a seat on the PPRC since its inception. The PPRC recommended sweeping changes in Medicare payment for physicians that were legislated in the Omnibus Budget Reconciliation Act of 1989 (OBRA-89).[16]

OBRA-89 established the Resource Based Relative Value Scale (RBRVS) fee schedule for Medicare payments. Payment under the RBRVS schedule is based on work effort, regardless of provider specialty.[22] Cognitive efforts, as well as specialized procedures, are recognized. The American Nurses Association (ANA), under the principle of equal pay for equal work, has lobbied for NP reimbursement under RBRVS to be the same as that of physicians.[3] Unfortunately, NPs do not currently receive direct reimbursement under Medicare unless they are working in rural areas. OBRA-89 mandates direct Medicaid payment to family NPs and pediatric NPs. New Medicaid managed care plans, however, do not always include NPs as directly paid primary care providers and gatekeepers.

Payment policies provide many of the incentives for patients and providers in health care. Historically, preventive services were separated from illness care and not readily reimbursed, therefore, they were seldom sought and seldom provided. The challenge today is to restructure both health care financing and delivery to integrate preventive and curative care. NPs and community health nurses, the original case managers, are well equipped for that challenge. Clinical partnerships between NPs and community health nurses are essential to the provision of coordinated, comprehensive care.

■ CASE MANAGEMENT AND CLINICAL PARTNERSHIPS

Case management is the gatekeeper activity required by primary care providers under managed care. It is central to the provision of continuous and comprehensive primary care, but it has been obscured by a focus on specialty medical care. The essence of case management dictates that a consistent provider coordinates a clinical data base to ensure follow-up, consultation, referral, and advocacy as needed for an individual client. Primary care NPs, with education in the principles of community health, communication skills, holistic assessment, and intervention techniques are extremely well suited to direct case management.

The major outcomes of case management are "(1) the integration of services across a cluster of organizations . . . ; and (2) achieving continuity of care"[19] (p 11). The goals of case management are "to provide quality health care, decrease fragmentation, enhance the client's quality of life, and contain costs."[1] There is tension inherent in case management between "dual sets of goals—one set related to service quality, effectiveness, and service coordination; and the other set related to goals of accountability and cost-effective use of resources"[31] (p 2). Clinical partnerships between community health nurses and NPs can ease this tension and provide an improved quality of care.

Besides case management skills, nurse practitioners have advanced preparation to provide primary care independently. NPs are educated to gather information from the patient and family, perform a physical examination, and interpret laboratory tests. Based on the information obtained, diagnoses and plans are made and implemented in collaboration with the patient and family. Interventions employed by an NP include treatment, education, counseling, and monitoring. Interventions over time are evaluated and adjusted as part of holistic case management that integrates the physical, psychosocial, and environmental realities facing the patient and family. The American Nurses' Association defines advanced practice nursing to include: nurse practitioners, nurse midwives, clinical nurse specialists and nurse anesthetists (Table 27-1).

NPs and nurse midwives in primary care provide care comparable in quality to physicians' care while offering superior health education and follow-up with significant cost savings.[10] Related costs of diagnostic tests and medications have been lower in NP care. Future costs savings were averted through prevention of repeat teenage pregnancies and low-birth-weight infants.[10]

A clinical partnership between community health nurses and NPs is a powerful strategy to promote high-quality health care delivery. To borrow

TABLE 27-1   Scope of Practice*

ACTIVITIES	PRIMARY CARE NP	COMMUNITY HEALTH NURSE
Community roles	Assessment; group education, support, and screening; collaborate with community agencies	Assessment; group education, support, and screening; collaborate with community agencies
Relationship with patient/family	First contact, comprehensive, coordinated, longitudinal, preventive/acute/chronic care	Home care—continuous through an illness episode; ambulatory care—longitudinal within a defined community
Assessment of patient/family	Comprehensive history and physical examination, medical and nursing diagnosis	Basic history and physical examination, nursing diagnosis
Intervention with patient/family	Prescribe medications, diagnostic studies, nonpharmacologic treatments; educate, counsel case management—refer to community nurse as needed monitor and evaluate treatment	Prescribe nonmedical treatments, educate, counsel, case management—consult with/refer to primary care nurse practitioner; monitor and evaluate treatment
Payment issues	Direct payment/reimbursement to individual provider; contract with agency	Indirect—payment/reimbursement to agency when authorized by primary care provider

*Overlap acknowledged

a phrase from Doris Haire, who questioned modern childbirth practices, we have experienced a "culture warping" of health care.[13] Expensive, specialized medical care has been paid for and used while primary care in the community has not. Most of the money is directed to the fewest people. About 70% of American physicians are specialists, while 85% of health care needs are for primary care services. The vast majority of these primary care needs can be met effectively by advanced practice nurses in community health.

▬ A NURSING MODEL OF HEALTH CARE DELIVERY

A restructured health care system will enhance consumer access to primary care nursing services in community-based settings. Funding advanced practice nurses to deliver primary care services and case management would increase care at the community level and provide continuity of care between levels. Figure 27-1 presents a graphic representation of a pyramid of primary health care delivery based on population needs for access to appropriate health care.

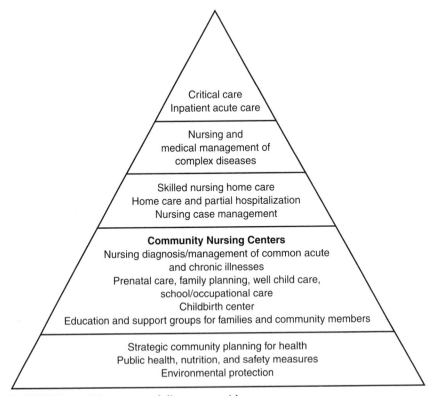

FIGURE 27-1   Primary care delivery pyramid.

Public Health Services

At the base of the pyramid are the elements of its foundation: public health nursing, epidemiology, primary prevention, community program planning, and a focus on the sociopolitical dimensions of illness. Environmental health and safety, occupational safety and health, planning for child health programs on a national level, planning interventions to decrease the disparities in infant mortality, and assuring more equal opportunity for health on behalf of all Americans are goals at this level. Strategic planning at community as well as state and national levels begins the journey to implement Healthy People 2000 objectives (Table 27-2).

Community Nursing Centers

At the second level of the pyramid are community nursing centers, the heart of primary care delivery. Case management of illnesses and health promotion are provided by community health nurses, NPs, psychiatric nurse specialists, nurse midwives, and a team of other professionals. Because most patients come to the nursing center when they perceive a problem, personal preventive health care is integrated with treatment of common acute and chronic diseases. Community education and support groups, such as Alcoholics Anonymous, could operate out of the nursing center. A childbirth center could be integrated into the center. Neighborhood resources such as day care, teen clubs, job training, and nutrition and social services should be available. When necessary, referrals and consultations, integral to case management, would be made to medical specialists, dentists, or crisis services (Table 27-3).

Community nursing centers are a base for traditional district nursing, which is population-based care for the healthy and the sick.[8] Local community control and a high level of nursing autonomy would conserve an integrated, comprehensive health service relevant to the population served.

A model nursing center in Philadelphia is Abbottsford Community Health Center, staffed by four primary care NPs, two community health nurses, three lay outreach workers, a psychologist, and support personnel. A pediatrician and internist provide consultation and medical back-up for family-centered care. The family nurse practitioners at Abbottsford are the

---

TABLE 27-2   Health Planning for Populations

Tasks:	Strategic planning at local level
	Environmental protection services
	Targeting vulnerable populations
	Health care for the societal good
Providers:	Primary care NPs
	Public health nurses

TABLE 27-3   Community Nursing Centers

Tasks:	Community education and support
	Individual health promotion and education
	Well-child care
	Prenatal care
	Nursing and medical intervention
	Case management/acute and chronic illness
Providers:	Family NP
	Community health nurse
	Nurse midwife
	Multidisciplinary nurse clinicians

---

first NPs in the state of Pennsylvania to be paid directly as primary care providers under capitated managed care insurance plans. The community health nurses provide home visits; administer programs, such as summer immunization clinics; and supervise outreach activities.

Abbottsford's outreach workers are neighborhood residents who have begun education and support groups for pregnant women, teenagers, grandparents caring for grandchildren, and those recovering from drug and sexual abuse. The tenant council of Abbottsford Homes, a predominantly African-American public housing development, requested the health center and remains actively involved in its activities.

Congress passed legislation in the Omnibus Budget Reconciliation Act of 1987 to "test prepaid, capitated payments to Community Nursing Organizations (CNOs) under the Medicare program"[23] (p 253). The two test sites are On Lok and Carondelet St. Mary's. In a model similar to district nursing, the On Lok program for frail elders integrates primary care, home health care, and day care.[4] Elderly citizens are given the opportunity to live at home while receiving skilled nursing care. The Carondelet St. Mary's project is a nursing HMO in which geriatric nurse practitioners, professional nurse case managers, and consumers forge a team to provide direct services to senior citizens in community health centers. Cost savings and quality care have been demonstrated through reductions in hospital admissions, length of stay, and emergency room visits.

Home Care, Partial Hospitalization, and Nursing Home Care

At the third level of the pyramid, case management by advanced practice nurses ensures continuity of care when the patient requires more intensive nursing care. Partnerships between NPs and home care nurses advance high-quality and holistic care for patients who are best supported in the context of home and family. Reduced in-hospital time, reduced symptom distress, and less social dependency in patients with progressive lung cancer visited at home by master's-prepared oncology nurses have been demonstrated.[17] Case studies show that primary care nurse practitioners working with visiting nurses enhanced home management of patients and reduced costs of care (Table 27-4).[22]

Proactive assessment and intervention on hospital discharge can be provided by community health nurses who coordinate care with family members, primary care NPs and a myriad of health care professionals. Especially for patients who lack primary care providers, direct coordination of care between primary care NPs, community health nurses, and home care NPs would enhance services for patients and families.[22] More research is needed to evaluate costs and outcomes of collaboration between a nurse providing primary care and a nurse providing home-bound services.

Modeled after the British day hospital and administered by the University of Pennsylvania School of Nursing, the Collaborative Assessment and Rehabilitation for Elders (CARE) program provides coordinated primary care and rehabilitation services for frail elders following acute illnesses. Funded by Medicare as a comprehensive outpatient rehabilitation facility (CORF), the aim of the program is to promote independence at home and reduce multiple hospitalizations while improving the individual's functional status through interventions coordinated by advanced NPs. Psychiatric partial hospitalization similarly has been used for many years to promote rehabilitation of the chronic mentally ill.

Skilled nursing homes are settings where nurse practitioners and geriatric nurse specialists manage chronic and acute conditions with a focus on the prevention of further problems.[12] As patients move from the community into institutional settings, the complexity of care increases.

Medical Management

Physician expertise is recognized at the next level of care for the management of complex medical, surgical, and psychiatric problems. A nurse-physician team approach could provide specialized care that is required by a small minority of the population with complicated problems. The evolv-

---

TABLE 27-4 Home Care and Long-Term Care

Short-stay hospitalization

Nursing case management

Home care partnerships

NPS and visiting nurses

Long-term care nursing facilities

Home health care

Visiting nurses

Family and primary NP

---

ing role of the tertiary NP as a high-technology specialist who coordinates medical and nursing care is an example of advanced NPs functioning at this level of care (Table 27-5).[15]

Acute and Critical Care

Inpatient acute and critical care, the top of the pyramid in Figure 27-1, is where most of the attention and financial payment is currently focused. Studies have documented reduced complications, reduced disease acuity, and shorter patient length of stay when quality inpatient nursing care is delivered.[10] Moreover, the scope of practice of critical care NPs is evolving to include management of high technology services within a nursing framework (Table 27–6).

Discharge planning and linkage to home or nursing home are key to appropriate and continuous care when the patient leaves the expensive acute care setting. Hospital and community nurses specialists must share information in order to facilitate the patient's transition to home and decrease rehospitalization.[20]

▬ FUTURE VISIONS

The Office of Technology Assessment recommended increased use of NPs and nurse midwives in primary care with direct reimbursement for their services in order to reduce health care costs.[24] Direct access to nursing services has been restricted for more than 50 years, however, largely because of lack of direct payment to nurses. Although NPs currently receive direct reimbursement for evaluation and management services from Medicaid and from Medicare (in designated rural areas), wide variations in reimbursement laws among states impede access to services provided by advanced practice nurses.[18]

Bowman[5] points out that "except for rare circumstances, most third-party payers still require physician orders for home care before payment is made for nursing visits. If payment is out of pocket and there are no regulations to the contrary, *nursing visits do not require physician authorization*"[11] [author's italics] (p 245). Imagine a health care delivery model that re-

---

TABLE 27-5   **Medical Management**

Tasks:	Outpatient medical management
	Complex medical and surgical case management
Providers:	Physicians
	Tertiary NP/CNs
	Home care nurses
	Speciality nurses
	Gerontology NPs

TABLE 27-6 Hospital Care

Tasks:	Inpatient acute care
	Critical care
	Discharge planning
Providers:	Critical care nurses
	Critical care NP and CNs
	Hospital nurses

---

moves the necessity of physician approval for payment of home nursing care or primary care nursing services. In this model, primary care NPs, community health nurse specialists, and home care nurses would coordinate care and refer between nursing systems for care focused on the patient, family, and community. Patients and society would benefit from a more efficient and meaningful systems of care.

CONCLUSION

Americans need to decide on a package of health care benefits that balances quality, cost, and access. Ethical discussions, development of quality standards, and outcome-based research are needed to identify the most cost-effective services. As accumulating evidence shows, the American health care system will be more equitable, cost-effective, and rational if it is restructed to include direct access to NPs. The task at hand is to promote the independent role of advanced practice nurses and to ensure direct payment for their services.

Primary care nurse practitioners in partnership with community health nurses, are ready to become the backbone of a coordinated, community-based health care system that will focus on prevention and early treatment of common problems. For any health reform package to cut costs in the long run, existing regulations that restrict independent advanced nursing practice must be removed. When advanced practice nurses are paid directly for services and financial incentives for health care delivery are redefined, Americans will reap the benefits of a cost-effective, coordinated nursing model of health care.

Acknowledgments

The Primary Care Delivery Pyramid was presented in 1989 in a doctoral seminar and in 1990 at the American Public Health Association Convention in New York City.

REFERENCES

1. American Medical Association: Current Procedural Terminology, ed 4. Chicago, American Medical Association, 1994.
2. American Nurses Association: Nursing Case Management (NS-32). Kansas City, American Nurses Association, 1988.

3. American Nurse Association: Testimony of the American Nurses' Association Before the Physician Payment Review Commission on Payment to Nonphysician Providers. Kansas City, American Nurses Association, 1990.
4. Ansak ML, Zawadski RT: On Lok CCO-DA: A consolidated model. Home Health Services Quarterly 4:147, 1983.
5. Bowman, RA: Nursing returns to the home health frontier: Markets and trends in home health care. *In* Aiken LH, Fagin CM (eds): Charting Nursing's Future: Agenda for the 1990s. Philadelphia, JB Lippincott, 1992, p 235.
6. Buhler-Wilkerson K: Left carrying the bag: Experiments in visiting nursing, 1877–1909. Nurse Res 36:42, 1987.
7. Buhler-Wilkerson K: Public health nursing: In sickness or in health? Am J Public Health 75:1155, 1985.
8. Dreher, M: District nursing: The cost benefits of a population-based practice. Am J Public health 74:1107, 1984.
9. Ethridge P: A nursing HMO: Carondelet St. Mary's experience. Nursing Management 22:22, 1991.
10. Fagin CM: Cost-effectiveness of nursing care revisited: 1981–1990. *In* Aiken LH, Fagin CM (eds): Charting Nursing's Future: Agenda for the 1990s. Philadelphia, JB Lippincott, 1992, p. 13.
11. Ford L: Advanced nursing practice: Future of the nurse practitioner. *In* Aiken LH, Fagin CM (eds): Charting Nursing's Future: Agenda for the 1990s. Philadelphia, JB Lippincott, 1992, p 287.
12. Garrard J, Kane RL, Ratner ER, et al: The impact of nurse practitioners on the care of nursing home residents. *In* Katz PR, Kane RL, Mezey MD (eds): Advances in Long Term Care, vol 1. New York, Springer, 1991, p 169.
13. Haire DB: The cultural warping of childbirth. Environmental Child Health 19:171, 1973.
14. Health Care Financing Administration: Proposed Rules. Federal Register, 58(133):38010, 1993.
15. Keane A, Richmond T: Tertiary nurse practitioners. Image 25:281, 1993.
16. Lockhart CA: Physician payment reform: Implications for nursing. *In* Aiken LH, Fagin CM (eds): Charting Nursing's Future: Agenda for the 1990s. Philadelphia, JB Lippincott, 1992, p 448.
17. McCorkle R, Benoliel JQ, Donaldson G, et al: A randomized clinical trial of home nursing care for lung cancer patients. Cancer 66:1375, 1989.
18. Mittlestadt P: Third-party reimbursement for services of nurses in advanced practice: Obtaining payment for your services. *In* Mezey MD, McGivern DO (eds): Nurses, Nurse Practitioners: Evolution to Advance Practice. New York, Springer Publishing Co, 1993, p 322.
19. Moxley DP: The Practice of Case Management. Newbury Park, CA, Sage, 1989.
20. Naylor MD, Brooten D: The roles and functions of clinical nurse specialists. Image 25:73, 1993.
21. Starr P: The Social Transformation of American Medicine. New York, Basic Books, 1982.
22. Sullivan EM: Nurse practitioners and reimbursement: Case analyses. Nursing & Health Care 13:236, 1992.
23. Sullivan EM, Fields B, Kelly J, et al: Nursing centers: The new arena for advanced nursing practice. *In* Mezey MD, McGivern DO (eds): Nurses, Nurse Practitioners: Evolution to Advanced Practice. New York, Springer Publishing Co, 1993, p 251.
24. US Congress, Office of Technology Assessment: Nurse practitioners, physician's assistants, and certified nurse midwives: A policy analysis (OTA-HCS-37). Washington, DC, US Government Printing Office, 1986.
25. Weil, M, Karls JA, et al: Case Management in Human Services Practice. San Francisco, Jossey-Bass, 1988.
26. Williams CA: Public health nursing: Does it have a future? *In* Aiken LH, Fagin CM (eds): Charting Nursing's Future: Agenda for the 1990s. Philadelphia, JB Lippincott, 1992, p 255.

Chapter 28

Computerized Documentation in Home Health

CATHERINE NOONE   JANICE CAVANAUGH   CATHY McKILLIP

New tools, brought about by advances in technology, are bringing many changes to nursing—within the acute care setting as well as in the community. One advance that affects practice in both settings in the same way are the changes brought about by the use of the computer and computerized client records. Physicians' orders, standardized nursing care plans, pharmacy, dietary, and laboratory data are all computerized along with computerized documentation by nurses. The authors explain one agency's experience with adapting a computerized clinical documentation system to the nurses' needs and the nurses' responses to the process.

In Home Health Services is a licensed, certified home care agency serving rural Sussex County, New Jersey. Nurses coordinate and deliver 48,000 visits annually in a 526-square mile area. The agency, an affiliate of Newton Memorial Hospital, is one of the first in New Jersey to use hand-held computers to fully automate its patients' records from admission through discharge. The agency chose Psion Series 3 palm-top computers initially because they were lightweight, could be easily transported in the nurse's bag, and were less expensive than lap-top computers.

Before in Home Health Services' electronic patient record adaptation, the manual charting system lacked consistency and did not include elements required by the Community Health Accreditation Program Standards of Excellence in evaluating client outcomes.[1] Improving the quality of documentation in the client's clinical record often is an overwhelming challenge for staff nurses and managers. The topic repeatedly came up at staff, utilization review, and quality management committee meetings.

The agency administrator recognized that the manual charting system was cumbersome, lacked consistency among nurses, and rarely included evaluation of client outcomes. Although the quality management committee was aware that the nurses provided high-quality patient care, they sought a tool to assist the nurse in documenting this care. The managers envisioned the computerized patient record as a tool for nurses to accomplish this goal.

From *Journal of Nursing Administration* 25(1):67–69, 1995. Reprinted by permission of Lippincott-Raven Publishers.

PROJECT DEVELOPMENT

To prepare for computerization, the management team formed a task force to implement the change to computerization. The 10-member task force consisted of 4 nursing staff members, 2 data processing staff members, 2 clinical support staff members, and 2 project directors. The task force met weekly to discuss the staff nurses' goals, which were to reduce paperwork time and meet agency standards for documentation. The task force also analyzed the impact of computerization on each support staff position and planned the steps necessary to adapt to the change. The support staff received reassurance that computerization would change some aspects their jobs, but not eliminate them. Working together, the task force began working toward the agency goal of fully automating the clinical record to reflect the high quality of care provided.

Four nurses, who were with the agency from 2 to 5 years, volunteered to be "pioneers" in the use of the hand-held computer. The data processing staff and clinical support staff had been with the agency from 1 to 5 years. This group's computer experience was much more extensive than the nurses', and they were committed to supporting the nursing staff with this exciting project.

The two project directors had different backgrounds. One had a clinical background and one had a management information systems background. Before implementation, the clinical project director adapted the manual charting system to mirror the computerized charting system. This was a transition step that assisted the nurses in learning the program and ensured that nursing care plans would be standardized throughout this agency. The clinical project director worked closely with the four nurses to develop manual home visit reports that could be used for documenting nursing visits by weekend nurses who were not using the computer. The technical project director educated the nurses on basic computer operation, data transfer, and support staff functions. She also acted as a resource to the nurses for troubleshooting any computer-related problems. The two project directors complimented one another's area of expertise to produce a successful outcome of the project.

IMPLEMENTATION
OF THE COMPUTERIZED RECORD

A week-long training session consisted of classroom and home visits with clinical trainers provided by the software vendor. During the 3-day classroom training, the nurses learned all aspects of system communications, including how to enter nursing assessments and other clinical information. After the training, the nurses were ready to use the computer independently in the patients' home with support from project directors as needed. The project directors or the clinical trainers accompanied each nurse on home visits on the first day of implementation. Initially, the agency was going to run parallel systems for 1 month, however, because there were so few problems, the agency decided to go "live" after the first day of implementation. This decision eliminated the need to duplicate every visit made during the test period.

Each nurse was assigned a member of the support staff to be her buddy, someone the nurse could contact throughout the day with any problems related to the system. For example, if a nurse received a program error message on her computer, she would call her buddy, and the support staff member would explain steps to resolve the problem. This enabled the nurse to continue visiting her patients with minimal interruption.

■ DESCRIPTION OF WORK FLOW

During home visits, the nurse accesses the hard drive of her palm-top computer, reviews information regarding diagnosis, short- and long-term goals, and enters updated information, such as vital signs, assessments, and medications. At the end of the nurse's day, all completed patient files are uploaded into the agency's main system via a telephone and modem hook-up. The data processing staff then prepares the reports for the nurse's review (Fig. 28-1) for the nurse to read and sign assessments and care plans.

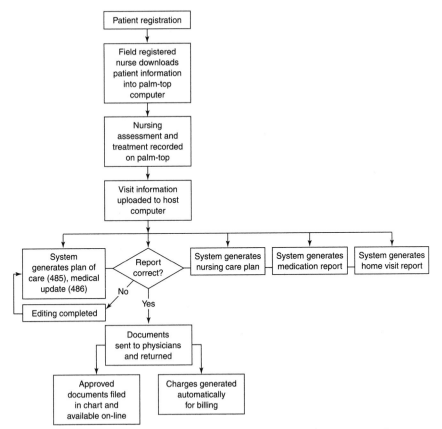

FIGURE 28-1   Flowchart of electronic clinical record with financial interface.

The nurse reviews and signs all reports that will become part of permanent record.

EVALUATION

After 3 months of using the system, the four nurses were surveyed to determine their opinions on using the computer for documentation (Table 28-1). The nurses thought that the system-generated prompts improved their nursing assessments. For example, in monitoring a patient's cough, the system prompted the nurse to assess onset, frequency, duration, and pain. If the cough is productive, additional prompts include assessment of color and consistency of sputum.

The management staff believes that the system has been implemented successfully. A camaraderie has developed between the nursing and clerical staff members, who appreciate each other's special area of expertise, creating a cooperative organization climate. The hand-held computers have increased the nurses job satisfaction. None of the four nurses would go back to the manual charting system. Comparisons will be done to compare the project goals at 6 months, 9 months, and annually as more nurses are added as users of the system.

The agency recently was surveyed by Community Health Accreditation Program, and the computerized clinical record system met all of the clinical and financial standards. The surveyor said the attempt by agency staff

TABLE 28-1   Staff Nurses' Opinions About the Use of Computers in Home Settings

WHAT I *LIKE* ABOUT THE COMPUTER FOR DOCUMENTATION	WHAT I *DO NOT LIKE* ABOUT THE COMPUTER FOR DOCUMENTATION
The *prompts* make you document more about your patient's status.	I'm frustrated when I'm not able to up or download because of program errors.
The home visit reports for admissions and revisits provide more information than the manual record did.	It is less personal—there is less eye contact during data entry.
There is less chance of omitting a problem, the assessment covers all body systems.	Initial assessments are time consuming—it takes longer to open a case.
It is more legible.	It is difficult for nurses to edit mistakes.
It is easy to add diagnosis and intervention as needed.	You need more windows for open text.
It is systematic approach to nursing process.	It sometimes is difficult to make charts individualized.
It prompts nurses to make more complete initial assessments.	
There is uniform charting.	
There are summary reports.	

was innovative in nursing and a "cutting-edge" concept adaptation. This was an important impetus to continue our project as designed and to prepare to integrate more nurses into the computerized system rather than manual recording of patient care.

REFERENCES

1. *CHAP Standards of Excellence.* New York: National League for Nursing; 1991.
2. Chu S, Thom J. Information technology as a proactive strategic weapon in healthcare. *J Nurs Adm.* 1994; 24(4):5–7.
3. National Association of Home Care. *Uniform Minimum Data Set.* Washington, DC: National Association of Home Care; 1994.

Chapter 29

The Omaha System: A Research-Based Model for Decision Making

KAREN MARTIN   GARY LEAK   CATHY ADEN

In this chapter Karen Martin, Gary Leak, and Cathy Aden describe the value, diversity, and potential benefits of the Omaha System of decision making in generalizing and manipulating client, clinical, and financial data. The Omaha System of collecting and analyzing essential client-focused data was developed by the Visiting Nurse Association of Omaha, Nebraska and provides agency administrators with a useful tool that is based on the nursing process and mutuality of the nurse–client relationship. A research-based model for decision making, this tool provides for day-to-day and long-range clinical and financial decision making in home health and community health agencies.

How can nursing administrators be certain that the number and preparation of staff fit the fluctuating service needs of their clients? How can they meet the escalating accreditation requirements and third party regulations for quantified client data? How can they address quality issues and the measurement of outcomes from the client's perspective? No single nursing strategy, management style, or system can ensure individual or collective nursing excellence and success. No simple answer exists for nursing administrators, regardless of their setting.[1-3]

Historically, healthcare services and reimbursement have been defined and driven by medical diagnoses. Although extremely important, medical diagnoses are not sufficient to explain clinical data in the community health setting. For example, when clients with newly diagnosed insulin-dependent diabetes are discharged from the hospital and referred for home health services, their nursing care requirements vary markedly. Significant variation is likely in the optimal number, length, and focus of the home visits to clients and the optimal assignment of agency personnel. To make informed decisions, agency administrators and staff need data in addition to medical diagnoses and demographic and health history information. Such data are needed to deliver high-quality home health services that produce the best possible client outcomes and to maximize the agency's personnel and financial resources.

From *Journal of Nursing Administration* 22(11):47–52, 1992. Reprinted by permission of Lippincott-Raven Publishers.

The Omaha System offers a method of collecting and analyzing essential client-focused data. When considered as a unit, the System's three schema provide a comprehensive, valid, and reliable framework to describe and measure clients' healthcare requirements and the services provided by direct delivery personnel.

■DESCRIPTION OF THE OMAHA SYSTEM

Early in the 1970s, the Visiting Nurse Association (VNA) of Omaha administrators and staff saw the need to develop a client-focused management information system. They believed that changes in regulation, reimbursement, and accreditation requirements and the demand for more detailed, client-specific data were imminent.

These changes ended an era when funds were allocated with minimal reporting requirements; instead, demands for accountability increased dramatically. To meet these demands, VNA administrators and staff needed a system capable of generating data to describe and quantify clients' care requirements and providers' services. Such a system must be functional even if competition among healthcare providers increased, revenue decreased, or costs increased. The VNA of Omaha staff channeled their concerns and energy into research that produced and refined the Omaha System.

The previous concerns prompted the VNA personnel to develop a model that is based on the nursing process and illustrates mutuality of the nurse–client relationship. The model consists of three schema that are amenable to automation.[4,5] The Omaha System is a simple, useful method for describing, organizing, enumerating, and measuring critical client-focused data. It is not a magical means of independently or instantly solving all data problems for administrators and clinicians. However, the Omaha System is designed to provide:

a framework for integrating a clinical practice and documentation system;

a method of organizing and entering client data into a manual, partially automated, or automated management information system.

The purpose of such a practice, documentation, and data management model are to help staff practice more efficiently, increase the quality of client services, focus and streamline recording, decrease costs, increase the potential for obtaining full reimbursement with minimal challenges, and generate single and aggregate client data for staffing decisions and program management.

■PROBLEM CLASSIFICATION SCHEME

The Problem Classification Scheme is a client-focused taxonomy of nursing diagnoses or health-related concerns. Client problems and nursing diagnoses will be used synonymously in this article. The Problem Classification Scheme includes 4 domains encompassing 40 problems, 5 problems modifiers, and clusters of problem-specific signs and symptoms. The language and codes of the Problem Classification Scheme are organized at four hierarchical levels with domains being the most general level. The four domains and a problem from each are: Environmental–Sanitation; Psychosocial–Caretaking/Parenting; Physiological–Circulation; and Health-Related Behaviors–Substance Use.

■ PROBLEM RATING SCALE FOR OUTCOMES

The Problem Rating Scale for Outcomes consists of three, five-point, Likert-type subscales. The subscales are designed to measure clients' knowledge, behavior, and status for specific problems. The Rating Scale is used by nurses at critical points of time such as when the client is admitted to service, at regular time intervals throughout the period of service, and when the client is dismissed. Ideally, ratings of clients improve over time. Although improvement in a newly admitted hospice client's respiratory knowledge and behavior ratings is a realistic goal, improvement in status is not anticipated when the client has a medical diagnosis of lung cancer. Detailed knowledge, behavior, and status criterion measures or patterns were developed to increase the usability and reliability of the Scale. The patterns consist of simulated client data and show the most negative to the most positive outcome ratings for every client problem.

■ INTERVENTION SCHEME

The Intervention Scheme is a taxonomy of nursing actions or activities with three distinct hierarchical levels. The first level includes four broad categories of interventions: Health Teaching, Guidance, and Counseling; Treatments and Procedures; Case Management; and Surveillance. The second level is comprised of 63 alphabetized targets of objects of nursing action. Finally, client-specific information provides details necessary for practice and documentation. A users' guide is available that suggests care planning/intervention guides for all Omaha client problems.[6]

■ PRACTICE AND DOCUMENTATION SYSTEM

Clinicians and administrators need accurate and timely descriptions of clients and the services those clients receive. Such data are required for accurate staffing and budgeting activities and for efficient use of resources. Furthermore, if a goal of the nursing profession is to develop a method of charging for nursing services, descriptions of clients, and the nursing services they receive will need to be quantified and easily retrieved.[7,8]

The Problem Classification Scheme provides a structure that drives and defines community health nursing services. It is a system that facilitates a thorough yet concise assessment of clients, assists staff nurses to focus and quantify clients' health-related concerns, and offers cues and clues to guide practice. The Scheme enables clinicians to identify essential admission and ongoing client data objectively and efficiently, organize and identify patterns in the data, and select problem-specific nursing interventions.

In many community health settings, administrators and their staff members have revised their client record forms to accommodate the Problem Classification Scheme. Because the language and organization of the Scheme are simple and standardized, it is being used by physical therapists, occupational therapists, social workers, speech pathologists, nutritionists, dentists, and physicians as well as nurses.

The Problem Rating Scale for Outcomes is a measurement instrument for quantifying client outcomes when used with specific Omaha nursing diagnoses. The ratings of the knowledge, behavior, and status subscales serve two purposes. First, the ratings help the clinician differentiate between problems of greater and lesser priority and to judge the severity of problems. Second, the ratings enable the clinician to clearly measure client progress throughout the period of service and communicate that progress to others. Evaluating progress involves noting numeric rating changes, assessing client willingness to address problems, and identifying others who can contribute to the client's improvement. As outcome effectiveness, quality improvement, and reimbursement issues continue to increase, both administrators and clinicians need tools, such as the problem rating scale for outcomes, to measure and document the impact of their services.

The Intervention Scheme provides a flexible system for healthcare professionals to use as they describe and quantify anticipated plans and completed interventions in relation to specific client problems. A universal goal of administrators and clinicians is to improve practice and streamline documentation. The brief categories, targets, and client-specific narrative of the Intervention Scheme can replace lengthy and disorganized progress notes. The problem-specific, organized, standard language and codes of the Scheme assist nurses and other users to create a concise data trail. That trail identifies the users' critical decisions and the type and frequency of selected strategies, especially when accompanied by clients' responses.

Benefits of the Omaha System

The primary benefits of the Omaha System have been systematically investigated, especially during the VNA's 1989–1992 research project. Because of widespread interest in the Omaha System, we felt it was necessary to conduct such research to 1) demonstrate the reliability, validity, efficiency, and utility of the model; and 2) increase the generalization potential for home health agencies.

A sample of recent VNA research and studies conducted by other service providers, educators, and students is included in this article. The purpose is to demonstrate the importance of the research process in selecting, implementing, and evaluating practices essential to the delivery of excellent nursing services.

▬ RELATED PRACTICE AND DOCUMENTATION RESEARCH

Numerous research projects have been conducted to investigate practice and documentation benefits of the Problem Classification Scheme, Problem Rating Scale for Outcomes, and Intervention Scheme. The three studies included in Table 29-1 and described below illustrate the diversity of such research.

Community health nursing leaders selected the Omaha Problem Classification Scheme as their model when they decided to introduce nursing diagnoses through New Jersey in 1981. Three agencies served as experimental sites and four agencies as control sites; all agencies provided home health and public health nursing services. Analysis using t-tests confirmed a statistically significant increase in the quality of client information and documentation practices of nurses in the experimental sites.[9,10]

Since 1982, faculty members and students in New Brunswick have used the Omaha Problem Classification Scheme at their screening and counseling clinic. The Scheme is part of the assessment procedure and the framework for the client's service record. Gilbey[11] used paired t-tests and Chisquare to evaluate the effectiveness of the clinic by exploring changes in 56 clients' health behavior during a 3-year period. The Omaha Scheme was determined to be a satisfactory tool for monitoring clients over time and evaluating clinic services.

The focus of the 1989–1992 VNA of Omaha study was home health clients served by four diverse agencies in Omaha and Beatrice, Nebraska, Trenton, New Jersey, and Balsam Lake, Wisconsin. Data were collected from over 2,000 client records, staff nurse–researcher shared home visits, and time studies. Descriptive and inferential data analyses included frequencies, t-tests, correlations, and discriminate analysis. The findings produced a comprehensive profile of clients' demographic and health history

TABLE 29-1   Omaha System Research Relevant to Nursing Administrators

RESEARCH STUDY	AUTHOR, YEAR	P*	D†	DM‡
Implement nursing diagnosis in New Jersey community health agencies	Cell, Peters & Gordon (1984);	X		
	Cell & Becker (1992)		X	
Evaluate the effectiveness of clinic services in New Brunswick	Gilbey (1990)	X	X	X
Develop the diagnosis, intervention, and outcome schema of the Omaha System	Martin & Scheet (1992)	X	X	X
Relate clinical data to reimbursement in Connecticut	Pasquale (1987)			X
Automate multidisciplinary client records for ambulatory care in Boston, Massachusetts	Zielstorff, Jette & Barnett (1990)	X	X	X
Explore relationships among nursing care requirements, selected factors, and home health nursing resource consumption	Hays (1992)	X	X	X

*P=practice.
†D=documentation.
‡DM=data management.

characteristics. Results indicated that the Omaha System offers nurses a useful model for describing and evaluating services. Furthermore, essential aggregate data were generated for agency administrators to use for management purposes, to demonstrate that nursing services make a difference, and to offer to policy makers as a means of describing clinical data in the community health setting. Detailed descriptions of the research methods and findings will appear in other publications.

■MANAGEMENT INFORMATION SYSTEM

Administrators and clinicians are recognizing the need for more sophisticated management information systems. During the last several decades, requirements for comprehensive, accurate, and timely health-related data have increased dramatically. Simultaneously, administrators recognize that they must rely on automated support systems to manage and control operations rather than increasing the time that clinicians and other personnel spend on documentation, data entry, and data management.

Four conditions have prompted many community health nursing administrators to develop management information systems. First, agencies must meet the detailed accountability demands of Medicare and other third party payors such as Medicaid, insurance companies, health maintenance organizations, and preferred provider organizations. If a home health prospective payment system is initiated, these demands will only increase. Second, the accounting practices of many agencies are struggling to meet current requirements. Automation of accounting procedures has become a necessity rather than a luxury. Third, clinical staff need automated systems to address the growing demands for documenting services. Romano suggests that " . . . the modern nursing role is to take the explosion of new information and find new and better ways to deliver care. Nursing has a role of innovator in the 1990s."[12](p.99) Finally, management information systems are needed for marketing decisions and strategic planning. Rapid changes in regulations, legislation, and political coalitions make past decisions obsolete.

A well-designed management information system offers these benefits to community health administrators and clinicians:

1. It facilitates organization and tracking of client care data.
2. It provides the statistical and predictive data base that can enable managers to make informed decisions.
3. It supplies a foundation for administrators to build a more powerful structure that can support growth in clients, personnel, and programs.
4. It expedites the agency billing process and reduces the number of errors.[4] (p.24,25)

The Omaha System provides a framework for integrating clinical data with other essential personnel and financial data in an automated management information system. Wise nursing administrators recognize that computerized management information systems, even those that include the Omaha System, do not automatically improve nursing practice and client outcomes, save time and money, and improve staff morale.[13,4] The Omaha System provides a beginning link between critical financial and clinical data. This link is especially important as the profession considers methods of costing out nursing services and mediating utilization of resources.[8,14–17]

RELATED MANAGEMENT INFORMATION SYSTEMS RESEARCH

Three related studies are shown in Table 29-1 and described below. They show interest in data management issues and the diversity of Omaha System research being conducted by nurses.

The Massachusetts General Hospital Coordinated Care Program for the elderly was funded and initiated in 1984 as part of a 4-year grant. Teams of nurses, social workers, and physicians provided services to high-risk elders at satellite health centers. The teams documented client services with a common automated record system that was based on COSTAR, developed at Massachusetts General Hospital (Boston, MA) and now available in the public domain. Although the COSTAR vocabulary was rich in medical diagnoses, it did not meet the assessment and documentation needs of the nurses and social workers. When the Omaha Problem Classification Scheme was added to the COSTAR vocabulary, the client record met the clinicians' flexibility and inclusive requirements and the researchers' validity and reliability vocabulary requirements.[18]

A retrospective review of client records was conducted during a pilot study in Connecticut. Relationships among Medicare-eligible home care clients' living arrangements, functional status, plan of care (independent variables), and consumption of home care resources (dependent variable) were explored. The plan of care portion of the data collection instruments was derived from the Omaha System. Multiple regression analysis showed that consumption of home healthcare resources could be reliably predicted from the variables in the Omaha System model. Within the limitations of the study, the findings established the ability of the client focused, Omaha nursing diagnoses to explain a significant amount of variance in resources consumption.[19]

A doctoral study was conducted to explore relationships pertinent to home health nurse administrators. Specifically, nursing care requirements, selected client and nurse factors, and resource consumption were examined. Using regression and multiple regression analyses, the Omaha client problems were found to explain a statistically significant amount of variation in hours of direct nursing care provided and of variation in nursing care requirements. Variation explained by problems with one modifier, actual, was compared to variation explained by the combination of actual, potential, and health promotion modifiers. Using a combination of the three modifiers explained more of the variation and produced statistical significance.[20]

SUMMARY

The Omaha System facilitates generation and manipulation of client, clinician, and financial data. These data are useful for diverse practice, documentation, and data management purposes in clinical settings and research. This article includes examples of such application at home health and public health agencies, colleges of nursing, and ambulatory care centers. Omaha System application and research support the value of the System to nursing administrators in general and community health administrators in particular.

Acknowledgment
This article is based on a study funded by the National Center for Nursing Research, NIH, grant #1 R01 NR02192-04 and a paper presented at the University of Iowa Fourth National Conference on Nursing Administration Research, Iowa City, Iowa, October 12, 1991.

REFERENCES
1. Barkauskas V. Home health care: Responding to need, growth, and cost containment. In: Chaska N, ed. *The nursing profession: Turning points.* St. Louis: CV Mosby, 1990:394–404.
2. Douglas D, Murphy E. Nursing process, nursing diagnosis, and emerging taxonomies. In: McCloskey J, Grace H, eds. *Current issues in nursing (3rd Edition).* St. Louis: CV Mosby, 1990.
3. Thomas J. Helping home health managers with hard data on staff productivity. *Home Health Line.* 1988;13:305–306.
4. Martin K, Scheet N. *The Omaha System: Applications for community health nursing.* Philadelphia: WB Saunders Company, 1992.
5. Weidmann J, North H. Implementing the Omaha classification system in a public health agency. *Nurs Clin North Am.* 1987;22:971–979.
6. Martin K, Scheet N. *The Omaha System: A pocket guide for community health nursing.* Philadelphia: WB Saunders Company, 1992.
7. Martin K, Scheet N. The Omaha System: Implications for costing community health nursing. In: Shaffer FA, ed. *Costing out nursing: Pricing our product.* New York: National League for Nursing, 1985.
8. McCloskey J. Implications of costing our nursing services for reimbursement. *Nursing Management.* 1989;20:44–49.
9. Cell P, Becker A. A framework for practice: New Jersey experiences. In: Martin K, Scheet N, eds. *The Omaha System: Applications for community health nursing.* Philadelphia: WB Saunders Company, 1922:23–24.
10. Cell P, Peters D, Gordon J. Implementing a nursing diagnosis system through research: The New Jersey experience. *Home Healthcare Nurse.* 1984;2:26–32.
11. Gilbey V. Screening and counselling clinic evaluation project. *Can J Nurs Res.* 1990;22:23–38.
12. Romano C. Innovation: The promise and the perils for nursing and information technology. *Comput Nurs.* 1990;8:99–104.
13. Hendrickson G, Kovner C. Effects of computers on nursing resource use. *Comput Nurs.* 1990;8:16–22.

14. Lundeen S, Kreuser N, Friedbacher B. Omaha System applications for the future. In: Martin K, Scheet N, eds. *The Omaha System: Applications for community health nursing.* Philadelphia: WB Saunders Company, 1992:321–322.
15. Marek K. Analysis of the relationships among nursing diagnoses, and other selected patient factors, nursing interventions and measures of utilizations, and outcomes in home health care. Doctoral dissertation, University of Wisconsin, Milwaukee, WI, 1992.
16. Williams C. The nursing minimum data set: A major priority for public health nursing but not a panacea. *Am J Public Health.* 1991;81:413–414.
17. Williams B, Phillips E, Torner J, Irvine A. Predicting utilization of home health resources. *Med Care.* 1990;28:379–391.
18. Zielstorff R, Jette A, Barnett GO. Issues in designing an automated record system for clinical care and research. *Advances in Nursing Science.* 1990;13:75–88.
19. Pasquale D. A basis for prospective payment for home care. *Image.* 1987;19:186–191.
20. Hays B. Nursing care requirements and resource consumption in home health care. *Nurs Res.* 1992;41.

Unit 5
Family Nursing

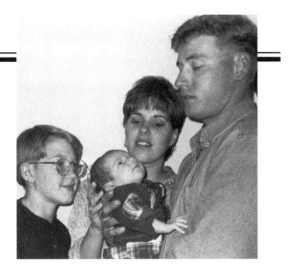

Community health nurses work with families. Three major reasons underlie the importance of the family for community health nursing. First, the family itself, not merely its individual members, needs service. Based on a growing body of research data, we now know that a family behaves as a unit and needs to be viewed in totality for therapy to be effective. Like an individual, a family grows through developmental stages, performs specific functions, and has many needs. Thus the total family can be viewed as a client. How well is the family functioning? What are its interrelationships? What is its stage of development? The nurse must be able to assess these dynamics. Understanding family development and the characteristics of healthy families enables the nurse to develop measures for preventing problems and promoting family health.

Second, individual health and family health are closely linked. A healthy, well-functioning family promotes the growth of its members. A family with limited capacity for problem solving and self-management, however, is often unable to promote the potential of its members or assist them in times of need. Consider a family in which abuse toward one or more members occurs—abused children, a battered spouse, an abused grandparent. That family's level of functioning is generally very low, and the physical, emotional, and social health of each member suffers as a result.

Third, families are smaller units of a larger system, the community, and the level at which each family functions determines the degree to which it promotes or detracts from a healthy community. A healthy family influences community health positively. Some families, for example, encourage actions, such as neighborhood cleanup, recreational development, or safety enforcement, to meet community needs. However, a family with a low level of health negatively influences community health. Consider families whose members have no concern for others, who engage in violent or criminal acts. Instead of contributing to community well-being, these families require the creation of special efforts and programs. They divert energy and resources away from other community needs and threaten community health.

Healthy families exhibit six important characteristics. First, they communicate well. There is a facilitative process of interaction among family members. They are able to share feelings, ideas, and concerns with one another, verbally and nonverbally, in a manner that promotes understanding and resolves conflict. Second, healthy families enhance the development of each member. They are responsive to each individual member's needs and provide the support and freedom necessary to promote each member's growth. Third, healthy families adapt roles and tasks to meet changing family needs over time. They are flexible. With changing developmental stages and external forces, such as economics, creating new family needs, they are able to adjust and develop new roles and tasks to meet those needs. Many women and men are single parents or a spouse retires and is at home all day, for example, requiring a change in family roles, relationships, and tasks to meet the demands of the situation. Fourth, healthy families actively attempt to cope with problems and issues. They assume responsibility for problem solving and seek energetically and creatively to meet the demands of the situation. When faced with a problem they cannot solve with their own resources, they seek and accept outside help. Fifth, healthy families exhibit a healthy home environment and life-style. They recognize the importance of such things as safety, good nutrition, exercise, and relaxation from stress and promote their practice among members. Finally, healthy families maintain regular ties with the broader community. They develop social networks and use external resources to meet the family's needs.

The cultural dimension is an important element in family nursing. Every family has its own cultural values and practices. These influence the way family members eat, dress, and live and what they believe. Practices that negatively affect health may be firmly entrenched in the family's cultural value system and may not be easily changed. For example, a child is severely injured in an accident and needs a blood transfusion. The parents refuse because receiving blood from another person violates their beliefs. The community health nurse must determine the family's cultural orientation; this will increase the nurse's understanding of the family and make nursing care planning and intervention more appropriate.

Various aspects of family-focused community health nursing are considered in Unit V. Each chapter describes a different facet of family care: family assessment, levels of family functioning, encouraging family self-help, and preventative work with families. Two specific issues in families are included: the challenges of single parenting and family violence as child abuse. Each is geared to increase the nurse's understanding of families and, in turn, the effectiveness of nursing services offered.

Chapter **30**

Family Health Assessment— An Integrated Approach

LINDA REUTTER

Within a community, families are subsystems whose health affects and is affected by the larger system. Accurate and thorough assessment of family health becomes essential, then, to promote the health of the community and to design appropriate community health nursing interventions. Linda Reutter has developed an approach to family assessment that integrates family systems theory and Orem's self-care nursing framework. In this comprehensive guide Linda Reutter uses five major assessment categories—environmental data, family structure, family function of self-care, family function of adapting to change, and family perception of health—which the community health nurse can use to assist families in promoting their health.

■COMMUNITY HEALTH NURSING

A major emphasis in community health nursing (CHN) is the interrelationship between individual, family and community health. Community health nursing, in its responsibility and commitment to the health of the total population has traditionally viewed the family unit as a primary focus for nursing intervention. In order to provide nursing care to families in the community, nurses need to integrate community health principles, family theory, and a conceptualization of nursing.

In this article the process of developing a family assessment guide is discussed. The guide is designed to help students integrate concepts from family system theory and Orem's self-care conceptual framework for the purpose of promoting family health in the community. It was developed to be used by baccalaureate students in an introductory community health nursing course, where the emphasis is on family health care.

Rationale for Approach

In recent years, two major areas have received increasing attention in nursing curricula: the use of nursing frameworks, and the emphasis on family-

From *Journal of Advanced Nursing* 9(4):391–399, 1984. Reprinted by permission of Blackwell Science, Ltd.

focused care. Nursing frameworks are used to assist students in conceptualizing the essence of nursing—in defining its parameters, and in identifying its unique focus. Family conceptual frameworks provide guidelines for operationalizing a family focus for health care. As the author attempted to help students incorporate these two approaches, it was necessary to consider several questions. If nursing frameworks or models provide a conceptualization of nursing, how can family health (a recognized focus of nursing) be promoted using a nursing model? Or, how can theories of family functioning be adapted for use in nursing? Further, what guidelines for family assessment will provide data which can be used to promote family health? In addressing these questions, it was necessary to analyse family and nursing frameworks in terms of their adequacy in providing guidelines for practice.

As existing theories of family functioning have been developed primarily within sociology and psychology they tend to reflect the point of view of these disciplines. The discipline of nursing has largely adopted these theories 'as is' and has not viewed them from the syntax of nursing theory (Whall 1980). In this regard, Murphy & Hoeffer (1982) emphasize the need to adapt to the perspective of nursing, concepts and theories from other disciplines. While existing family frameworks are useful to nurses in understanding and working with the family, it is the author's contention that these frameworks fail to adequately emphasize or give direction for those areas of health promotion that are nursing's domain. While it is generally recognized that the family is the major unit through which health care is organized and carried out, many existing family frameworks do not focus on the *health care function* of the family (Pratt 1976). Recently, nurses have begun to incorporate the health care function into a family framework (Friedman 1980; Leonard & Erickson 1983). It is the author's belief that the use of a nursing model combined with a family framework would more clearly emphasize the nurse's role in assisting families with their health care needs.

In evaluating nursing models for their utility for family nursing, it is apparent that most models emphasize care directed toward the individual, rather than the family unit (Stevens 1979), and hence, focus on assessment of individual health. Recently, nurses have applied these models to the nursing of families (Clements & Roberts 1983; Mermel & Congdon 1977). While the use of one nursing framework throughout the nursing student's undergraduate programme has been advocated (Stevens 1979), there has been concern expressed regarding the 'carte blanche' acceptance of nursing models for all areas of nursing practice (Hardy 1982; Hamilton 1983). That adaptation of models for various areas of practice may be required and should be encouraged has been emphasized by these authors. Such adaptation may be necessary for family nursing and could result from integrating concepts from both family and nursing frameworks. The family assessment guide developed by the author is one example of such a synthesis, designed to provide a meaningful, holistic framework for nursing of families.

▬THE FAMILY AS A SYSTEM

In integrating concepts to form a family/nursing model with utility for CHN, the initial task was one of choosing a conceptualization of family which reflects the basic philosophy of community health nursing. One of the major premises in community health nursing is the inter-relationship of individual/family/community health. When the focus of intervention (i.e., the client) is the family the framework guiding assessment would necessarily need to emphasize both internal and external influences on family health. General systems theory appeared to provide an appropriate basis for such a framework. General systems theory has been adopted as the most commonly used theoretical framework in the family process movement (Clements & Roberts 1983); at the same time it has been regarded as an especially useful theory in the area of family/community health (Freeman & Heinrich 1981; Helvie 1981; Braden & Herban 1978; Clemen et al. 1981). Clemen et al. (1981) emphasize the importance of examining the multiple aspects of internal family functioning *as well as* the family's relationship with other social systems in the community. Helvie (1981) argues that in order to assist members in health matters, it is important not only to look at the family as a unit, but at the individual members and the community and how they influence the family's behaviour and health.

The conceptual framework for family used in the development of this family assessment guide is adapted from Friedman (1980). The family is conceptualized as a system with structure and function. For Friedman, structure is the organization of the family members *and* the patterns of relationships among them. Structural dimensions are delineated as communication patterns, role relationships, value systems and power structure. Friedman views function as the purposes or goals of the family system. Functions of the family have been discussed by numerous authors. In developing this guide, the author has categorized these functions into two main areas: (a) promoting individual growth and development and (b) adapting to internal and external demands in order to remain a viable unit. Clemen et al. (1981) incorporate the two broad functions in their definition of family health, stating that family health is oriented toward maximizing individual potential, and maintaining the integrity of the family as a system.

▬OREM'S SELF-CARE MODEL

The conceptualization of nursing which has been used in developing the family assessment guide is Orem's (1980) self-care framework. The faculty adopted this framework for use throughout the undergraduate programme. Students in the family nursing course have used this framework for the previous 3 years, largely with individuals in acute-care/extended-care settings. In order to develop a guide for family assessment it was necessary to assess Orem's framework for its compatibility with family systems theory, and for its usefulness in CHN practice.

The presuppositions underlying the self-care philosophy have been embraced by CHN for years, and indeed are necessary when working with individuals in the area of health promotion. The perception of man as a decision-making being accomplishing goals through deliberate action is reflected in the basic principles of CHN: active client participation in all phases of the nursing process, the client's right to self-determination, and increased client self-responsibility and independence (Clemen et al. 1981). The importance of self-care principles in the field of health promotion has been well presented by Pender (1982). There is widespread acceptance that the major health problems in our society are related to life-style and environment. Prevention and reduction of these problems require that individuals assume responsibility for engaging in positive health behaviours (therapeutic self-care actions) designed to meet universal self-care requirements. Orem (1980) defines self-care actions as those activities performed which will contribute to human structural integrity, human functioning and human development. Universal self-care requisites (requirements) are those basic human needs that must be met by everyone in order to maintain health. According to Orem (1980), effectively meeting the universal self-care requisites is health care at the primary level of prevention.

While Orem's framework focuses primarily on the individual rather than the family unit, the significance of the family in meeting individual self-care requirements is presented. Orem views the family as a developmental environment for individual growth and development, maintaining that an organized cooperative effort is required to meet the self-care demands of individuals within the group, and to promote the well-being of the group as a unit. This reflects the two broad functions of family previously discussed.

In this family assessment guide, Orem's (1980) universal self-care requisites have been adapted to reflect the major focuses of CHN, as self-care actions are assessed within these categories. The family is viewed as existing for the purpose of meeting individual self-care requisites. Developmental and health-deviated requisites are incorporated within the universal categories as appropriate. Although CHN offers a broad range of services on all levels of prevention, its major focus (and that of this course, and the agency in which students do their clinical practice) is on health promotion and illness prevention, rather than on health restoration. Orem acknowledges that CHN situations have a health focus oriented toward the life cycle. She suggests that health care needs of clients would include periodic health evaluation; health maintenance and health promotion adjusted to the specific phase of the clients' life cycle; protection against environmental factors; and assistance to the patient and family in assuming self-care. The appropriate nursing system (as classified by Orem) to meet these needs would generally be the supportive-educative one, where clients' self-care limitations are overcome with education and supportive counselling interventions. As well, strengths and self-care assets are reinforced for health maintenance.

■ASSESSMENT CATEGORIES

Five major areas for data collection were developed. Each area will be briefly discussed, together with the rationale for its inclusion. A detailed list of data to be collected under each category is found in Appendix 1.

Environmental Data

In community health nursing practice, the influence of the environment (physical and social) is recognized as a crucial determinant of health and health practices. Environmental factors which impede or facilitate health are viewed not only as influencing elements but as potential targets for nursing intervention. Community health nursing interventions are aimed at mobilizing both personal and environmental resources to increase the level of the health of the total community. The importance of studying the environment (community) as it relates to family/individual health is emphasized by many authors (Friedman 1980; Archer 1982; Dreher 1982; Stein & Eigsti 1982). Unfortunately, nursing models devote little attention to this concept (Flaskerud & Halloran 1980). Orem does not emphasize environment as a potential focus of intervention but acknowledges that the ability to perform self-care can be influenced by environmental change, and that nursing requires knowledge of the 'social and economic forces affecting the individual and family, and the influence of physical, biological, and social agents in the environment on individual, family and community health.'

Family Structure

The structural characteristics assessed are those adapted from Friedman (1980); communication, role relationships, power structure and value systems. The rationale for assessing these is two-fold: to determine if they are 'functional/dysfunctional', and to work 'with' the family more effectively, based on a knowledge of these dimensions. Guiding questions in this category will yield data that can be validated using 'healthy' characteristics of family structure as documented in the literature (Pratt 1976; Otto 1973). As determinants of family health, these structural dimensions have important implications for CHN. The importance of communication in assisting individual members to grow and in maintaining the family as a unit is undisputed. Role relationships are accepted as a crucial assessment area, as it is through family roles that family functions are fulfilled. This is a particularly significant area for CHN because of various societal changes affecting families. In the growing number of single-parent families, role overload is not uncommon. Those families facing role transition (e.g. new parents, elderly) may experience role conflict due to the acquisition of new roles and/or relinquishing of former ones, and to incompatible expectations of self and others. Nurses, when helping the family to effect change, must be cognizant of the family's power and authority structure as reflected in its decision-making behaviour. Awareness of family values is beneficial, if not essential, in relating services to family goals.

Family Function: Meeting Self-Care Requisites
of Family Members

Family functions have been broadly divided into two main categories to incorporate the two major tasks of a family system: (a) meeting self-care requirements of individual members, and (b) adapting to change.

AIR, FOOD, WATER, ELIMINATION, REST, AND ACTIVITY. Within each of these five requisites it is necessary to gather data to ascertain if individual needs are being met, the resources available (within and outside the family system), how the family organizes itself to meet the requisites, as well as individual health deviations and their effect on other family members. In gathering data, one must be cognizant of actual and potential health risks due to both life-style behaviours and environmental influences.

All of the requisites incorporated within this category are 'common' areas of community health nursing interventions. Students will analyse the data collected keeping mind the developmental stage of family members.

PROMOTING HEALTHY PERSONALITY DEVELOPMENT AND MEETING PSYCHOSOCIAL NEEDS OF ALL MEMBERS. Although physical and socio-emotional needs of members cannot be arbitrarily divided into mutually exclusive categories in the real world, in this guide psychosocial needs have been delineated as a separate category for emphasis. This category incorporates Orem's (1980) categories of 'solitude and social interaction' and 'promotion of normalcy.'

In the area of solitude and social interaction, family and individual interaction in the broader community is emphasized, as this has been implicated as a 'healthy' family characteristic (Pratt 1976; Otto 1973). The availability of resources is assessed as community health nurses are often involved not only in working with available resources, but in attempting (and encouraging families) to influence policy which will improve their availability, accessibility, and acceptability (e.g. recreation, child care).

The 'promotion of normalcy,' not well developed by Orem (1980), is expanded to include those self-care practices which foster optimum development of individuals within the family, especially in terms of emotional and intellectual growth. A section on developmental tasks has been included to provide a measure of individual and family task accomplishment. CHN emphasizes the provision of anticipatory guidance to families in the area of child growth and development. This section also serves to emphasize the internal changes in the family brought about by individual growth and maturation which will place demands on the family system as it progresses through the life cycle. Mental health promotion and the concomitant affective function of the family is of crucial importance to the effective personality, development and maintenance of family members. Most current discussions of family functions emphasize the importance of the affective function for the survival and functional of the family as a whole and of its individual members (Pratt 1976; Smilkstein 1978; Friedman 1980; Duvall 1977). The sub-categories which expand on the fostering of social, cognitive and spiritual growth are important considerations in assisting families in childrearing and socialization functions. Parenting education is a major component of family health care and of CHN's role.

PROTECTION FROM HAZARDS. This requisite was left as a separate category to emphasize its importance to CHN. Its 'risk reduction' emphasis includes not only self-care practices aimed at primary prevention, but actions which serve to detect early any health deviations (e.g. Pap smear, breast self-examination). The specific data collected would be in part determined by the 'common health problems' of the age of individual members. Because of their high incidence in the population at large and their deleterious effects on individual/family and community health, specific areas have been singled out, i.e. prevention of accidents in the home and on the road, substance abuse, and communicable disease. Because the workplace has been increasingly implicated as a potential source of hazards, both to the worker and his/her family, occupational stressors are emphasized to increase student and family awareness of this environmental influence on health.

Family Function—Adapting to Change
The second major function of the family emphasizes the characteristic of the family system to grow while maintaining itself as a viable unit by adapting to internal and external demands for change. This is a very relevant area in CHN where many clients are experiencing role transitions due to maturational and/or situational events. Data collected in this category should enable students to analyse situations using the components of crisis as described by Aguilera & Messick (1978): events, perception of events, and resources. Internal and external resources of the family are assessed not only to assist clients in their present use, but also to strengthen and develop these in anticipation of future events, thereby preventing crisis situations. Helping families to develop and use social support systems and problem-solving skills are frequent CHN interventions.

Family Perception of Health Situation
This last category is an often neglected, but important aspect of data collection. Eliciting from the family their perception of both strengths and perceived areas for further development involves the family as an active participant in its own care, beginning at the data collection phase of assessment. It acknowledges that the family is the primary source of knowledge of its unique situation. Awareness of the family's knowledge of its strengths can assist the nurse and client in planning of care. Reinforcement of these strengths by 'an outsider' is often reassuring to clients. Strengths not recognized by the family can be pointed out as pertinent areas for continued development. Sharing with clients their self-care competencies enhances self-awareness, self-esteem, and feelings of control. By pointing out to clients what they do well, interest can be stimulated in developing further self-care assets (Pender 1982).

The family's perception of areas needing further development provides nurses with the client's knowledge of deficits. This may help to determine client priorities, and provide a basis for contracting in areas where motivation may be high. It also enables the nurse to increase client awareness of those areas requiring a need for change of which the client may be unaware. Systematically reviewing areas in which self-care could be improved assists the client in making choices about those areas he will concentrate on, providing freedom for the client to determine the direction he will proceed to improve health status (Pender 1982).

▬SUMMARY

Very little mention has been made throughout this discussion regarding methods of data collection. These will necessarily vary, depending on the nurse, client, and family situation. The family assessment guide is intended to outline the information needed to adequately assess family health, and not to describe how this will be collected. Various techniques—tools, interviews, observation—can be utilized for this purpose.

Analysis of the data will include statements of family strengths and areas for further development. The self-care practices of the family will be analysed using 'healthy' characteristics of families, and validated self-care practices viewed within the family's cultural milieu and its perception of its unique situation. With a systems perspective, it is necessary to look at intervention in terms of the individual, family and community, keeping in mind the inter-relationship between these levels.

The family assessment guide was developed for use in community health nursing, using a combined family systems and nursing conceptual framework. It was developed as a learning tool for students, to assist them in the synthesis of concepts of health promotion, community health nursing and family theory, and to facilitate their understanding of the family's (and nurse's) role in promoting the health of its members.

As more of the helping professions direct their attention to the family unit, and inter-disciplinary teamwork becomes necessary, it is beneficial, if not crucial, that nurses articulate aspects of family care which are appropriate for nursing interventions. This will hopefully result in more coordinated, comprehensive health care.

▬REFERENCES

Aguilera D. & Messick J. (1978) *Crisis Intervention* 3rd edn, C.V. Mosby Co., St. Louis.

Archer S. E. (1982) Synthesis of public health science and nursing science. *Nursing Outlook* 30, 442–446.

Braden C. J. & Herban N. L. (1978) *Community Health—A Systems Approach.* Harper & Row, New York.

Clemen S. A., Eigsti D. G. & McGuire S. L. (1981) *Comprehensive Family and Community Health Nursing.* McGraw-Hill, New York.

Clements J. W. & Roberts F. B. (eds) (1983) *Family Health—A Theoretical Approach to Nursing Care.* John Wiley & Sons, New York.

Dreher, M. C. (1982) The conflict of conservatism in public health nursing education. *Nursing Outlook 30*, 504–509.

Duvall E. M. (1977) *Marriage and Family Development*, 5th edn. J. B. Lippincott, New York.

Flaskerud J. H. & Halloran E. J. (1980) Areas of agreement in nursing theory development. *Advances in Nursing Science 3*, 1–7.

Freeman R. B. & Heinrich J. (1981) *Community Health Nursing Practice*, 2nd edn, W.B. Saunders Co., Philadelphia.

Friedman M. M. (1980) *Family Nursing—Theory and Assessment*. Appleton-Century-Crofts, New York.

Hamilton P. (1983) Community nursing diagnosis. *Advances in Nursing Science 5*, 21–36.

Hardy L. K. (1982) Nursing models and research—a restricting view? *Journal of Advanced Nursing 7*, 447–451.

Helvie C. O. (1981) *Community Health Nursing—Theory and Process*. Harper & Row, Philadelphia.

Leonard L. G. & Ericksen J. (1983) A framework for family nursing. *Nursing Papers 15*, 34–50.

Mermel V. & Congdon A. (1977) *Assessment Tool for Universal Self-Care Requirements of a Family*. Georgetown University School of Nursing, Washington, D.C. unpublished manuscript.

Murphy S. A. & Hoeffer B. (1982) Role of the specialties in nursing science. *Advances in Nursing Science 4*, 31–39.

Orem D. E. (1980) *Nursing: Concepts of Practice* 2nd edn, McGraw-Hill, New York.

Otto H. A. (1973) A framework for assessing family strengths. In *Family-Centered Community Nursing* (Reinhardt A. M. & Quinn M. D. eds), C. V. Mosby, St. Louis, pp. 87–94.

Pender N. (1982) *Health Promotion in Nursing Practice*. Appleton-Century-Crofts, Norwalk, Connecticut.

Pratt L. (1976) *Family Structure and Effective Health Behavior: The Energized Family*. Houghton-Mifflin, Boston.

Smilkstein G. (1978) The family apgar: a proposal for a family function test and its use by physicians. *The Journal of Family Practice 6*, 1231–1239.

Stein K. Z. & Eigsti D. G. (1982) Utilizing a community data base system with community health nursing students. *Journal of Nursing Education 21*, 26–32.

Stevens B. J. (1979) *Nursing Theory—Analysis, Application, Evaluation*. Little, Brown & Co., Boston.

Whall A. L. (1980) Congruence between existing theories of family functioning and nursing theories. *Advances in Nursing Science 3*, 59–67.

■ APPENDIX 1: FAMILY ASSESSMENT GUIDE

I. Environmental data

A. Characteristics of home
- Type of dwelling
- General condition
- Ventilation, heating, lighting, furnishings
- Facilities for toileting, laundry, garbage disposal

B. Characteristics of neighbourhood
- Condition of dwellings and streets
- Incidence of crime and safety problems
- Presence and types of industry
- Demographic characteristics of community
- Availability and accessibility of health and other basic services and facilities

C. Family's geographic mobility
- How long has family lived in the area?
- What is their history of geographic mobility?

II. Family structure
    A. Communication patterns
        1. Communication *networks* in the family
            • direct, intermediaries, coalitions
            • communication lines between and among subsystems
        2. *Content* of communication
            a) *Instrumental* messages—how do members communicate about instrumental activities?
            b) *Affective* messages
                • what types of emotions are communicated?
                • how are feelings expressed?
                • how is expression of feelings received?
            c) Are there any areas not open to discussion/difficult to discuss?
        3. *Method* of communication
            • clear *vs* marked
            • open *vs* closed
            • specific *vs* general
        4. Is communication appropriate for age and development of members?
        5. Family's perception of and satisfaction with its communication patterns
    B. Role relationships
        • Positions and roles assumed by members
        • Are roles and associated tasks acceptable to those involved?
        • Presence of role conflict/strain
        • Is there role flexibility and flexible task assignment as situation demands?
        • Family's perception of and satisfaction with role relationships and role behaviour
    C. Decision-making behaviour
        • Who makes what decisions in the family? Consider areas of health care practices, household matters, childrearing
        • Method of decision-making
        • Method of conflict resolution
        • Family's perception of and satisfaction with the decision-making process
    D. Patterned values
        • Goals/aspirations of the family
        • Presence of value conflicts
            • within family system
            • with those outside of family system
        • Importance of specific values to family:
           e.g. Education
               Work ethic
               Family
               Health
               Religion

- Family's view of health/illness
  - what does it mean to be 'healthy'?
  - how is illness viewed?

III. Family function: meeting self-care requisites of family members
A. Air, food, water, elimination, rest and activity
  1. Air
     - Factors in home and community influencing quality of air intake
     - Do any individuals have difficulties in meeting requirement for air?
       - effect on family
       - how is this managed?
  2. Food and water
     - Usual diet for individuals of family
     - Family's knowledge of balanced diet
     - Patterns of eating
     - Resources for obtaining, storing and preparing of food
     - Sources of food supply—availability, accessibility, acceptability
     - Source of water supply—adequacy, safety, chemical content, fluoridation
     - Allocation of division of labour re: meeting nutritional needs of family
     - Social, cultural, or religious factors influencing nutrition
     - Dental practices of members
     - Do any members have difficulty nutritional requirements?
       - effect on family
       - how is this managed?
  3. Elimination of family wastes
     a) Body wastes
        - hygiene of family members
        - availability and adequacy of facilities for personal hygiene
        - do any members have difficulty with elimination?
        - effect on family
        - how is this managed?
     b) Other organic, inorganic wastes
        - methods of garbage disposal
        - general cleanliness of household
        - hygienic care of pets
  4. Maintaining a balance of activity and rest
     a) Rest
        - Sleep and rest patterns of family members
        - Environmental factors affecting rest and sleep patterns
        - Do any members have difficulty meeting requirements for rest and sleep?
          - effect on family
          - how is this managed?

- adequacy of amount of sleep and rest as perceived by members
  b) Activity
  - Activities engaged in by individual members (occupational pursuits, home tasks, school and other intellectual pursuits, leisure time activities, relaxation)
  - Do members regularly participate in physical activity?
  - Is provision made for periods of rest and relaxation?
  - Do any members have difficulty in achieving relaxation?
  - Availability, accessibility, acceptability of facilities and resources to pursue activities
  - Members' perception of balance of activity and rest for themselves; for rest of family
B. Promoting healthy personality development and meeting psychosocial needs of all members
  1. Solitude and social interaction
    a) Solitude
      - Adequacy of solitude and privacy as perceived by members
      - Resources available to meet requirements
    b) Social interaction
      - Activities engaged in within the family group
      - Interaction among family members
      - Individual and family involvement with others outside the home
        - friends
        - extended family
        - participation in community activities, clubs, organizations
      - Availability, accessibility and acceptability of resources to meet needs:
        - recreational
        - cultural
        - transportation
        - child care, babysitting
      - Do any members have difficulty in achieving a balance of solitude and social interaction?
        - effect on other members
        - how is this managed?
      - Family's satisfaction with balance of solitude and social interaction
  2. Developmental needs of individual family members
    - Identify the developmental stage of the family life cycle
    - To what extent are the developmental tasks of individual family members being achieved?
    - Family's knowledge of growth and developmental needs of individual members
  3. Family's affect

- Family's sensitivity and response to concerns, interests and needs of family members
- Mutual respect among family members
- Opportunities provided to foster autonomy
- Is individuation appropriate for age and needs of members?
- Opportunities provided to foster 'belongingness'
- To what extent do family members provide support and nurturance to each other?
- How well do members 'get along'?
- Members' perceptions of how family meets emotional needs of its members
4. Behaviour control
   - Standards of behaviour: clarity, appropriateness for age and development of members, flexibility, enforcement
   - Methods of responding to unacceptable and acceptable behaviour
   - Are there specific behaviour concerns in family?
     - how is this managed?
5. Provisions for cognitive development
   - Family's knowledge of intellectual needs of members
   - Methods of promoting cognitive development
   - Appropriateness of intellectual activities for age and development of members
   - Availability, utilization, and acceptability of resources:
     - school
     - opportunity for self-study
     - appropriate 'play' material
   - Are family members developing normally in this area?
6. Provision for spiritual and moral development
   - Family's beliefs regarding moral and spiritual education
   - Utilization of outside resources:
     - schools
     - religious institutions
7. Sexuality
   - What education is being provided in this area?
   - Family planning practices
   - Are there any specific concerns any family member has? How is it managed?
C. Protection from hazards
   1. Family self-care practices in relation to:
      a) accident prevention in the home
         - hazards identified
      b) motor vehicle accident prevention and protection
         - hazards identified
      c) protection from acts of violence—crime, child safety
         - hazards identified
      d) prevention of substance abuse

- use of medications—prescription and nonprescription
- use of alcohol
- use of tobacco

    e) protection from communicable disease—immunization status of family members

2. Presence of hazards in the workplace and environment
   - provisions made to prevent ill effects
3. Family's use of preventive health measures (appropriate for age group)—e.g. Pap smear, breast self-examination, dental/medical exams
4. Family's utilization of health care resources
   - services utilized
   - purpose

IV. Family function—adapting to change

  A. Major events (situational and maturational) which have occurred during past year
   - methods of adjusting to change

  B. Family's perception of present sources of stress or worry
   - methods of dealing with stress

  C. *Internal* and *external* resources available to cope with stress and change:
   - Problem-solving skills of family
   - How do family members aid each other in time of need?
   - Social support systems and purpose for which they are utilized

  D. Is family able to seek and accept help when required?

  E. Does the family anticipate change, and plan for same?

V. Family perception of health situation

  A. Perception of the family's strengths to engage in self-care

  B. Area of health for further development

Chapter 31

The Nursing Process in Family Health

JAYNE ANTTILA TAPIA

> Jayne Tapia developed a systematic approach to assessing a family's level
> of functioning which is shared in this classic writing. Her Model for Family
> Nursing is based on a continuum of five levels of family functioning and
> the nurse's skills, attributes, and activities which are appropriate to each
> level in order to meet family goals. Knowing how to work effectively with
> families is important for several reasons. First, as our health care delivery
> system continues to undergo changes, more family care is being delivered
> in the community. Second, nontraditional family structures place new
> stressors on the family unit. Third, nurses are leaving the acute care setting
> and are beginning to work with families in a variety of community settings.
> How families perceive the role of the nurse and the focus of the nurse's
> work with families functioning at different levels are described in Tapia's
> Model—a useful tool for the new as well as the experienced community
> health nurse.

Public health nurses have long believed that the family is the unit of community nursing service; there is nothing new about this concept. What *is* new, however, is that more and more nurses are beginning to realize that they are not always able to describe accurately what nursing service to the family means, nor have they been able to render this kind of service consistently.

Yet, the need for coordinated, ongoing, comprehensive health and illness care for all members of the family, as a group and as individuals, is all too evident today in our fragmented health delivery system. Community health nurses can and should play an important part in providing this type of care in the newly emerging health delivery systems. But, to do this, they must have a clearer idea of what they mean by working with a family, rather than just with individual members.

They must be able to diagnose specific health problems of the family, prescribe a nursing approach to the family, carry it out, and evaluate its outcome just as they now do with individuals. Their goal should be to help the family grow in its ability to meet its needs and fulfill its functions in a

From *Nursing Outlook* 20(4):267–270, 1972. Reprinted by permission of Mosby-Year Book, Inc.

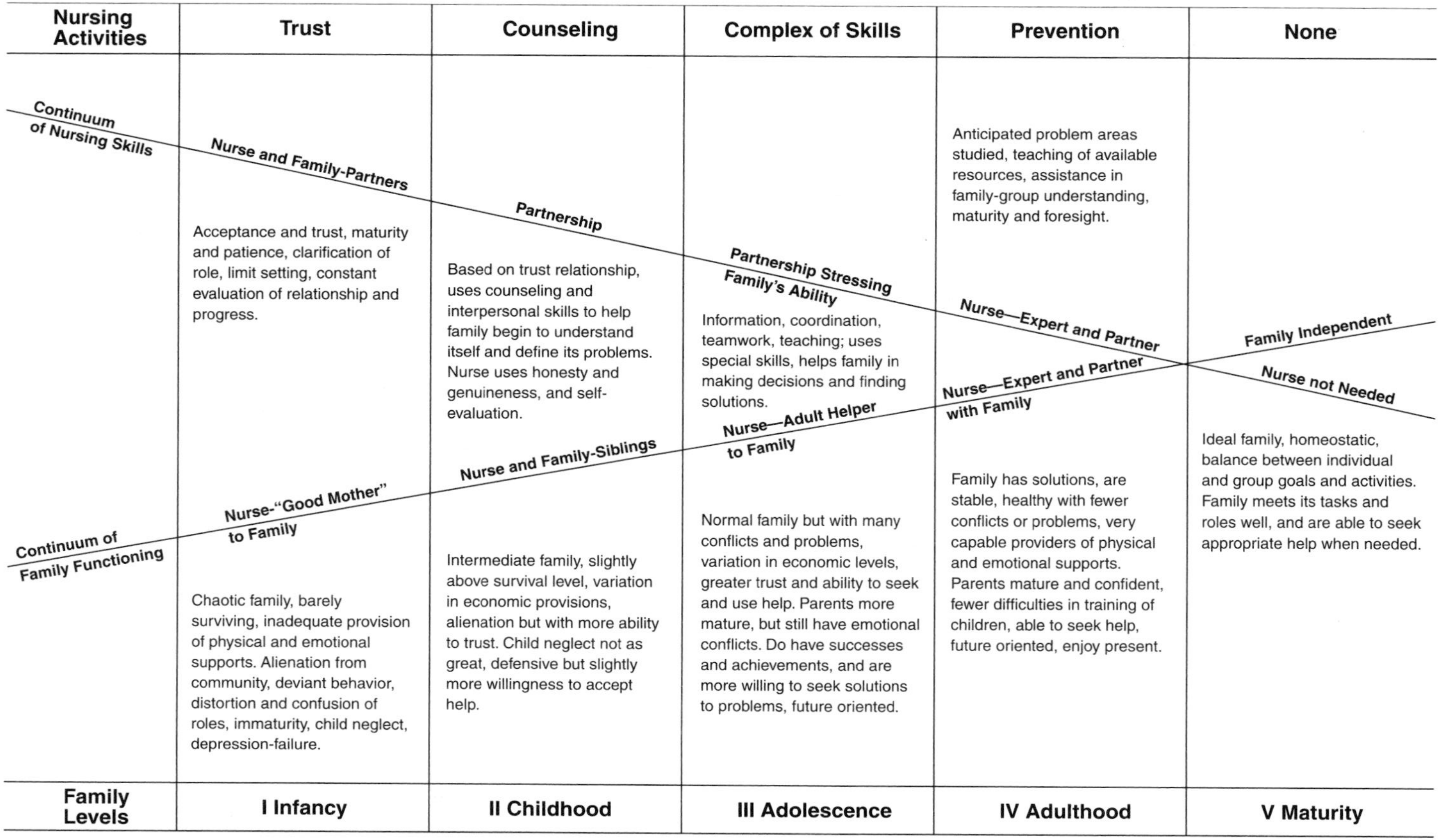

Nursing Activities	Trust	Counseling	Complex of Skills	Prevention	None
Continuum of Nursing Skills	Nurse and Family-Partners	Partnership	Partnership Stressing Family's Ability	Nurse—Expert and Partner with Family	Family Independent — Nurse not Needed
	Acceptance and trust, maturity and patience, clarification of role, limit setting, constant evaluation of relationship and progress.	Based on trust relationship, uses counseling and interpersonal skills to help family begin to understand itself and define its problems. Nurse uses honesty and genuineness, and self-evaluation.	Information, coordination, teamwork, teaching; uses special skills, helps family in making decisions and finding solutions.	Anticipated problem areas studied, teaching of available resources, assistance in family-group understanding, maturity and foresight.	Ideal family, homeostatic, balance between individual and group goals and activities. Family meets its tasks and roles well, and are able to seek appropriate help when needed.
Continuum of Family Functioning	Nurse-"Good Mother" to Family	Nurse and Family-Siblings	Nurse—Adult Helper to Family	Nurse—Expert and Partner	
	Chaotic family, barely surviving, inadequate provision of physical and emotional supports. Alienation from community, deviant behavior, distortion and confusion of roles, immaturity, child neglect, depression-failure.	Intermediate family, slightly above survival level, variation in economic provisions, alienation but with more ability to trust. Child neglect not as great, defensive but slightly more willingness to accept help.	Normal family but with many conflicts and problems, variation in economic levels, greater trust and ability to seek and use help. Parents more mature, but still have emotional conflicts. Do have successes and achievements, and are more willing to seek solutions to problems, future oriented.	Family has solutions, are stable, healthy with fewer conflicts or problems, very capable providers of physical and emotional supports. Parents mature and confident, fewer difficulties in training of children, able to seek help, future oriented, enjoy present.	
Family Levels	I Infancy	II Childhood	III Adolescence	IV Adulthood	V Maturity

FIGURE 31-1 Family nursing model.

more healthful way, while, at the same time, using their own talents and time most effectively.

▬ PAST DEFINITIONS

Several attempts have been made to clarify and define family nursing service. Mickey described it as being called for in situations in which an individual or a family has a health problem requiring nursing assistance of the kind that might include therapeutic care, health teaching, counseling, or guidance.[1] The assumptions underlying this definition were that the family did not have prior knowledge or competence to meet the situation and that the provision of nursing service would produce change.

Freeman and Lowe devised a form to systematize the process by which a nurse judges family nurse competence, and Lee and Frazier tried to differentiate family group service from such concepts as "the family as a unit of service" or "family health service."[2,3]

I propose another means of determining family nursing needs and related nursing activities: the study of the tasks of the nuclear family and the family's ability in accomplishing these tasks. According to Feldman and Scherz, the four main tasks of the nuclear family are to provide for security and physical survival, emotional and social functioning, sexual differentiation and training of children, and growth of individual members.[4] Families, however, differ in their ability to carry out these tasks and, thus, have different levels of family functioning. In order to provide nursing service appropriate to the needs of a particular family, the community health nurse must be able to assess the family's level of functioning.

Using the above tasks as guidelines, I have developed a model for family nursing based upon a continuum of five levels of family functioning. Level I is the chaotic family—at the infancy stage of development; Level II is the intermediate family—at the childhood stage; Level III is the normal family with many conflicts and problems—at the adolescent stage; Level IV is the family with solutions to its problems—the adult stage; and Level V is the ideal independent family—at full maturity.

Nursing services and activities appropriate to each level of family functioning can also be put on a continuum. The major focus of the nurse's work with a Level I family is to develop a trust relationship; with a Level II family, to help the family begin to define problems; a Level III family will require a complex of nursing skills; and prevention will be the point of emphasis in working with a Level IV family.

All of these nursing activities are inherent in the nursing process, but they will be more effective if the nurse can concentrate her efforts on the nursing activity appropriate to the family's level of functioning. In doing so, the nurse will initiate nursing measures that are meaningful and economic in time and effort, and this in turn will lead to greater success in helping families reach their highest level of functioning.

Since the family's level of functioning is an indication of its state of health, any change in that functioning level also indicates a change in its health status. Thus, the degree of family movement from one level to another can serve as a yardstick whereby the nurse can measure and evaluate the effect of her nursing intervention and service.

■INFANCY OR CHAOTIC FAMILY

The lowest level of family functioning is characterized by disorganization in all areas of family life.[5] The family barely meets its needs for security and physical survival; members are characterized by their inability to secure adequate wages or housing, to budget money, or to maintain adequate nutrition, clothing, heat, and cleanliness. This family lives from day to day without orientation to the future.

These lacks increase the family's inability to provide for healthy emotional and social functioning of its members, and this is reflected in the family members' apparent alienation from the community. They distrust outsiders, are unable to utilize community resources and services, and become hostile and resistant to offers of help. The immaturity of the parents is shown in their inability to assume responsible adult roles—a factor that often results in socially deviant behavior, including child abuse and neglect.

The children suffer in other ways, too, because their parents are unable to act as the role models that the children need if they are to mature into capable, socialized, adult men and women. There is consequently much distortion and confusion of roles in the family. The children, sometimes at a young age, may even have to take over many of the tasks and roles of their nonfunctioning parents. Such situations perpetuate the family's pattern of chaos and disorganization into the next generation.

This type of family also fails in providing for support and growth of its individual members. The family exhibits depression and a feeling of failure, with no hope of success either for individual members or the family group. The basic insecurity of the family members prevents change: defensiveness and distortion are used as devices to keep people from getting near enough to cause change.

Establishing a trusting relationship with this type of family is the most important nursing activity in the therapeutic process, yet a most difficult one. The nurse must develop a caring, freeing relationship with one more members of the family and help the family to feel that she cares about them, accepts them as they are, and understands their difficulties. If she cannot establish this relationship with them, she cannot help them to grow. While this activity is basic for a level one family, it is difficult for them to accept because of their fear and distrust of people outside of the immediate family.

The task will demand much of the nurse—maturity, patience, endurance, limit setting, and clarification of her role. The family will see the nurse as a good mother and will test her for consistency and try to be dependent on her. The nurse, seeing herself as a partner working with the family, cannot allow the dependency to go beyond the trust relationship. She must be constantly alert to the factors operating within herself, the family, the community, and environment in order to evaluate progress toward the development of mutual trust. When the nurse has ascertained that this relationship is developing, and that the family, like the newborn infant, has had its need to security met within an interpersonal relationship, she and the family can then move into level two activities.

▬CHILDHOOD OR INTERMEDIATE FAMILY

The second level of family functioning is characterized by a somewhat lesser amount of disorganization than the first level family. Members are slightly more able to meet their need for security and physical survival. Although still alienated from the community, they have more ability to trust and, subsequently, have more hope for a better way of life.

The parents are immature, and socially deviant behavior may occur. Distortion and confusion of roles exist but the parents are more willing to work together for the benefit of the whole family. The children are not neglected to the extent that they must be removed from the home, as is often the case in a level one family.

However, this type of family is still unable to support and promote the growth of its members. Members appear unable to change, are defensive and fearful, and lack the resources to gain a sense of accomplishment. This family does not seek help actively and requires much assistance before the members are able to acknowledge their problems realistically.

With this level two family, the nurse will continue to maintain the warm accepting support of the trust relationship, but now she uses it as a stepping stone to help the family begin to understand itself more clearly. Because of the trust established between the two, the family can begin to venture forth in self-discovery, with help from the nurse who will clarify and reflect their words, actions, thoughts, and responses. The nurse is honest in sharing her observations and personality with the family in order that they may feel more willing to be honest with themselves. By her actions, she demonstrates various roles and tasks to the family and uses these actions to further increase the family's understanding of itself.

This counseling relationship demands even more of the nurse than the previous trust relationship, as her interpretations and diagnoses must be accurate, her behavior consistent, and her concerns genuine. She must understand her feelings and relationship with the family very accurately. Her goal is to help this family grow to the point (level three) where they can work on solutions to some of their problems.

Progress is seen when members begin to feel more like a family and experience the nurse as a sibling—that is, they will vacillate between dependence and independence and compete for attention and control. The nurse, acting as a partner with this family, helps them to understand that she shares her thoughts and actions with them so that they may further understand themselves and their interaction as a family group.

▄ADOLESCENT OR FAMILY WITH PROBLEMS

The level three family is essentially normal but has more than the healthy and usual amount of conflicts and problems. As a unit, it is more capable of physical survival and of providing security for its members, but these abilities may vary greatly. Socially and emotionally, this family functions better than either previous types. Members demonstrate greater trust in people, have the knowledge and ability to utilize some community resources, and are less openly hostile to outsiders. Usually, one parent is more mature than the other, and the children have less overall difficulty adjusting to changes in the family, school, and environment.

This family, however, may have more difficulty in the task of providing sexual differentiation and training of children, than they have in the first two tasks. Although the children are cared for physically, there may be more emotional conflicts, resulting in much confusion for the children. In addition, because one parent may be quite immature, difficulties for one or more of the children may result. Very often individuals in the family experience successes and achievements outside the family, and members may even deliberately seek outside achievements to replace some missing satisfaction within their family life.

On the positive side, this family shows an increasing ability to face some of its problems and to look for solutions. They may seek and use outside help much more effectively and appropriately than a level one or two family. Members are future oriented, even though the present may be painful.

A complex of nursing activities is required to help the level three family solve its recognized problems. The nurse assists them by providing teaching, information, coordination, referral, team-work, or special technical skills such as those involved in performing complicated nursing care activities. Often she must move backward to a previous level of nursing activities and then forward again as more and more difficulties are looked at and worked on. In order to facilitate success, the family should be encouraged to start with the easiest of the most pressing problems.

Working with this family demands of the nurse a wealth of technical and interpersonal skills as well as knowledge of community resources and the ability to lead, coordinate, and cooperate with other team members. The nurse is seen by the family as an adult helper with expertise in the solution of problems. The nurse provides the needed teaching, referral, and coordination to assist the family, but she continually emphasizes the importance of their making their decisions; she helps them to do so, to try out their decisions, and to evaluate outcomes. Thus, she helps them improve their ability to manage their roles and tasks as they proceed from one problem to another.

▄ADULTHOOD OR FAMILY WITH SOLUTIONS

A family at this level may be described as normal, stable, healthy, and happy with fewer than the usual number of problems or conflicts. This is because they are able to handle most problems as they arise. This family capably provides for physical security and emotional and social functioning. The parents are usually quite mature and confident in their roles as mates, parents, wage earners, and members of society. They have fewer difficulties in providing for sexual differentiation and training their children.

Their main problems center around stages of growth and various developmental tasks. If problems in this area arise, very often the parents refer themselves to outside sources for help. However, they may show excess anxiety over these problems. Individual members and group needs and goals are usually brought into harmony by this family. Although crisis may immobilize this family, they have the ability to adapt and change, enjoy the present, and plan for the future.

The main nursing activity with this family is preventive health teaching to enable the family to maintain its health. The nurse helps the members to anticipate problem areas, to work through possible alternatives, and then to study the consequences of these alternatives. As she stresses prevention, she teaches the family about all the resources that are available in time of crisis or need. The nurse is also in a unique position to help this family grow and to increase the members' self-understanding and effectiveness in group functioning.

Such nursing activity requires much maturity, foresight, and experience. If the nurse is able to serve the family at this level, she knows that they will be functioning on a higher level than previously, and that they will use community services more appropriately when there is a need. This family sees the nurse as an expert teacher and partner and is able to utilize this partnership until it moves to level five.

▬MATURITY OR IDEAL FAMILY

This is only a short step above level four. Here the family can be described as truly homeostatic, with a healthy balance of individual and group goals, activities, participation, and concerns. All tasks are met by this family, and all supplies are provided. The only exception is in times of extreme or multiple crises, when the family is immobilized but can still ask for help from appropriate sources and use it.

Nursing activity is not necessary for this family unless there is a crisis, and at such times the family would seek help from the appropriate community source. If nursing services are required, the nurse would probably use nursing activities appropriate to the situation—either level III or IV—in assisting the family to regain its equilibrium.

The proposed model of family nursing attempts to explain how community health nurses view and work with families, what goals they set for the family, and what skills and attributes they need to accomplish their objectives. The model is based on an existential philosophy of man and the concept that health is a dynamic term which encompasses all aspects of a person's life and being—physical, psychological, emotional, social, environmental, spiritual, and cultural.

▬ REFERENCES

1. Mickey, Janice E. Studying extra-hospital nursing needs; a preliminary report. *Am. J. Public Health* 48:881, July 1958.
2. Freeman, Ruth B., AND Lowe, Marie. Method for appraising family public health nursing needs. *Am.J.Public Health* 53:47–52, Jan. 1963.
3. Lee, M. J., AND Frazier, D. M. Recognition of family-group problems by public health nurses. *Am.J.Public Health* 53:932–940, June 1963.
4. Feldman, F. L., and Scherz, F. H. *Family Social Welfare; Helping Troubled Families.* New York, Atherton Press, 1967, pp. 68–71.
5. Geismar, L. L., and La Sorte, M. A. *Understanding the Multi-problem Family.* New York, Association Press, 1964.

Chapter 32

A Family Caregiving Model for Public Health Nursing

JOYCE V. ZERWEKH

The absence of clear definitions of community health nursing competency have plagued efforts to demonstrate the need for community health nursing programs. Offered here is a practice model for community health nursing which presents a clear picture in explaining expert nursing solutions to high-risk parenting situations. Joyce Zerwekh bases this model on 16 family caregiving competencies identified and described by experienced community health nurses. The relationships between competencies are presented in the Family Caregiving Model. She challenges others to contribute to the continued development of this model by sharing their stories of expert practice and explains why public health nursing services should be integral to the public agenda.

Seeking to illustrate the need to fund nursing visits for high-risk mothers, a public health nurse in eastern Washington took her state legislator on home visits. After two hours of witnessing her exquisitely delicate work to reweave the fabric of the life of a parenting teenager, the policymaker concluded that the visit had been "a waste of time" and that the teen could have done just as well with some photocopied handouts! He had not appreciated what to look for and literally did not recognize her subtle expert competencies. Indeed, the absence of clear definitions of public health nursing competency have plagued efforts to articulate the need for public health nurse positions and programs.[1-3] Expert practice remains shrouded in vague generalizations because it is superficially documented, inadequately funded, and lacks descriptive models.

Robert Coles, the psychiatrist and social activist, proposes "the call of stories" to elicit colleagues' tales of practice wisdom.[4] Likewise, Schultz and Meleis recommend understanding practice knowledge by bringing to consciousness the practice experiences of nurses.[5] Patricia Benner was the first to elicit and interpret the practice stories of hospital nurses.[6] She asked them to tell anecdotes of their outstanding clinical practice experiences. Interpreting these, she uncovered richly descriptive portraits of hospital nursing and the names of twenty-one competencies. In like manner,

From *Nursing Outlook* 39(5):213–217, 1991. Reprinted by permission of Mosby-Year Book, Inc.

Hamilton and Bush recommend examining the stories of practicing public health nurses to elucidate practice knowledge.[2]

▬THE HUB OF FAMILY CAREGIVING: ENCOURAGING FAMILY SELF-HELP

Toward this end and inspired by Benner, the author interviewed 30 western Washington public health nurses who had a mean of 20 years nursing experience and 14 in public health. They were asked to tell "anecdotes [about those instances] when you believe that your home visiting really made a difference in the outcome with maternal/child clients." Ninety-five anecdotes were recorded and transcribed. Using a qualitative constant comparative methodology, the text was interpreted by continually asking the question, "What is the nurse doing here?" Employing the language of the nurses themselves, 16 family caregiving competencies were identified and explained using multiple excerpts from the nurses' own words.[7] To make sense of the nonlinear relationships between competencies, a Family Caregiving Model was drawn (see Figure 32-1). The remainder of this article briefly describes each competency in the model and illustrates these explanations with excerpts from the nurses' anecdotes.

The primary focus of public health nurses' visits to vulnerable families is to develop their personal capability to take charge of their lives and make their own choices. The experts repeatedly emphasize that it is the client rather than the nurse who is responsible to make changes in the client's life. Determining how much is done for the family and how much the family is expected to do for itself is learned through experience. Nurses struggle to determine when to take the initiative and when to wait for the family to take the initiative. Many clinical examples involve backing away so that independent choice is possible. To *Encourage Family Self-Help,* four strategies are intrinsic to the competency:

1. *Believing* in the clients' ability to make choices and helping the clients believe in themselves,
2. *Listening* to what the clients want and starting there,
3. *Expanding* families' vision of options, and
4. *Feeding back reality* to help them see the patterns of their lives and the implications of unhealthy choices.

▬LAYING THE GROUNDWORK: LOCATING AND BUILDING TRUST

Three competencies are essential to build groundwork before self-help can be encouraged. This foundational phase of public health nurse family caregiving is brief and straightforward with stable families who are easy to locate, readily trusting, and sure of their own strengths. However, with a growing caseload of highly disturbed and distressed families, the groundwork competencies assume a larger and larger proportion of nurse effort. Historically, these competencies have been implied but not emphasized or

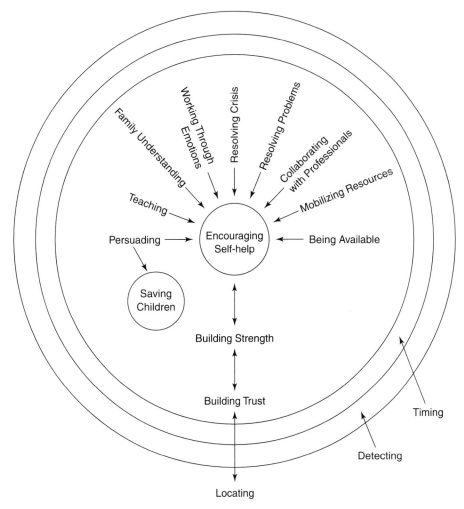

FIGURE 32-1   Family caregiving model.

documented. The uninitiated nurse, supervisor, or policymaker does not understand that the groundwork cannot be skipped in order to get on with the "real business" of Encouraging Family Self-Help.

Locating vanishing families is a taken-for-granted aspect of the public health nurse's day. Young, unstable families disappear frequently due to eviction, loss of work, broken families, or problems with the law. The nurses can knock on many doors before finding the family at home. Even when the client does not move, the Locating challenge for the nurse may be lack of a telephone or an unclear address or broken appointments. The nurses use extensive metaphorical language to describe Locating: "sniffing them out," "tracking them down," "keeping a watch out," "putting out feelers," "keeping ears to the neighborhoods," "putting out a bulletin." The competency of Locating requires persistence and expert networking skills. Success comes through the trusted community contacts that the expert nurse has developed over time.

Building Trust is foundational for all helping relationships, but is a difficult proposition when not even family or friends are trusted, much less human service professionals. The nurses describe strategies to build trust among the untrusting. *Getting through the door* involves behaving like a respectful guest and "meeting them at their level. Do not take over." *Backing off* and not pressuring is often needed when expert scrutiny reveals withdrawal clues, such as lack of eye contact. *Listening* is central to discover the families' main concerns. "Just being there" with a listening presence develops trust. Careful listening involves finding out something to "hook them," visible practical help that really interests the family. Trust building also involves *discovering and affirming strengths*, "finding the positive." *Not judging* is integral to building trust. Nurses seek to present themselves as accepting, despite the shocking, self-destructive behaviors which are often revealed. Finally, experts develop trust by *persisting* to make home visits over time.

Building Strength develops the foundation for a vulnerable family developing the capacity to help themselves. Developing strength begins with discovery and validation of existing capacity. "My gosh, do you know how infrequently so many of our clients ever hear anything positive about themselves!" In particular, *women are strengthened as persons and as mothers.* Affirming what the woman does well and the validity of her emotions and views, the nurse then encourages her to believe that she can make choices to move toward a more positive future. "Look at what's positive, while pointing out wider possibilities." Finding strengths to build upon in very dysfunctional circumstances can be "a stretch" for even the most expert nurse. The nurses share a common maxim, "build up the mother so she can care for the baby." Strengthening the woman as parent begins by searching for ways to praise positive aspects of parenting. Nothing is taken for granted so that even the most basic parenting behaviors are affirmed. The mothers begin to see themselves as able to undertake self-help. Growing self-esteem promotes the process of taking charge of one's life.

▬THE ENCOMPASSING COMPETENCIES: TIMING AND DETECTING

The *Timing* competency envelopes and informs all family caregiving activities. The expert public health nurse regulates the speed of her interventions to produce the best results. "Tincture of time: describes the developmental process needed for a public health nurse to learn Timing so that she matches her speed in pushing for change with that of the family's movement toward change. Timing has three dimensions. First, *detecting the right time* involves picking up clues that the time is right to initiate an approach. "Catch them when they're ready." Second, *persisting* involves continuing to visit in order to be there when the Timing is right, adjusting to slow progress, one step at a time. Third, *futuring* is an aspect of Timing in which the nurse experts time their intervention based on their vision of future problems and possibilities. For instance, they anticipate child development challenges, prenatal and postpartum needs, and family crises. They try to "catch things before they get out of hand." "I am standing by with my fire hose in hand in case the sparks ignite again." Futuring also involves guiding young mothers who live only in the present to plan for a positive future "to improve their lives."

Like Timing, *Detecting* is an ongoing competency that determines how all other competencies are implemented. The experts describe themselves as detectives looking for clues, evidence, signals that indicate what's really happening in the home. They believe that a clear sense of family circumstances affecting health can only be discovered by gaining entrance to the home to see how people live their lives. Public health nurse detectives begin with broad investigation and then narrow their inquiry based on their sense of timing and level of trust. The client's concerns must first be heard and she must have a sense of control rather than intrusion. Experts are wary of using structured assessment protocols too early. However, evidence is eventually gathered through a wide variety of systematic assessments including physical examination of mother and children, child behavior and development screening, scrutiny of parent-child interaction, family system assessment, nutritional assessment, safety investigation, and determination of possible domestic violence and chemical abuse.

In this natural setting, the nurse discovers incapacitating living environments, dysfunctional family interaction, troubling child behavior, mother's concerns, and physiological alterations. *Environment discoveries* might include households without food, cooking facilities, bathing facilities, sanitation; or those unsafe due to fire hazards, drug traffic, or violence. *Family dynamics* discovered through an inside look at the family system could include destructive patterns between parents, between parents and children, and within the extended family. Examples of troubling discoveries about *children at home* might include a child left alone in a walker all day, a sibling failing to thrive, a so-called colicky baby whose actual problem is difficulty sucking. Clues about *mother's needs* might range from misunderstanding how to mix the formula to suicidal ideation. Finally, a home visiting nurse may be the first to detect evidence of *Physiological alterations* and problems with prescribed medical regimens.

▬FOSTERING COMMUNITY: BEING AVAILABLE, MOBILIZING, AND COLLABORATING

Expert nurses *Being Available* to clients encourages self-help. Three different facets of nurse availability emerge from anecdotes. First, the public health nurse may be the only care-giving option available for some families who cannot access assistance with health care and parenting due to inadequate community resources, poverty, distance, and lack of child care. "If the public health nurse isn't advocating for most of these children, there would just be nothing." Second, *persisting in being available* is essential to Encouraging Self-Help. The nurse becomes a stable force who can be counted on over time. "The thing that really makes a difference is always being there for them."

The third facet of Being Available is a striking contrast to contemporary health care practice. These expert public health nurses strongly encourage calling them with problems. At a time when most health care providers seek to detour calls from the worried well, and consumers have been conditioned to avoid bothering the busy provider, public health nurses urge their clients to call. With a population who frequently wait until they are overwhelmed by immobilizing crises, experts emphasize calling as a strength, a self-aware health seeking behavior. Calling implies recognition of need and choosing support rather than isolation.

Likewise, *Mobilizing Resources* further affirms the nurses' belief that self-help and responsibility are enabled through community support, not further isolation. The individual's ability to make healthy decisions is strengthened when adequately sustained by others. To mobilize resources, the expert nurse carefully develops a network of connections. "Get to know every agency, every professional, every volunteer, every banker, every gas station attendant who might speak Spanish . . . Our job is pulling in an incredible network." The nurses commonly used "hooking them up" to refer to the process of "arranging the nuts and bolts of services." Public health nursing "is directing and being the maestro for my clients . . . I am willing to pull all the different resources and services together and stroke my wand to get things done." Hooking them up varies on a continuum from nurse-initiated to client-initiated contact based on the public health nurse's judgment of client strengths and the accessibility of the resource.

Finally, *Collaborating with Professionals* emphasizes the public health nurses working in partnership with many community professionals on behalf of the client. It is particularly common to develop partnerships with hospital and clinic nurses, physicians, counselors, Child Protective Service caseworkers, and teachers. Sometimes expert competency requires working through divergent opinions that occur when different disciplines approach common problems.

■RESOLVING PROBLEMS AND RESOLVING CRISES

Expert public health nurses are competent in *Resolving Problems* that are everyday in the lives of vulnerable families and which might appear unresolvable to the novice. Openness and flexibility are considered essential. Nurses try to create solutions where none are obvious as they help parents with matters such as finding food and transportation, caring for children in adverse environments, and dealing with a wide variety of infant and child problems. The nurses stand behind mothers and work through issues of child management, family management, and self-care management for the mother. The nurse takes greater initiative as mothers' problem solving skills are impaired by developmental disability, drugs, or psychiatric illness. However, every effort is made to develop parent skills in resolving problems. Nurses target everyday problems identified by the parent and work on prioritizing. Helping parents make decisions is guided by the four strategies identified under Encouraging Self-Help.

Resolving Crises is an overlapping competency. Public health nursing is an ongoing process of facing unexpected problems, which either nurse or client may perceive as crises. Many families "are in regular and continuing crisis." Once crises are resolved, "that's not to say that things won't fall apart." Practicing futuring, the nurses consistently recognize potential for disaster and try to avoid it.

▬ WORKING THROUGH EMOTIONS AND FOSTERING FAMILY UNDERSTANDING

"The strong people skills are always focused back to parenting issues." For broader counseling issues, public health nurses refer to counseling professionals when accessible. *Working Through Emotions* that impair parenting includes exploring feelings about pregnancy, children, and relationships; grief work; focusing on reality; and encouraging emotional self-help. The nurses continually describe "being there emotionally" for parents. "They've never really had a caring person sit down long enough to listen." "I've had many women tell me of abuse or a great pain or grief they've never sat down and discussed." *Grief work* is emphasized following death or when a child or relationship is not what the parent anticipated. *Focusing on reality* rather than denial of feelings is stressed. Clients are often immobilized by denial and cannot make change until they face their own reality. Clients are urged "to be a real person with real emotions." Having expressed and gained insight into their feelings, the clients are encouraged to apply self-help and problem-resolving approaches to their own healing. Frequently they are assisted to develop self-assertion and to set boundaries to protect their feelings.

Fostering Family Understanding is the competency in which the nurse promotes family insight and accord. Unfortunately, nurses seldom work with a functional mother-father dyad as heads of household. Mothers are commonly raising children alone, perhaps with the assistance of grandmothers or other female relatives. Fathers are frequently not supportive, absent, and/or abusive. Fostering family understanding is practiced when the nurses assist mothers to work out their relationships with other adult family members, including family of origin and husbands or lovers. Experts promote insight into family patterns, such as histories of chemical abuse, and accord between the generations. Often they mediate differences between grandmothers or great grandmothers and mothers. Sometimes they have the opportunity to promote extended family understanding of health and "get the whole family squared away with their health care."

Fostering Family Understanding also includes the nurses' support of functional male-female relationships and fathers' relationships with children. In the case of domestic violence, the paramount goal becomes promoting safety of mother and children rather than promoting unity of the couple. The nurses advocate escape from the cycle of violence. As nurses' caseloads are increasingly composed of multiproblem dysfunctional families, the possibility of fostering family understanding declines.

■PARENT EDUCATION: THE TEACHING COMPETENCY

Nurses instruct families so that they can develop the knowledge and skill to care for themselves. Effective teaching requires expert building of trust and timing to match teaching to client emotional and intellectual readiness for learning. The absence of readiness in families who are heavily drug-involved means "we can't do our usual parenting education because they are so uniterested." The nurses prefer to engage in a dialogue, with parents asking questions and nurses responding. Teaching high-risk parents requires flexibility, adjusting to concrete rather than abstract thinking, repetition, focusing on one goal at a time, asking for feedback on knowledge and return demonstration of skill, and role modeling. "We demonstrate hugging the baby, talking to the baby, playing with the baby, picking up on the baby's cues." With an increasing proportion of learning impaired parents, the nurses are struggling to develop special expertise. They believe strongly in the effectiveness of group teaching through community parenting and support groups, which many public health nurses lead.

The nurses focus their teaching on the child and on the mother. For the young mothers isolated from functional extended family, the nurses often need to teach basic child care that would normally have been learned from their mothers. "Help her with the nitty gritty child care issues. How do you fix formula? How do you wash diapers? How do you bathe a baby?" Understanding and responding to child behavior, particularly infant cues, is an integral aspect of teaching. Parents are taught to understand child development. "Try to keep one step ahead of the baby in letting mom know that he'll be doing next." They are assisted to see the child as an individual and to have age-appropriate expectations. Likewise, public health nurses advise and demonstrate positive disciplining techniques geared to developmental level. Teaching about safety is a vital agenda, including standard recommendations about accident prevention as well as coping with hazards discovered in home visits. Finally, nurses teach mothers to recognize illness in healthy children and to manage common child health problems as well as the complex regimens of children with chronic illness and disability.

Teaching focuses on the mother through educational strategies that prepare her for pregnancy and childbirth and postpartum, as well as learning life skills such as time management, assertiveness, and decision making.

■FORCEFUL COMPETENCIES:
PERSUADING AND SAVING CHILDREN

When a nurse finds that children are at risk which is not reduced by the competencies that promote family self care and autonomous choice, she redefines her authority to convince the parents of the need for change. In other words, the nurse uses the force of social authority to oppose the parents' expressed wishes. She does this by three types of *Persuading*. Persuading through reasoning involves using a logically developed argument to convince family they must change. Persuading through confronting involves a face to face statement opposing parent's wishes and behaviors. This is not done if there is any threat to the nurse's physical safety. Confrontation boldly opposes denial and blaming to name and face extreme health hazards such as drug abuse or domestic violence. Most coercive is persuasion by threatening action such as removing a child or calling the police.

Saving Children contrasts with Encouraging Family Self-Help and emphasizes nurse accountability for child protection. On behalf of children judged to be in great peril, the nurse believes child well-being is a higher priority than continued respect for parental authority. The nurses detect the level of risk to children by visiting the home regularly. Often they must witness and document marginal abuse and neglect for years before "the straw that breaks the camel's back." In cases where they are not already working with Child Protective Services, they judge whether to notify authorities. At some point in their effort to strengthen and develop the parent, emphasis swings to protecting the child. They struggle with divided loyalties as they try to stand by both the vulnerable child and the vulnerable but abusing parent. Divided loyalties has been described in the child protection literature as a "schizophrenic exercise" to try to be both parents' accuser and counselor.[8] In Saving Children, the nurses not only represent authority but become authority.

◼ CONCLUSION

The credibility of qualitative description is tested by subjecting conclusions to those whose reality is being described.[9] This practice model, the competencies, and their interpretation have been repeatedly confirmed in sessions with practicing nurse experts in Western Washington. However, readers are reminded about the limits of generalization from this initial investigation. Each is invited to validate selectively and transfer information relevant to her own context. The model will be clarified, expanded, and modified with additional qualitative studies of public health nurse experts. It needs to be replicated in other parts of the country. In particular, participant observations, group interviews, and multiple investigators would assure a comprehensive descriptive portrait of practice.

Immediate implications for this practice model include the advantage of presenting a clear picture that explains expert nursing solutions to high-risk parenting situations. The model can be used for teaching nursing students and novice public health nurses. It can be a framework for agency practice. And in conclusion, it can be used to explain the role of public health nurses to policymakers, such as the ignorant legislator mentioned at the beginning of this article. Services that can be defined can be marketed using the model and illustrative local stories about nurses making a difference. As the public is finally becoming concerned with the plight of vulnerable families and children, the model is suitable to explain why public health nursing services should be integral to the public agenda.

■ REFERENCES

1. Erickson, G.P. Public health nursing initiatives: guideposts for future practice. *Public Health Nurs.* 4:202–211, Dec. 1987.
2. Hamilton, P.A., and Bush, H.A. Theory development in community health nursing: issues and recommendations. *Sch. Inq. Nurs. Pract.* 2:145–165, Summer, 1988.
3. Oda, D.S., and Boyd, P. Documenting the effect and cost of public health nursing field services. *Public Health Nurs.* 4:180–182, Sept. 1987.
4. Coles, R. *The Call of Stories: Teaching and the Moral Imagination.* Boston, Houghton Mifflin, 1990.
5. Schultz, P.R., and Meleis, A.I. Nursing epistemology: traditions, insights, questions. *Image J. Nurs. Sch.* 20:217–221, Winter, 1988.
6. Benner, P. *From Novice to Expert.* Menlo Park, CA: Addison-Wesley, 1984.
7. Zerwekh, J.V. *Qualitative Description of the Competencies of Expert Public Health Nurses.* Seattle, Seattle University, 1990. (Unpublished doctoral dissertation)
8. Silverman, P. *Who Speaks for the Children? The Plight of the Battered Child.* Don Mills, Ont.: Musson Publishing, 1978.
9. Lincoln, Y.S., and Guba, E.G. *Naturalistic Inquiry.* Beverly Hills, CA: Sage, 1985.

Chapter 33

When A Woman Heads the Household

MARY E. DUFFY

Single-parent families are increasing in number, and the majority of these families remain headed by women. The unique physical, emotional, and economic stresses experienced by single parents and their concomitant effects on the rest of the family are not often understood or addressed. Community health nurses are in a unique position to provide service to this important population as they work with families in the community. In this chapter, Mary Duffey offers a challenging look at the needs of single-parent families, particularly at the needs of women who are single parents. She describes nursing's responsibilities in prevention, intervention, advocacy, and research.

Nursing is a female profession that, ironically, often seems to ignore the health care needs of women. Many nurses have been accused of being "deaf, dumb, and blind to the needs of women."[1] A recent analysis of four leading nursing journals found that 81 percent of the clinical nursing research published was unrelated to the health needs of women themselves or to their maternal role.[2] The apparent dearth of nursing research concerning women's health and the maternal role becomes poignant when addressing the health care needs of single-parent families.

According to the U.S. Census (1981), in the U.S. there were 79.1 million households of which 60.3 million had children under the age of 18. These households represent a variety of traditional and nontraditional family structures.[3] Of these almost nine million are single-parent families and over 80 percent of these are headed by women.[4] The number of single-parent households has increased dramatically over the last few years.

Although the number of single-parent families, mainly female headed, represent a significant and growing population in our society, this family structure is not awarded equal status with the two-parent family. Labels such as "broken home" and "latch-key children" are indiscriminately attached to the single parent family.

Societal expectations, as we know, are based upon labels. "Broken home" conjures up fantasies of unruly children deprived of a father or any

From *Nursing Outlook* 30(8):468–473, 1982. Reprinted by permission of Mosby-Year Book, Inc.

consistent male role-model. "Latch-key children" insinuates that the parent is frequently absent from the home, leaving the children unsupervised.

These stereotypes may be somewhat exaggerated, but they generally reflect how the female headed, single-parent family is perceived. The values and norms of this culture reinforce the myth that the traditional nuclear family is the only healthy environment in which to raise children. Yet, in the U.S. only seven percent of the families are traditionally composed of both a male and female parent and children.[5]

Single-parent families emerge from all socioeconomic classes for a multitude of reasons: divorce, death, never married, or desertion. The meaning of being a single-parent family for each of its members and the reactions of society to that family will be influenced by the factor(s) that precipitated the single-parent status.

Divorce, for instance, implies failure in a controllable situation. Death, on the other hand, elicits sympathy because of the helplessness of the family in an unpreventable situation.

Regardless of the cause, the single-parent family is considered a transitory stage and tolerated only as a temporary arrangement. Remarriage is thought to be the appropriate solution to an "undesirable" state. These perceptions can only place the single-parent in double jeopardy.

Remarriage, due to pressure and undertaken hastily, will probably result in divorce. Another marriage is entered before the loss and conflicts from the previous relationship have been resolved. The adult who delays remarriage or chooses to remain a single-parent is placed in perpetual limbo. This family system remains a deviation from the so-called "norm."

As Smith says, "this traditional perspective is dangerous. It could result in our deemphasizing the conditions in one-parent families as 'only' short-term conditions. Also, it could result in our overlooking the needs of those who head one-parent families over a longer period of time."[6] The pressure to marry and raise children in two-parent families is felt by both sexes. Alternative family forms are viewed as deviations from the norm and less adequate as an environment to socialize future generations.

▬ IS IT EASIER AS A MAN?

The single-parent family headed by either a male or female may be considered to be a deviant family form, but society's expectations are quite different for the male assuming a dual parent role than for his female counterpart. Less attention is focused on these families because: 1) the male is the "natural" head of a family, 2) the number of male headed, single-parent families is significantly smaller, approximately 20 percent of all single-parent families, and 3) society's expectations of a man in the home are minimal.

The male head of a single-parent family is unconditionally admired for adding to his primary role, as breadwinner, tasks of less value such as housekeeping and child-care. Men, by nature, are considered so inept at woman's work that any accomplishment in this role is received with amazement and given positive reinforcement by onlookers. There is a difference throughout all socioeconomic levels between the male and the female headed, single-parent family.

The parent is a pivotal family member whose own mental and physical health will be instrumental in influencing the health needs of the children. The family unit is viewed as a system, with the parent retaining primary control over the actions of the system. A parent unable to cope with the loss of a spouse and fearful of the responsibilities as head of a household will be unable to assist the children in coping with their loss.

Do the health care needs of the female headed, single-parent family differ from those of the two-parent or even male headed, single-parent family? Certainly the stresses placed on a female head of the family in a male dominated society would suggest that they do. The experiences of a woman in this role determine the family's status within society and impact on the family both internally and externally.

■WHAT ARE THE ODDS FOR A WOMAN ALONE?

Woman are neither prepared nor expected to assume the role of head of the household. The economic, legal, political, and religious systems discouraged women, once forced to assume this role, to attempt to succeed at it.

Women from childhood are socialized into dependence, passivity, and submissiveness. Female child's play is usually restricted to tasks and games which prepare the girl for marriage and children. The myth purports that women are innately driven to this domestic role and unfulfilled without it. Another explanation might be that the cultural meaning of this role is so deeply ingrained in girls and women that options are essentially unavailable. Some recent changes have occurred through the feminist movement but this traditional pattern remains dominant.

In marriage, the custody of the woman is transferred from her father to her husband. The husband is now the woman's protector, economic provider, and buffer in negotiating between the family unit and the patriarchal society. His identity becomes hers and the woman continues to live through and from a "dominant other."[7] The "dominant other" relationship is seen when she is at home with her husband and follows the woman to work. For instance, the nurse-physician relationship in a hospital has been pointed out to be analogous to the wife-husband interaction in the family unit.[8,9]

Women are relegated to secondary positions in society and according to the historical myth, shielded from the stresses of the world. As a result, women are unprepared, both financially and emotionally, to cope with their situation as head of a household in a male-dominated society. Women are accustomed to negotiating through men and must confront a disapproving society directly without many of the resources needed.

The immediate consequence of being a woman alone is a loss of her identity. The married woman's identity comes from her husband's occupational status and social position in society. In a 1981 pilot study that I conducted, 17 single mothers who were either divorced or widowed were interviewed. Each woman shared the significance of establishing her own identity, independent of any dominant person. The woman's identity, independent from a man, could only develop during this period in which she was unmarried.

■ WHAT SATISFACTION IS THERE?

Socialized to be housewives and to reject the notion of a career, with the fantasy of being married happily ever after, women are denied the preparation needed to support themselves and their families. Also, the full-time homemaker has only one source of satisfaction—her family. If she is dissatisfied with her home life, she has no source for positive reinforcement from her life and career. Men, on the other hand, having an occupation in addition to a family, can absorb themselves in their work achieving rewards from their careers.

Housework is unpaid, devalued, and invisible labor. The result for the woman can be very little else besides low self-esteem and she is at a greater risk for mental illness, specifically depression.[10-13] Being at high risk with low self-esteem intensifies when a woman faces the stresses and uncertainties of single parenthood.

Even employed women rarely have a career. Employment is undertaken as a part-time or temporary endeavor and carries a different meaning from the husband's job. The married woman is rarely labeled the breadwinner and expected to fulfill that role. For example, the married woman who puts her husband through college will frequently wait to obtain an education herself until after his career is established.

The woman's employment and household responsibilities must be coordinated; she needs to be available to care for a sick child or manage a household crisis. The husband is not expected to take time off from his work for domestic needs. His career cannot tolerate such interruptions.

This does not imply that women take off more days than men; but rather that the domestic reasons causing women to be absent from their job will carry negative connotations in an office environment. As a result, women are perceived as unreliable employees, motivated to work out of financial necessity and not career interest.

In the male-dominated work outside the home environment there is an incompatibility between society's definitions and expectations for a woman and the characteristics required for pursuing a career. Society not only has low expectations for women outside the home in contrast to men, but the rewards and reinforcements will tend to become negative once the woman begins to achieve beyond her expected and accepted level.[13]

This scenario for the woman who becomes the head of a household dooms her to an economic crisis. A comparison of the Census Bureau's median annual incomes provides evidence of the discrepancies.* The sin-

---

*The median income for all families in 1980 was $21,020, the median income for the male, single-parent family was $17,519; whereas the female single-parent's median income was as little as one-half this: $10,408.[2]

gle father, with greater financial resources and flexibility than the single mother, can relieve some of the stress of the dual-parent role by purchasing help needed to perform tasks created by the extra responsibilities.

More devastated economically is the single mother with children under the age of 6 years. In 1979, this woman's annual income was $4,500 per year. Another prevailing myth about the financial resources available to the single mother is child support, payment by the noncustodial parent for *part* of each child's care. The average annual child support payment in 1979, however, was no more than $1,800 per child.[14]

The reality is that approximately 3 million female headed, single-parent families live on incomes below poverty levels. Many more exist at near poverty level.

▬WHAT IS THE EFFECT?

The treatment of women who are single parents has an impact on the health of all members of her family. Society, in attempting to deny the phenomenon of the female headed, single-parent family unit, refuses to facilitate the integration of women heads of households into the structural and functional aspects of society.

As a result, the family experiences a multitude of stresses related to: 1) the loss of the spouse/parent; 2) the loss of status which is reserved for the two-parent family; and 3) the position of women in society. The female headed, single-parent family, especially with the woman at the helm, suffers an increased risk for physical and mental health problems.[15-18]

The stresses generally resulting from the single-parent experience can be grouped into three categories: 1) pragmatic concerns; 2) interpersonal and social problems; and 3) family related stressors.[17] Pragmatic concerns relate to the daily activities of a family including job, money, child care, household tasks, legal concerns, and economics of time. Support systems, family and community reactions to the changes in marital status, the parents' intimate personal relationships, loss of role and social status are examples of the interpersonal and social problems. Family related stressors are dominated by the adjustment to the loss of the spouse/parent, parent-child relationships, and resolution of custody.

Leavell and Clark's natural history of disease paradigm, delineating three levels of prevention provides a framework to analyze the potential health risks and hazards of these families.[19] Although in reality, any one of these three levels may be dominant at a given time, the process of assessing and intervening at each level is continual whenever the family comes in contact with the health care delivery system.

▬IDENTIFYING THE PROBLEM BEFORE IT IS A CRISIS

Primary prevention is the assessment of and intervention with potential or actual stressors which threaten health prior to the onset of illness. These stressors are both internal and external factors including the entire family's total health habits. The family experiencing loss from a separation, divorce, or death is in a time of crisis and this family relies on the previously developed strengths of its members to lessen the impact.

For primary prevention, health professionals need to work with women and their families who are not yet experiencing a crisis in order to strengthen their individual abilities and the family unit. Ideally, this level of prevention should occur during the time that the family is a two-parent family. Unfortunately, the medical model that begins intervention only after illness is diagnosed has been the paradigm for the health care delivery system. Primary prevention rejects the traditional approach to health care and focuses interventions on strengthening individuals and groups who are not in crisis. For example, learning effective family communication patterns, particularly between the spouses, may prevent communication breakdown and eventual divorce.

For the woman, development of an independent self-identity and positive self-esteem needs to be her primary concern. Low self-esteem can result from a lack of a clearly defined personal identity. And it can be the cause of depression, a condition more frequently diagnosed in women than men. A woman who knows her own identity as differentiated from her husband's cannot be stripped of an identity when she is no longer married.

Families should be encouraged to take care of themselves, physically and emotionally, prior to the onset or expectation of a crisis. Individuals who have practiced primary prevention behaviors—stress reduction, exercise, good nutrition, development of a support system, etc.—will be more resilient physically and mentally and able to call upon these resources for support.

Finally, women must learn to take responsibility for themselves. The myths of marital bliss and growing old together must be reassessed. Society and women must realize that women may not be cared for and protected in the family haven throughout their life span. Girls need to be socialized from childhood into accepting the reality that they will probably be responsible for their own and, perhaps, their family's financial support. Society must set higher expectations for women and learn to reward them, positively reinforcing female achievement.

The ultimate reward for women will be a break in what is referred to as "a vicious cycle": learned helplessness, low self-esteem, and depression.[13] The outcome of strengthening women, as a group, must be a lessening of the current, overwhelming secondary and tertiary health effects of single parenthood on female headed families.

■FATIGUE, DEPRESSION, AND PSYCHOSOMATIC ILLNESS

Recognizing the existence of female headed, single-parent families and responding with appropriate interventions are the crucial elements of quality secondary prevention. Secondary prevention is the call for early diagnosis of and intervention in health disruptions. In this case, depression and the physical problems resulting from emotional stress are major illnesses experienced. The accumulative effects of multifaceted stressors are exacerbated and manifested in mental and/or physical illness.

The uniqueness of the female headed, single-parent family—lack of financial resources, existence in a male dominated society, and so forth—contributes to the health problems and the difficulties resolving them. The characteristics of the female headed, single-parent family seem to be those contributing to high risk factors for depression. The individual most likely to be depressed is a poor, unemployed, working-class woman living alone with three or more children who does not have an intimate personal relationship and possesses a low self-esteem.[12]

Strengthening both the family's resources and the mother's self-esteem will help the family towards independence, decrease the risk of prolonged and severe depression, and avoid family chaos. The women interviewed in my pilot study cited the development of their own identity, and the recognition of their ability to make independent decisions as the major factors in reorganizing their lives and those of their families. The women stated when they felt better about themselves they took better care of their health and consequently that of their children, more so than during the time when they were married. These responses were consistent regardless of economic status and whether the loss of the spouse was through death or divorce.

Support systems and resources are another concern. Support systems frequently change with the change in marital status as married friends slowly withdraw from the single person. The woman must be helped to make new friends and to identify and utilize new sources of support. The woman's emotional need is further complicated if her family is either unavailable or unwilling to help her. The latter situation will often accompany divorce.

Resources, namely money, are greatly limited and this usually remains a stressor. Limited income decreases the family's ability to purchase help and to engage in social activities. An inverse relationship has been found between the parent's social participation and adjustment to single-parent status.[16]

The "superwoman syndrome" is created as a no-win situation which reinforces the myth that women are incapable of being the heads of households and assuming adult responsibilities. The superwoman is expected to harmoniously coordinate and synthesize the roles of two parents into one in a society that denies the long-term existence of the female headed, single-parent family and does not establish mechanisms to facilitate her integration into the existing economic and social spheres. Her role overload can result in fatigue, guilt, and psychosomatic illness.

▬NURSING PREVENTION: PUBLIC AWARENESS AND ADVOCATE POSTURE

Rehabilitation is the goal of tertiary prevention in the Leavell and Clark paradigm.[19] For the single-parent family, rehabilitation is *not* a hasty remarriage. Instead, rehabilitation is the continuance of the interventions begun during the crisis and the teaching of basic preventive health behaviors. The family unit and each of its members is strengthened by the development of new behaviors and the encouragement for each family member to enhance their potential.

Depending on the family's health status prior to the loss of the spouse, tertiary prevention may require prolonged intervention. Family and individual therapy, disciplining, job training, and general health education are some of the interventions that may be necessary. Health care must be planned to meet the needs of each female headed, single-parent family.

Tertiary prevention is also public education. Health professionals, especially nurses, must become activists in changing the position of women and single-parent families in this society.

Strengthening the family unit through the parent will result in a beneficial, long-term investment. Children, as well as their parents, are vulnerable to physical and mental health problems when faced with increased and prolonged stress. Health care professionals intervening with children from a single-parent family need to recognize that there is just one primary parent and they need to be sensitive to the unique needs of this family unit.

The health problems threatening the female headed, single-parent family are complicated by their treatment in the health care delivery system. Health professionals, influenced by societal values, either ignore the single-parent family, treat them as deviants, or perceive them as a two-parent family.[15] This latter perception allows the health care professional to place the same expectations on the single-parent family as on the two-parent family. This prevents fair, nondiscriminating treatment.

Nurses, predominantly women, must emerge as the advocates of women and their families in health care research and practice. The norms of male health are the criteria by which clients of both sexes are evaluated. Male values, affecting male and female clients, are steeped in objectivity, technical competence, and universality. Female values emphasize individualism and personal relationships. Nurses, in the struggle to attain professional recognition by male-dominated professions such as medicine, seem to be abandoning female values and clients.[1]

Our incapacity to care for women plus the devaluing of the single-parent family unit means female headed, single-parent families are deprived of the quality of care that recognizes them as legitimate people and part of a legitimate family unit. Nurses should be outraged to see female headed families, often their own, treated in a system which in essence denies their existence.

◼ RESEARCH: AN IMPORTANT BEGINNING

What can nurses do to alter this skewed system? In both research and practice, the issues of health needs and care of women and women with their children (the single-parent family) must become a priority. Nurses must learn to care for and nurture women and realize the potential of women in all aspects of our society.[1,20]

Research is a preliminary step to fully addressing these issues in the delivery of health care. Yet, less than one-fifth of all nursing research is directed at women and the maternal role issues, despite the fact that the majority of nurses are women, and women and their children are more frequent clients than men.[2]

Research is the foundation of nursing practice. Each step of the nursing process when applied to female headed, single-parent families is devoid of nursing research. The nursing process delineates a framework for potential research: 1) assessment of the health care needs of women and their children particularly in the single-parent family; 2) effective planning and implementation of health care services designed to meet these needs; and 3) evaluation research to assure that the needs are being met by quality care and with dignity. The nursing process applied to all three levels of prevention provides a framework for the holistic investigation of the health care of female headed, single-parent families.

Practice should then implement the nursing research findings. Until adequate data is available and theories developed, nurses in practice can assume the advocate role for women and female headed, single-parent families through their individual care and as political proponents in policy issues at all levels.

If women nurses begin by listening to women clients, the necessary data for planning individualized and quality care will be available. These clients will begin to get the attention and care they deserve and women nurses will be using their natural strengths.

Politically, nurses have the unique opportunity to create change in society through the health care delivery system. Nurses have the numerical strength to redefine the norms upon which health care delivery is based. Women—nurses, clients, and their children—would be the primary beneficiaries of such changes.

▬ REFERENCES

1. Ashley, J. A. Power in structured misogyny: implications for the politics of care. *ANS* 2:3–22, Apr. 1980.
2. Dunbar, S. B., and others. Women's health and nursing research. *ANS* 3:1–16, Jan. 1981.
3. U.S. Census Bureau. *Money, Income and Poverty Status of Families and Persons in the U.S.* (Ser. P. 60; No. 127) Washington, D.C., U.S. Government Printing Office, 1981.
4. ———. *Statistical Abstracts of the United States.* Washington, D.C., U.S. Government Printing Office, 1978, p. 454, table 751.
5. Rich, A. *Of Women Born.* New York, W. W. Norton and Company, 1976.
6. Smith, M. J. The social consequences of single parenthood: a longitudinal perspective. *Fam. Relations* 29(1):75–81, 1980.
7. Arieti, Silvano. Roots of depression: the power of the dominant others. *Psychol. Today* 12:54–55ff, Apr. 1979.
8. Lovell, M. C. Silent but perfect 'partners': medicine's use and abuse of women. *ANS* 3:25–40, Jan. 1981.
9. Ashley, J. A. *Hospitals, Paternalism, and the Role of the Nurse.* New York Teachers College Press, 1976.
10. McGrory, A. Women and mental illness: a sexist trap? Part 1. *J. Psychiatr. Nurs.* 18:13–19, Sept. 1980.
11. ———. Women and mental illness: a sexist trap? Part 2. *J. Psychiatr. Nurs.* 18: 16–22, Oct. 1980.

12. Jacobsen, A. Melancholy in the 20th century: causes and prevention. *J. Psychiatr. Nurs.* 18:11–21, July 1980.
13. Beck, C. T. The occurrence of depression in women and the effect of the women's movement. *J. Psychiatr. Nurs.* 17:14–16, Nov. 1979.
14. U.S. Census Bureau. *Child Support and Alimony.* (Ser. P. 23; No. 106) Washington, D.C., U.S. Government Printing Office, 1980.
15. Horowitz, J. A., and Perdue, B. J. Single-parent families. *Nurs. Clin. North Am.* 12:503–511, Sept. 1977.
16. Price-Bonham, Sharon, and Balswick, J. O. Noninstitutions: divorce, desertion, and remarriage. *J. Marr. Fam.* 42:959–972. Nov. 1980.
17. Berman, W. H., and Turk, D. C. Adaptation to divorce: problems and coping strategies. *J. Marr. Fam.* 43:179–189, Feb. 1981.
18. Herman, S. J. Women, divorce, and suicide. *J. Divorce* 1(2):107–117, 1977.
19. Leavell, H. R., and others. *Preventive Medicine.* 3rd ed. New York, McGraw-Hill Book Co., 1965.
20. Kjervik, D. K. Women, nursing, leadership. *Image* (NY) 11:34–36, June 1979.

Chapter 34

Child Abuse and the Community Health Nurse

JANICE MAE RYAN

Family violence continues to be a significant public health issue. It appears in many forms. Child abuse, battered women, battered elderly—we read about, hear, and see these and other evidence of dysfunctional lives every day in the media. What causes family members to engage in violent acts toward one another? Can it be stopped? Can it be prevented? Unhealthy families have not learned the basic functions essential to good health; instead they have developed inadequate patterns of coping, making the stresses of daily living more than they can handle. Inadequately equipped, they act in inappropriate and often harmful ways to themselves, to family members, and to society. Community health nurses see many such families. Their challenge is to understand the causes of family dysfunction and to design useful intervention and preventive strategies. Janice Ryan describes a moving case study of child abuse prevention which provides important insights and suggestions for nursing action. Principles drawn from this chapter can be applied to other forms of family violence as well.

Rarely does a day go by that the newspaper does not carry an article on child abuse. The article may present an actual case, recent statistics, or an interview with an expert on child abuse. In 1986 in one major city, 830 children were treated for child abuse (Child Abuse Team, Children's Hospital, Columbus, Ohio), and 3,396 children were removed from homes in which abuse actually occurred or was suspected (Franklin County Children's Services, Franklin County, Ohio).

A review of the community health nursing texts on this subject reveals that the chief focus is on physical symptoms that appear after the child abuse has occurred and on the public laws that require reporting of child abuse.[1-4] Although state laws require professional nurses and others to report child abuse, the area of prevention is almost completely neglected. While further abuse has undoubtedly been prevented in those children who are reported, it appears that little is done in assessing families with potential for abuse.

From *Home Healthcare Nurse* 7(2):23–26, 1989. Reprinted by permission of Lippincott-Raven Publishers.

371

Why is it that child abuse is not prevented but only discovered after the fact, when parents bring the child in for treatment or the coroner is called? Shamansky and Clausen[5] define primary prevention as that which "precedes disease or dysfunction and is applied to a generally healthy population." The purpose of primary prevention is to safeguard a population against a disease or problem by removing or reducing risk factors. Prevention is the very heart of community health nursing and has been practiced by nurses in the community for years.

This paper presents an actual case of a family at risk for abuse, discussing the factors that placed the family at risk and summarizing the nursing interventions that can effectively reduce such risk.

▬THE GREEN FAMILY

At 10 A.M. one morning a visit was made to the Green family to determine how the family was benefiting from the county health department's Women, Infants and Children program (WIC). The city health department in whose jurisdiction this family resided was not regularly visiting the Greens for any services. Once a month, the mother went to the county health department for renewal of the WIC service, where she spoke only with a nutritionist.

The home was located on a corner in a deteriorating neighborhood. Houses were in need of paint and repair. A trucking firm located adjacent to the house caused increased traffic and noise at the nearby intersection. Cars seemed to be exceeding the 35-mph speed limit.

The Greens' front door opened directly into a dimly lit kitchen. The screen door had most of the upper screen hanging free and it swung back and forth as the door was opened. The lower screen was missing altogether.

A small black and white kitten bounced into view, with a toddler not far behind. The child was dressed in diapers and a colored T-shirt. Although it was only late September and the sun was shining, the nights had been cold and there was a chill in the house.

The mother motioned for the visitor to go into the far room, where her 6-month-old daughter lay in a baby carriage that was barely large enough to hold her. As the visitor entered the room, the husband was just getting out of a bed on the far side of the room. He had a heavy beard and thick, black hair and seemed menacing at first glance. He said nothing to the greeting offered, and left the room. The visitor picked up the baby from the carriage and found that she had soaked through all her clothes, including the thin blanket wrapped around her. The visitor also discovered that the mother had only two diapers, one of which was being dried with a hair dryer. There was no pail or other receptacle in which to soak diapers. There was no hot water because the gas had been turned off.

There were no toys in evidence. The toddler slept in a crib in another room on a bare mattress that had a large gaping hole from which the stuffing bulged. The baby carriage was the only sleeping equipment for the infant.

Once the baby had on the dry diaper and clean clothes, the visitor held her for a while and learned the following facts. The family was subsisting on welfare, Social Security disability benefits, and Aid to Dependent Children. The father was unemployed, having quit his job in an adjoining county because he could not get along with his boss. He could find no employment as an unskilled laborer. The couple's inability to pay the gas bill at their previous residence in another county was their reason for moving. Unfortunately, the same gas company serviced the new residence and refused to turn on the gas.

The husband returned and joined in the conversation. His tone and manner were indicative of frustration and despair. When the visitor placed the child in his arms, he held her for about 2 minutes and then placed her in the carriage, saying that he did not want to spoil her. A discussion began about spoiling children. The father firmly believed that parents spoil children by holding them. The visitor discussed how words of caring say one thing but that actions convey much more—for example, telling a spouse he or she is loved versus holding the spouse in one's arms. The husband stated that he and his wife did not love each other and were considering divorce.

In planning to assist this family, the visitor mentally reviewed what is normal about families and parent–child relationships. It is well known that the addition of a new member to any family system is a stressor. The coping skills used by a family to assimilate the new member into the system determine whether or not a persistent stressful situation will develop. Stress in a family system can often erupt in the form of abuse of the most vulnerable member.[6]

Among others, the local League Against child Abuse had named stress of a financial nature as first in a list of stressors contributing to abuse (League Against Child Abuse, Columbus, Ohio). The limited income of this family could easily become stressful to the point of fostering abuse. Having appropriate resources to give adequate care to a new baby is essential. Further, the emotional climate in which the family as a whole functions is a contributing factor to the overall well-being of children. Support systems should be available to the family. These systems consist of immediate family, relatives, friends, neighbors, and the community at large. It has been found that families in which abuse occurs are likely to be isolated from the larger community and without support systems.[7]

In the Green family the lack of significant material and psychological resources could easily lead to abuse. There were no relatives or friends who could help this family. The absence of support people to assist with caring for the children denied the parents occasional respite from parenting, and opportunities for recreation were nonexistent. The only resource this family used in the larger community was the Women, Infants and Children program. As for material resources, there were not enough clothes—especially diapers—for the infant. The toddler had no toys, the sleeping facilities were cramped or dangerous with loose bed stuffing, and without gas service, neither child had adequate warmth. There was the potential for ill health since without hot water, neither dishes nor diapers could be made adequately clean. The father was very discouraged and lacked the motivation to even look for employment. The emotional climate of the possible divorce of this couple further complicated the situation.

The above factors are stressors in any family. If there was a history of abuse (that is, if either parent had been abused as a child), one or both of the children would probably have shown signs of abuse. Fortunately, these children were not found to be abused at the initial home visit, although it could be said that they suffered from neglect. Given that various sources[5–8] have indicated that there is a high correlation between poverty and abuse, and that abusive families have "closed boundaries," this family could be diagnosed as "a family with potential for abuse."

Once a community health nurse diagnoses a family with potential for abuse, further assessment is needed. The nurse needs to identify how the family solves problems and what the family perceives as problems. It is very important for the nurse to ascertain whether or not any of the children are considered a problem.[9] Through no fault of their own, certain types of children have been perceived as problems and therefore abused. If the infant is premature, will not cuddle, has a developmental disability, has a congenital defect, does not eat or feed easily, is unwanted, unplanned for, places a financial drain on the family system, or is an overactive child, that child may be the victim of abuse. The nurse needs to listen to ways in which the mother describes the child. Is it a "special child" often referred to by "He's not like the rest of my kids," "She's always been different," or even referred to as "it" rather than by the child's given name?

The coping skills of the new mother need to be assessed by asking appropriate questions. For instance, the nurse can ask, "How is the baby sleeping during the night?" "Tell me how he eats?" "Does he cry a lot? When? What do you do when he cries?" "How does it make you feel when he will not stop crying?"[10]

The nurse further needs to determine how the family uses the larger system, the community. Are there relatives with whom the family spends time and shares goods and services? Or is this a family that prefers to remain alone? Closed boundaries by families are often an indication of a system in stress. Stress within a system strives for release. Without outside contact with the support elements of the larger community, the stress is often released by abusing family members.[7]

It is a foregone conclusion that those who were abused as children will abuse their child or children.[6,7] The community health nurse needs to ask the parents if they were abused as children. The nurse needs to remember that not all individuals perceive themselves as having been abused. Therefore, asking them to describe what happened to them as children if they did something wrong is often helpful. One young man described how he had to stand on a hot radiator with his bare feet. He was adamant in his statement that he was bad and deserved that kind of treatment.

▬THE NURSING INTERVENTIONS

The unemployment of the father as well as the outstanding gas bill placed great stress upon this family, and financial assistance was the first priority. With the help of community nurses, money was secured from Catholic Social Services to make some payment on the gas bill, and soon the gas company was providing warmth and hot water for the family.

Disposable diapers for the baby and clothes for both children were the next priority, and these too were obtained from Catholic Social Services. Faculty members in the nursing program at the college in the area donated toys, considered necessary to provide diversion for the toddler as well as to foster developmental skills.

The nurses of the county health department discussed the Green case with the community health nurses of the city health department. The nurses from the city department made weekly visits for approximately 2 months, then monthly for about 4 to 5 months. Thereafter they visited every 3 months. This occurred over a 2-year period. Their visits assured that the level of stress had continued to decrease—a process that had begun almost immediately on the second visit, which took place after the gas had been turned on, and when the husband was found to be less depressed and actively seeking employment.

Linkage with the larger community was provided through professional counseling offered to the couple by the local area mental health center. The counseling also helped to improve the emotional climate in the family.

The county health department referred the Green family to Children's Services. The children were never removed from the home, but the caseworker monitored them closely.

About two years after the potential abuse was discovered, the Green family moved and came under the jurisdiction of the county health department for home health visits.

▬WHAT NURSING NEEDS TO DO

Increased case finding of potentially abusive families is needed so that interventions can prevent child abuse at the primary level. Services of a home health aide to assist with child care and teach parenting skills may have a significant effect on decreasing child abuse. In addition, community health nursing texts that address prevention of child abuse at the primary level are needed. The literature is full of examples of types of families in which abuse occurs, as well as data about "special children."

Continuing education programs about abuse in children also need to address prevention. Finally, community health nurses should explore the feasibility of securing grants from appropriate agencies to assist with prevention of child abuse through home visits. Home visits, as well as work in schools and clinics, place community health nurses in key positions to assess potential abuse and to have a profound impact on prevention.

■CONCLUSION

Reimbursement for home visits to "healthy" individuals and families is a rarity for home health agencies. The unfortunate implication of the Green family case study was that much of this information would never have been gained if a professional home visit had not been made. This visit was happenstance, made at a time when a lull in more pressing tasks had occurred.

The visit to the Greens was made also at a time when the community health nurses in the county were already involved with a case of actual child abuse. The child in that case never recovered from the brain damage, and the father served a jail sentence. The nurses were especially enthusiastic about the opportunity to monitor and assist the Green family so that in this family child abuse would not occur.

Since then, one health department in the area has received a sizable grant from the county child protective agency to allow home visits to families in the hope of preventing child abuse (Nursing and Rehabilitation Service, Columbus City Health Dept, Columbus, Ohio). Other public agencies should follow this example.

A postscript: It has been over 5 years since the potential for abuse in the Green family was discovered. The family continues to manage on a meager income. No abuse to the children has occurred. In 1986 the county health department's nurses familiar with their situation provided clothes and toys for the children's Christmas.

■REFERENCES

1. Archer S, Fleshman R: *Community Health Nursing Patterns and Practice,* ed 2. North Scituate, Mass, Duxbury Press, 1979.
2. Jarvis L: *Community Health Nursing: Keeping the Public Healthy.* Philadelphia, FA Davis, 1981.
3. Logan B, Dawkins C: *Family-Centered Nursing in the Community.* Reading, Mass, Addison-Wesley, 1986.
4. Spradley B: *Community Health Nursing Concepts and Practice.* Boston, Little, Brown, 1981.
5. Shamansky S, Clausen C: Levels of prevention: Examination of the concept. *Nurs Outlook* 1980; 28(2): 104–108.
6. Janosik E, Davies J: *Psychiatric Mental Health Nursing.* Boston, Jones & Bartlett, 1986.
7. Stuart G, Sundeen S: *Principles and Practice of Psychiatric Nursing.* St Louis, CV Mosby, 1983.
8. Campbell J, Humphery J: *Nursing Care of Victims of Family Violence.* Reston, Va, Reston Publishing, 1984, pp 361–362.
9. Pillitteri A: *Child Health Nursing,* ed 2. Boston, Little, Brown, 1981, pp 912–913.
10. Leahy K et al: *Community Health Nursing,* ed 4. New York, McGraw-Hill, 1982, p 151.

Chapter 35

Preventive Work with Families:
Issues Facing Public Health Nurses

LINDA J. KRISTJANSON   KAREN I. CHALMERS

Public health nurses function as advanced generalists across different system levels. Much of this work is with healthy families and families dealing with early health changes. Nurses must have the skills necessary for effective family nursing. This chapter examines the issues nurses experience when entering the family system to work preventively. In order to develop a knowledge base for practice, the theoretical basis of family-centered nursing is analyzed and the need for empirical work is identified. The unique characteristics of the public health nursing role are discussed with emphasis on territorial issues, power relationships, and accountability problems. However, the authors support the general structure of public health practice as of value for preventive work and call for a collaborative approach with families.

■ INTRODUCTION

For years public health nurses have recognized that 'community' care is usually 'family' care and that the family is the primary unit of health care. Over the past decade there has been an increasing emphasis in the literature on 'family-focused care', 'family-centered nursing' and 'family interventions' (Barnes 1985, Garrett 1985, Gilliss *et al.* 1989, Pesznecker & Zahlis 1986, Sullivan 1982, Wright & Leahey 1984). These writings have been helpful in understanding how families contribute to or restore health and prevent illness. This literature has widened the conceptual lens through which health problems are assessed and managed.

A second theme in the public health literature is the need for preventive health care (Breslow 1978, Pender 1987). The aim of reducing and eliminating health problems through early detection and intervention is recognized by many health professionals as a priority for health care (Canada Health Survey 1981).

This paper is designed to contribute to the understanding of how public health nurses can work preventively with families to promote their

From *Journal of Advanced Nursing* 16:147–153, 1991. Reprinted by permission of Blackwell Science, Ltd.

health. Although we agree with the 'expanded lens' approach to community health care that includes the family, we share concerns about the
methods used in this care, the theory base for this practice, and obstacles
to family-centered care that may be inherent in

1. That the nursing literature, to date, lacks a theory base to direct fam-
    ily health-care practice. Most literature currently used by nurses has
    been 'borrowed' from the social sciences and family therapy and has
    not been tested for its 'fit' within family nursing contexts.
2. That much of the family theory used by nursing is based upon a
    male-dominated systems view that does not recognize that the major-
    ity of family health care is given by women.
3. That there is a related need to develop an empirically based theory
    to explain and predict effective public health nursing with families.
4. That there are unique features of the public health role that are
    both an advantage and disadvantage to the nurse interested in pro-
    viding family-centred nursing. Some of these influences come from
    the historical public health role and the power relationship between
    public health nurses and their clients.
5. That the most appropriate level for public health nursing interven-
    tion may vary. It is recommended that in some instances greater ben-
    efit might be attained from intervening at the macro-system level
    rather than at the family level.
6. And finally, that the skills required by public health nurses who work
    preventively with families are varied and complex, requiring that
    these individuals are prepared as advanced generalists.

▄THEORY BASE OF FAMILY NURSING

There is a lack of clearly documented theory related to how to nurse families in the community. The knowledge that does exist includes authors'
opinions or anecdotal experiences about individual family nursing incidents. Community health textbooks describe the importance of family-
centered nursing and identify key times to include the family in health
care, but are rather non-specific about actually how to work with families.

In a search for a theory base to guide practice, nurses have often looked
to other disciplines for assistance. This is not unusual, as many disciplines
share aspects of theoretical knowledge. However, to adopt a body of theory from a neighbouring field without careful analysis and testing of its
'fit' to nursing practice is a serious error (Fawcett 1984, Hardy 1978).
Using theory from another discipline may be entirely legitimate; but
nurses must evaluate the conditions unique to nursing practice which alter
other disciplines' generalizations. As well, nurses may also find that they
need to expand the original theory.

These theories were developed by social scientists to explain and predict patterns of family functioning (Ackerman 1938, Bateson *et al.* 1956,
Bowen 1976, Duvall 1971). In recent years, nurses have looked to the field
of family therapy as a theoretical source of direction. Much of this theoret-

ical writing originated from the work of family therapists who developed their theory from clinical work with specific population groups. For example, Minuchin's structural theory was developed from his work with low-income families with disturbed adolescents, and was later expanded and tested with families with anorexic members (Minuchin *et al.* 1967, Minuchin *et al.* 1978). Indeed, the reference population of most family therapists is families with entrenched patterns of dysfunction.

The population that public health nurses encounter, however, is not the same population from which family therapists developed their theories. Many family issues that public health nurses encounter involve families considered to be generally healthy. Some might be experiencing health concerns in the early phases of a problem, requiring more straightforward preventive and supportive interventions. As well, the context in which public health nurses work is quite different from that of family therapists. For the most part, family therapy is conducted in the health professional's territory for a recognized family problem. In public health nursing, family-centred care occurs in the family's territory, most often initiated by the nurse for a health concern that may or may not be obvious to the family. Public health nurses need a theory base that helps them understand how to approach families in their territory, how to assess potential or actual health concerns from a family perspective, and how to intervene most effectively with families to prevent and manage health concerns. Although some family theory developed in other disciplines may be appropriate to community nursing contexts, such as family developmental theory, more research is needed to test these theories in family nursing settings and isolate important theoretical constructs and propositions that may be unique to family health care nursing.

Nursing Women in Families
Although the literature in public health nursing frequently refers to family nursing, the majority of this health care is directed at women as the recipient of services such as maternal health care, preventive paediatric care, and management of home care for the elderly and chronically ill. The family caregiving literature documents that much of the nurturing and health care provided to children, elderly and the chronically ill is provided by wives and daughters (Brody 1981, Brody & Lang 1982, Burke 1987, Mace & Rabins 1981, Heckerman 1980, Smoyak 1987).

In addition, family theory has been criticized for presenting a male-dominated definition of the family. This criticism has been directed particularly at structural–functional family therapy because of the emphasis on the importance of conventional family roles and boundaries. Feminist critics of family theory literature (Bogdan 1984, Braverman 1986, Goldner 1985, 1987, 1988, Oakley 1980) have been quick to argue that the concept (gender) influences family dynamics in relation to power, privilege and fairness and is of profound importance to effective intervention with families. These authors point out that an analysis of gender issues is notably absent in the theoretical writing about families, limiting understanding by the practitioner who employs these theories. Public health nurses who adopt or borrow this body of literature without careful examination of the biases inherent in the work, may be applying theory inappropriately in client contexts. The fact that women form the major group of family care-givers, and are most frequently the recipient of public health nursing ser-vices, necessitates careful attention to these issues.

The Need for a Research Basis for Practice

Another issue related to the theory basis of family-centred community health nursing is the research base that underlies the theory and direct practice. With some exceptions, nursing's current theory is rationally or deductively arrived at, with few empirical verifications. It is essential in the development of a scientific theory base that these modes of inquiry inter-face so that logical explanations are rooted in observed phenomena (Gort-ner 1983).

> *Nursing has a mandate from society to use its specialized body of knowledge and skills for the betterment of humans. The mandate implies that knowledge and skills must go in such a way as to keep up with the changing health goals of soci-ety. (Hardy 1978)*

There has been a tendency to base nursing actions on tradition, routine and intuition (Hamilton & Bush 1988). According to Hardy (1978), these sources of knowledge may give nurses a sense of security in what they do but they remain in the realm of myth and non-scientific knowledge.

A particular example of the need for research in family community health practice relates to the timing and amount of nursing intervention provided. A popular assumption in health care is that early intervention will prevent later health problems. For example, early detection of cancer will lead to longer survival rates. The literature related to child abuse de-scribes the importance of preventive work to decrease the likelihood of abuse (Campbell & Humphreys 1984). However, it is also known that some health care interventions are more effective if applied later in the dysfunctional process. Cataracts, for instance, are best treated when suffi-cient lens damage is present that the person is almost blind. It may also be true that certain family problems are more effectively managed when in-tervention is applied late in the course of the problem, making preventive efforts inappropriate. At present, there is little empirical knowledge in the community health nursing literature related to the success and timing of interventions with families. Research is needed to test the effectiveness of the application of different strategies at various points in the development of family problems.

As well, the 'dosage' or amount of intervention is another variable that may require study. The current practice in public health is to visit families according to a routine schedule, the nurses' sense of completion of goals, or, in some cases, according to a nurse–client contract. How often do nurses need to visit families to prevent or intervene in family health prob-lems? Effective use of nursing time and energies could be enhanced by evaluative research that addresses this issue. As well, it might be important to ask if there is such a thing as an 'overdose' of family nursing interventions? To assume that nurses enter family systems and effect only benevolent results is naive and professionally arrogant. Therefore, clinical research is required to explore these important questions.

It appears that the study of preventive interventions with families has been particularly neglected. Part of the reason for the paucity of research in this area is that evaluative research related to family work is fraught with complexities. It is difficult to control the multiple variables that impinge on a family and simply measure the effect of the timing or type of preventive nursing interventions. However, despite the challenges of this type of research it is important to evaluate systematically the process of nursing care to community health families in order to build a scientific knowledge base to direct practice.

▬WHAT MAKES PUBLIC HEALTH NURSING WITH FAMILIES UNIQUE?

Public health nurses are in a unique position because they are the professional group that has the opportunity to visit families in their own homes to detect health concerns and prevent problems before they become serious. This role is not performed by other health or social service professions. In other instances, families seek out health professionals because a health or family problem is of sufficient severity to prompt families to find external resources. If a family does not comply with or follow through with ongoing interventions the helping relationship, in most instances, dissolves.

One exception might be the social worker who visits families in their homes to assess family functioning with respect to child welfare concerns. In these instances, however, there is a specific risk in the family's mind of the child being apprehended or some mandatory intervention or treatment being imposed. The relationship here occurs in the family's territory, but the professional clearly holds the balance of power and the reason for contact is not a positive health-promoting one. In contrast, the public health nurse is the ambassador of the health care system who enters family territory to promote health and prevent problems. The nurse is a 'guest in the house' and offers a service that may or may not be received by the family.

In any professional–client relationship, the issue of power emerges as a potential block. Public health nurses enter family territory often as uninvited guests. For example, they often initiate contact with families because of a routine visiting requirement to postpartum families. Families' receptiveness to the nurse will vary depending upon their previous perceptions of public health nurses and their understanding of the reason for the visit. Some families may be influenced by notions of public health nurses that arise from historical public health practices.

Public health practice was based on the public health model developed in the nineteenth century, when the major threats to health were communicable disease and malnutrition. For a nurse practicing within this model, the focus was on screening the population for early detection of disease or detection of individuals at high risk for developing problems (Pender 1987). Case finding was carried out so that interventions could be applied early and the disease process arrested or slowed down. With the passage of time, and as many communicable disease were brought under control, public health nurses have addressed the prevention of chronic illness, often through lifestyle risk reduction, and the social health problems of high-risk families. The predominant interventions, however, have remained active case finding through assessment and screening procedures, and ongoing surveillance and monitoring. The public health model places strong emphasis on the nurse as the definer of the health problem. The nurse frequently detects the problem, seeks out the family and attempts to intervene. The client may or may not be aware or interested in the health concern as the nurse defines it, and may not be wanting service. The nurse appears to justify her attempts to engage the client based on her concept of health (Chalmers 1984).

Problems

The influence of the earlier public health role may result in a number of problems related to family-focused community-health nursing today. The historical stereotype of a public health nurse may be held by families who see the nurse as someone coming to 'check' on them and report them to some unknown authority. Indeed, recent experiences with public health nurses may have led families to expect nurses to perform in this way. Although a more collaborative approach to working with people is being used to some extent currently and is recommended in the more recent public health literature (Baum 1988, Kickbusch 1987, Labonte 1989, Martin & McQueen 1989), some nurses may see themselves as authority figures who can define the family's problem and give advice and teaching. This may be perceived as unhelpful or intrusive and also may not be aimed at concerns that families may be experiencing.

Public health nurses need to be aware of how some perceptions of the public health role may disadvantage them in their work with families. On the other hand, the preventive perspective and concern for health of groups that this history also emphasizes are aspects that should be retained and fostered. However, in family-focused community nursing there may need to be more specific efforts to establish collaborative relationships with families and communicate purposes for contact and establishment of mutual goals for health. In these ways, counterproductive 'ghosts' that represent a more authoritarian style of public health protection may be erased in nurse–family interactions.

Another control-related issue is the nurse's accountability. The nature of public health work makes the nurse accountable to the community as a whole, as well as to the individual or family being nursed. This responsibility to the aggregate may be in conflict with the nurse's responsibility to the professional ethics by which he/she practices. Codes of ethics of nursing practice emphasize the individual's right to autonomy, self-determinism, privacy and the nurse's requirement to respect these rights (Canadian Nurses Association 1989, Fry 1983). These rights may be violated under existing public health practices such as universal follow-up of all postnatal clients, or discussion of children with school officials without parental consent, or seeking out special groups for assessment and teaching.

Although policies are set by public health administrators, it is the nurse in the field who must resolve this conflict of initiating contacts with clients who have not requested service. Clients may react with anger, indifference or passivity, all difficult positions on which to base a collaborative working relationship. When adults alone are involved, nurses may resolve this dilemma more easily and remove themselves from unwanted client interactions. However, when young children in high-risk families are involved, nurses find themselves in deeper conflict. Should nurses press for involvement with unwilling families and risk intruding on rights to autonomy and self-determination, or withdraw and live with the uneasiness that these children may at some point be abused or neglected (Chalmers 1984)?

In these instances, public health nurses' primary responsibility is to protect the health of the children. Here, the purpose of the visit may not be made explicit to parents. This may be necessary and prudent. However, in the majority of instances this vagueness is not appropriate. A large part of the difficulty associated with effective family nursing stems from a lack of clarity about the reason for public health contact. In general, much more attention needs to be given to the process of referral to the community and nurses' entries into family systems. Mechanisms need to be developed so that clients are aware of the rationale for nurses' contacts by referring sources. Sometimes, families are unaware of the referral source or reason for referral to public health nurses. When concerns exist, the referring person needs to articulate clearly these to clients, and some level of consensus for follow-up needs to be reached prior to initiation of the referral to the nurse. This clarity would facilitate entry of the nurse into the family territory and set the stage for a collaborative relationship based on a more balanced and clearer understanding of the purpose of the contact.

▬ LEVEL OF INTERVENTION

An additional problem exists concerning the application of current family theory to nurses' work with families. It could be argued from a systems perspective that the family's problem is based at the macro level (e.g. poverty) rather than within the family system. While system theory may be used by public health nurses in their work with families, interventions usually are aimed at family processes rather than at external stressors. This may be helpful and appropriate. However, nurses working with families in the community also often need to work at the macro system level with the external stressors; as an advocate for families. For example, a problem that might be identified by a public health nurse would be poor nutritional practices of a low-income family. A nurse could work with the family to increase their knowledge of good nutrition and help them plan their budget to allow for nutritious meal planning. However, upon further analysis the nurse might also decide to use a macro system approach to address the problem by advocating for an increased food budget for the family at the welfare office, or working with an Anti-Poverty Coalition to improve the standard of living for those on low fixed incomes.

It is argued that to be effective in dealing with many potential health concerns, public health nurses need to be able to work at various levels of the system. This notion is exemplified well by the story of the nurse standing by the river who sees a man floating face down in the water (McKinlay 1979). She quickly pulls the man out of the water and begins to resuscitate him, when she notices a second man floating face down in the water. She pulls the second man out of the water and then sees a third and a fourth person floating downstream. The nurse becomes so busy pulling nearly drowned bodies out of the river, that she has no time to run upstream and see who is pushing the people into the river.

This story illustrates that over-attention to one level of action may limit effective management of a problem. Nurses are usually less confident at intervening at macro or sociopolitical levels of the system and feel more comfortable 'downstream' dealing with individuals/families who are in distress. Yet they often express frustration that they are performing 'band-aid' types of interventions that do not really address the sources of family health concerns. Nurse educators and public health administrators are encouraged to examine ways that are helpful in preparing and supporting public health nurses to intervene at this level. As a collective, public health nurses could play a much more active role at this level.

Necessary Skills

Nurses require special skills to 'enter' a family. Usually the family has not sought the nurse's services and therefore may not welcome the nurse easily into their territory. Nurses need to have 'engaging' skills or social skills that convey interest in and acceptance of the family. Authoritarian or heavy-handed approaches that presume automatic entry into the family will more than likely result in passive if not active rejection of the nurse.

Usually, nurses enter the family system because of a recognized health concern. The concern is most often focused on one individual family member. Upon further assessment, the problem may be identified by the nurse as rooted in the family and therefore successful work on the problem necessitates a shift from an individual to a family level. The family may not see the need for the nurse to meet, let alone work with, the whole family. Therefore, access to the entire family may be limited, as nurses find themselves talking to mothers and babies only. Tangles of contracting to work often begin here.

Nurses need the skills to be able to contract with families clearly and openly in order to clarify the purpose of visits and the usefulness of family involvement in discussion of health concerns. Nurses need to meet families to assess the impact of one family member's health on the other members, and vice versa. Once a family assessment has been conducted, nurses have the further task of helping families explore actual and potential health problems, learning new ways of dealing with situations, or changing potentially hazardous health behaviours. This is when the ability to contract is essential. The problem or potential problem must be mutually recognized and the family should be included in determining their own goals for health. It is evident that communication skills are central to effective family work, as nurses need to negotiate and interact with a variety of families who may have different perceptions and expectations of the nurse's role. Nurses also need to examine their own value systems and look critically at their styles of practice. Do they hold on to power and control? Do they like to be the authority and the expert? Can they work in a non-judgmental way with different families? To work effectively and collaboratively with families, nurses must be willing to be a 'guest in the house'. They must accept that although they have expert power in terms of their general knowledge base, there is much that they do not know about the uniqueness of the particular family they are visiting.

This combination of knowledge and abilities is extensive and many public health nurses would identify these skills as part of the usual repertoire of a competent generalist. However, based upon our own practice experience, observations of nursing students and research with community health nurses (Kristjanson & Chalmers 1987, 1990), it appears that the complexity of community situations and family dynamics in this context requires that the public health nurse be prepared as an advanced generalist. This would require a clinical major in advanced community practice with families, either as an internship or elective, or advanced study at the master's level of community health practice.

■CONCLUSION

Public health nurses could choose to go the route of many other helping professions and have the system within which they work restructured so that families come to them, thus eliminating the frustrations of working with families who may not wholeheartedly welcome nurses into their homes. On the other hand, if this restructuring were to occur, nurses would miss opportunities to see health problems early, offer anticipatory teaching and support to families and help a family mobilize resources that they might not otherwise locate. The risk of intruding into family territory is still present, and nurses must be sensitive and cautious so as not to invade. However, the potential benefits to families and to society appear to warrant this risk. The important issue is that nurses acknowledge that a risk exists and make efforts to minimize it. In most instances, except for the few health problems that legally require the nurse to contact the family, the family should be in control as to whether or not the nursing service is accepted. Prevention of health problems in families is an important role for public health nurses to assume. Waiting for a family to recognize a health problem may be too late in the process to work preventively. Therefore, the 'door-to-door' approach of public health nursing fills an important void in the family health system.

The literature indicates that several factors influence a person's decision to seek preventive health services (Murray & Zentner 1979, Pender 1987, Pratt 1976, Ramsay 1985). First, the person may seek health care because of family encouragement. Second, patterns of using preventive services are learned in the family. Third, expectations of friends are powerful motivators to seek preventive health care. Fourth, information and respectful care from health professionals also increases the readiness to engage in preventive health behaviour, especially if the health professional is seen as knowledgeable and caring.

Further empirical research is needed to clarify the processes that public health nurses carry out that lead to improved health outcomes with families. However, in the meantime nurses need to analyze and assess their day to day work with families. Family-focused community nursing provides an excellent opportunity to promote health practices, understand family processes that affect health, and intervene in a meaningful way at a preventive level. Public health nurses can be strong influences in promoting positive health outcomes for families by helping them make knowledgeable choices about their health.

▄▄REFERENCES

Ackerman N. (1938) The family as a social and emotional unit. *Archives of Pediatrics* **55**, 51–61.

Barnes A. (1985) The continuity of care in the family. *Nursing* **36**, 1051–1054.

Bateson G., Jackson D.D., Haley J. & Weakland J. (1956) Toward a theory of schizophrenia. *Behavioral Science* **1**(4), 251–264.

Baum F. (1988) Community-based research for promoting the new public health. *Health Promotion* **3**(3), 259–268.

Bogdan J.L. (1984) Family organization as an ecology of ideas: an alternative to the reification of family systems. *Family Process* **23**, 375–388.

Bowen M. (1976) Theory in the practice of psychotherapy. In *Family Therapy* (Guerin Jr P.J. ed.), Gardner Press, New York.

Braverman L. (1986) Beyond families: strategic family therapy and the female client. *Family Therapy* **8**, 143–152.

Breslow L. (1978) Prospects for improving health through reducing risk factors. *Preventive Medicine* **7**, 449–458.

Brody E.M. (1981) 'Women in the middle' and family help to older people. *Gerontologist* **21**(5), 471–480.

Brody E.M. & Lang A. (1982) 'They can't do it all': aging daughters with aging mothers. *Generations* **7**, 18–20.

Burke S.O. (1987) Assessing single-parent families with physically disabled children. In *Families and Chronic Illness* (Wright M. & Leahey M. eds), Springhouse, Springhouse, Pennsylvania.

Campbell J. & Humphreys J. (1984) *Nursing Care of Victims of Family Violence*. Reston, Reston, Virginia.

Canada Health Survey (1981) *The Health of Canadians: Report on the Canada Health survey* (No. 82–538E). Health and Welfare Canada, Ottawa.

Canadian Nurses Association (1989) *Code of Ethics for Nursing*. Canadian Nurses Association, Ottawa.

Chalmers K.I. (1984) Family nursing: the need for clearly defined frameworks for practice. *Proceedings of the Conference 'Expanding the Scope of Nursing Practice: Development of Theoretical Frameworks'*. College of Nursing, University of Saskatchewan, Saskatoon, pp. 276–287.

Duvall E.M. (1971) *Family Development*. J.B. Lippincott, Philadelphia.

Fawcett J. (1984) *Analysis and Evaluation of Conceptual Models of Nursing*. F.A. Davis, Philadelphia.

Fry S.T. (1983) Dilemma in community health ethics. *Nursing Outlook* **31**(3), 176–179.

Garrett G. (1985) Family care and the elderly. *Nursing* **36**, 1061–1063.

Gilliss C., Highley B., Roberts B. & Martinson I. (1989) *Toward a Science of Family Nursing*. Addison-Wesley, Don Mills, Ontario.

Goldner V. (1985) Feminism and family therapy. *Family Process* **24**, 31–47.

Goldner V. (1987) Instrumentalism, feminism and the limits of family therapy. *Journal of Family Psychology* **1**, 109–116.

Goldner V. (1988) Generation and gender: normative and covert hierarchies. *Family Process* **27**, 17–31.

Gortner S.R. (1983) The history and philosophy of nursing science and research. *Advances in Nursing Science* **5**(2) 1–8.

Hamilton P. & Bush H. (1988) Theory development in community health nursing: issues. *Scholarly Inquiry for Nursing Practice* **12**(2), 146–160.

Hardy M.E. (1978) Perspectives on nursing theory. *Advances in Nursing Science* **1**(1), 37–48.

Heckerman C. (1980) *The Evolving Female: Women in Psychosocial Context*. Human Sciences Press, New York.

Kickbusch I. (1987) Issues in health promotion. *Health Promotion* **1**(4), 437–442.

Kristjanson L.J. & Chalmers K.I. (1987) Nurse–client interactions in community based practice. Unpublished research report.

Kristjanson L. & Chalmers K. (1990) Nurse–client interactions in community based practice: creating common meaning. *Public Health Nursing* **7**(4).

Labonte R. (1989) Community health promotion strategies. In *Readings for a New Public Health* (Martin C. & McQueen D. eds), Edinburgh University Press, Edinburgh, pp. 235–249.

Mace N.L. & Rabins P.V. (1981) *The 36-Hour Day*. Johns Hopkins University Press, Baltimore.

Martin C. & McQueen D. (1989) Framework for a new public health. In *Readings for a New Public Health* (Martin C. & McQueen D. eds), Edinburgh University Press, Edinburgh, pp. 1–10.

McKinlay J.B. (1979) A case for re-focusing upstream: the political economy of illness. In *Physicians and Illness* 3rd edn (Jaco E. G. ed.), The Free Press, New York, pp. 9–25.

Minuchin S., Montalvo B., Guerney B.G. Jr., Rosman B.L. & Schumer F. (1967) *Families of the Slums: An Exploration of Their Structure and Treatment*. Basic Books, New York.

Minuchin S., Rosman B. & Baker L. (1978) *Psychosomatic Families*. Harvard University Press, Cambridge, Massachusetts.

Murray R.B. & Zentner J.P. (1979) *Nursing Concepts for Health Promotion*. Prentice-Hall, Englewood Cliffs, New Jersey.

Oakley A. (1980) *Women Confined: Towards a Sociology of Childbirth*. Martin Robertson, Oxford.

Pender N.J. (1987) *Health Promotion in Nursing Practice*. Appleton-Century-Crofts, Norwalk, Connecticut.

Pesznecker B.L. & Zahlis E. (1986) Establishing mutual-help groups for family-member care givers: a new role for community health nurses. *Pubic Health Nursing* **3**(1), 29–37.

Pratt L. (1976) *Family Structure and Effective Health Behaviour: The Energized Family*. Houghton Mifflin, Boston.

Ramsay J. (1985) Health behavior and compliance. In *Community Health Nursing in Canada* (Stewart M., Innes J., Seal S. & Smillie C. eds), Gage, Toronto, pp. 437–461.

Smoyak S.A. (1987) Assessing aging families and their caretakers. In *Families and Chronic Illness* (Wright M. & Leahey M. eds), Springhouse, Springhouse, Pennsylvania.

Sullivan J.A. (1982) *Directions in Community Health Nursing*. Blackwell Scientific, Oxford.

Wright L. & Leahey M. (1984) *Nurses and Families: A Guide to Family Assessment and Intervention*. F.A. Davis, Philadelphia.

Unit 6

Community Health Nursing With Populations and Groups

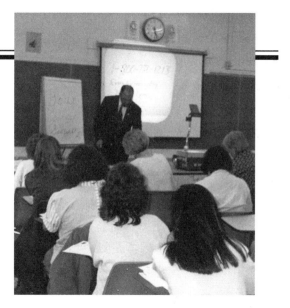

The primary dimension of community health nursing service is to populations. New populations needing health services are emerging. Consequently, we must identify the groups that can benefit from health services, learn to assess their needs, design effective intervention strategies, and evaluate the contributions of the programs and services.

Frequently reaching the high-risk populations, such as children in a Head Start Program, sexually active teenagers, immigrant farm workers, the incarcerated, and people with Alzheimer's disease, in their entirety happens mainly through group effort. Surprisingly, however, these groups are much more accessible and in need of health education, information, or appraisal than we might believe. Innovative and assertive nurses can work with groups under a variety of circumstances. Sometimes, a captive population that we traditionally think of as well groups—students in a high school, workers in a factory, or participants in a senior center—can be anxious recipients of a community health nurse's services. In settings such as these, many groups have formed to learn about and improve their health status by participation in family planning seminars, weight-control classes, and groups dealing with parenting, retirement, and grief and loss.

At other times, the population that is in need of service is scattered throughout a community or is located in a less accessible area. These people are equally, if not more, in need of the services of a community health nurse than the more readily visible groups. Teaching safety practices to farmers or emergency care to women in a homeless shelter, conducting hypertension screening in a shopping mall, providing emotional support to family members of people living with AIDS, and empowering residents in an urban neighborhood to improve their safety from gangs are a few examples of group services offered by nurses in community health.

Because a population has different needs, the nurse must assess its needs and interests and plan with the group before mutually setting goals and objectives. Commonly identified community health groups consist of learning groups, support groups, socialization groups, psychotherapy groups, and task-accomplishment groups. Learning groups, such as teen parenting classes, try to change and/or reinforce behaviors to meet perceived health needs. Support groups, for example, a group of new retirees, form to promote healthy behavior and prevent maladaptive coping patterns. Socialization groups are formed to assist clients such as refugees to learn new social roles and adapt to unfamiliar cultural patterns. In addition, clients newly released from confined subcultures, such as psychiatric centers, or prisons, also must learn new roles and ways of behaving. Psychotherapy groups treat the needs of people with emotional disturbances. At times the community health nurse may colead a group with an interdisciplinary team member, such as an adolescent health educator, social worker, or mental health therapist. Finally, task-accomplishment groups are those groups with which the community health nurse works to perform some predetermined task. An occupational health nurse may work with a group of employee representatives and the safety officer to plan and implement a safety program for newly hired staff; another nurse may serve on a school's health planning committee.

Working with groups requires that the community health nurse have specialized knowledge and skills. Whether being a part of planning a new group or a leader or member of an existing group, the nurse must have a working knowledge of group dynamics to facilitate the group process and achieve desired outcomes. The nurse who has developed these skills and is comfortable with group work is able to positively influence group action and uses the vehicle of groups to promote the health of populations.

Once community health nurses recognize the variety of ways they can influence people through group work, they will not be limited by group size. They will be able to extend their range of influence from small groups such as the family in home health nursing, to large groups such as a parent–teacher association meeting. Nurses are challenged to identify the possibilities of change within a variety of groups and develop them in collaboration with other community health professionals. To assist the community health nurse in this challenge, selected examples and discussions of successful nursing interventions with populations-at-risk are included in Unit VI.

Chapter 36

Healthy Children Ready to Learn: An Essential Collaboration Between Health and Education

ANTONIA C. NOVELLO   CHRISTOPHER DEGRAW

DUSHANKA V. KLEINMAN

All children have a right to be healthy and ready to learn. Families must receive the support and assistance they need to raise healthy and educated children. To reach the National Education Goals and the goals of "Healthy People 2000," the critical systems of education and health services need to work collaboratively with social services. Community health nurses focus their attention on prevention with aggregates. They work to promote heathy pregnancies, reduce infant mortality, and provide for nutrition, oral health, immunizations, safety, protection from infections, toxic substances, and sound emotional development. The authors reinforce these needs and stress collaboration among the larger systems to achieve the goal of healthy and educated children—the foundation of our society.

Society is slowly coming to the realization that the health status of children and their educational development are inextricably linked. A child must be physically and emotionally healthy in order to learn, and a child and the child's family must be educated in order to stay healthy.

While this is true for children of all ages and at all stages of development, it is particularly apparent in early childhood. Concurrent with this realization, national goals to be achieved by the year 2000 were set recently for education as well as for health *(1,2)*. If taken together, activities directed toward the first National Education Goal and the related National Health Promotion and Disease Prevention Objectives can advance progress toward school readiness, focus attention and resources on needed programs and services, and help the nation to achieve its goal of having all children arriving at school each day healthy, well nourished, and ready to learn.

The President and the State Governors have set six National Education Goals to be reached by the year 2000 *(1)*. The first is "By the year 2000, all children in America will start school ready to learn." Three objectives de-

From *Public Health Reports* 107(1):3–10, 1992.

fine the components of this readiness goal (Box 36-1). Two critical and interrelated factors, health and education, are implicit or explicit in this goal and in each of the three objectives.

The health component of the first National Education Goal transcends all three readiness objectives. In order for parents to participate as their children's first teacher, their own health and education needs must be addressed as well. All children, including the disadvantaged and those with disabilities, must have their health and education needs assessed throughout their growth and development years. This should allow them not only to realize their full developmental potential, but to keep incipient disabilities or pathological conditions from progressing. Throughout their lives, the health and education needs of children should be addressed in tandem.

▬HEALTHY PEOPLE 2000

A set of 300 national health promotion and disease prevention objectives to be achieved by the year 2000, called Healthy People 2000 *(2)*, has been developed under the leadership of the Public Health Service. Of these, more than 170 objectives relate to the health of mothers, infants, children, adolescents, and youth *(3)*. Similarly, many of the Healthy People 2000 objectives complement the National Education Goals. Achieving national health promotion and disease prevention objectives is basic to advancing progress toward the school readiness goal.

The national health objectives highlight important problems affecting the health of young children that are amenable to preventive measures and that relate to school readiness. Among them are

- maternal health and prenatal care;
- immunization;
- access to high quality and developmentally appropriate preschool programs;
- nutrition issues, including iron deficiency, breast feeding, nutrition education, and nutritious child care food services;
- exposure to tobacco smoke;
- mental health;
- the importance of assessment by providers of primary health care of the child's cognitive and emotional development, and parent-child functioning;
- violence and child abuse;
- injury prevention;
- reducing mental retardation;
- persistent environmental problems, such as lead poisoning;
- oral health;
- asthma;
- screening for impairment of vision, hearing, speech, or language, developmental milestones, and chronic disease; and
- financing of preventive services.

(Text continues on page 401)

BOX 36-1   *Healthy People 2000 Objectives and the National Education Goals*

National Education Goal 1: By the year 2000, all children in America will start school ready to learn.

National Education Objective—All disadvantaged and disabled children will have access to high quality and developmentally appropriate preschool programs that help prepare children for school.

RELATED NATIONAL HEALTH PROMOTION AND DISEASE PREVENTION OBJECTIVE:
  8.3: Achieve for all disadvantaged children and children with disabilities access to high quality and developmentally appropriate preschool programs that help prepare children for school, thereby improving their prospects with regard to school performance, problem behaviors, and mental and physical health.

National Education Objective—Every parent in America will be a child's first teacher and devote time each day helping his or her preschool child learn; parents will have access to the training and support they need.

National Education Objective—Children will receive the nutrition and health care needed to arrive at school with healthy minds and bodies, and the number of low birthweight babies will be significantly reduced through enhanced prenatal health systems.

Children will receive the nutrition and health care needed to arrive at school with healthy minds and bodies. . . .

RELATED NATIONAL HEALTH PROMOTION AND DISEASE PREVENTION OBJECTIVES:

Nutrition
  2.4: Reduce growth retardation among low-income children aged 5 and younger to less than 10 percent.
  2.5: Reduce dietary fat intake to an average of 30 percent of calories or less and average saturated fat intake to less than 10 percent of calories among people aged 2 and older.
  2.10: Reduce iron deficiency to less than 3 percent among children aged 1 through 4 and among women of childbearing age.
  2.11: Increase to at least 75 percent the proportion of mothers who breastfeed their babies in the early postpartum period and to at least 50 percent the proportion who continue breastfeeding until their babies are 5 to 6 months old.
  2.12: Increase to at least 75 percent the proportion of parents and caregivers who use feeding practices that prevent baby bottle tooth decay.
  2.17: Increase to at least 90 percent the proportion of school lunch and breakfast services and child care food services with menus that are consistent with the nutrition principles in the Dietary Guideline for Americans.
  2.19: Increase to at least 75 percent the proportion of the Nation's schools that provide nutrition education from preschool through 12th grade, preferably as part of quality school health education.

(continued)

BOX 36-1   *Healthy People 2000 Objectives and the National Education Goals (continued)*

2.21: Increase to at least 75 percent the proportion of primary care providers who provide nutrition assessment and counseling and/or referral to qualified nutritionists or dietitians.

Tobacco

3.8: Reduce to no more than 20 percent the proportion of children aged 6 and younger who are regularly exposed to tobacco smoke at home.

Mental Health and Mental Disorders

6.3: Reduce to less than 10 percent the prevalence of mental disorders among children and adolescents.

6.14: Increase to at least 75 percent the proportion of providers of primary care for children who include assessment of cognitive, emotional, and parent-child functioning, with appropriate counseling, referral, and followup, in their clinical practices.

Violent and Abusive Behavior

7.1a: Reduce homicides among children aged 3 and younger to no more than 3.1 per 100,000.

7.4: Reverse to less than 25.2 per 1,000 children the rising incidence of maltreatment of children younger than age 18.

7.13: Extend to at least 45 States implementation of unexplained child death review systems.

7.14: Increase to at least 30 the number of States in which at least 50 percent of children identified as physically or sexually abused receive physical and mental evaluation with appropriate followup as a means of breaking the intergenerational cycle of abuse.

7.15: Reduce to less than 10 percent the proportion of battered women and their children turned away from emergency housing due to lack of space.

Education and Community-Based Programs

8.4: Increase to at least 75 percent the proportion of the Nation's elementary and secondary schools that provide planned and sequential kindergarten through 12th grade quality school health education.

Unintentional Injuries

9.3a: Reduce deaths caused by motor vehicle crashes to no more than 5.5 per 100,000 among children aged 14 and younger.

9.5a: Reduce drowning deaths to no more than 2.3 per 100,000 among children aged 4 and younger.

9.6a: Reduce residential fire deaths to no more than 3.3 per 100,000 among children aged 4 and younger.

9.8a: Reduce nonfatal poisoning among children aged 4 and younger to no more than 520 emergency department treatments per 100,000 children.

9.12a: Increase use of occupant protection systems, such as safety belts, inflatable safety restraints, and child safety seats, to at least 95 percent of children aged 4 and younger who are motor vehicle occupants.

9.13: Increase use of helmets to at least 80 percent of motorcyclists and at least 50 percent of bicyclists.

BOX 36-1   *Healthy People 2000 Objectives and the National Education Goals*

9.15: Enact in 50 States laws requiring that new handguns be designed to minimize the likelihood of discharge by children.

9.18: Provide academic instruction on injury prevention and control, preferably as part of quality school health education, in at least 50 percent of public school systems (grades K through 12).

9.21: Increase to at least 50 percent the proportion of primary care providers who routinely provide age-appropriate counseling on safety precautions to prevent unintentional injury.

9.22: Extend to 50 States emergency medical services and trauma systems linking prehospital, hospital, and rehabilitation services in order to prevent trauma deaths and long-term disability.

Environmental Health

11.1b: Reduce asthma morbidity, as measured by a reduction in asthma hospitalizations, to no more than 225 per 100,000 among children aged 14 and younger.

11.4: Reduce the prevalence of blood lead levels exceeding 15 micrograms per deciliter and 25 micrograms per deciliter among children aged 6 months through 5 years to no more than 500,000 and zero, respectively.

11.4a: Reduce the prevalence among inner city low-income black children (annual family income less than $6,000 in 1984 dollars) to no more than 75,000 and zero.

Oral Health

13.1: Reduce dental caries (cavities) so that the proportion of children with one or more caries (in permanent or primary teeth) is no more than 35 percent among children aged 6 through 8 and no more than 60 percent among adolescents aged 15.

13.2: Reduce untreated dental caries so that the proportion of children with untreated caries (in permanent or primary teeth) is no more than 20 percent among children aged 6 through 8, and no more than 15 percent among adolescents aged 15.

13.8: Increase to at least 50 percent the proportion of children who have received protective sealants on the occlusal (chewing) surfaces of permanent molar teeth.

13.9: Increase to at least 75 percent the proportion of people served by community water systems providing optimal levels of fluoride.

13.10: Increase use of professionally or self-administered topical or systemic (dietary) fluorides to at least 85 percent of people not receiving optimally fluoridated public water.

13.12: Increase to at least 90 percent the proportion of all children entering school programs for the first time who have received an oral health screening, referral, and followup for necessary diagnostic, preventive, and treatment services.

13.15: Increase to at least 40 the number of States that have an effective system for recording and referring infants with cleft lips and/or palates to craniofacial anomaly teams.

(continued)

**BOX 36-1   *Healthy People 2000 Objectives and the National
Education Goals (continued)***

Maternal and Infant Health

14.15: Increase to at least 95 percent the proportion of newborns screened by
State-sponsored programs for genetic disorders and other disabling
conditions and to 90 percent the proportion of newborns testing
positive for disease who receive appropriate treatment.

14.16: Increase to at least 90 percent the proportion of babies aged 18 months
and younger who receive recommended primary care services at the
appropriate intervals.

Chronic Disabling Conditions

 17.4: Reduce to no more than 10 percent the proportion of people with
asthma who experience activity limitation.

 17.8: Reduce the prevalence of serious mental retardation in school-aged
children to no more than 2 per 1,000.

17.15: Increase to at least 80 percent the proportion of providers of primary
care for children who routinely refer or screen infants and children for
impairments of vision, hearing, speech and language, and assess other
developmental milestones as part of well-child care.

17.16: Reduce the average age at which children with significant hearing
impairment are identified to no more than 12 months.

17.20: Increase to 50 the number of States that have service systems for
children with or at risk of chronic and disabling conditions, as required
by Public Law 101-239.

Immunization and Infectious Disease

 20.1: Reduce indigenous cases of vaccine-preventable diseases as follows:

Disease	1988 baseline	2000 target
Diphtheria among people 25 and younger	1	0
Tetanus among people aged 25 and younger	3	0
Polio (wild-type virus)	0	0
Measles	3,058	0
Rubella	225	0
Congenital Rubella Syndrome	6	0
Mumps	4,866	500
Pertussis	3,450	1,000

 20.7: Reduce bacterial meningitis to no more than 4.7 cases per 100,000 people.

 20.8: Reduce infectious diarrhea by at least 25 percent among children in licensed child care centers and children in programs that provide an Individualized Education Program (IEP) or Individualized Health Plan (IHP).

 20.9: Reduce acute middle ear infections among children aged 4 and
younger, as measured by days of restricted activity or school
absenteeism, to no more than 105 days per 100 children.

20.10: Reduce pneumonia-related days of restricted activity as follows:
children aged 4 and younger, 24 days per 100 children.

20.11: Increase immunization levels as follows: basic immunization series
among children under age 2 to at least 90 percent; basic immunization
series among children in licensed child care facilities and kindergarten
through post-secondary education institutions to at least 95 percent.

BOX 36-1   *Healthy People 2000 Objectives and the National Education Goals*

20.13: Expand immunization laws for schools, preschools, and day care settings to all States for all antigens.
20.14: Increase to at least 90 percent the proportion of primary care providers who provide information and counseling about immunizations and offer immunizations as appropriate for their patients.
20.15: Improve the financing and delivery of immunizations for children and adults so that virtually no American has a financial barrier to receiving recommended immunizations.

Clinical Preventive Services
21.2a: Increase to at least 90 percent the proportion of infants up to 24 months who have received, as a minimum within the appropriate interval, all of the screening and immunization services and at least one of the counseling services appropriate for their age and sex as recommended by the U.S. Preventive Service Task Force.
21.2b: Increase to at least 80 percent the proportion of children 2-12 years who have received, as a minimum within the appropriate interval, all of the screening and immunization services and at least one of the counseling services appropriate for their age and sex as recommended by the U.S. Preventive Services Task Force.
21.3: Increase to at least 95 percent the proportion of people who have a specific source of ongoing primary care for coordination of their preventive and episodic health care.
21.4: Improve financing and delivery of clinical preventive services so that virtually no American has a financial barrier to receiving, at a minimum, the screening, counseling, and immunization services recommended by the U.S. Preventive Services Task Force.
21.5: Assure that at least 90 percent of people for whom primary care services are provided directly by publicly funded programs are offered, at a minimum, the screening, counseling, and immunization services recommended by the U.S. Preventive Services Task Force.

. . . and the number of low birthweight babies will be significantly reduced through enhanced prenatal health systems.

RELATED HEALTH PROMOTION AND DISEASE EVALUATION OBJECTIVES:

Nutrition
3.7: Increase smoking cessation during pregnancy so that at least 60 percent of women who are cigarette smokers at the time they become pregnant quit smoking early in pregnancy and maintain abstinence for the remainder of their pregnancy.

Maternal and Infant Health
14.1: Reduce the infant mortality rate to no more than 7 per 1,000 live births.
14.2: Reduce the fetal death rate (20 or more weeks of gestation) to no more than 5 per 1,000 live births plus fetal deaths.
14.3: Reduce the maternal mortality rate to no more than 3.3 per 100,000 live births.

(continued)

BOX 36-1   *Healthy People 2000 Objectives and the National Education Goals (continued)*

14.4: Reduce the incidence of fetal alcohol syndrome to no more than 0.12 per 1,000 live births.

14.5: Reduce low birth weight to an incidence of no more than 5 percent of live births and very low birth weight to no more than 1 percent of live births.

14.6: Increase to at least 85 percent the proportion of mothers who achieve the minimum recommended weight gain during their pregnancies.

14.7: Reduce severe complications of pregnancy to no more than 15 per 100 deliveries.

14.8: Reduce the cesarean delivery rate to no more than 15 per 100 deliveries.

14.10: Increase abstinence from tobacco use by pregnant women to at least 90 percent and increase abstinence from alcohol, cocaine, and marijuana by pregnant women by at least 20 percent.

14.11: Increase to at least 90 percent the proportion of all pregnant women who receive prenatal care in the first trimester of pregnancy.

14.12: Increase to at least 60 percent the proportion of primary care providers who provide age-appropriate preconception care and counseling.

14.13: Increase to at least 90 percent the proportion of women enrolled in prenatal care who are offered screening and counseling on prenatal detection of fetal abnormalities.

14.14: Increase to at least 90 percent the proportion of pregnant women and infants who receive risk-appropriate care.

National Education goal 2: By the year 2000, the high school graduation rate will increase to at least 90 percent.

National Education Objective—The nation must dramatically reduce its dropout rate and 75 percent of those students who do drop out will successfully complete a high school degree or its equivalent.

RELATED NATIONAL HEALTH PROMOTION AND DISEASE PREVENTION OBJECTIVE:

8.2: Increase the high school graduation rate to at least 90 percent, thereby reducing risks for multiple problem behaviors and poor mental and physical health.

National Education Goal 6: By the year 2000, every school will be free of drugs and violence and will offer a disciplined environment conducive to learning.

National Education Objective—Every school will implement a firm and fair policy on use, possession, and distribution of drugs and alcohol.

RELATED NATIONAL HEALTH PROMOTION AND DISEASE PREVENTION OBJECTIVES:

Tobacco

3.5: Reduce the initiation of cigarette smoking by children and youth so that no more than 15 percent have become regular cigarette smokers by age 20.

> **BOX 36-1   *Healthy People 2000 Objectives and the National Education Goals***
>
> **3.9:** Reduce smokeless tobacco use by males aged 12 through 24 to a prevalence of no more than 4 percent.
> **3.10:** Establish tobacco-free environments and include tobacco use prevention in the curricula of all elementary, middle, and secondary schools, preferably as part of comprehensive school health education.
> **3.11:** Increase to at least 75 percent the proportion of worksites (includes schools) with a formal smoking policy that prohibits or severely restricts smoking at the workplace.
> **3.12:** Enact in 50 States comprehensive laws on clean indoor air that prohibit or strictly limit smoking in the workplace and enclosed public places (including health care facilities, schools, and public transportation).
> **3.13:** Enact and enforce in 50 States laws prohibiting the sale and distribution of tobacco products to youth younger than age 19.
> **3.14:** Increase to 50 the number of States with plans to reduce tobacco use, especially among youth.
> **3.15:** Eliminate or severely restrict all forms of tobacco product advertising and promotion to which youth younger than 18 are likely to be exposed.
> **3.16:** Increase to at least 75 percent the proportion of primary care and oral health care providers who routinely advise cessation and provide assistance and followup for all of their tobacco-using patients:
>
> *Alcohol and Other Drugs*
> **4.5:** Increase by at least 1 year the average age of first use of cigarettes, alcohol, and marijuana by adolescents aged 12 through 17.
> **4.6:** Reduce the proportion of young people who have used alcohol, marijuana, and cocaine in the past month.
> **4.7:** Reduce the proportion of high school seniors and college students engaging in recent occasions of heavy drinking of alcoholic beverages to no more than 28 percent of high school seniors and 32 percent of college students.
> **4.11:** Reduce to no more than 3 percent the proportion of male high school seniors who use anabolic steroids.
> **4.12:** Establish and monitor in 50 States comprehensive plans to ensure access to alcohol and drug treatment programs for traditionally underserved people.
> **4.14:** Extend adoption of alcohol and drug policies for the work environment to at least 60 percent of worksites (includes schools) with 50 or more employees.
>
> *National Education Objective—Every school district will develop a comprehensive K–12 drug and alcohol prevention education program. Drug and alcohol curriculum should be taught as an integral part of health education. In addition, community-based teams should be organized to provide students and teachers with needed support.*
>
> (continued)

***BOX 36-1   Healthy People 2000 Objectives and the National
Education Goals (continued)***

*RELATED NATIONAL HEALTH PROMOTION AND DISEASE
PREVENTION OBJECTIVES:*

Alcohol and Other Drugs

4.9: Increase the proportion of high school seniors who perceive social
disapproval associated with the heavy use of alcohol, occasional use of
marijuana, and experimentation with cocaine.

4.10: Increase the proportion of high school seniors who associate risk of
physical or psychological harm with the heavy use of alcohol, regular
use of marijuana, and experimentation with cocaine.

4.13: Provide to children in all school districts and private schools primary
and secondary school educational programs on alcohol and other drugs,
preferably as part of quality school health education.

Education and Community-Based Programs

8.4: Increase to at least 75 percent the proportion of the nation's elementary
and secondary schools that provide planned and sequential
kindergarten through grade 12 quality school health education.

8.9: Increase to at least 75 percent the proportion of people aged 10 and
older who have discussed issues related to nutrition, physical activity,
sexual behavior, tobacco, alcohol, other drugs, or safety with family
members on at least one occasion during the preceding month.

*OTHER NATIONAL HEALTH PROMOTION AND DISEASE
PREVENTION OBJECTIVES RELATED TO NATIONAL EDUCATION
GOAL 6:*

Violent and Abusive Behavior

7.1: Reduce homicides to no more than 7.2 per 100,000 people.

7.2a: Reduce suicides to no more than 8.2 per 100,000 youth aged 15–19.

7.3: Reduce weapon-related violent deaths to no more than 12.6 per
100,000 people from major causes.

7.4: Reverse to less than 25.2 per 1,000 children the rising incidence of
maltreatment of children younger than age 18.

7.6: Reduce assault injuries among people aged 12 and older to no more
than 10 per 1,000 people.

7.7: Reduce rape and attempted rape of women aged 12 and older to no
more than 107 per 100,000 women.

7.9: Reduce by 20 percent the incidence of physical fighting among
adolescents aged 14 through 17.

7.10: Reduce by 20 percent the incidence of weapon-carrying by adolescents
aged 14 through 17.

7.16: Increase to at least 50 percent the proportion of elementary and
secondary schools that teach nonviolent conflict resolution skills,
preferably as a part of quality school health education.

7.17: Extend coordinated, comprehensive violence prevention programs to at
least 80 percent of local jurisdictions with populations over 100,000.

The two sets of national goals and objectives provide guidance for identifying, prioritizing, and addressing health problems at the national, State, and community levels. In order to realize the goals and objectives, two critical systems—those providing health services and those providing education—need to collaborate, not only among themselves, but also with social services. Historically they have not always done so. Today, however, health care providers are increasingly focusing on prevention as well as treatment of disease and disability, and on the developmental as well as the physical needs of their young patients. Similarly, educators are recognizing that many additional factors, such as social, economic, health, and nutrition factors, affect their students' abilities to learn.

▬ THE NEED FOR COLLABORATION

Health, education, and social service professionals increasingly recognize that they must collaborate closely to meet the needs of the children and families they serve. A team that consists of parents and providers of other relevant services as full partners is needed to provide a continuum of services that fosters optimal development of the child from the prenatal period through early school years.

Many factors, such as economics, come to bear on a child's health, development, and nutritional status, and consequently on the child's readiness for school. The National Center for Health Statistics data shows that in 1988, 12.6 million children younger than 18 years were living in poverty; with black and Hispanic children three times more likely than white children to be living in poverty. In 1989, more than 24 percent of all children younger than18 years lived with one parent only. Data show that black children are three times more likely than white children to be living with a single parent *(4)*.

Single parent living arrangements also directly affect family income, as evidenced by findings for 1989, when 44.7 percent of children living only with their mothers were poor. Studies show that children whose families earn less than $20,000 per year had fewer physician contacts than those whose families earn more. Children from families earning less than $20,000 had 40 percent more hospital days, suggesting that children from poorer families do not receive health care until later in the course of their illnesses and as a result require more hospitalizations *(4)*.

▬ THE IMPORTANCE OF PRENATAL CARE

The process of ensuring that a child arrives at school healthy, well nourished, and ready to learn begins with the health of the child's parents. Today, however, more than 14 million women of reproductive age have no insurance to cover maternity care *(5)*. Early, high-quality prenatal care, including attention to maternal nutrition, illness, smoking and alcohol or other drug use, psychological health, and other risk factors, is critical to improving pregnancy outcomes, especially low birth weight. While necessary for all pregnant women, prenatal care is especially important for women at increased medical or social risk. Maternal characteristics associated with receiving late or no prenatal care include low socioeconomic status, less than a high school education, teenaged pregnancy, or high parity *(6)*. Women who are substance abusers also are less likely to get prenatal care *(7)*.

Between 1970 and 1980, there was a significant trend toward increasing early entry into prenatal care for the groups with the lowest levels of care. Since 1980, among all racial and ethnic groups, however, the proportion of women who begin prenatal care in the first trimester of pregnancy has reached a plateau *(2a)*. The increase between 1982 and 1987 in the proportions of women not receiving care until their third trimester or receiving no care has been of particular concern. According to 1987 data, nearly 40 percent of pregnant black women and 39 percent of Hispanic women failed to receive early prenatal care *(2a)*. Recent congressional mandates expanding Medicaid eligibility have resulted in more women being eligible for prenatal and postpartum care *(8,9)*. Yet persistent barriers, including a growing shortage of obstetrical care providers, as well as language and cultural barriers remain.

▄INFANT MORTALITY AND RELATED RISKS

Although gains have been made in recent years and infant mortality is steadily improving, it still remains a problem here in the United States. In 1988, a total of 38,910 infants died before their first birthday, and the infant mortality rate for blacks remains twice as high as the rate for white infants *(10)*. In the presence of these disparities, the problem must be addressed.

While not all babies of normal birth weight are automatically healthy, and not all low birth weight babies are automatically at a disadvantage, the evidence shows that being born at low birth weight places a baby at greater risk. When babies of normal birth weight are compared with low and very low birth weight babies, they have 7 to 10 times the risk of severe developmental problems, such as severe cerebral palsy, blindness, deafness, and retardation. They also have two to three times the probability of poor school performance as they are more likely to have chronic health problems. In essence, when low birth weight is combined with poverty, the child faces what has been referred to as "double jeopardy" *(11)*.

▄ADEQUATE NUTRITION AND ORAL HEALTH

Pregnant women and their children will require adequate nutrition if the children are to grow and develop normally. It has been shown that when infants and young children lack adequate nutrition, their growth can be slowed, they may be more susceptible to illness, and, as a consequence, they can be at greater risk of neurodevelopmental problems that impair learning *(12)*. Undernutrition and inadequate food intake, primarily among low-income and certain minority populations, still exist in this country *(13)*. Nutritional problems, such as iron deficiency anemia, are known to affect pregnant women and children and are frequently associated with poverty.

While there is debate over the prevalence of childhood hunger in America, with estimates of the number of children who experience hunger ranging from 2 to 5.5 million, the National Commission on Children found that the problem has increased during the past decade *(12)*. Programs such as the Special Supplemental Food Program for Women, Infants, and Children (WIC) and the nutrition components of the Head Start Program can play an important role in addressing the problem of inadequate nutrition during pregnancy and early childhood, and have the potential to link nutrition to other important health services affecting young children and their families.

Similarly, the pain and suffering some children undergo due to untreated extensive dental caries is unnecessary. Unfortunately, early and regular dental care among children is far from universal. In 1986, only 25 percent of children aged 2 years had ever visited a dentist *(14)*. Early and periodic assessments of oral health are necessary not only for diagnosis and treatment of existing disease but for the delivery of primary preventive services such as fluorides and sealants. Equally important is the accurate and early diagnosis and prompt treatment of congenital anomalies, such as cleft lip or palate, to minimize disability and other adverse sequelae.

■ TIMELY AND APPROPRIATE IMMUNIZATIONS

Health care in early childhood has emphasized the prevention and control of infectious diseases through timely immunization. The current measles epidemic provides an indicator that the nation's provision of this traditional and key preventive service needs to be reexamined. The recent report of the National Vaccine Advisory Committee points out that the majority of the cases of measles occurred among unimmunized preschool children who came primarily from minority communities in inner cities *(15)*. That report clearly demonstrates that the principal cause of this rise in childhood measles has been the fact that children are not receiving immunizations on time. The National Vaccine Advisory Committee reports that many opportunities for vaccination are lost when children do not receive all vaccines they need at a single visit or are sent home without vaccination because of invalid contraindications, such as a minor illness.

Innovative ways to ensure that all children are immunized on time are needed. As an example, many unvaccinated children could be reached through a strengthened emphasis on immunizations in such public programs as WIC and Aid to Families with Dependent Children. Out-of-home child care, which encompasses an increasing number of infants and young children, offers another potential opportunity to improve immunization rates.

▬INJURY PREVENTION

In 1988, injuries, many of them preventable, remain the leading cause of death in childhood, claiming the lives of more than 22,400 children ages 19 years and younger in the United States *(16)*. It is estimated that more than 30,000 children suffer permanent disabilities from injuries each year, many resulting in subsequent learning problems and school difficulties. For young children between the ages of 1 and 4 years, injuries claim more lives than all other causes combined, requiring about 65,000 annual hospitalizations among those in this age group. Increased awareness of the preventable nature of many injuries long referred to as accidental, and the adoption of proven measures to prevent and minimize injury, are becoming a necessity. Healthy People 2000 objectives call for increased efforts in reducing the growing burden on children of violence and intentional injuries, including child abuse and homicide.

▬HIV INFECTION AMONG CHILDREN

New issues are emerging to challenge the health and education systems. Through August 1991, 3,253 children with acquired immunodeficiency syndrome (AIDS) who were younger than 13 years were reported to the Centers for Disease Control. Of them, 84 percent were infected perinatally, and 52.5 percent have already died *(17)*. These figures do not reflect the even larger number of children infected with HIV, many of whom are symptomatic but do not yet meet reporting criteria for AIDS. In addition, while 20 to 30 percent of all children born to women infected with HIV will go on to be infected themselves, the 70 to 80 percent who are spared infection will, nevertheless, suffer from the devastating impact of losing their mother, father, or siblings to the HIV infection, and will carry the stigma of the disease as if they were infected with the virus themselves.

▬DRUG-EXPOSED INFANTS AND CHILDREN

Schools and health care providers already are beginning to deal with the effects of crack cocaine and other substance abuse by pregnant women. While recognizing that determination of the true substance exposure rates among pregnant women is difficult, current estimates of the number of crack- or cocaine-exposed newborns range from 30,000 to 100,000 or greater annually *(18)*. Prenatal cocaine exposure can lead to premature birth, low birth weight, birth defects, and respiratory and neurological problems *(19)*. In addition to these biological vulnerabilities, the social environment to which these infants are exposed postnatally can affect subsequent development and educational potential *(20)*.

As the results of long-term studies on drug-exposed infants begin to emerge, researchers are predicting that older children who were exposed to drugs prenatally may need specialized educational services that cannot be provided by the average day care facility, preschool, or kindergarten *(21)*. Even more prevalent than the effects of cocaine abuse, each year fetal alcohol syndrome affects nearly 5,000 babies and is the third leading cause of birth defects associated with mental retardation. Thousands more children are born with fetal alcohol effect, a milder form of fetal alcohol syndrome but no less devastating *(22)*.

A General Accounting Office report notes that drug-exposed infants have more health problems and higher medical costs than infants not exposed to drugs. In addition to costly medical treatment, the impact of these drug-exposed infants on the social welfare system is high. The report notes that without intervention, such children may be expected to have major problems in school and high dropout rates *(23)*. Clearly, primary prevention measures are needed, as well as measures to prevent the health, educational, and social sequelae of maternal drug use on exposed infants.

■EMOTIONAL AND MENTAL DEVELOPMENT

Increasingly, attention is being paid to the healthy emotional and mental development of infants and young children. New knowledge about the earliest years of life tells us some important things about infants. Infants learn, respond, and interact from the earliest moments of their lives and are even more vulnerable than older children to emotional and social deprivation, as well as to physical injury. Development in the early years is too important to leave to chance.

Factors such as poverty, abuse, or neglect, and disturbed family relationships are known to increase the risk of emotional dysfunction and mental disorders in infants and young children. Yet their obvious consequences are not always documented until children's learning or behavioral problems are noticed when they reach preschool or school *(24)*. The emotional and mental disorders of early childhood need to be addressed before they lead to school failure and behavioral problems.

The Office of Technology Assessment of the Congress estimates that of the 7.5 million children of all ages who need mental health treatment, only about 2 million actually receive it. Increasing the understanding of how biological, psychological, and social factors interact in children's development is likely to lead to many more specific measures that can be used to prevent, in a timely fashion, delays and impairments in young children's cognitive, social, and emotional development *(25)*.

■CHILDREN WITH DISABILITIES

While all infants and young children potentially can have health needs affecting their subsequent school readiness, the needs of children with disabilities or chronic illnesses require particular attention. They are especially at risk of school failure. Such children and their families have special health care needs requiring early identification, diagnostic and evaluation services, treatment services, habilitation and rehabilitation services, dental services, nutrition services, and family and child education and counseling services.

In the past, education and health professionals have seen themselves addressing different needs of these children, joined at times only by the fact that they were serving the same population. Now the education and health systems, one primarily public and tax-supported and the other supported by a complex mix of public and private resources, struggle with a common set of problems and barriers as they seek to enhance the services provided to these children and families *(26)*. Public Law 94-142, the Education for All Handicapped Children act, and Public Law 99-457, the 1986 amendments to this act, which establishes programs of early intervention for infants and young children, have laid the groundwork for collaboration, resulting in improvements in services to these children and their families.

The health, education, and social service needs of children with disabilities and those at risk for disabilities have helped the health care community to identify deficiencies in services. We now realize better the importance of ensuring the availability of coordinated, comprehensive, community-based, family-centered, and culturally sensitive services for these children and their families. A continuum of appropriate, accessible services must be available in the community for this to succeed.

■ AN INTEGRATED APPROACH

Programs such as Head Start, that concurrently address the health and education needs of children, are examples of an integrated approach to both health and education services that have been known to work. The demonstrated long-term benefits of quality early childhood programs on school achievement, graduation rates, and participation in the work force emphasize the importance of this approach. In addition to Head Start, WIC, coordinated early intervention services being developed under Public Law 99-457, and specific projects, such as the Chicago Beethoven project, the Perry Preschool Project in Michigan, and Project Giant Step in New York City, provide other examples of this integrated approach.

■ THE INITIATIVE

The Administration, cognizant of the need to link education and health, has asked the Surgeon General to "mobilize the nation" toward realizing the health component of the first national education goal. With the help of an ad hoc group of Federal leaders from the Presidential staff offices, and the Departments of Health and Human Services, Education, and Agriculture, the Surgeon General has initiated several key activities establishing the basis for the Healthy Children Ready to Learn Initiative. Starting with the underlying concept that health is a critical partner to optimum education, three operating principles for this initiative have been advanced.

To start, all children have a right to be healthy. At a minimum, this includes promoting optimum use of available and effective preventive measures, such as ensuring compliance with immunization recommendations;

promoting measures to prevent injuries; ensuring opportunities to identify disease and disabilities early; and providing prompt treatment when needed.

Second, a "good science, good sense" approach is needed. Promising program options need to be identified and evaluated and effective models disseminated for replication.

Third, healthy children, ready to learn, come from healthy families. Educated men and women form the basis for a healthy nation, a nation ready to be productive and innovative. Families must receive the support and assistance they need to raise healthy and educated children. Furthermore, the needs of special populations, whose children may inadvertently be at increased risk for disease and disability, also must be addressed. Communities must be encouraged to promote health and emphasize disease prevention.

Initial steps toward successful achievement of the readiness goal require identification of health, education, and social service programs serving young children and their families, and creating a climate that fosters innovative and effective collaboration between programs at the Federal and State levels, and especially at community levels. Policies and programs should be built around the needs of families. In this regard, the critical role that parents play in shaping a healthy environment conducive to school readiness must be recognized as a key element of strategies to achieve the readiness goal. It is important to engage professional organizations and other private sector groups involved with health, education, and other children's issues to work with government and families to achieve the school readiness goal and its related health objectives.

▬NOT JUST FOR YOUNG CHILDREN

While being healthy and ready to learn is especially true for young children, it is also crucial that children of all ages move toward the same goal. Every child, throughout their school career, should have the opportunity to arrive at school healthy and ready to learn each day. School programs need to recognize the bidirectional connection between health and education—children must be healthy in order to be educated and children must be educated in order to stay healthy. This connection should be fostered through educational curriculums and by the provision of a safe and healthy school environment conducive to learning.

National Education Goals 2 and 6, and the related National Health Promotion and Disease Prevention Objectives, support this vital health and education connection for children of all ages (see Box 36-1).

▬CONCLUSION

The interface between the National Education Goals and the National Health Promotion and Disease Prevention Objectives points out the close interrelationship between health and education and their critical link to related social services. The development of these goals and objectives represents a consensus that these are matters of importance to the nation, and they present a road map for change and an impetus toward improvement. The Department of Education, working with the Department of Health and Human Services, recently developed guideposts for achieving National Education Goal 1 *(27)*.

Collaborations such as this must be fostered. The goal is too large to be left to single entities. Organizations, government agencies, communities and persons dedicated to achieving each of these sets of goals and objectives must find a way to work together. The health, education, and related social service needs of children and their families can no longer be approached categorically.

When the day comes that all children in America start school healthy and ready to learn, it will be because of the success of these partnerships and collaboration between the health, education, and social services communities and the parents of America's children.

■ REFERENCES

1. Department of Education: America 2000: An education strategy source book. Washington, DC, 1990.
2. Public Health Service: Healthy people 2000: national health promotion and disease prevention objectives. DHHS Publication No. (PHS) 91-50212. Office of the Assistant Secretary for Health, Office of Disease Prevention and Health Promotion. U.S. Government Printing Office, Washington, DC, 1990; (a) p. 381.
3. Health Resources and Services Administration: Healthy children 2000: national health promotion and disease prevention objectives related to mothers, infants, children, adolescents, and youth. DHHS Publication No. HRSA-MCH 91-2. Public Health Service, Washington, DC, 1991.
4. Health Resources and Services Administration: Child health, USA, 1990. Public Health Service, Washington, DC, 1990.
5. Alan Guttmacher Institute: Blessed events and the bottom line: the financing of maternity care in the United States. New York, NY, 1987.
6. Singh, S., Torres, D., and Forrest, I. D.: The need for prenatal care in the United States: evidence from the 1980 national natality survey. Fam Plann Perspect 17: 118–124 (1985).
7. Kith, L. G., McGregor, S. N., and Sciarra, I. I.: Drug abuse in pregnancy. *In* Drugs, alcohol, pregnancy and parenting, edited by I.I. Chasnoff. Kluwer Academic Publishers, Bingham, MA, 1988, pp. 17–44.
8. 101st Congress: Omnibus Budget Reconciliation Act of 1989 (Public Law 101–239). U.S. Government Printing Office, Washington, DC, 1989.
9. 101st Congress: Omnibus Budget Reconciliation Act of 1990 (Public Law 101–508). U.S. Government Printing Office, Washington, DC, 1990.
10. National Center for Health Statistics: Health, United States, 1989. DHHS Publication No. (PHS) 90-1232. Public Health Service, Centers for Disease Control, Hyattsville, MD, 1990.
11. National Health/Education Consortium: Crossing the boundaries between health and education. National Commission to Prevent Infant Mortality, Washington, DC, 1990.
12. National Commission on Children: Beyond rhetoric: a new American agenda for children and families. U.S. Government Printing Office, Washington, DC, 1991, p. 124.
13. Splett, P. L., and Story, M.: Child nutrition: objectives for the decade. J Am Diet Assoc 91: 665–668, June 1991.
14. Use of dental services and dental health, United States, 1986. Vital Health Stat [10] No. 165 (1986).

15 National Vaccine Advisory Committee: The measles epidemic: the problems, barriers, and recommendations. Public Health Service, Centers for Disease Control, Atlanta, GA, 1991.

16. Children's Safety Network: A data book of child and adolescent injury. National Center for Education in Maternal and Child Health, Washington, DC, 1991.

17. Centers for Disease Control: HIV/AIDS surveillance report. Atlanta, GA, 1991.

18. Gomby, D. S., and Shiono, P. H.: Estimating the number of substance-exposed infants. *In* The future of children: drug exposed infants, vol. 1, no. 1, spring 1991. Center for the Future of Children, The David and Lucile Packard Foundation, Los Altos, CA, pp. 17–25.

19. Kusserow, R. P.: Inspector General's report on crack babies. Report OEI-03-89-01540. Department of Health and Human Services, Washington, DC, June 1990.

20. Zuckerman, B.: Drug-exposed infants: understanding the medical risk. *In* The future of children: drug exposed infants, vol. 1, no. 1, spring 1991. Center for the Future of Children, The David and Lucile Packard Foundation, Los Altos, CA, pp. 25–35.

21. Subcommittee on Human Resources of the Committee on Ways and Means, U.S. House of Representatives: The enemy within: crack-cocaine and America's families. U.S. Government Printing Office, Washington, DC, 1990.

22. Select Committee on Children, Youth, and Families: Women, addiction, and perinatal substance abuse fact sheet. U.S. House of Representatives, Washington, DC, 1990.

23. U.S. General Accounting Office: Drug-exposed infants: A generation at risk. GAO/T-HRD-90-46. U.S. Government Printing Office, Washington, DC, 1990.

24. National Center for Clinical Infant Programs: Infants can't wait. Washington, DC, 1986.

25. National Advisory Mental Health Council: National plan for research on child and adolescent mental disorders. DHHS Publication No. (ADM) 90-1683. Public Health Service, Alcohol, Drug Abuse, and Mental Health Administration, Rockville, MD, 1990.

26. The American Association of Colleges for Teacher Education: The health/education connection: initiating dialogue on integrated services to children at risk and their families. Summary of a symposium sponsored by the American Association of Colleges for Teacher Education, the American Academy of Pediatrics, and the Health Resources and Services Administration, Maternal and Child Health Bureau, Alexandria, VA, March 5–6, 1990.

27. U.S. Department of Education: Preparing young children for success: Guideposts for achieving our first national goal. Washington, DC, 1991.

Chapter 37

Public Policy and Adolescent Pregnancy: A Reexamination of the Issues

ADA CATHERINE MONTESSORO   CAROL E. BLIXEN

Adolescents in the United States are becoming parents in increasing numbers even though this issue was termed an "epidemic" 20 years ago. The complex problem of adolescent pregnancy and childbirth lie at a crossroads. A variety of legislative and judicial events and social trends complicate simple solutions. Montessoro and Blixen present a comprehensive examination of the issue in the context of historical patterns and current trends on a national and international level. The authors also offer recommendations for a solution that focuses on the societal level through consistent policies and coordination of efforts supported by adequate funding.

For the past two decades the issues of adolescent pregnancy and childbirth—along with attendant issues of adolescent sexual behavior, contraceptive use, and abortion—have occupied the public agenda in the United States. The discussion has focused on morality and parental involvement, the health status of both the adolescent and infant, and on resulting public and personal costs. In 1976 adolescent pregnancy was termed an "epidemic" by the Alan Guttmacher Institute, and legislation on the federal level was passed during both the Carter and the Reagan Administrations to address various facets of the issue.

Despite the programs that evolved out of this legislation and the subsequent state and local programs that have been developed, the issues of adolescent pregnancy and childbirth continue to be prevalent ones. Critics of the programs claim that the United States has no coherent policy on this issue, that there is confusion over exactly what the problem is—morality, fertility, or poverty. In the past few years a body of revisionist discussion has grown that challenges the original data and assumptions and the conclusions that were drawn from them. From this new interpretation of the problem alternative strategies for solutions are evolving. In this article we examine the issues and identify various factors involved in the original public policy solutions directed toward the problem of adolescent preg-

From *Nursing Outlook* 44(1):31–36, 1996. Reprinted by permission of Mosby-Year Book, Inc.

nancy. In addition, we reexamine statistical data on this problem and recommend policy alternatives.

■ SCOPE OF THE PROBLEM

In the United States it is estimated that 45% of all female adolescents engage in premarital sexual behavior; this represents an increase of 15% over the last decade. Forty percent of female adolescents will become pregnant at least once before reaching the age of 20, because most do not consistently use contraception, and approximately four-fifths of these pregnancies will be unintended.[1] The influential 1976 publication by the Alan Guttmacher Institute, *11 Million Teenagers: What Can Be Done about the Epidemic of Adolescent Pregnancy in the U.S.,* stated that each year 1 million adolescents will become pregnant, that adolescents account for a third of all abortions that are performed in the United States, and that 9 of 10 adolescents who give birth choose to keep their baby rather than choose adoption.[2] In addition, one in five adolescents will have more than one child before reaching age 20, and more than four of five will be unmarried at the time of the birth.[3]

It is not just these large numbers that are seen as the problem; rather, it is what these numbers mean, the consequences, both for the adolescent and the nation. Adolescent pregnancy has been associated with increased health risks for the teen mother and her infant. The adolescent is 1.3 times more likely to suffer from nonfatal anemia or toxemia as a result of the pregnancy or birth than older women, and infants born to adolescent mothers are twice as likely to be premature and be of low birth weight than infants born to older mothers.[2] These health complications are seen to result from postponed (or nonexistent) prenatal care, poor nutrition, and other lifestyle factors. Additionally, only 6 in 10 adolescent mothers will graduate from high school, compared with 9 in 10 of their peers who delay parenthood.[3] This incomplete education will have a long-term effect on the adolescent's employment future, bringing a lifetime of underemployment or unemployment, as well as other diminished life options. Many adolescent mothers are choosing not to marry, and the resulting increase in the number of single-parent families has contributed significantly to the increase in child poverty rates, from 15% in 1960 to 20.3% in 1988.[4] Studies indicate that being from a single-parent family also puts a child at risk for emotional and behavioral problems and learning problems at school, and this contributes to a cycle of poverty.[4]

In addition to the high costs that are borne by the adolescent mother, the American taxpayer also pays a price for the high rate of early childbearing. Burt[5] cites a study, produced by SRI International in 1979 for the Population Resource Center, that estimated that the family begun by each first birth to a teenager in that year would eventually cost taxpayers $18,710 (in 1979 dollars). Further, it was estimated that all such families begun by first births to teenagers in 1979 would eventually cost at least $8.3 billion (in 1979 dollars). Included in these public costs were Aid to Families with Dependent Children funds (AFDC, also known as welfare), medical assistance, and other social services. According to the Alan Guttmacher Institute, teenagers who become mothers are disproportionately poor and dependent on public assistance for their economic support.[6]

AFDC is a federally funded program that provides income support to the custodial parent of dependent children. It began as a program to provide benefits to the children of widowed mothers but was expanded in 1950 to its current coverage. For most of its existence, AFDC has been controversial. Ozawa[7] reported a study that indicated that AFDC payments are significantly and inversely related to the birth rate and that increasing the household's income level results in greater security and an improvement in the quality of life for the children in the family. AFDC, however, has drawn criticism for "perpetuating the dysfunctional families that make up America's underclass."[4] No distinction is made between children born within a marriage and those born outside of one. By providing slightly more benefits than those of a minimum-wage job, a working mother appears to be penalized. Feminists also object to AFDC rules that require the female adolescent to remain the responsibility of her parents, thus perpetuating the status of the female adolescent as a child.[8]

The presentation of the data on pregnancy rates and costs, and their projected effects, led to several legislative efforts in the 1970s and early 1980s at the federal level aimed at decreasing the rate of adolescent pregnancy and childbirth. One such effort was the Adolescent Health, Services, and Pregnancy Prevention Act of 1978, which intended to provide federally funded contraceptive services to adolescents. This measure has drawn criticism as being only minimally effective because of limited funding.[9] The perception among policymakers and the general public today, however, remains that the pregnancy and birth rates among adolescents are still too high and the resulting consequences are still too dear. Because the problem has not been solved by previous strategies, the issue and past data have been reexamined.

▬A SECOND LOOK

According to Vinovskis,[10] a reexamination of the statistics on adolescent births shows that the rates had declined during this recent period of increased public concern. Data from the National Center for Health Statistics show that the rate of teen childbearing had increased sharply after World War II and reached a peak of 97.3 births per 1000 women aged 15 to 19 in 1957. By 1977 the rate had declined to 52.8 births per 1000 in this age group, and during the 1980s there were 51.8 births per 1000 in each year. Vinovskis states that if the Adolescent Health, Services, and Pregnancy Prevention Act, enacted in1978, was truly a response to demographic trends among adolescents, it should have been passed 20 years earlier, during the Eisenhower, not the Carter, Administration.

Rather than an increase in the childbearing rates among adolescents, policymakers and the general public were responding to the effects of the legalization of abortion and several separate social trends that were converging during the 1970s and 1980s. These trends include the growing acceptance of nonmarital sexuality and cohabitation and the increase in nonmarital birthrates among all women, but particularly among adolescents. Humenick et al.[11] state that during the 1950s and early 1960s a high proportion of teenagers who gave birth were already married or got married to legitimate the birth or gave up their babies to adoption. Beginning in the mid-1960s the social climate began to change. The growing acceptance of out-of-wedlock births led to an increase in the nonmarital birthrates among all women, and the legalization of abortion in 1973 had a major effect on the resolution of adolescent pregnancies. The nonmarital childbearing rate for all women increased from 11% in 1970 to about 28% in 1990.[12] This is an increase of 61%, but the rate among women under age 20 is even higher—a 127% increase, from 30% in 1970 to 68% in 1990. In addition, it is estimated that 90% of unmarried adolescents who currently give birth choose to keep their babies, compared with 10% in 1970.[13] It is clear that the increased concern over adolescent childbearing occurred during a period when birthrates among all teenagers were continuing a pattern of decline but when nonmarital teen birthrates were increasing. Thus feminists view the recent concern as a response to a "challenge to the prescribed norms of marriage and motherhood" and think that the real issue is "single-parenting females living and surviving economically without men."[8]

Through the 1950s rates for adolescent pregnancy and nonmarital adolescent births were relatively low among the white population, compared to rates in minority populations.[11] Since the 1960s, however, there has been a faster increase in the rates of early sexual activity, pregnancy, birth, and nonmarital birth among white adolescents than in the African-American and Hispanic populations. In 1955 only 6% of white teens gave birth while not married, compared with 41% of African-American adolescents. In 1985 the figures were 42% for white adolescents and 90% for African-Americans. Currently in the United States, white teens account for about 68% of all adolescent births and 52% of births to unmarried mothers. Only 16% of adolescent pregnancies occur to unmarried African-American or Hispanic teens under age 18.[1] While African-Americans and Hispanics continue to have disproportionately high rates of pregnancy and birth, an increasing number of white adolescents are following the pattern of early nonmarital childbirth that once was largely limited to minority communities. Given these statistics it is hard not to reach the conclusion that the intense concern for adolescent childbearing reflects a feeling that the problem is now effecting "us," rather than only "them."

▬ HISTORICAL CONTEXT OF THE PROBLEM

Vinovskis[10] states that the framers of policy during the 1970s did not have an understanding of the historical pattern of adolescent sexual behavior and childbearing and that this limited the options that were explored. In colonial America adolescent sexuality, pregnancy, and childbearing were not a problem. During that time pregnancy among adolescents was rare, because the average age of puberty was 15 years or older.[9] Up until the nineteenth century American attitudes toward early childbearing were relatively permissive and intimacy was often permitted during courtship.

However, there were wide fluctuations in rates of premarital sexual activity among both adolescents and adults and in rates of premarital pregnancy over time and between regions of the country. For example, an increase in rates at the end of the eighteenth century was attributed to increased geographic mobility, the breakdown of stable communities during and after the American Revolution, and an increased legal tolerance for bastardy and fornication.[9] During the mid-nineteenth century the successful efforts to discourage adolescent sexual activity grew from the various religious revival and moral reform movements and the influence of Victorian ideology.[10] The increased rates during the 1920s was attributed to the liberalization of sexual mores and urbanization occurring after World War I.[9] Thus attitudes regarding adolescent sexual behavior and childbearing have varied throughout our history and functioned to influence the rates of such behavior. However, even though early sexual activity and childbearing has, at times, been seen as an area of concern, it was only in the last 25 years that the federal government became involved in attempting to provide solutions for these problems.

▬INTERNATIONAL CONTEXT

Statistics show that, compared with their counterparts in other industrialized countries, adolescents in the United States do not have higher levels of sexual activity but they do have higher rates of pregnancy, abortion, and childbirth.[14] All Western European countries have lower rates than the United States, and the only developed countries that have higher rates than that of the United States are Bulgaria, Cuba, Puerto Rico, Rumania, and Hungary.[14] The higher rates for adolescent pregnancy and childbirth in the United States mimic those societies that have an agricultural pattern of early family formation, socially approved early childbearing, and increased levels of religiosity. Analysis indicates that those developed countries with lower rates of adolescent pregnancy and childbirth have achieved them by having a consistent policy of sex education and contraception for adolescents, an accessible and affordable health care delivery system, and a relatively equitable distribution of income and opportunities.[11]

In those countries with lower birth rates, the attitudes held by adults about sexuality, sexual behavior among adolescents, and how those attitudes are passed on to adolescents is very different from the pattern and attitudes in the United States. Adolescent sexual behavior is not universally approved of, but it receives greater acceptance than in the United States. In addition, while there continues to be efforts in these countries to further decrease the birth rates among adolescents, "the problem" there is defined as one of adolescent pregnancy and birth, which contrasts with the United States, where the problem is defined as inappropriate adolescent sexual activity. This contributes to the controversial nature of sex education and health clinics in public schools and results in inconsistent and inadequate programs and compounds the misunderstanding and misinformation that may characterize discussions in the home between parents and adolescents. Forrest[14] states that when compared with other developed countries, the United States is more "societally and individually ambivalent on sexuality issues" and that this significantly contributes to the higher rates of adolescent pregnancy and childbirth.

In addition to the statistics that indicate stable childbirth rates but increasing nonmarital childbirth rates among adolescents, these attitudes are amplified by the rapid pace of social change that began to occur in the United States in the late 1950s and early 1960s. Tremendous changes took place in American culture, in the American family, and in the social and sexual relationships between males and females in this period. Important among these changes are the rise of feminism, which led to increased political activity and research on issues pertaining to women, the development of oral contraceptives, and the 1973 legalization of abortion. The demographic data show that over the past few decades there has been a rising rate of abortion, as well as a rising nonmarital birth rate.[14] Feminists explain this apparent incongruence as evidence of a "rejection of early marriage as the defining objective in women's lives."[15] This interpretation acknowledges a profound change occurring in American culture, whereas arguments between liberals and conservatives have focused on sexual behavior, contraception, and morality.

Petchesky[15] states that controversy has artificially separated such issues as abortion, contraception, and nonmarital or adolescent pregnancy and that it is more correct to understand the hysteria over them as a distillation of a much larger issue—that of women's sexuality. For her and other feminist researchers and theorists, human sexuality is a social activity, rather than a biologic one, and therefore gets its meaning from the social and cultural setting. Such events as abortion and adolescent pregnancy make sex visible and "the idea of women as sexual agents . . . is still a dangerous one."[15] And so the phenomenon of adolescent pregnancy needs to be viewed within the context of an increasing female independence challenging traditional social norms and expectations about appropriate female behavior.[15]

In addition to this double standard concerning female morality, American culture presents adolescents with a double message about sexuality. It is very clear that whatever their rate of sexual activity, adolescents are able to effectively use birth control to a remarkable degree and to avoid pregnancy in a culture that presents them with widely conflicting cultural and ideologic pressures. On the one hand, responsible reproduction is urged, by which is typically meant delaying childbearing until reaching emotional maturity and economic independence. On the other hand, sexuality is used by the media as a marketing device.[11] Currently in television commercials young, female sexuality is alluringly portrayed in the effort to sell automobiles, but ads promoting healthful sexual behaviors to avoid transmission of HIV are so controversial they may be presented only infrequently and in the off-peak hours.

■ECONOMIC CONTEXT

Over the past few decades, the U.S. economy has become technologically sophisticated and has acquired a growing need for educated and technically competent workers. The lack of a high school education became a serious barrier to economic self-sufficiency, and teenage mothers and their infants face a much more uncertain economic future than was once the case. In addition, "acquiring economic, social and technical independence in this environment requires an extensive training period for young people, thus prolonging the period of dependence on their families."[11]

The dependence has also often meant a reliance on AFDC by young, single mothers and their children. The data and the various interpretations of the data are conflicting, but the issue of welfare reliance has become intertwined with those of adolescent pregnancy, contraception, and abortion. Critics have claimed that young women have used the financial support of AFDC to be able to move out of their parents' homes and thus avoid parental supervision. At the national level, recent proposals by President Clinton to reform the welfare system include regulations requiring unmarried adolescent mothers under age 16 to live with their parents in order to receive welfare payments.

■PUBLIC POLICY

Thus there is substantial evidence for defining adolescent pregnancy and childbirth as problematic. However, there has not been a consensus on the solution. As is apparent, the issue has become blended with several other controversial ones and over the last 20 years become politicized. Liberals, who had extensive political influence during the 1960s and 1970s, have felt that the solution lies in sex education and greater access to contraceptives. Conservatives, who gained power and influence in the late 1970s and early1980s, want efforts directed at programs that reduced adolescent sexual activity. This difference is exemplified by a statement by Connaught Marshner, chairman of the National Pro-Family Coalition: "They [liberals] begin with the premise that teenagers should not have babies. We begin with the premise that single teenagers should not have sex."[16] What has resulted, however, were programs that focused assistance on young women who were pregnant or were already mothers, rather than on programs to prevent the pregnancy.

The civil rights movement and the Great Society programs of the 1960s had identified early childbearing as contributing to a cycle of poverty, thus linking it to economic issues and making it amenable to federal solutions.[13] These programs provided services to minority or poor populations in the area of medical and family-planning services. During the 1980s and the Reagan Administration the issues of birth control and sex education became linked with the issue of abortion, primarily through the efforts of the growing New Right conservatives who focused on social issues rather than the traditional conservative interest of foreign policy. This removed the issue of adolescent pregnancy from the public health and social service arena and brought it into the political one.

Originally the only services for pregnant adolescents were residential maternity homes operated by the Child Welfare League (known as Florence Crittenden Homes), the Salvation Army, and other religious groups. Adolescents who became pregnant were required to drop out of school because it was felt that they would corrupt other students.

However, Title IX of the Education Amendments, passed in 1972 (but not in effect until 1975), prohibited school discrimination on the basis of sex and required that any separate instructional programs that were often established by local school districts now be optional as well as comparable in quality to those for nonpregnant students. This provision led to increased numbers of pregnant adolescents remaining in school, but other legislation directed at adolescent pregnancy reflects the discomfort and ambivalence that legislators and the public feel about this issue. Policymakers have felt the issue of adolescent sexuality to be controversial and politically dangerous, and, consequently, legislation has centered variously on family planning and on alternatives to abortion.[10]

The primary source of public funding for pregnancy prevention is the Family Planning Services and Population Research Act of 1970 (Title X of the Public Health Services Act). This act increased funding for family planning programs from $80 million in 1971 to $197 million in 1975. Despite continued funding cuts during the Reagan and Bush Administrations and efforts to abolish it entirely, funding under this legislation still helps to support 4500 family planning clinics around the country.

The Adolescent Health Services and Pregnancy Prevention and Care Act of 1978 was the first legislative initiative to focus on adolescent sexual behavior. The legislation had both "pro-choice" and "pro-life" support, which made it easy for those in Congress to vote in favor it it.[10] This act established in 1979 the Office of Adolescent Pregnancy Programs (OAPP), within the U.S. Public Health Service, to coordinate all programs in the Department of Health and Human Services that deal with adolescent pregnancy. The OAPP developed and administered programs in various states to offer education, counseling, and social and medical assistance to adolescents, either throughout pregnancy or through the first year or two of parenthood. Originally $60 million was to be made available, but only $7.5 million was allocated during the first year. Funding levels continued to limit those who were eligible, but the effort has been credited with a number of successful intervention strategies.[17] However, this legislation was repealed in 1981 by the Omnibus Reconciliation Act because it was felt the "emphasis should be on strengthening family commitment and encouraging postponement of sexual activity rather than providing more money for the mechanics of birth control or more value-free sex education."[11]

In 1981 another political compromise was passed to replace this repealed law. Passed with great pressure from conservatives, the Adolescent Family Life Act was first proposed to address birth control education and services, but in the end it was focused on services to those adolescents who were already pregnant. Again, limited funds were available, and programs established by the act focused on encouraging chastity rather than on providing contraceptive services. Under this act the use of federal funds for abortion counseling was banned. One provision of this legislation began its life titled as the Chastity Bill and was aimed at promoting self-discipline and chastity and a family-centered approach to "the problems of adolescent promiscuity and pregnancy."[13] This section awards grants to community programs that emphasize both sexual abstinence by the adolescent and parental involvement in pregnancy prevention.

During the 1980s there was a national political shift toward a "New Federalism," emphasizing state and local initiatives rather than federal ones and resulting in attempts to switch responsibility for adolescent pregnancy from government to private initiatives and the family.[13] The role of government in this area then became the coordination of a network of local initiatives and programs. The result has been a variety of state and local programs with a variety of policies and regulations leading to great inconsistency throughout the country and no central entity to coordinate and focus the effort. Individual states can limit their commitment to what is often seen as controversial programs simply by limiting the funds available.

In addition to these legislative programs that focus on adolescent sexual behavior and contraception, the U.S. government provides a broad range of health, welfare, and social service programs to individuals and families in need. Initially these programs were created to assist the poor, but like AFDC were extended to include pregnant adolescents.[10] The Special Supplemental Food Program for Women, Infants, and Children (WIC), part of the Child Nutrition Act of 1972, provides food vouchers for pregnant women and for children up to age 5. AFDC recipients are also eligible to participate in the federal Food Stamp Program, established in 1977, and to receive health care benefits through Title XIX of the Social Security Act (Medicaid).

▬ALTERNATIVE RECOMMENDATIONS

The pattern of public policy and legislation on adolescent pregnancy has been too narrowly focused at the individual, on adolescent behavior, rather than focusing at the societal level. The assumption of all policy has been that adolescent pregnancy and childbirth result in decreased education, decreased employment opportunity, and low self-esteem and perpetuate a cycle of poverty. It is now coming to be understood that poverty is a cause of early childbearing, rather than its consequence. Males[18] states that poverty is actually a key predictor of early pregnancy and cites a 1988 study showing the state of Louisiana had a teen pregnancy rate 2.5 times higher than Minnesota and a poverty level among teens of 31.2%, as compared with 12.4% in Minnesota. A solution to the problems of early childbearing will require a multifaceted approach, and it is linked to the larger issues of welfare, racism, unemployment, child care, the minimum wage. Attention to these concerns will have many positive effects on adolescent pregnancy prevention, but efforts to address adolescent childbearing do not have to wait until those larger issues are solved.

Both primary and secondary prevention strategies may be used to approach a solution. Primary prevention, which focuses on the delay or abstention from sexual activity or the practicing of effective contraception is far more cost-effective than secondary prevention, which involves interventions that take place at the point of pregnancy resolution and may involve abortion, giving birth, or adoption. Primary prevention, however, is very controversial, and there is ambivalent support for these strategies.[5]

Existing programs that provide sex education in schools and family planning services need to be adequately funded, but an expansion above what is provided at the present will be required. Caldas[12] states that current programs are piecemeal "basic plumbing" instruction. Realistic sex education should offer honest information about reproduction and contraception, be part of a total approach to human sexuality, and start earlier in the school curriculum than is now common. Age-appropriate material should be presented at the early elementary level, and sex education should be provided before the initiation of sexual activity, rather than after a pregnancy has occurred.

Most previous education attempts have been directed toward adolescent females. Lawson and Rhode[1] state that in addition to changing gender norms that link masculinity with dominance and femininity with passivity, sex education needs to address male behavior and responsibility. And, according to Males,[18] such efforts also need to be directed toward adult males, because California Vital Statistics show that men older than high school age account for 77% of all births among women of high school age (ages 16 to 18).

Positive health practices, critical thinking on methods to avoid risk-taking behavior, and discussion on postponing sexual activity until the person is emotionally and psychologically ready—all should be components of the program. In addition, self-esteem issues and assertiveness skills need to be included, as well as a focus on personal development, which is consistent with the task of adolescence.[11] To see a benefit to postponing early pregnancy and childbearing, adolescents need improved educational and employment opportunities that give them hope for the future and goals to work toward.

Health clinics need to be available to adolescents. These can be located in the schools or readily available in the nearby community. In addition to general health information and care, counseling and treatment for sexually transmitted diseases and the provision of contraceptives should be included. Studies have shown that the provision of such information does not increase the level of sexual activity. And two successful school clinic programs in Minneapolis–St. Paul and in Baltimore show reduced pregnancy rates among sexually active teenagers.[11] Additionally, prenatal care should be provided to adolescents early in pregnancy. It has been shown that the negative health effects of adolescent childbearing are due more to the lack of prenatal and postnatal health care and to poverty-level economic status rather than the age of the mother.[6,18]

The cost for comprehensive programs are estimated to be high. Some current multi-service community programs cost $1400 per participant per year, whereas school-based health services can be as low as $250.[17] However, these costs are much lower than those that would result if the adolescent mother and her child required social service support. The Alan Guttmacher Institute estimates that in 1990 the government spent more than $25 billion for social, health, and welfare services to families begun by teenage mothers and that babies born to teenagers in 1990 will cost U.S. taxpayers more than $7 billion over the next 20 years.[6]

Ideally it would help to remove politics from the solution process. Liberals and conservatives need to realize that there is common ground between them. It seems to be a universal belief that early sexual activity and early childbearing are not good things. However, it is a fact that in this century the age of menarche has decreased. Public expectations and public policy need to acknowledge that. Campaigns such as that recently run by the Children's Defense Fund that targets "children having children" perform a disservice to teenagers by treating them as children rather than emphasizing responsible sexual behavior.[8]

To allow for a less emotional look at the issue and a solution to the problem, policymakers must reexamine adolescent pregnancy by placing available statistical examination in the context of historical patterns and current social trends. A consistent policy, a coordination of efforts by educators, parents, and health professionals, and the adequate funding of programs are necessary to give adolescents incentives and hope for the future.

■REFERENCES

1. Lawson A, Rhode DL. Introduction. In: Lawson A, Rhode DL, eds. The politics of pregnancy: adolescent sexuality and public policy. New Haven: Yale University Press, 1993:1–19.
2. Alan Guttmacher Institute. 11 Million teenagers: what can be done about the epidemic of adolescent pregnancy in the US. New York: Alan Guttmacher Institute,1976.
3. Children's Defense Fund. A vision for America's future—an agenda for the 1990s: a children's defense budget. Washington: Children's Defense Fund, 1989.
4. Magnet M. The American family: 1992. Fortune 1992;126 (Mar):42–7.
5. Burt MR. Public costs and policy implications of teenage childbearing. In: Stiffman AR, Feldman RA, eds. Advances in adolescent mental health: contraception, pregnancy, and parenting. London: Jessica Kingsley, 1990: 265–80.
6. Alan Guttmacher Institute. Facts in brief: teenager sexual and reproductive behavior. New York: Alan Guttmacher Institute, 1993.
7. Ozawa MN. Social policy and out-of-wedlock births to adolescents. In: Stiffman AR, Feldman RA, eds. Advances in adolescent mental health: contraception, pregnancy, and parenting. London: Jessica Kingsley, 1990: 281–99.
8. Pearce DM. Children having children: teenage pregnancy and public policy from the woman's perspective. In: Lawson A, Rhode DL, eds. The politics of pregnancy: adolescent sexuality and public policy. New Haven: Yale University Press, 1993:46–57.
9. Rhode DL. Adolescent pregnancy and public policy. In: Lawson A, Rhode DL, eds. The politics of pregnancy: adolescent sexuality and public policy. New Haven: Yale University Press, 1993:301–35.

10. Vinovskis MA. An "epidemic" of adolescent pregnancy?: Some historical and policy considerations. New York: Oxford University Press,1988.
11. Humenick S, Wilkerson N, Paul N. Adolescent pregnancy: nursing perspectives on prevention. White Plains, New York: March of Dimes Birth Defects Foundation,1991.
12. Caldas SJ. Teen pregnancy: why it remains a serious social, economic and educational problem in the U.S. Phi Delta Kappan 1994;75(May):402–5.
13. Rothenberg R, Sedhom L. Teenager pregnancy. In: Natapoff IN, Wieczorek RR, eds. Maternal-child health policy: a nursing perspective. New York: Springer, 1990:131–52.
14. Forrest JD. Adolescent reproductive behavior: an international comparison of developed countries. In: Stiffman AR, Feldman RA, eds. Advances in adolescent mental health: contraception, pregnancy and parenting. London: Jessica Kingsley, 1990:13–34.
15. Petchesky RP. Abortion and woman's choice: the state, sexuality, and reproductive freedom. Revised ed. Boston: Northeastern University Press, 1990.
16. Marshner CC. The new traditional woman. Washington: Free Congress Research and Education Foundation, 1982.
17. Brindis C. Antecedents and consequences: the need for diverse strategies in adolescent pregnancy prevention. In: Lawson A, Rhode DL, eds. The politics of pregnancy: adolescent sexuality and public policy. New Haven: Yale University, 1993:257–83.
18. Males M. Poverty, rape, adult/teen sex: why pregnancy prevention programs don't work. Phi Delta Kappan 1994;75(May):407–10.

Chapter 38

Mutual Support Groups

LIZBETH A. DRURY-ZEMKE

The knowledge that mutual support groups exist and their value for others are among the resources community health nurses have available for their clients. Nurses may think of mutual support groups for their clients, but not for themselves. By revealing the details of a personal tragedy, Lizbeth Drury-Zemke recounts how she started a mutual support group to meet a need she and others in the community had. She identifies the steps needed to begin a successful program of support by collaborating with others from many disciplines and peppers this chapter with humor as she comes to terms with her loss. Readers are exposed to her self-care and adaptive approach to holistic recovery through a mutual support group that is complementary to medical care—a much needed service, but one that may be overlooked.

▬THE ACCIDENT

A devastating experience in my life made me aware that the formal health care delivery system in the United States is, at times, not enough. Even though I am a community health nurse with over 20 years of experience, until two and one-half year ago I had very little experience with self-help groups. I was aware of groups such as Alcoholics Anonymous, Reach to Recovery, and Parents Without Partners and referred my clients to them, but felt no need to become involved in any such group. I had experienced life situations that might have warranted attending such groups, but, because I have always been strong, independent, adaptable, and optimistic, I viewed attending these groups as a possible sign of weakness or "sickness." I didn't want to attend and possibly feel worse than before I attended. After all, I knew that they worked for some people; they just didn't seem right for me.

Then one day in 1993, while driving to a rural clinic site, a man driving on the wrong side of the road hit my car head on and my healthy and busy life abruptly came to a halt. I was unconscious for 20 minutes or so. When I was able to speak, I naturally asked, "What happened?" I was told by the life-flight crew that I had a big laceration on my head and that my right leg was badly broken. In my nurse's brain, I thought to myself, at least I'm

This chapter was especially written for this edition of this book.

alive!—six to eight weeks in a cast and I'll be all better and back to work. Weeks became months, and the realities of the extent of the injuries became depressingly evident: a head injury resulting in cognitive damage requiring therapy and retraining; a vestibular disorder and a central auditory processing deficit that I was told would not improve; and, basically, a right foot and knee that were no longer functional. These injuries would require multiple surgeries and, eventually, after two years, amputation of my right leg below the knee.

While I was in cognitive therapy, the rehabilitation facility asked if I wanted to attend a head-injury support group consisting of varied participants with brain injuries from motor vehicle accidents, strokes, brain tumors, and other causes. Although I felt uncomfortable at first (indeed, I didn't mention it to anyone, including my family), it now seems, after almost three years, that they have become a second family to me. After attending this group for almost a year, I wanted to find out more about my vestibular disorder, mild as it seemed. I wrote to VEDA (the Vestibular Disorders Association) and ordered all their educational materials. Soon after, I was contacted by the local vestibular disorders support group and began attending their meetings, sharing the tapes and materials I received from VEDA. Then March, 1995 arrived. Along with my health care providers, I accepted the fact that amputation was necessary so that I could begin my recovery and close that chapter in my life devastated by the horrible accident. I just wanted to get on with my life to the best of my abilities.

I had many questions! And, as I discovered answers to these questions, more questions and concerns arose—questions my doctors could not answer. Whom was I to ask? My physicians referred me to a few amputees, and they also told me about a support group. As a result, I joined the American Coalition of Amputees (ACA) and, again, sent for educational materials and tapes, making a great decision—to attend the annual meeting of the ACA, five weeks before the scheduled amputation. There, I received answers to my many questions—new questions to research and think about. At the same time I received warm, understanding support. Oh, did I get support! I went into surgery, feeling as ready for it as anyone possibly could. Being a nurse in this situation is not always a benefit. Sometimes you know too much! But this is when I included humor in my treatment. At times you hear about surgeons making mistakes—removing the wrong limb—and I didn't want that to happen to me. So I got off the gurney right before I was wheeled into the operating suite, ducked into the restroom, and wrote on my left leg, "Not this one, please." Then, I went rolling into the operating room singing a rendition of "All of Me," but I changed the words to, "Part of Me, Why Not Take Part of Me?" I felt more relaxed and the operating staff were "in stitches." Throughout this entire process, I had my head-injury group to provide support and help me through this situation. Also as important, I had the support, comfort, and prayers of my family and friends. The amputee support groups, although they were very helpful, were three and four hours away from home, not plausible because of the distance. Why, in a city of 300,000 people, was there not an amputee support group, where there are hundreds of amputees who could benefit from one?

▄ SELF-HELP GROUPS

Millions of people all over the world have experienced problems for which there are no easy answers. When problems and needs are not met through formal health care, social services, and counseling programs, hope and personal support can be found in mutual-help or support groups. It is within these groups, whose members share common concerns, that people are offered what is important to their recovery: the understanding and help of others who have gone through similar experiences. Social support helps healthy people stay well, speeds the recovery of people who are ill, and improves the quality of life for those for whom full recovery is not possible. Despite the diversity of the thousands of self-help groups that exist in the United States, the basic purposes of all self-help groups are the same: to provide mutual aid and emotional support for people who share the same predicament (ACA, 1994). People who have struggled long and alone to cope with a personal problem or tragedy feel great relief and security when they discover others who know exactly what they are experiencing because they are in the same situation. In this accepting environment where there is empathy, people can express their feelings and know they are understood; through mutual help the members also can develop more effective ways to cope with the problems they share. Also, when people help others, they help themselves, and that can be a happy discovery. Len Borman, founder of the Illinois Self-Help Center, says "Self-help is barn raising revisited. In the old days, when neighbors came together to build a barn, they not only accomplished a task but also enjoyed themselves and gave and received emotional support. This tradition continues today as people gather in self-help groups to help each other deal with shared concerns" (ACA, 1994).

Emotional support in times of trouble is a basic need, and human beings have traditionally received it from family and community. But there have been profound changes in the nature of family and community life in recent history that have made those sources less available or less reliable for many people. Community life can be practically impossible in a society that is as mobile and fragmented as ours. One other factor is that there are always going to be situations and problems that we can't (or don't want) to share with our family members. Therefore, the personal support we receive from family and friends is only one part of the support network that helps sustain us through life. Despite these changing social patterns, our needs for stability and support remain constant. More than ever, we are faced with pressures and demands that produce anxiety and leave little time for relaxation. In an attempt to keep pace with an ever-changing society and to exercise more control over the quality of our lives, increasing numbers of people are turning to the resources of shared experience and support found in self-help or mutual support groups (US Dept. HHS, 1987).

These groups provide an effective and rewarding alternative to coping with serious problems alone. Members help each other cope with or overcome health problems or other kinds of problems they all share. Nearly one-half million self-help groups exist in the U.S. today, serving some 10 million people (ACA, 1994). There are basically three kinds of groups. The National Institute of Mental Health (1980) classifies them as follows:

1. Groups for people with a physical or mental illness, with groups in existence for practically every known disorder
2. Recovery groups for people with problems with compulsions and addictions
3. Groups for certain minorities such as persons with disabilities

In addition to serving the primary member, most groups also serve family members, caretakers, and/or professionals who deal with the interest of the group.

For these groups emotional support is the central purpose; but advocacy for changes in policies, laws, and practices, and psychological, educational, recreational, social and financial support are also extremely important reasons for these groups to form. Therapeutic community groups are a vital link for healthy recovery from major illness, physical conditions, or life crises, often preventing and alleviating further emotional distress. Unrelieved distress can often lead to pathology. Mutual support groups provide an outlet to relieve the distress.

Support groups, then, are formed to develop a network of others who understand the person's problems and the effect of these problems on the family. They deal with feelings of helplessness and provide moral, emotional, psychological, recreational, educational, and social support to members and their families. Self-help principles are highly adaptable to different sexual, racial, cultural, and demographic groups. The group can serve as a tool for resolving sensitive issues and conflicts in life situations and a tool for coping with one's responses to disability, isolation, powerlessness, and hopelessness. Health information, when it is delivered by a person who has experienced a health problem first hand and can share personal experience, is of more value. An important function of these groups is to supplement and humanize treatment services by serving as adjuncts to treatment and to provide social support and help that is not available within the professional milieu. Self-help groups have demonstrated an ability and effectiveness in providing aftercare that reduces recidivism, reinstitutionalizing, and readmission to the health care system, demonstrating their cost-effectiveness and financial worth.

The importance of self-help and mutual support groups to individuals cannot be over-emphasized. However, it is necessary to correlate the importance of self-help and mutual support groups to providers within our health care system. There is an ever-present challenge to health care systems and providers today—to provide effective, quality services when resources are limited and needs for those services often exceed an organization's capacity to respond. Self-help and mutual support presents an opportunity to meet this challenge. It is extremely important that partnerships are developed between the self-help movement and the health care delivery systems. These partnerships will have significant impact on public and community health.

This partnership provides opportunities for providers to share their knowledge and expertise in a receptive and non-threatening environment. Self-help groups should be used as a tool by professionals to promote health and wellness, with additional benefits of improving communication among staff, enhancing sensitivity and responsiveness to clients/participants, and improving staff–client communication. Partnerships help to break down communication barriers between providers and clients by creating an atmosphere where greater trust is possible: they provide a process for translating technical health and medical information into an understandable form. Also, the partnership builds bridges between public and private health and the community and provides a mechanism to access hard-to-reach groups and populations. Providers, as well as clients, learn additional ways of coping and they can often gain insight into issues causing "non-compliance." Perhaps one of the most important benefits of a partnership between self-help or mutual support groups and the health care delivery system lies in referrals to the group from the community and endorsement of the group's benefits by providers. To develop a self-help or mutual support group, it is most helpful to secure health professionals on advisory boards, etc.

GETTING STARTED

It is possible, as it was for me, to start a self-help group. The first step includes a needs assessment. Talk to others with the same problem and professionals in the specialty area. It is important to find out their needs and wants. Discuss the idea of a support group with them and also with professionals in the field. (In the case of amputees, this includes prosthetists, physicians, social workers, physical therapists, and rehab counselors.)

How does one find others with like problems and the appropriate professionals in the first place? Here are a few suggestions: Submit press releases to all local papers and send short announcements for the community bulletin boards of TV, radio, and newspapers in your area. I designed flyers and distributed them personally to all appropriate professionals (found in the Yellow Pages of your telephone book). In addition, meet with other support groups and find out the particulars of their organization, such as how they started and how they run their organization and how they recruit and retain membership. In my case, there wasn't an amputee support group in Central California between Sacramento and Los Angeles; and frankly I was tired of traveling to either one of these locations on a regular basis. Also, many of the amputees are just not capable of traveling such distances; therefore, they learn through trial and error and by what little information is given through their prosthetists' office or Physical Therapists during their hospital stay. I have found most people, including me, are not receptive physically or emotionally for the barrage of information which follows in the first days following surgery. Information, then, generally needs to come to patients through an ongoing, repetitive process. Needless to say, this information must be given not only by professionals but by persons from a support group or organization and must be provided at the opportune times when the clients need the specific information and when they can assimilate it. What is this specific information that only people with like problems can share with you? For instance, what problems will you encounter by just taking a shower? How do you get out of bed at night to go to the bathroom? How do you face those thousands of everyday things that you can no longer do as you did before? What if you can't do your job anymore? Could you deal with not being able to touch or feel as you did before? How do you deal with the attitudes of spouses, children, loved ones? What about sex, positions, awkwardness, discomfort? How do you accept your limitations? These are the questions an amputee may have and why support groups are a must as an adjunct to the care given by health professionals.

During my needs assessment, I was directed to a gentleman who tried to get a support group going for amputees many years ago, without success. But he did continue to visit new amputees in the hospital and developed a small network of other amputees willing to make hospital and home visits. I quickly became involved in this project and found that I could make a full-time job of just volunteering to visit new female amputees. My case manager, a rehabilitation professional, had many clients who could use an amputee support group, and amputees and their family members were calling me from all over our area, wanting more information on a support group. I also realized that many amputees mainstream, return to their jobs and their lifestyles, and do not want anything to do with a support group. But I needed to reach this group to invite them to attend for the educational presentations and, perhaps, to help those that still needed support. However, this project was growing into a bigger project than I could handle. Therefore, the logical solution was to get help!

▬GETTING HELP

Every semester at Central Valley Indian Health, Inc., where I have been the Nursing Outreach Director and Public Health Nurse for nine years, we host nursing students in their fifth semester of the nursing program at California State University, Fresno, for their community health clinical laboratory experience. One requirement of the class is the organization and implementation of a group project. Projects have varied from health fairs to community assessments to newly designed forms for improving health care delivery. In the Fall 1995 semester, the class chose to help three of us (a rehabilitation nursing consultant, the gentleman who tried to get the support group going before, and me) develop and launch the Central California Amputee Education and Support Group.

▄THE PLANNING PHASE

To develop such a group, a plan of action with goals must be developed. First, define your group's shared concern (in this case, amputees). Second, decide who your group's members will be. We decided that amputees, family members and caretakers, prosthetists, physical therapists, and others caring for amputees could attend. Third, define the group's initial focus. For example, we decided that we wanted a forum where participants could share feelings and experiences, where participants could share information and resources, where we could exchange new ways to solve old problems, and where we could reduce stress and anxiety by having a good time. We wanted to develop an environment where empowerment, participation, and recovery could take place. The following prototype, our program, might be helpful to your implementation of a like program.

We decided on a date for the first meeting. We allowed ourselves three or four months to plan the initial meeting. The students made assignments among themselves and set a time log with deadlines, etc. One student designed the flyer, which we distributed at least one month prior to the first meeting. Of course, there were numerous steps of preparation prior to that point. First, I secured the speaker and financial support for the first meeting. We felt that if a lunch and good speaker were provided free, it would be a "drawing card"—we were right! Next, the students secured a location for the meeting and made all the arrangements for set-up and clean-up. They also developed a questionnaire to hand out at the first meeting, addressing such topics as meeting times, days, topics, and speakers desired. Because we didn't want to name the group, the members selected their own name for the group after the first two meetings. We discussed topics such as incorporation and dues collection; we also obtained product samples such as Oil of Olay Moisturizing Body Wash and cleansing puffs, Palmolive Dish Washing Liquid (used for cleaning prosthetic liners), and Q-Tips to hand out at the meeting. In addition, we were able to obtain free copies of the book, *You Can't Afford a Negative Thought*, for distribution. Most importantly, the students developed a press release and notified all the major newspapers, radio and TV stations, and places where amputees visit—the physical therapists, prosthetists, etc. We were fortunate that a public relations employee who had previously worked at one of the local TV stations also wrote and released press releases. This was just the preliminary planning.

▄STEPS TO SUCCESS

The following steps are extremely important to guarantee a positive outcome:

1. Define your relationship with professionals whose expertise can be beneficial. (The group's leaders must be sensitive to the competition present among the professionals participating. They cannot view this group as threatening to their business and livelihood.)
2. Use business and community support to provide paid advertising, financial aid and grants, and sponsorship of events.
3. Establish levels of anonymity and confidentiality which is vital for some groups, such as AA, etc.
4. Consider the methods of gaining financial support to carry on the group's activities: dues, advertising, donations, fund-raising events, grants, etc.
5. Decide the logistics of the meeting place.
   a. Decide on a meeting day satisfactory to the members of the group.
   b. Choose a site appropriate for a varied group.
   c. Set a time when the majority of members can attend.
6. Determine frequency of meetings.
7. Determine status of the group—formal incorporation, non-profit, or informal group which will determine whether elections, bylaws, etc. are necessary.
8. Decide on provision of refreshments and social protocol.
9. Design a questionnaire to poll members on the above issues and design members' profile to gain information for a future directory.
10. Ask the local newspapers and TV stations to provide coverage of the meetings and to further support the activities of the group. Send press articles to national publications, newsletters, etc.

Remember, don't reinvent the wheel. Instead, obtain "how-to" packets from established organizations such as self-help clearinghouses, national associations, etc. And, delegate responsibilities. **Remember, you are not alone!**

▬THE FIRST MEETING

The above preparations complete, we are ready for the first meeting of the Self-help or Mutual Support group. From the beginning, an atmosphere of acceptance and welcome must be established.

Structure the group so that every member feels important and involved. Encourage participation (no one knows the potential that everyone has). Peer visitation, hospital and home visits to new amputees, and telephone calling to homebound clients are vital components of many support groups, and are ways for members to be involved. Make sure that everyone knows everyone else—nametags are not enough. Prepare an agenda for the meeting. Have an activity or speaker that is meaningful to the members; this is a strong motivation for recruitment and retention of members. For instance, at our first meeting, we had a state-of-the-art prosthetics display, a nationally known motivational speaker, and a neuropsychologist known for his work with support groups. At the close of the meeting, it is absolutely necessary to discuss the particulars of future meetings and to encourage continued support by those in attendance.

▬ INTEGRATING SELF-HELP GROUPS INTO THE HEALTH CARE DELIVERY SYSTEM

This paper has advocated that health care delivery systems must integrate self-help and mutual support groups to ensure quality care. Often the motivation to establish a mutual support group may come from the community health nurse who visits the person in the home, the hospital, or the clinic setting, or from the client. Some necessary steps to ensure this integration should be followed:

- Information provided to health care providers by self-help groups (meeting dates and times, contact persons, and appropriate referral information)
- Establishment of a peer visitation program by self-help groups to provide intervention
- Provision of an ongoing support network by both self-help organizations and the health care system (home health, rehab specialist, case managers, etc.)
- Assessment of self-help groups by discharge planners, case managers, etc. concerning the appropriate referral for their individual clients
- Compilation of resource information by both self-help and health care provider available as a vehicle for improved communication that ensures continuity of care
- Visitation of other support groups by both support group leaders and health care providers to gain insight concerning the effectiveness of their organization

▬ EVALUATION

The mechanics of a self-help group have been presented and have been put into action. Evaluation of this process is an important step and should not be overlooked or deemphasized. What outcome criteria measure the success of the integration of the self-help/mutual support groups with the health care delivery system? The following criteria may be indicators of how the successful program has achieved its purpose:

1. Is the group receiving referrals from all appropriate sources?
2. Is the volunteer system adequate and active enough to fulfill the needs?
3. Are members giving and receiving support on a regular basis?
4. Is the atmosphere of emotional support present?
5. Is this group dynamic and fluid in that the older members can help the newer members achieve their own level of improvement? Do some members no longer need the group, physically and emotionally?
6. Is the group able to retain members and recruit new members?

The purpose of and need for self-help and mutual support groups is clear. However, their function in the whole health picture needs to be clarified: they do not replace physicians, therapists, and other skilled professionals. Rather, they are an extension of the physical and mental support needed and often the only venue of continuing care available. That clients choose to participate in a mutual support group is not an indication of failure on the health care provider's or caretaker's services; it is merely the recognition that they need more help and support from the group and its participants than they are presently receiving from the health care delivery system.

SUMMARY

People need to take more responsibility for self-care; mutual support groups can provide the tools, not only for survival, but for enriching their lives. Furthermore, these groups are one of the keys to the survival of the health care delivery system now and in the future. Both the groups and the professionals involved must recognize the necessity and benefits of partnerships and of one anothers' roles. Without this cooperation it is the client who suffers from the lack of cooperation of these two factions. If the client has a successful experience in a mutual support group, as I have, outcomes are generally more positive. Although I was a community health nurse, an RN with my master's degree in health care administration, and working in the field, I was still reluctant to attend a support group. I had no idea of the value they would have for me. I am thankful that my providers recognized the need for integrating mutual support groups into my total rehabilitation program. Hopefully, through mutual cooperation, experiences such as mine will be the standard of care for all clients who can benefit from such programs.

REFERENCES

Mutual Help Groups: A Guide for Mental Health Workers. US Dept. of Health and Human Services Publication Number ADM. 80-646, National Institute of Mental Health, Rockville, Md, 1980.

Organizing a Successful Amputee Support Group: A Start-up Guide. Amputee Coalition of America, Rosemont, Illinois, 1994.

The Surgeon General's Workshop on Self-Help and Public Health. US Dept. of HHS Publication No. 224-250-88-1, Public Health Service, Health Resources and Services Administration, and Bureau of Maternal and Child Health and Resource Department, Rockville, MD, 1987.

Chapter 39

Acquired Immunodeficiency Syndrome and Social Dis-ease

JO ANNE BENNETT

The social construct of diseases have influenced how they are "treated" by society. Over the years diseases carried with them the stigmas of myths, prejudices, and values. Existing beliefs affected national policies hindering expedient research on treatments and cures. Nurses, a part of the larger society, also have their mythology which affects caregiving. Jo Anne Bennett describes the AIDs pandemic as today's social *dis-ease*. Dr. Bennett suggests that responses to people with AIDS include blaming and stereotyping and is tied in with attitudes about sexual diversity and addictions. These stigmas influence advocacy for people with AIDS and research directions among nurses. She proposes a holistic focus by placing AIDS in a larger social context which broadens the potential scope of prevention efforts.

What can be known of caring . . . is essential knowledge for practice . . . [including] the unique perspective of particular situations.[1(p153)]

Social responses to any specific disease, and to disease in general, reflect the nature of society and are shaped by political and economic realities. Responses can be analyzed on many levels: the organized responses of governments, scientific communities, service institutions, and professional groups as well as the individual and aggregate social treatment of infected persons. Nursing and nurses are not separate from the larger society or immune from its myths, prejudices, and values. At the same time, nursing has its own mythology, ethical code, and traditions of service and compassion. Understanding these social contexts, both within and outside the profession, is important to understanding the nature of caring and the caregiving relationship in nursing.

In the voluminous literature on acquired immunodeficiency syndrome (AIDS) since 1981, there has been considerable attention to nurses' (and other health care workers') attitudes about people with AIDS (PWAs) and

From *Holistic Nursing Practice* 10(1):77–89, 1995. Reprinted by permission of Aspen Publishers, Inc.

caring for them. There has also been substantial discussion about the social construction of disease in general[2,3] and of AIDS in particular.[4,5] Researchers and other observers have suggested that both public and individual professional responses to AIDS and people affected by human immunodeficiency virus (HIV) are related to and influenced by negative judgments about certain groups, behaviors, and/or life styles.

▰FRAMING AIDS: THE SOCIAL CONSTRUCTION OF A LATE-20TH CENTURY PANDEMIC

The US AIDS epidemic has challenged American security in scientific progress and disturbed the collective perception of society's capacity to meet public health threats. In some ways, this challenge has almost catapulted us back to the pre–antibiotic era's sense of vulnerability. Responses also demonstrate that our scientific literacy is less than we might expect (or take for granted) in the midst of the 1990s' high-technology standard of living.

The AIDS epidemic arrived during a time of intense cultural transformation and diversification, which continues to challenge America's self-perception as a melting pot with a prospering economy able to support its can-do philosophy and status as a global economic and political leader. Moreover, the pandemic's very etiology lies in the sociocultural dynamics of the mid-20th century world: intense urbanization in Africa, unprecedented intercontinental mobility by people from diverse social strata for both business and pleasure, and both local and global revolutions in sexual behavior reflected in changing marriage and fertility patterns, more explicit sex in diverse entertainment media, younger age at first coitus, and more sexual partners. Indeed, HIV infection is only one of at least two dozen sexually transmitted diseases (STDs) that exhibited an epidemic rise in incidence in the United States from the 1970s through the 1980s.

As a new disease about which information has evolved rapidly, AIDS can be daunting to the nurse who is trying to keep up with the headlines. Today's truth may be tomorrow's half-truth. It is easy to feel unsure about one's knowledge base and competence and, with so much media emphasis on AIDS' uniqueness, to wonder how well basic education and previous experience have prepared one for AIDS care.

Bean and colleagues[6] suggested that AIDS-related social behavior (ie, responses to AIDS and PWAs) reflects a complex of beliefs, attitudes, and values surrounding the disease, its causes, symptoms, associated illnesses, treatments, preventive measures, and those affected. They suggested that the complexity of this AIDS attitude system and the overall accuracy of beliefs within it will be greater for those who are more involved with the disease: patients, their families and friends, professional and nonprofessional care providers, health care policymakers, researchers, community leaders, and government officials. They posited that avoidance behavior, including patterns of stigma, reflects fear of and discomfort in associating with AIDS-involved people and that this anxiety-induced social behavior represents an attempt to execute health-protective behavior.

Conceptions of Disease Causality

Health risk assessments often reflect counterintuitive "gut feelings" about contagion that run along a continuum from metaphoric to magical thinking, the latter of which holds that positive and negative physical, psychologic, or moral qualities can be transferred from person to person through direct or indirect contact.[6-9] Illogical and superstitious though it may be, some degree of adherence to a "magical law of contagion"[7] is ubiquitous, although unconscious. This type of thinking is reminiscent of disease conceptions that predated 19th century bacteriology,[10] yet its focus on life style and spiritual energy also reflects modern, so-called New Age, perspectives.

Brandt[4] noted that AIDS arrived during an era of decline in the authority of experts. He called the disasters with the Challenger space shuttle and at the Three Mile Island and Chernobyl nuclear plants building blocks of distrust in both official reassurances and scientific authorities. Thus it may not be surprising to find that even nurses and physicians in a 25-state sample[11] lacked trust in AIDS experts' estimates of occupational HIV infection risk: Only 36% agreed that these estimates were "about right," 44% indicated that they thought they were too low, and 19% said that they had no idea how accurate they might be. These findings may be an example of what Bean and colleagues[6] have called AIDS social paranoia: distrust in authority, belief in conspiracies, and reliance on folk beliefs about prevention and treatment instead of the recommendations of scientists and the medical establishment.

Such distrust can only be augmented by news stories about researchers not collaborating or misappropriating one another's specimens, government scientists' colluding with drug companies for personal profit, and findings unearthed in congressional hearings and by presidential commissions of diverse inadequacies in the government's own research efforts. Acute mistrust, according to Dalton, frequently manifests itself as resistance to recommendations for prevention, or "buying time until we are sure we are safe."[12(p212)] An example among health care professionals is the use of irrational rituals along with, or instead of, reliable precautions against transmission. Ritual actions can carry both psychologic and social meaning: Some are individual and group attempts to allay anxieties provoked by encounters with human suffering; others are general expectations prescribed by social and cultural dynamics rather than precautions that are relevant to the health-specific context of caregiving or infection control.

Chapman[9] distinguished between irrational and nonrational ritual practices and suggested that rituals can, to some extent, be simultaneously nonrational and rational. The rationale for infection control procedures is technical: breaking a (putative or demonstrated) chain of infection. The nonrational aspect reflects cultural values: Action and purpose are linked by beliefs and affect, with or without a technical relationship. For example, like the concealment rituals surrounding death in a hospital, isolation measures can also serve to conceal and thus to protect the unaffected from exposure to more than just contagion.[9] Specialized AIDS-dedicated units or residential facilities can also serve this function.

Who Gets AIDS and Why

In Africa, AIDS is a disease of the majority,[13] but the mounting number of PWAs in the United States has remained invisible to the majority except in headlines. Despite a changing epidemiologic profile, the media continue to herald the higher risk among injecting drug users and men who have sex with men, thus emphasizing categorization and marking these people (and their lives) as different. People belonging to these groups are seen as sources of contagion not by way of activities in which all people participate but simply because they are in these groups, whose integral overlap with the community at large is somehow disregarded.

As recently as the fall of 1994, extensive national press coverage of a survey[14] of sexual behavior focused on how conservative "most" Americans' sexual behavior is and emphasized that people tend to choose partners from within a relatively narrow geographic and social network. The stated implication was thus how unlikely it is for the majority to be exposed to HIV. (What was ignored was how mobile people are across networks over time, the many bridges between apparently discrete reservoirs of infection, and the marked differences between older, middle-age, and young adult cohorts.) Likewise, the heretical view remains popular that so-called heterosexual AIDS is rare, if not a myth altogether,[15] despite the growing incidence of sexual transmission between heterosexuals in the United States and the predominance of this transmission category in AIDS incidence worldwide.[16]

Altman[5] attributed the "hysteria around AIDS" in the United States to irrational fears of "otherness" and sexuality. Defining serious illness as afflicting only others and assigning specific character flaws to affected individuals are common ways to distance oneself from death.[17] With AIDS, however, it has been more common to blame the groups to which most people with AIDS belong.[18] Watney suggested, "The presence of AIDS in these groups is generally perceived not as accidental but as a symbolic extension of some imagined inner essence of being."[19(p8)] The sense of otherness "makes it possible to cut funding for AIDS research because only *they* get the disease" and we don't realize *they* are us.[20] Yet "the only way civilization prospers and progresses is through commonality."[20(p11)]

■ RESPONSES TO PWAS

Herek and Glunt identified AIDS-related stigma as "a socially constructed reaction to a lethal illness most prevalent among groups that already were targets of prejudice."[18(p886)] They suggested that it interacts with preexisting stigma in complex ways. As a disease of marginal groups (groups viewed as different from the norm, and therefore on the periphery of a hypothetical societal center, on the basis of their identities, associations, experiences, or environments[21] who already are targets of prejudice), AIDS provides "a convenient hook on which to hang hostility toward outgroups."[18(p889)] Dalton described how racial prejudice and homophobia can activate or reinforce each other: "Someone who is viewed as an 'other' along one dimension will more easily be viewed as an 'other' along a second and third. . . . Even the originator of the hostility may not know where one motivation ends and the other begins."[12(p214)] Indeed, racism and homophobia correlate empirically.[22]

It has frequently been suggested that AIDS prevalence in marginal groups (gay men, drug users, non-drug-using Black and Hispanic women and children, and the poor) and its relative absence in the larger middle-class, white population influenced the US government response to the epidemic. Once AIDS was identified as a "gay disease," the political response to it was characterized as a response to the gay community,[5(p191)] leading some to suggest that political deference or even catering to the gay community led to AIDS policy detrimental to public welfare (eg, lack of mandatory testing or quarantine) and others to maintain that the government's slow response and limited funding of research, service, and prevention programs were due not merely to neglect but also to deliberate disregard for those affected (ie, an unstated official assessment that marginal groups, already socially dispossessed, are disposable).

Certainly there is a stark contrast between the American government's response and that of almost every other industrialized nation.[23] The different responses (and responsiveness) reflect differences among nations and across cultures in tolerance, differences in health care and social service systems, and differing emphases on public health and prevention. Indeed, AIDS has highlighted many problems in the US health care system.

Blaming

The placing of blame has been a pervasive theme in popular discourse on AIDS.[17] There is a subtle distinction between assigning responsibility for actions and assigning liability and blame for outcome, however. Blaming emphasizes why, not how. Blaming carries a connotation that the affected person deserves the problem and is somehow not so deserving of relief or help with problem solving. The problem and its related suffering are seen as just punishment for deviance rather than part of the human condition. This view was even an argument put forth against disease prevention efforts in earlier times.[3] The idea that disease should be used to discourage selected risky behaviors persists.[3] Thus explanations of disease often become means to define appropriate and moral behavior or to justify outcasting and other social policies.[17]

Before concepts of contagion were understood, disease was viewed as a result of both original sin and transgressions against nature (ie, as punishment). Those who became ill were viewed as predisposed to illness "because of certain unholy habits."[5(p775)] Some see AIDS "in a purely moral light . . . [as a] disease that occurs among those who violate the moral order . . . a fateful link between social deviance and the morally correct."[17(p62)] Children with AIDS and adults infected through transfusions have frequently been called innocent victims, implying that others may be deserving of illness and suffering.

Inferences about another and attributions of the cause of a need or problem have been shown to influence a potential helper's perception of the person and the inclination to help.[24,25] Considering a problem as being within a needy person's control (ie, blaming the victim) may elicit disgust instead of sympathy. Disgust, in turn, can distance potential helpers, including health care professionals, from the person in need. Indeed, researchers have found that nurses and physicians differentially attribute responsibility for illness according to diagnoses, disease etiology, and various patient characteristics, including sexual orientation, compliance with medical regimens, risk-taking and/or health-seeking behavior, and presumptions about patients' promiscuity.[26] With devaluation of a person in need, there is unsympathetic interpretation of that person's distress.

Blaming both creates and reflects psychologic and social boundaries, including class stereotypes and political biases.[17] Marginal social groups often carry the burden of blame for disease and other social ills. Throughout history, disease has been attributed to particular racial and/or national groups, social stereotypes, life styles, immoral behavior, and sources of power and status. Assignment of responsibility for actions, however, can be without apparent censure and blame (ie, without suggesting that the person deserves to be ill or to suffer or does not deserve care).[27,28]

Stereotyping

Labels tend to evoke stereotypical categories, whereas relationships depend on people perceiving each other's humanity and individual uniqueness.[29] Stereotypes can lead to misperceptions, which in turn may be accepted as evidence of the stereotype,[30] compounding the problem. With AIDS, for example, selective attention to media messages may occur such that only negative news reports are remembered and counteractive messages are discounted because information sources are not trusted.[6] Sensational, sometimes outright erroneous, presentations of the facts in reports about AIDS can further distort perceptions. Even the nursing and medical literature, while clearly specifying that sexual orientation per se is not the source or basis of differential risk (risk factor), often refers to homosexual and heterosexual intercourse as distinct modes of transmission instead of pointing to population subgroups as different reservoirs of infection. Thus the stereotype of an essential difference between affected and unaffected people is reinforced instead of the basic commonality that underlies the viral spread. Meanwhile, the basis for differential risk is confused.

Herek[31] highlighted the social context in which various forms of prejudice, including homophobia, develop. He pointed out that social categories can be so deeply ingrained in one's understandings of the world that they appear to be natural rather than products of social interaction. Perhaps more important, they are functional. They maintain self-esteem, reduce anxiety, secure social support, and guide behavior relative to a categorized object: We approach, favor, praise, cherish, and protect those in a favorable class; we avoid, disfavor, blame, neglect, and even harm those in unfavorable classes.[30] In turn, these courses of action become problem-solving strategies in relevant situations:

> By assigning negative values to marginalized persons and groups, those at the [conceptual center of a homogeneous majority] reinforce their sense of belonging and belief in a singular, moral " reality." The dynamics of scapegoating has a long history in which selected "victims" who symbolically embody the sins of the majority are driven out of the societal center.[21(p27)]

Researchers have found that homophobia is part of a larger belief system that supports cultural stereotypes about homosexual behavior.[31,32] Weinberg[33] suggested that homophobia is a form of acute conventionality. He posited that the most important unstated (perhaps unconscious) assumption shared by people who shun homosexuals is that "something is frighteningly wrong when a human being diverges from the standardized pattern of existence. . . . Ultimately it condemns because of difference."[33(p21)]

Homophobic affect may be more relevant than beliefs and intolerance. Interacting with homosexual persons could produce anxiety and lead to social distancing or avoidance altogether. Homophobia may have less impact overall on these attitudes than knowledge and attitudes about sex, however, which accounts for substantial variance in homophobia.[27]

▬ATTITUDES ABOUT SEX

The likes and dislikes implied by attitudes are not determined by systematic thinking and evaluation of relevant information.[30] Attitudes, however, predispose to actions and/or ways of acting. The Institute of Medicine Committee on a National Strategy for AIDS noted how AIDS has magnified previous perceptions of the dangers of sexual freedom and anonymous sex.[34] Confronting the potential negative implications of such perspectives, DeMayo[35] emphasized the importance of making HIV prevention programs sex positive and urged health educators to take care not to convey the message that sex, rather than a virus, is the problem.

Attitudes provide a heuristic for making sense of the social world.[30] Sexual attitudes express values important to one's self-concept and tend to be consistent with a larger ideology supported by important reference groups. Sexual values usually reflect cultural, religious, and class norms. As such, people with different values are perceived not only to hold a different opinion or viewpoint but also somehow to represent a fundamentally different social norm, perhaps even to threaten a community's moral fabric. Sexual activity is not so morally laden in all cultures, however. Neither sexual taboos nor the bases underlying them are universal.

Sexual expression is related to social networks and factors such as gender, education, class, occupation, marital status, religion, and ethnicity. The interpersonal meanings attached to sexual interaction range from the emotional to the ritual, including reproduction, recreation, dominance, finance, libido, taboos, and duty. Individual behavior (eg, practices, frequency, number of partners, and places of partner contact), however, also reflects more personal attitudes, such as prudishness, sexual shyness, fear of intimacy, erotophobia, and permissiveness.[36]

Strongly held beliefs and values about sex are almost always present, and attitudes about sexual behavior are not readily dissolved by scientific evidence and rational thinking.[37] Perceptions of people with different sexual values are colored by emotional knowledge. When confronted by personal and interpersonal value conflicts, a nurse may develop a protective shell, choosing detachment and avoidance as ways to avoid his or her own and others' distress.[29] Thus attitudes about sex, sexuality, and sexual behavior may influence nurses' orientation to health care situations involving sexual function or dysfunction and may impede communication about related concerns. Indeed, in one study nurses' practice in situations related to sexual function correlated with their attitudes about sex, regardless of how they prioritized the importance of attending to sexual concerns.[38] Attitudes about sex also influence perceptions of, and attitudes toward, victims of sexual assault[24] and PWAs[27]: Conservative attitudes correlate with judging the victim or patient to be more responsible for what happened to him or her.

▬STDS

Along with differences in psychological investments in sexual behavior, the social and psychologic associations with STDs differ across cultures. Medical historians suggest that assessments of most STDs in the 20th century have rested on the simplistic view that the problem would be solved if individuals conducted their lives more responsibily.[3] Ross[39] posited that the meaning an STD has for a patient and, to a lesser extent, for a health care professional will affect patients' adherence to treatment and risk reduction recommendations and also psychologic sequelae of the STD experience. Clearly, it also affects approaches to prevention and related health education.

Ross[39] proposed five possible attributions for STDs, ranking them according to blame:

1. STDs are a deserved outcome of indiscriminate sexual behavior and punishment for sexual sins.
2. STDs are a consequence of individual inadequacy that leads to sexually indiscriminate behavior.
3. STDs are a consequence of a breakdown in traditional social values and rapid social change.
4. STDs are the result of an individual coming into intimate contact with a virulent pathogen.
5. STDs are a sign of being sexually active and are a matter of pride.

He suggested that concomitant with this hierarchy of blame is a similar hierarchy of responsibility and that health care professionals' approach to patients reflects an attitudinal continuum—from seeing gonococci as "God's little helpers" through approaching STDs as just a part of infectious disease management—that corresponds to the five attributions.

▬ATTITUDES ABOUT DRUG USE AND CHEMICAL DEPENDENCY

Substance abuse continues to be one of the most devastating problems faced by our society. Attitudes about both drug use and addiction differ sharply across cultures, as evidenced by differences in tolerance, the relative investment in health and social services for this population, and approaches to addiction treatment and also to AIDS prevention programs that target those who use drugs. Underlying these variations are essentially dichotomous perspectives on drug use, dependency, and its consequences: the criminal and health perspectives.

Criminalization generates "no tolerance" approaches, further marginalizes those who are most seriously affected, and potentially aggravates less severe problems, directing resources toward supply and related transactions rather than treating demand (ie, dependency itself) and its antecedents and consequences. These approaches limit (or preclude) AIDS prevention programs that support, much less promote, safer drug use. In such a social climate, a user's involvement in treatment is often intertwined with involvement in the legal and penal systems, and relationships with health care providers may reflect reciprocal mistrust rather than therapeutic alliance. Indeed, attitudes about addiction, along with misunderstanding of the physiology involved, often obstruct the most basic caregiving goal: pain relief.[40]

Sociopolitical and economic characteristics of American society have contributed to the ongoing epidemic of substance abuse.[41,42] Telashek et al[41] suggested that it is a predictable consequence of a culture that emphasizes consumerism, immediate gratification, and a pain-free, pleasurable life. They pointed out how drinking, smoking, and drug taking are supported through advertising, public policies, and ready availability. Certain aspects of substance abuse are common across population groups (ethnic minorities, adolescents, elderly, gays and lesbians, and adult children of the addicted), but other aspects are specific.

Prevention and treatment programs must be based on an understanding of cultural influences. These influences are not static, however, and should not be used to stereotype. Thus, rather than focusing on a group identity or label, assessment should examine related behavior. For example, the incidence of problem drinking is lower in cultures with high alcohol consumption, where drinking is introduced as part of daily life at a young age in the context of eating.[41] In contrast, when alcohol is emphasized for relaxation and stress relief, it is associated with drunkenness and high-risk behavior. Excessive drinking is also associated with tight social controls over sexual behavior and marital roles.

Drug users may be seen as more marginal than other PWAs, there being stereotypical perceptions of their lives. Their social and psychologic complexity and diversity as individuals and as a group are often overlooked, and their links to conventional social networks may not be appreciated.[42] Whereas some people may view drug users as even more unlike themselves than middle-class gay men, to others the problems associated with drug use and dependency may seem more threatening to their community and family than AIDS. This has been suggested as a reason for resistance to safer drug use initiatives in urban Black and Hispanic communities, where other drug-related problems may seem more immediately tangible, and more threatening, than AIDS.[12,43]

■RISK TAKING AND RISK PERCEPTION

Risk discourse is layered with ethical, political, and moral subtexts whose ideologic rhetoric extends beyond quantitative estimates. Implications for public and personal health are often ambiguous.[44,45]

In many social and professional situations, we applaud risk taking. We recognize it as an essential leadership characteristic. We admire and reward those who risk personal safety in sports competition even though there is no benefit to be accrued beyond winning a competition or furthering one's personal best.

In most situations, the threshold of acceptable-unacceptable risk is not clearly demarcated. Risk acceptability relates to the value or utility that individuals attach to the various costs and benefits involved in an action. The higher the potential benefits and the lower the potential costs, the more acceptable the risk. The perception of benefit and cost, however, depends on the cultural context. An action may entail potential long- or short-term adverse effects on values other than life and health. Actions thus have multiple potentials that are not easily quantified. Psychologic, social, institutional, and cultural processes can interact in ways that may amplify or attenuate responses to perceived risks.[46]

An individual's intention vis-à-vis an action generally reflects an emphasis on goal attainment, not hazard avoidance. When harm potential is considered, behavior is influenced more by the acceptability of perceived risks than by risk appraisal, which is related to both the magnitude and the likelihood of an outcome. Perception is influenced by characteristics of a hazard. We tend to conflate magnitude and probability so that low, even negligible, risk is overshadowed by immense consequences (such as mortality). We also tend to perceive risks to be greater than they actually are when the consequence is regarded as uncontrollable and inevitable. Familiar risks are accepted more readily (ie, with less outrage) than the less familiar, detectable risks are accepted better than undetectable risks, risks that are better understood by science are accepted more than those that are not, and risks that seem fairly distributed are also more easily accepted.[46]

To reduce our perception of risk and increase our sense of control, we use various forms of denial. Victim blaming, as discussed above, is an example. Ironically, it serves to heighten individuals' actual risk. At the same time, by making it seem more remote, it diminishes its acceptability and relieves the community's sense of responsibility to care for those affected, further magnifying the catastrophe associated with the illness experience.

Clustering PWAs on specific units can also magnify unfamiliarity, implying that specialized nursing knowledge or skills are required, which can foster nurses' feelings of incompetence or fear of the unknown.[26,45] It may be more useful to emphasize how similar AIDS is to other diseases and the potential benefits of basic nursing interventions.[27,47,48]

IMPLICATIONS FOR NURSING

The current extent and expected reach of the AIDS epidemic, along with the continued rising epidemics of other STDs and morbid substance use, presage a soaring demand for nursing resources, both person power and skills. To meet emerging demands for care, we must be able to "reach out in solidarity with diverse communities to meet the health needs of the most vulnerable."[21(p33)] To do so, we must recognize how the fragmenting and isolating effects of stigma, secrecy, and mistrust are intertwined with barriers to health-promoting and care-seeking behavior. We need to recognize how health transitions can be openings for further marginalization, magnifying the potential for negative outcomes.[21]

Advocacy for Health

Access is only part of the struggle. Many lack not only economic resources but also the respect and social and political legitimacy to make decisions about their health and other basic needs.[21] Nurses can support their interests by working to change the practices and images of health care institutions that deter people from using available services. This requires efforts to encourage community involvement and to influence providers to accept and welcome community-based initiatives to redesign delivery structures.

Controlling the HIV epidemic requires clinicians' attention to discussing sex-related health risks at length, repeatedly, in explicit detail, and with people who may themselves be uncomfortable with the topic in general, with specific aspects of it, or with discussing their own sexuality and sexual behavior. If nurses are to contribute effectively, we must be able to initiate frank, nonjudgmental discussions of sexual topics with different types of people (peers and people older and younger than ourselves, people of the opposite sex, people of different sexual orientation and experience, etc). A recent survey of 1520 nurses in 25 states, however, found that less than 5% ask new patients about the number of recent sexual partners compared with more than 70% who inquire about cigarette smoking.[11]

Prevention programs must incorporate values of the intended audience, not sell new values. Presumed differences in values may not, in fact, be real. Common values need to be recognized and presented so that audiences (individuals and groups) can identify with them. Too often, values are used to divide audiences. Devaluation of people's choices and preferences can close off communication. Conversely, victim blaming precludes client-centered approaches to problem solving. Both force clients to tailor their needs to the framework of service providers (ie, to adapt themselves to available services). By contrast, health problems can be defined from potential clients' viewpoint(s), and health messages can be framed within their value systems. For example, safe-sex messages about condom use have been framed by family values and even so-called macho themes that are often used as arguments against safe-sex teaching.

Nurses can help raise public awareness about the social complexities underlying substance use and abuse, support public policies designed to modify attitudes and practices (including harm reduction intervention strategies), make drug use assessment a routine part of health screening and history taking, identify codependency, and develop more aggressive outreach, particularly to new drug users and youth at high risk.

Research

Nurses' attitudes about AIDS and caring for PWAs have been the most frequent focus of AIDS-related nursing research. Empirical investigations have focused on individual nurses, whereas attitudes and behavior both emerge in the reality of social situations. Actions, including the expression of attitudes, result from both personal predispositions and situational factors. Thus it might be more advantageous to explore attitudinal variations within social contexts, the ways in which caring (and perhaps not so caring) communities evolve, and the influence of organizational culture on nurse–patient relationships and interactions in diverse health care settings, including the home and community.[27]

By incorporating the concept of marginalization as basic to empirical and theoretical activities, nurses' knowledge development can be better grounded and more meaningful to diverse groups and may more accurately explicate the complex linkages between vulnerability and health. We should also ask whether AIDS care education that emphasizes sensitivity and consciousness raising about groups at higher risk perpetuates misperceptions or corrects myths and improves knowledge about sexual diversity and addictions.

A holistic focus places a disease, its etiology, and its course in a larger social context. It directs us to review the HIV pandemic's emergence and progression not only as a bioecologic phenomenon but also as a consequence of broad (global and local) social changes. This view, in turn, can broaden the potential scope of prevention efforts. It challenges us to reconsider how risk appraisal and public policy debates are framed, for it is the framework that shapes, perhaps even confines, community and professional responses to the disease and to those affected.

■ REFERENCES

1. Boykin A, Schoenhofer S. Caring in nursing: Analysis of extant theory. *Nurs Sci Q.* 1990;3:149–161.
2. Rosenberg CE. The definition and control of disease—An introduction. *Soc Res.* 1988;55:327–330.

3. Brandt AM. *No Magic Bullet: A Social History of Veneral Disease in the United States since 1880.* New York, NY: Oxford University Press; 1987.
4. Brandt AM. AIDS and metaphor: Toward the social meaning of epidemic disease. *Soc Res.* 1988;55:413–492.
5. Altman D. *AIDS in the Mind of America.* New York, NY: Anchor; 1986.
6. Bean J, Keller L, Newburg C, Brown M. Methods for the reduction of AIDS social anxiety and social stigma. *AIDS Educ Prev.* 1989;1:194–221.
7. Rozin P, Nemeroff C, Markwith M. Magical contagion beliefs and fear of AIDS. *J Appl Soc Psychol.* 1992;22:1081–1092.
8. Nemeroff CJ, Brinkman A, Woodward C. Magical contagion and AIDS risk perception in a college population. *AIDs Educ Prev.* 1994;6:249–265.
9. Chapman GE. Ritual and rational action in hospitals. *J Adv Nurs.* 1983;8:13–20.
10. Kleinman LC. To end an epidemic: Lessons from the history of diphtheria. *N Engl J Med.* 1992;326:773–777.
11. Colombotos J, Messeri P, Burgunder M, Elinson J, Gemson H, Hymes M. *Physicians, Nurses, and AIDS: Preliminary Findings from a National Study.* New York NY: Columbia University of School of Public Health, Division of Sociomedical Sciences; 1991.
12. Dalton HL. AIDS in blackface. *Daedalus.* 1989;118:205–227.
13. Simpson MA. The malignant metaphor: A political thanatology of AIDS. In: Corless IB, Pittman-Lindeman M, eds. *AIDS: Principles, Practices and Politics.* New York, NY: Hemisphere; 1988.
14. Laumann EO, Gagnon JH, Michael RT, Michaels S. *The Social Organization of Sexuality.* Chicago, Ill.: University of Chicago Press,; 1994.
15. Centers for Disease Control and Prevention. *HIV/AIDS Surveillance Report, February 1995.* Atlanta, Ga: US Public Health Service; 1995.
16. Fumento M. *The Myth of Heterosexual AIDS.* New York, NY: Basic Books; 1989.
17. Nelkin D, Gilman SL. Placing blame for devastating disease. *Soc Res.* 1988;55:360–378.
18. Herek GM, Glunt EK. An epidemic of stigma: Public reactions to AIDS. *Am Psychol.* 1988;43:886–891.
19. Watney S. *Policing Desire: Pornography, AIDS and the Media.* Minneapolis, Minn: University of Minnesota Press; 1987.
20. Quinlan A. The rising tide of otherness. *Volunteer.* January 1995:11.
21. Hall JM, Stevens PE, Meleis AI. Marginalization: A guiding concept for valuing diversity in nursing knowledge development. *Adv Nurs Sci.* 1994;16:23–41.
22. Larsen KS, Cate R, Reed M. Anti-Black attitudes, religious orthodoxy, permissiveness, and sexual information: A study of the attitudes of heterosexuals toward homosexuality. *J Sex Res.* 1983;19:105–118.
23. Sepulveda J, Fineberg MD, Mann J, eds. *AIDS—Prevention through Education: A World View.* New York, NY: Oxford University Press; 1992.
24. Weidner G, Griffitt W. Rape: A sexual stigma. *J Pers.* 1983;51:152–166.
25. Barnett MA, Howard JA, King LA, Dino GA. Helping behavior and the transfer of empathy. *J Soc Psychol.* 1981;114:125–132.
26. Klonoff EA, Ewers D. Care of AIDS patients as a source of stress to nursing staff. *AIDS Educ Prev.* 1990;2:338–348.
27. Bennett JA. *The Effects of Knowledge and Attitudes about Sex, Empathy, and Homophobia on Nurses' Attitudes about AIDS Care: An Exploration of Orem's Concept of Nursing Agency Using Propositions from Travelbee's Theory of Interpersonal Aspects of Nursing.* New York, NY: New York University; 1992. Thesis.
28. Kelly JA, St Lawrence JS, Hood HV, Smith S, Cook DJ. Nurses' attitudes towards AIDS. *J Cont Educ Nurs.* 1988;19:78–83.
29. Travelbee J. *Interpersonal Aspects of Nursing.* 2nd ed. Philadelphia, Pa: Davis; 1971.
30. Aronson E. *The Social Animal.* 6th ed. New York, NY: Freeman; 1992.
31. Herek GM. Can functions be measured? A new perspective on the functional approach to attitudes. *Soc Psychol Q.* 1987;50:285–303.
32. Crawley DM. *Attitudes and Personal Anxiety about Homosexuality.* Ithaca, NY: Cornell University; 1983. Thesis.
33. Weinberg G. *Society and the Healthy Homosexual.* New York, NY: St Martin's; 1972.

34. Institute of Medicine Committee on a National Strategy for AIDS. *Mobilizing against AIDs.* Cambridge, Mass: National Academy of Sciences; 1986.
35. DeMayo M. The future of HIV/AIDS prevention programs: Learning from the experiences of gay men. *SIECUS Rep.* 1991;20:1.
36. Eysenck HJ. *Sex and Personality.* London, England: Abacus; 1978.
37. Lief HR. Why sex education for health practitioners? In: Green R, ed. *Human Sexuality: A Health Practitioner's Text.* Baltimore, Md: Williams & Wilkins; 1979.
38. Wilson ME, Williams HA. Oncology nurses' attitudes and behaviors related to sexuality of patients with cancer. *Oncol Nurs Forum.* 1988;15:49–53.
39. Ross W. Psychovenereology: Psychological aspects of AIDS and other sexually transmissible diseases. In: Ostrow DG, ed. *Behavioral Aspects of AIDS.* New York, NY: Plenum; 1990.
40. Friedman D. Perspectives on the medical use of drugs of abuse. *J Pain Symptom Manage.* 1990;5(suppl 1):S2–S5.
41. Telashek ML, Gerace LM, Starr KL. The substance abuse pandemic: Determinants to guide interventions. *Public Health Nurs.* 1994;11:131–139.
42. Waterston A. *Street Addicts in the Political Economy.* Philadelphia, Pa: Temple University Press; 1994.
43. Herek GM, Capitano JP. AIDS-related stigma persists in the United States. Presented at the 8th International Conference on AIDS; July 1992; Amsterdam, The Netherlands.
44. Lupton D. Risk as moral danger: The social and political functions of risk discourse in public health. *Int J Heal Serv.* 1993;3:425–435.
45. Bennett JA, DeMayo M, Saint Germain M. Caring in the time of AIDS: The importance of empathy. *Nurs Adm Q.* 1993;17:46–60.
46. Heffern MK. While the world waits. *Am J Nurs.* 1987;87:932.
47. O'Brien ME, Pheifer WG. Physical and psychosocial nursing care for patients with HIV infection. *Nurs Clin North Am.* 1993;28:303–315.
48. Orem DE. *Nursing: Concepts of Practice.* 4th ed. St Louis, Mo: Mosby Year Book; 1991.

Chapter 40

A Nursing Model for Addressing the Health Needs of Homeless Families

ANDREA S. BERNE   CANDY DATO

DIANA J. MASON   MARGARET RAFFERTY

Homelessness in the United States continues to be a major social issue. Presently, the largest growing segment of the homeless population is women with children, once a group not seen among the homeless. The authors chronicle the conditions in which the homeless family lives and the significant health and mental health problems this group experiences. Pesznecker's Model of Poverty is used to design effective interventions of which addressing health care needs is only a part. Homeless families respond best through strategies that empower them to develop self-esteem and skills that overcome the shackles of poverty. Major changes are needed in policies that deal with homeless families. Community health nurses have a role in influencing and shaping the policies through political advocacy.

Homelessness in the United States is a major social problem, directly affecting an estimated three million persons, of whom 30 percent are families. Of these families, 85 percent are headed by single women, a disproportionate number of whom are minorities. While families were the last subgroup to join the ranks of the homeless, they are now the fastest growing segment of that population. It is projected that in the near future a majority of the United States' homeless will be single m others with children (City of New York Human Resources Administration, 1986a, 1986b; Institute of Medicine, 1988; Molnar, 1988).

▄ETIOLOGY OF FAMILY HOMELESSNESS

Homelessness is a relative condition that exists worldwide in both developed and underdeveloped countries, although it expresses itself differently in different parts of the world (Patton, 1988). It encompasses Britain's growing poor who are housed in the bread and breakfast rooms in London that have been described as the equivalent of third-world shantytowns (Clines, 1987). It includes the Etiopian refugees in the Sudan and

From *Image—Journal of Nursing Scholarship* 2(1):8–13, 1990. Reprinted by permission of Sigma Theta Tau International.

other countries where war and politics have uprooted entire communities (Smith, 1989). It can be seen in the increasing number of young adults sleeping in hostels and shelters in Denmark, Austria and Belgium (Hope & Young, 1987a; Tennison, 1983; Thomas, 1985). It is evident in the explosion of slums in the cities of developing nations such as the Philippines, Mexico and India (Busuttil, 1987). And it can be seen in the so-called hidden homeless in Hungary—the growing number of people who are doubled-up in the dwellings of friends or families who are living in decrepit housing (Hope & Young, 1987b). In 1985, the United Nations reported that 100 million people worldwide had no shelter, and it proclaimed 1987 as the International Year of Shelter for Homeless (Ramachandran, 1988).

Homelessness used to occur predominantly in third world countries where material resources were underdeveloped or scarce. Its rise in developed countries suggests a maldistribution of existing resources. Nowhere is this more evident than in the United States, where homelessness is primarily caused by the lack of affordable housing and increasing poverty.

The lack of affordable housing in the United States is the result of several factors:

- Gentrification, or a process in which low-income housing is replaced by middle-income and high-income housing.
- A freeze on the welfare shelter allowances in most states, resulting in an allowance that has not kept pace with the rising cost of renting an apartment.
- The Reagan Administration's decision to withdraw the federal government from its prior commitment to build and maintain low-income housing (Report of the Committee on Legal Problems of the Homeless, 1989; Institute of Medicine, 1988).

Since most of the homeless would not be without permanent housing if they could afford to pay the rents on the housing that is available, homelessness in the United States is largely a by-product of the increasing gap between the rich and poor. From 1980 to 1984, family income for the poorest 20 percent of the population declined by almost 8 percent, while that of the wealthiest 20 percent of families increased by almost 9 percent (United Auto Workers, 1985). The poorest three fifths of all families received only 32.7 percent of the total national income, while the wealthiest two fifths received 67.3 percent of the income; these were, respectively, the lowest and highest percentages recorded since 1947 (Bureau of the Census, 1985). The relative nature of poverty that is associated with homelessness is illustrated by data indicating that 35 percent of homeless mothers and fathers outside of New York City work, but their incomes are insufficient to pay for the rising cost of housing (Schmitt, 1988). Indeed, a recent study found that the poor are paying an increasing percentage of their income on housing—now 63 percent, as opposed to the standard of 30 percent that is deemed the "affordable" limit by the Department of Housing and Urban Development (Dionne, 1989).

▬FAMILY HOMELESSNESS AS POVERTY: A MODEL FOR NURSING

Pesznecker (1984) synthesized the literature on poverty and delineated an interactional, adaptational model of poverty (see Fig. 40-1). It postulates that one develops health-promoting or health-damaging responses to the stress of poverty, which are shaped by interactions between the individual/group and the environment—interactions that are further mediated by factors such as public policy. It presents the poor as individuals and groups who are continually faced with multiple and chronic stressors, including frustration over few employment options, inadequate and unsafe housing conditions, repeated exposure to violence and crime, inadequate child care assistance and insensitive attitudes and responses of social service and mental health agencies. The coping abilities of the poor are strained by the unpredictable and unrelenting accumulation of these stressors. Mastery may be diminished so that a sense of helplessness develops

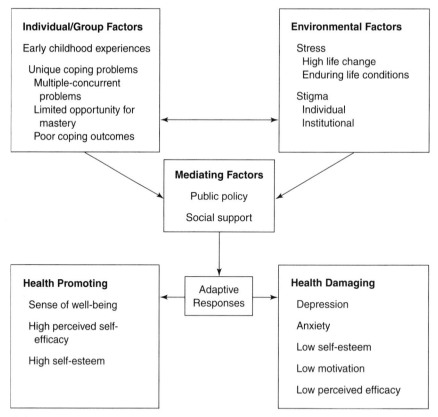

FIGURE 40-1   Adaptational model of poverty. From Betty L. Pesznecker, "The Poor: A Population at Risk," *Public Health Nursing, Vol. 1* (No. 4), December 1984, pp. 237–249. Reprinted by permission of Blackwell Scientific Publications, Inc.

with the resulting decrease in motivation as well as a sense of helplessness and hopelessness. The stigmatization of being poor in a society that measures one's worth by income only adds to the stress of poverty and makes it difficult to maintain any semblance of self-esteem or self-efficacy. Anxiety, depression and feelings of powerlessness are thus predictable concomitants of poverty.

The experience of homeless families can be described within this context. Pesznecker's (1984) model provides a basis for being particularly concerned about the children of these families and the bleak present and future they face. It incorporates the effect that the stigmas of poverty and homelessness can have on people who are often stigmatized also by their race and gender in a society that continues to contain covert and overt sexism and racism. It also provides a basis for nurses to incorporate social activism in their role as advocates and providers of care for homeless families.

■ HOMELESS CHILDREN

The research on homeless children is limited, but the data that are available suggest that homelessness is not an experience to which one can adapt positively. Wright and Weber (1987) reported that 16 percent of the homeless children have various chronic physical disorders, double the rate among patients in the general population. Asthma, anemia and malnutrition were among the most common. In the same study, many common acute pediatric problems were reported at inordinately high rates (upper respiratory infections, skin ailments, gastrointestinal problems, ear infections, eye disorders and dental problems). Data from Bellevue Hospital in New York City revealed that 50 percent of homeless children living in welfare hotels had immunization delays (Acker, Fierman & Dreyer, 1987).

Homeless infants living in welfare hotels in New York City had an infant mortality rate of 24.9 per 1000 live births in 1985. This was twice the overall city rate of 12.0/1000. Pregnant women living in welfare hotels in New York City were twice as likely to give birth to low-weight infants than were women living in the "city projects" (Chavkin, Kristal, Seabron & Guigli, 1987).

However, the effects of homelessness are even more profound on the mental health of the children. Bassuk and Rubin's (1987) study of children in Massachusetts shelters found that 47 percent of preschool children were delayed in at least one area of language, gross motor, fine motor and personal/social skills and development. One third of these children demonstrated problems in more than two areas. Almost half of the school-age children showed depression and anxiety, with the majority voicing suicidal ideation. The children were also noted to have sleep problems, shyness, withdrawal and aggression. Gewirtzman and Fodor (1987) reported that children in families left homeless after fires often exhibit these symptoms as well as isolation, disorientation, confusion, grief, psychosomatic complaints and regression. These problems are similar to those found in children of migrant workers and refugees and have been described as manifestations of posttraumatic stress disorder (PTSD) (Eth & Pynoos, 1985). PTSD is a reaction to some kind of psychological trauma and until recently was described mostly among war veterans. A psychologist in New York City reported that PTSD is the most common diagnosis among homeless children that she encounters (J. LeClair, personal communication; May 15, 1989).

Shelter life is stressful and shameful, compounding the children's problems. All school children are sensitive to dressing below peer standards, but homeless children may also face discriminatory remarks made by teachers and classmates, making them a "minority within a minority" (Gewirtzman & Foder, 1987). Poor attendance and truancy are major problems for this population. School attendance among 10-year-olds to 16-year-olds at the Martinique Hotel, the largest welfare hotel in New York City, was less than 40 percent. In one study, 43 percent of the children had failed at least one grade; 24 percent were in special education classes; 50 percent were failing (Bassuk & Rubin, 1987).

Children without parents in New York City fare worse than do homeless children with parents. Instead of being placed in individual foster homes, these children increasingly are housed in congregate shelters—dormitory-like facilities—that have recently been critically exposed and condemned in a study by the Public Health Interest Consortium of New York City (Brooklyn Health Action Committee, 1989). Unsanitary conditions, spoiled food, blatant fire and safety hazards and inadequate staffing predominate in these facilities. The "orphans" are shuffled from shelter to shelter, their emotional needs are ignored and they endure conditions that are often debilitating and sometimes life-threatening. The study reports that in one review of childhood immunizations, only 22 percent of the children were adequately immunized. Some of the children were HIV-positive and are at great risk for communicable diseases that easily spread in the congregate facilities:

> *The children in the shelters then are in profound psychological distress, and the custodial care they receive fails to lessen their pain. The harm to these children goes beyond their immediate suffering, however. It extends to their longterm emotional development. (p. 10)*

The data on homeless children suggest that predominant responses of homeless children to their experience with poverty are ones that Pesznecker categorizes as health damaging. The future for these children may be short-lived and without much hope for a better life. Longitudinal studies are needed to examine the long-term effects of a childhood experience with homelessness and the extent to which homelessness is an experience that precludes health-promoting responses to poverty.

HOMELESS MOTHERS

There is a paucity of research on the health problems of homeless mothers. They are a neglected population. The experience of one of the authors (A. B.) is that the mothers wait for health care until they are so acutely ill that they need emergency treatment. They may not seek health care for themselves since they tend to view themselves as the least important person in the household. Their schedules may also preclude attendance at clinics.

When the homeless mothers are seen, as they were in the Health Care for the Homeless Demonstration Project from June 1985 to September 1987 (Wright & Weber, 1987), it was confirmed that they suffer from most physical disorders at higher rates than do the general population. In addition to numerous chronic illnesses, the rate of tuberculosis among the homeless exceeds that of the general population by a factor of 25 to perhaps several hundred. Anecdotal reports from public health nurses in New York City suggest that AIDS is increasingly prevalent among homeless families and progresses more rapidly in these poor women. The overcrowded conditions of shelters and welfare hotels clearly impact on the health of the homeless mothers, as does inadequate diet, substandard bathing facilities and multiple chronic stressors.

It is evident that these same stressors contribute to the mental health problems of homeless mothers, although there is little research in this area as well. The research that has been done coincides with studies of poverty that repeatedly describe an increase in mental health problems—particularly anxiety and depression—with increasing poverty (Belle, 1982; Dohrenwend & Dohrenwend, 1974; Hollingshead & Redlich, 1958). Bassuk's (1986) study of 82 families in 14 Massachusetts shelters reported that the majority of the mothers had a limited number of relationships, with 43 percent reporting no or minimal support, and 24 percent seeing their children as their major emotional support. Of the 82 families, 18 were being assessed for potential child abuse. As children, one third of the mothers had suffered physical abuse, while one in every nine were victims of sexual abuse. The mothers' histories showed a significant amount of major family disruption, loss of parents, lack of work skills and residential instability (Bassuk, Rubin & Lauriat, 1986). The data suggested intergenerational aspects of family disruption and emotional difficulties. Another study estimated that 24 percent of homeless families in New York City were victims of domestic violence (Victim Services Agency, 1989).

Homeless mothers need to be distinguished from another subgroup of the homeless, the homeless mentally ill. Homeless mothers are not psychotic any more frequently than is the general population, and the etiology of their homelessness lies in poverty rather than a combination of poverty and mental illness. Bassuk's (1986) study did find 71 percent of homeless mothers had personality disorders; however, both advocates for the homeless and Bassuk herself criticized this finding as being an exaggeration of the degree of psychopathology. The diagnostic labels do serve to indicate severe functional impairment and the need for help.

One of the health-damaging responses that some of these mothers may have to coping with homelessness is substance abuse, although documenting the prevalence of the problem and whether it is antecedent to or a product of homelessness is difficult. The study of the foster children in New York City (Brooklyn Health Action Committee, 1989) identified parental drug abuse as "the single biggest underlying factor in child abuse and neglect" (p. 34) that results in children being removed from their families. Bassuk (1986) found 10 percent of the mothers to be substance abusers, while New York City public health nurses have estimated that between 80 percent and 90 percent of the mothers in some shelters use crack. Crack has intensified the problem of drug abuse because of its high potency and rapidly addictive qualities. Crack has become a cause of homelessness in New York City, as addicts use money for the drug instead of housing. Other health and mental health problems are expanded with substance abuse, and one would suspect that some of the character disorder problems seen in Bassuk's study were drug related.

As with homeless children, the data suggest that homelessness is a correlate of poverty that overwhelms the physical and emotional resources of homeless mothers. Pesznecker (1984) noted that poverty involves an interplay between environmental and individual factors. The poor encounter more stressors, especially surrounding money, social isolation, stigmatization and parenting, all of which can be exacerbated by homelessness. Coping positively with this multiplicity of persistent stressors becomes increasingly difficult, particularly if one is repetitively unable to change them. Depression, anxiety and feelings of powerlessness readily ensue. Under Pesznecker's model, the mental health problems of homeless mothers are most appropriately viewed as health-damaging responses to harsh environmental conditions that breed demoralization, hopelessness and despair. The model also suggests points of intervention that can foster health-promoting responses to homelessness.

▬HEALTH CARE SERVICES FOR HOMELESS FAMILIES

Access to health care has been a major problem for homeless families (Institute of Medicine, 1988). For example, a survey of sheltered children in Seattle revealed that 59 percent of the children had no regular care provider. The same group used emergency rooms at a rate of two to three times the rate of the general pediatric population in the United States (Miller & Lin, 1988). Although substance abuse appears to be a growing problem among homeless mothers, there is a paucity of drug treatment programs in the United States, particularly those that provide long-term treatment with a family focus.

Three traditional approaches that have been used to provide health care services to homeless families are the traditional out-patient department (OPD) or clinics, onsite services and comprehensive outreach.

The Clinics

Ambulatory care for the poor is generally delivered in "clinics." While funding from the national government and a nationwide grant from a private foundation have resulted in some outreach services to homeless families, most continue to lack access to anything except emergency room care. This has resulted in a woeful lack of prenatal care for homeless women who then present at the emergency room in labor and are at greater risk for maternal and infant morbidity and mortality (Chavkin et al., 1987).

Even homeless people who do have access to routine health care services often have difficulty negotiating the system. Families are usually sheltered outside their neighborhood of origin so that they are unfamiliar with and apprehensive about new health care providers. For families that are moved multiple times, it is difficult, if not impossible, to establish a stable relationship with a primary provider. Many hospital clinics have long waits for appointments, lack continuity of care and often are understaffed. There have been many reports of families with "hotel addresses" being treated poorly. The clinic staff may blame the homeless for lack of immunizations and records and missed appointments, labeling them "noncompliant." In addition, families often do not keep appointments because of fear of being reported to the Child Welfare Bureau for neglect and/or abuse related to being homeless. For these reasons, the clinic system increases the stressors and stigma with which homeless families must cope and fosters health-damaging responses such as anxiety, low self-esteem and low motivation.

On-Site Services

In some settings, visiting health teams have set up shop. The goal of many of these projects is to mainstream the families into existing clinics. While this is conceptually pleasing and congruent with the goal of establishing coordinated comprehensive care for all, this approach has limitations. The efforts of two or three health providers on site are inadequate to offset the stress and stigma of this extreme level of poverty. On-site providers have become frustrated by some of the same problems that the families are up against with the system as it presently exists, as they try to refer the families to existing services. There are transportation problems, delays in getting appointments and inadequate care. "Homeless providers" fall victim to the same discrimination that the homeless themselves face. The level of effort is inadequate to make a significant difference, but it is often used by politicians to demonstrate that they are "doing something" when, in fact, they are not. On-site services are too often a bandaid approach to the health problems of homeless families.

Comprehensive Mobile Outreach Services

One model program has enough resources to mitigate some of the effects of the poverty that underlies homelessness. The New York Children's Health Project has expanded on the concept of on-site services by providing comprehensive pediatric care with mobile medical units to children living in hotels and shelters in New York City. This project works collaboratively with the public health nurses and city social workers who are on-site at the hotels five days a week doing intake and casefinding. The public health nurses visit the families are they enter the system and take an initial health assessment. They identify children in need of immunizations, mothers in need of prenatal care and a wide variety of other acute and chronic health care needs. By knocking on doors, they attempt to cross the impenetrable boundary that exists between the family and the outside world.

Acute and chronic medical problems are diagnosed and treated by nurse practitioners and physicians. School, day care and camp forms and Women, Infants and Children certifications are frequently completed by the nurses, which has made an enormous impact on enrollment in such programs. In addition, nurses discuss routine health maintenance issues such as growth and development and nutrition as well as strategies for hotel living.

This project essentially provides "middle-class" pediatric health care to the poorest of the poor. Because of the intensive supports built into the

---

BOX 40-1   *Imagine You Are Homeless . . .*

Imagine you are a 33-year-old woman with three children. Your apartment burned down six months ago. You and your children had been living with your sister in her cramped apartment until she had another baby, and now there simply was not enough room for everyone.

You sleep in your car at night. During the day, you walk the streets with your children trying to find an apartment you can afford. Finally, you go to the department of social services to try to find shelter for the night and are told that your children may have to be placed in foster care if a place cannot be found for all of you. Knowing that the foster care system in this city is unreliable and sometimes unsafe, you agree to spend the first night in an overcrowded warehouse-type shelter, where you end up sleeping on the floor.

You and your children have no privacy here. Many of the children and adults have colds and you hear that tuberculosis has been an increasing problem among the homeless. When the opportunity arises, you agree to move into one of the single-room occupancy hotels that the city is using to house homeless families "temporarily." That temporary shelter becomes your home for 13 months.

The temporary shelter consists of one 10 by 10 ft. room. You have no kitchen, no refrigerator, no stove or cooking facilities. There is one bed for you and your three children.

You pull the mattress off the bed at night to make room for all of you to sleep and then pull the sheets off the bed in the day to eat on the floor.

You use running water to keep your baby's milk cool and you do the dishes in the tub where you bathe and store things.

There is no place for your children to play, no place to sit, no place to do homework. When they try to play in the hall, they are approached by drug dealers and sometimes even pimps.

This is what life is like for you and your children. Imagine the gradual dissipation of your own and your children's self-esteem and the isolation and depression that eventually overwhelm you. Imagine having a future without space, without privacy, without hope.

program, there is a 70 percent to 80 percent compliance rate, which is comparable to middle-class compliance. The project demonstrates the mitigating effects that public policy and social support—the mediating factors in Pesznecker's model—can have on the ongoing stressors confronting homeless families.

▬DESIGNING EFFECTIVE INTERVENTIONS FOR HOMELESS FAMILIES

This is not to suggest that comprehensive health services for the homeless are the magic tonic for the problems of homelessness. These families have an enormous number of problems of which health problems are only one small part. Indeed, nursing interventions with homeless families must reflect an understanding of the connections between health and other life and societal conditions. Pesznecker's Adaptation Model of Poverty reflects this understanding. It also is distinguished from most poverty frameworks that actually "blame the victim"—an approach that is contrary to nursing's view of health as a human-environment interaction (Mason, 1981). Her model provides direction for interventions with homeless families that address both the individuals and families and the environment and society.

Pesznecker's model suggests that homeless families can best be assisted through strategies that empower them to develop the skills and self-esteem to recognize and act on opportunities for moving out of homelessness and poverty as well as to cope more positively when those opportunities are not present. Approaching the homeless mothers and children with caring and respect is prerequisite to countering the stigmatizing attitudes that they face in other encounters with society. Additionally, homeless families need tangible and intangible support to cope with the multiple stressors in their lives. Such supports range from adequate public assistance and shelter subsidies to having a network of friends and professionals who will provide both mental and material support during times of crisis. In many communities, homeless families are removed from their community of origin and may be moved through a variety of communities during their experience with homelessness. Maintaining relationships with friends or providers becomes almost impossible. Policies that required each community to have a plan for maintaining families who need emergency housing would enable the maintenance and development of such support systems.

There has been a tendency for health care providers to view psychotherapy as a necessary intervention for homeless families, particularly given the mental health problems outlined earlier. Pesznecker's model suggests that stress management training may be an instrumental intervention. Support for this proposition is evident in two stress reduction projects with women in the United States and Canada who were on public assistance (Resnick, 1984; Tableman, Feis, Marciniak & Howard, 1985). Unfortunately, these approaches are seldom included in the health and social services that are available to homeless families.

Several model projects such as the Henry Street Settlement House in New York City and Trevor's Place in Philadelphia provide safe, clean shelter and supportive onsite services to families. These supportive services include 24-hour on-site staff, day care, after-school tutoring, job training for mothers, assistance with entitlement, and assistance with relocation. These projects have found that the mental outlook of both parents and children improves dramatically under these stable conditions. Children start attending school again; grades and behavior improve. This approach to homelessness both increases coping options and provides some stability so that referrals for self-help groups, stress reduction techniques or traditional psychotherapy services for the homeless who have major functional psychiatric disorders can have some hope for success.

Most health care services for the homeless are really secondary and tertiary prevention. True primary prevention of homelessness demands social policies that call for:

- Affordable housing
- Education and job training
- Meaningful work at an adequate wage
- Adequate levels of public assistance for families that cannot sustain themselves including adequate shelter allowances
- Accessible and adequate child care
- Access to health prevention and promotion including education about preventing pregnancy and substance abuse and coping with stress
- Drug treatment on demand

And if homelessness on an international level is considered, nursing's advocacy for primary prevention of homelessness would include efforts to promote world peace and improved means for resolving intranational and international political disputes.

Nurses can influence and shape policies that deal with homeless families through political advocacy. The American Nurses' Association has included homelessness among the issues it advocates in Washington, D.C., and many other state nurses' associations have done likewise. In New York City, the local district nurses' association adopted a position on homelessness that calls for affordable housing, adequate temporary shelter and accessible health care services.

If the nursing community is committed to primary prevention for homeless women and children, then we must participate in the debate regarding whether or not housing is a human right (Burns, 1988) and recognize the connections between the health of homeless women and children and the broader social, economic and political issues of our times. Such a perspective demands that we also understand that we truly are one world community and that these connections extend beyond geographic boundaries. We challenge the nursing community worldwide to join together in calling for conditions and policies that are health sustaining instead of health damaging, that are supportive and nurturing of families and that make housing a basic human right, without which one cannot ensure health.

■ REFERENCES

Acker, P., Fierman, A. H., & Dreyer, B. P. (1987). Health: An assessment of parameters of health-care and nutrition in homeless children (abstract). *American Journal of Diseases of Children, 141,* 388.

Bassuk, E. (1986). Homeless families: Single mothers and their children in Boston shelters. In E. Bassuk (Ed.), *The mental health needs of homeless persons: New directions for mental health services.* San Francisco: Jossey-Bass.

Bassuk, E., & Rubin, L. (1987). Homeless children: A neglected population. *American Journal of Orthopsychiatry, 57*(2), 279–286.

Bassuk, E., Rubin, L., & Lauriat, A. (1986). Characteristics of sheltered homeless families. *American Journal of Public Health, 76,* 1097–1101.

Belle, D. (1982). *Lives in stress: Women and depression.* Beverly Hills: Sage.

Brooklyn Health Action Committee. (1989). *Inexcusable harm: The effect of institutionalization on young foster children in New York City.* New York: Public Interest Health Consortium of New York City.

United Auto Workers of America. (1985). *Building America's future.* Detroit: UAW.

Bureau of the Census. (1985). *Money income and poverty status of families and persons in the United States: 1984.* Washington, DC: The U.S. Government Printing Office.

Burns, L. S. (1988). Hope for the homeless in the U.S.: Lessons from the Third World. *Cities, 5,* 33–40.

Busuttil, S. (1987). Houselessness and the training problem. *Cities, 4,* 152–158.

Chavkin, W., Kristal, A., Seabron, C., & Guigli, P. (1987). The reproductive experience of women living in hotels for the homeless in NYC. *New York State Journal of Medicine, 371,* 10–13.

City of New York Human Resources Administration. (1986a, October). *A one-day "snapshot" of homeless families at the Forbell Street Shelter and the Martinique Hotel.* New York: The Administration.

City of New York Human Resources Administration. (1986b, October). *Characteristics and housing histories of families seeking shelter from HRA.* NY: The Administration.

Clines, F. X. (1987). For poor, bed and breakfast at $34 million a year. *The New York Times,* October 22, 3.

Dionne, E. J. (1989). Poor paying more for their shelter. *The New York Times,* April 17, A18.

Dohrenwend, B. S., & Dohrenwend, B. P. (1974). *Stressful life events: Their nature and effects.* New York: John Wiley and Sons.

Eth, S., & Pynoos, R. (1985). *Post-traumatic stress disorder in children.* Washington, D.C.: American Psychiatric Association.

Gewirtzman, R., & Fodor, I. (1987). The homeless child at school: From welfare hotel to classroom. *Child Welfare, 66*(3), 237–245.

Hollingshead, A. B., & Redlich, F. C. (1958). *Social class and mental illness: A community study.* New York: John Wiley and Sons.

Hope, M., & Young, J. (1987a, August). Homelessness in Austria rising, although social programs help. *Safety Network, 4*(12), 2.

Hope, M., & Young, J. (1987b, December). Housing privatization in Hungary—Will it cause more homelessness? *Safety Network, 5*(3), 2.

Institute of Medicine. (1988). *Homelessness, health, and human needs.* Washington, D.C.: National Academy Press.

Mason, D. (1981). Perspectives on poverty. *IMAGE, 13,* 82–85.

Miller, D. S., & Lin, E. H. B. (1988). Children in sheltered homeless families: Reported health status and use of health services. *Pediatrics, 81*(5), 668–673.

Molnar, J. (1988). *Home is where the heart is: The crisis of homeless children and families in New York City.* New York: Bank Street College of Education.

Patton, C. V. (1988). *Spontaneous shelter: International perspectives and prospects.* Philadelphia: Temple University Press.

Pesznecker, B. (1984). The poor: A population at risk. *Public Health Nursing, 1*(4), 237–249.

Ramachandran, A. (1988). International Year of Shelter for the Homeless. *Cities, 5,* 144–162.

Report of the Committee on Legal Problems of the Homeless. (1989). *The Record of the Association of the Bar of the City of New York, 44*(1), 33–88.

Resnick, G. (1984). The short and long-term impact of a competency-based program for disadvantaged women. *Journal of Social Service Research, 7*(4), 37–49.

Schmitt, E. (1988, December 26). Suburbs cope with the steep rise in the homeless. *The New York Times*, 1.

Smith, S. (1989). People without land. *American Journal of Nursing, 89*(2), 208–209.

Tableman, B., Feis, C. L., Marciniak, D., & Howard, D. (1985). Stress management training for low-income women. *Prevention in Human Services, 3*(4), 71–85.

Tennison, D. C. (1983). Homeless people grow numerous in Europe, despite welfare states. *The Wall Street Journal, 80,* April 25, 1 +.

Thomas, J. (1985). The homeless of Europe: A scourge of our time. *The New York Times,* October 7.

Victim Services Agency. (1989). *The screening and diversion of battered women in the New York City emergency housing system.* New York: The Agency.

Wright, J. D., & Weber, E. (1987). *Homelessness and health.* New York: McGraw-Hill.

Chapter 41

Wellness for Elders

SUSAN NOBLE WALKER

Dramatic population shifts are occurring. People age 65 today can expect to live to age 80. In the next 30 years one in five Americans will be over the age of 65, with the fastest growing group those over age 85. One in three female children born today can expect to see her 100th birthday. How do community health nurses promote wellness among these elders? What can be done to help elders achieve their wellness potential? Susan Walker suggests a life style for wellness. This concept involves health responsibility, nutrition, exercise, stress management, interpersonal support, and self-actualization. Through a combination of being a role model for a wellness life style, educating groups of elders, and facilitating positive behavior changes, the community health nurse can promote wellness in elders.

Dr. Seuss wrote of a fanciful land called Fotta-fa-Zee where all remain healthy at the age of 103—apparently because they breathe clean air and eat nutritional foods.[1] Although such a universal state of health among centenarians goes beyond the bounds of reality, it is consistent with Dunn's concept of high level wellness, defined as "an integrated method of functioning, which is oriented toward maximizing the potential of which the individual is capable. . . . within the environment where he is functioning."[2(p447)] Dunn was the first to use the term wellness nearly two decades before the concepts of high level wellness and holistic health were popularized by Ardell,[3] Travis,[4] and others. His writing[5] reflects and acknowledges the ideas of thinkers such as Abraham Maslow, Carl Rogers, Erich Fromm, and Hans Selye, who also were concerned with how individuals might achieve their full potential within their world. Major threads running throughout the literature on high level wellness and holistic health are the integration of body, mind, and spirit, the ethic of self-responsibility and choice, and the interdependence of individual, social, and environmental wellness.

▬WHY WELLNESS?

Our society is now faced with both the opportunity and the challenge presented by escalating growth of the older population. Elders aged 65 and over constituted 12.4% of the US population in 1988, and that proportion

From *Holistic Nursing Practice* 7(1):38–45, 1992. Reprinted by permission of Aspen Publishers, Inc.

will grow to 22% by 2030. The most rapidly growing segment of elders is the group aged 85 and older, it is projected to increase from the current 9.6% of those older than 65 to 15.5% in the next 20 years.[6] Human life expectancy has increased dramatically, and people who reach the age of 65 today can expect to live into their 80s—another 16.4 years on average. However, it is likely that only 12 of those will be years of healthy life.[7] As more people live to older ages, it becomes essential to consider how the quality of life can be enhanced and maximized during those added years.

The notion that health promotion is something that goes on only in spas for the wealthy or in fitness centers for the beautiful youth is as far from reality as Dr. Seuss' fanciful land of Fotta-fa-Zee.[1] High level wellness is both a process and a goal that can be chosen by anyone of any age, in any setting, and with any condition of illness or disability. It is as relevant for the old as for the young, for the nursing home resident as for the marathon runner. Indeed, Dunn's description of high level wellness has many similarities to a definition of health proposed for older adults at the 1981 White House Conference on Aging as "the ability to live and function effectively in society, to exercise self-reliance and autonomy to the maximum extent feasible—but not necessarily total freedom from disease."[8(p4)]

Older adults themselves are concerned with achieving wellness. Contrary to popular belief, most older adults remain in their own homes rather than requiring caretaking in the homes of children or in nursing homes. The vast majority of adults older than 65 (95%) continue to live in the community, with 77% maintaining their own households (51% living with a spouse, and 26% living alone) and 18% residing with other family members or friends.[9] Only 5% of older adults live in institutions at any one time. The risk of institutionalization increases markedly with age; whereas only 2% of persons aged 65 to 74 lived in nursing homes in 1980, 23% of those 85 and older resided there.[10]

It is important to most elders to be able to function at a level that will preclude dependence on others and avoid institutionalization if possible. Whereas 80% of those older than 65 have one or more chronic illnesses, many fewer have any associated functional limitation. Only 20% of older adults living in the community in 1982 required assistance to perform either selected personal-care activities or home-management activities. Among those aged 85 and older, more than half still required no functional assistance.[10] Although older adults do express concern about health care costs and about being incapacitated and alone, they also are positively health-oriented and interested in working toward remaining well.[11] In a study conducted within the framework of Smith's four models of health[12] to determine what health meant to a sample of community-living elders, we found that they agreed most strongly with the functional or role-performance definition of health as being able to do what was important to them each day and to perform their expected roles. Second, they subscribed to the eudaimonistic definition of health as exuberant well-being or high level wellness that incorporates movement toward the individual's intrinsic potential for fulfillment and development. They were less likely to agree with the adaptive definition of health as flexible adjustment to changing environmental circumstances, and least likely to subscribe to the clinical definition of health as the absence of disease and associated symptoms.[13] They clearly preferred the positive, growth-oriented definitions of health to one oriented to the absence of disease; it is evident that elders perceive the possibility for movement toward wellness despite the presence of disease and disability. It is essential that health care providers recognize that potential as well.

TOWARD THE PROMOTION OF WELLNESS

American health care policy is not yet concerned with the achievement of high level wellness for the citizenry, but some progress has been made within the past decade toward incorporating a health promotion and illness prevention focus and extending that focus to older adults. The growing awareness of the importance of health promotion with older adults was evident in the far-reaching recommendations of the US Surgeon General's 1988 Workshop on Health Promotion and Aging,[14] the delineation of the National Health Promotion and Disease Prevention Objectives for the year 2000,[7] and the Institute of Medicine's call for health providers to look beyond curing and preventing disease to promoting health and preventing disability in the second 50 years of the human life span.[6]

Gerontological nursing has always been concerned with, indeed defined by, a focus on promoting health and function with older adults. Whereas geriatric medicine is concerned with the prevention, treatment, and cure of the diseases of the aged, gerontological nursing practice emphasizes "maximizing functional ability . . . ; promoting, maintaining and restoring health . . . ; preventing and minimizing the disabilities of acute and chronic illness; and maintaining life in dignity and comfort until death."[15(p23)] Several years after the American Nurses' Association (ANA) adopted a definition of nursing as "the diagnosis and treatment of human responses to actual or potential health problems,"[16(p9)] an ANA task force composed of gerontological nurses identified the limitations of such a definition for nurses concerned with helping their clients to achieve higher levels of health and wellness. They declared that the model provided for nursing instead should be a health model and suggested that a more appropriate definition would be, "nursing is concerned with the phenomena of human responses to illness and health."[17(p319)] They emphasized the importance of conceptualizing nursing within a health framework that views clients in terms of their strengths rather than their limitations. Hall and Allan point out that this is particularly important when working with older people, who so often are the victims of distorted evaluations of their capabilities.[17] A nursing focus on health allows us to separate individuals from their diseases and to view them as whole persons interacting with significant others and with the environment. Gerontological nurses see older people as having a potential for wellness and employ a holistic approach that looks beyond the diagnosis of chronic illness and symptomatology to seize opportunities for realizing potential and enhancing function—to help elders become the best they can be within their setting and circumstances.

▬LIFE STYLES FOR WELLNESS

In assisting elders to achieve their wellness potential, it is useful to consider the dimensions of a health-promoting life style, encompassing behavior that serves to maintain or enhance the wellness and fulfillment of the individual.[18] Those dimensions include health responsibility, nutrition, exercise, stress management, interpersonal support, and self-actualization. Each dimension will be addressed in this article. Although health-protecting behaviors that serve to reduce the elder's risk of encountering illness or injury are also relevant for wellness, they are not so central and will not be discussed here because of space limitations. Health-protective behaviors recommended for elders include obtaining influenza and pneumonia vaccinations, wearing automobile seat belts, installing smoke detectors and taking measures to prevent falls in the home, using medications safely and in an informed manner, using alcohol in moderation if at all, and not smoking; they are addressed elsewhere.[6,7,14,19] It is hoped that such a life style has been followed throughout life; if not, it is never too late for elders to initiate behavioral change and to reap the benefits of health-enhancing behavior.

Health Responsibility

Acceptance of self-responsibility for health is the cornerstone of a wellness life style. Travis and Ryan assert that self-responsibility along with love and compassion form the foundations of wellness by creating a context for all other choices,[4] and Ardell emphasizes that an active sense of accountability for one's own well-being provides the necessary motivation to pursue a health-enhancing life style.[20] Accepting responsibility for one's own health implies more than assuming an attitude; it involves becoming educated about health and health-enhancing behavior, avoiding high-risk behavior and adopting desirable behavior patterns, observing one's body and attending to its messages, and seeking advice and care from health professionals when indicated. Nurses can play a vital role in educating elders to understand the difference between normal bodily changes associated with aging and the symptoms of disease, the benefits and the process of behavior change, and how to access the health care system and interact effectively with health care providers without relinquishing decision-making power. It is essential that nurses view older adults as competent decision makers and help them to recognize the many options available to make personal choices for health enhancement.

Nutrition

The nutritional status of elders may be influenced by a complex interaction of physiological, psychological, economic, and social factors in addition to personal choices. Chronic diseases and their treatment, in particular the extensive use of prescription and over-the-counter drugs, may influence appetite, food tolerances, and nutrient absorption and utilization. Diminished acuity of smell and taste and dental problems may reduce food intake, and decreased metabolic rate and/or sedentary life style may reduce energy needs. Loneliness and untreated depression may alter eating patterns. Low income, impaired functional ability too shop or prepare food, and lack of availability of community support services may limit access to nutritious meals.

It has been recommended that primary care providers in both community and institutional settings provide nutrition assessment and counseling for older adults or refer them to qualified nutritionists or dietitians.[7,14] However, very little substantive information is available about elders' specific nutritional requirements. The widely used Recommended Dietary Allowances (RDAs) that were developed based on data collected from healthy younger people have been extrapolated to older age groups; few differences in standard nutrient and energy requirements are now identified between adults aged 23 to 50 and those older than 50, who are included in a single group encompassing a span of more than 50 years.[14,21] Although surveys of dietary intake suggest that many adults fall below the RDA for intake of energy and various nutrients, anthropometric measurements indicate that obesity as currently defined is a significant problem. These contradictions and other problems in evaluating the nutritional status of older persons are discussed and documented in the *Surgeon General's Report on Nutrition and Health*.[21] As our knowledgebase develops, we will be better able to provide clients with informed nutritional guidance.

Because both energy intake and energy expenditure appear to decline with aging, it is important that the nutrient density of the diet be high. It is recommended that dietary fat intake should not exceed 30% of calories, and saturated fat intake should provide less than 10% of calories for all adults.[7] Sufficient protein intake is necessary to maintain nitrogen balance. The year 2000 objectives target an increase in daily dietary intake of complex carbohydrate and fiber-containing foods to five or more servings of vegetables and fruits and six or more servings of grain products.[7] These foods are generally low in fat and may provide health benefits that include enhanced digestive function and reduced constipation, as well as prevention of common intestinal disorders and some cancers.

Although many elders take vitamin supplements, there is no indication that they are needed when dietary intake is adequate. Older people, particularly those not exposed to sunlight, do tend to have lowered vitamin D levels. Because of the role of vitamin D in calcium absorption, at least 10 to 15 minutes of sun exposure two or three times weekly is recommended, and supplements up to the RDA may be needed.[21] Much is yet to be learned about calcium requirements to prevent osteoporosis, but it is recommended that two to three servings of foods rich in calcium be consumed daily to achieve at least the RDA of 800 mg.[7] Older people may reduce intake of calcium-rich dairy products because of lactose intolerance; it is therefore important that they be aware of other calcium sources such as dark green vegetables, legumes, and calcium-enriched grain products.

There is considerable evidence that prevention of osteoporosis among post-menopausal women also requires hormonal replacement therapy and regular weight-bearing exercise, which together are more effective than simply increasing calcium intake.[7,22]

Exercise

Physical activity and nutrition are closely tied in achieving wellness by contributing to the maintenance of energy levels and prevention of disability among older adults. Benefits of exercise for elders include enhanced physiological, psychological, and cognitive functioning.[22,23] It has been estimated that 50% of the physiological decline observed among older people is caused by disuse rather than by disease or aging processes.[24] Through regular physical activity, older adults can maintain a high level of function throughout their eighties and perhaps beyond. Data from the 1985 National Health Interview Survey revealed that a sedentary lifestyle—physical activity less than three times per week and/or for less than 20 minutes at a time—is more common among women and that nearly half of the age group older than 65 is sedentary.[6] Fewer than one third of elders participate regularly in moderate physical activity, and fewer than 10% exercise vigorously on a routine basis.[7]

The year 2000 objectives seek to increase the proportion of adults, including elders, who engage regularly (preferably 30 minutes daily) in light to moderate physical activity equivalent to sustained walking, such as swimming, recreational cycling, dancing, gardening, and yardwork or other domestic or occupational activities.[7] The benefits of regular light to moderate physical activity, which most people can do, have only recently been acknowledged and publicized. Elders who have been sedentary should be encouraged to start slowly and gradually increase the frequency and duration of activity over a period of time to develop endurance and avoid injury. Such an approach is more likely to achieve sustained behavior change that will be incorporated into life style. The year 2000 objectives also target an increase in those who engage in vigorous physical activity to promote cardiorespiratory fitness 3 or more days per week for 20 minutes per occasion. Evaluation by a physician is recommended before an older adult increases activity to the vigorous level. Many elders are capable of engaging in vigorous exercise and may elect to participate in activities such as brisk walking, lap swimming, rowing, stair climbing, jumping rope, jogging or running, racquet sports, basketball, or cross-country skiing. The Senior Olympics provide opportunities for elders who are motivated by competition or the challenge of improving their own performance, or simply enjoying the camraderie of activity with their peers.

Stress Management

It has been suggested and supported by some research that the way in which individuals appraise and cope with the stressors encountered in life influences their state of health and well-being.[25] Three kinds of stressors that may be encountered have been classified as chronic stressors, major life events, and acute daily hassles.[26] Chronic stressors are generalized and long-lasting phenomena that are endemic in the life of an individual. Major life events are more discrete occurrences that may or may not be expected and that may have negative or positive consequences.[27] Daily hassles also are discrete events, generally negative but of lesser magnitude and duration of impact, that disturb equilibrium and require coping.[25] For older adults, major life events may include retirement, death of a spouse, birth of a grandchild, major surgery or sudden catastrophic illness, or revocation of a driver's license; daily hassles may include the loss of a pension check, being kept waiting 2 hours for a clinic appointment, damage to the garden by a neighbor's dog or children, or a plugged sink drain.

To achieve high level wellness, individuals must be able to achieve peace of mind, to recognize and manage their stress rather than letting it control and distress them. Awareness of the stressors in one's life is the first step to achieving such control. Various instruments, including the recently developed *Stokes/Gordon Stress Scale,*[28] designed to assess both major life events and daily hassles evaluated as stressful by older adults, may be useful in assisting elders to identify the sources of stress in their lives. Coping mechanisms that have been effective throughout a lifetime can be drawn on, and new management techniques to deal with stress can be learned. Although some techniques such as meditation, yoga, guided imagery, or biofeedback may be unfamiliar to the present cohort of older people, many are interested in and receptive to learning them when given an opportunity.

Interpersonal Support

Healthy interactions with others also are a component of a wellness life style. In particular, it is important to maintain relationships involving a sense of intimacy, warmth, and closeness. People need to have someone in whom they can confide and with whom they can share both personal joys and concerns. They need to experience the pleasure and sense of connectedness associated with touching and being touched. Older people may have lost their usual confidantes as a result of the death of a spouse and/or lifelong friends and of the distant relocation of children. Impaired mobility or hearing may reduce contacts and communication with supportive others. Many elders will tell you that they are not touched by others as often as they were when younger, and that they miss the contact—from the grasp of a friendly hand to the sexual embrace of a lover. It may be necessary to develop new sources of support as familiar and established ones are lost. Opportunities may be available through senior centers, church groups, community volunteer opportunities, and educational programs for older adults or for those of any age.

In addition to more intimate supportive relationships, both formal and informal social support networks are critically important to sustaining the independence of older adults.[6] The health, personal care, and social services delivered by the agencies of the aging network to community-living elders are vital to enhancing wellness by increasing the options available for personal life style choices.

Self-Actualization

Of all the dimensions of a health-promoting life style, self-actualization or spiritual growth may be most central to wellness. It involves having a sense of purpose in life, experiencing awareness of and satisfaction with self, and continuing to grow and develop as a person. The later years are a time to look back over one's life and review what one has accomplished; reminiscing is one mechanism often employed for that purpose. Those years are also a time to reevaluate and to establish new goals—albeit of a short-term nature—that will provide direction for the rest of life. As the burdens of earlier responsibilities are lightened, new horizons emerge and new opportunities present themselves. For instance, Grandma Moses began to paint. Persons seek fulfillment and actualization of their potential in unique ways. As elders of the tribe, they can share their wisdom gained through experience as part of the legacy they leave for those in younger generations who are open and willing to learn.

Elders have a potential for wellness that nursing can help them to recognize and achieve. Nurses do this by providing role models for a wellness life style, by educating older individuals and families about health-promoting options available, and by facilitating attempts at behavior change. Nurses do this through caring, empathy, and love.

■REFERENCES

1. Seuss, Dr. *You're Only Old Once.* New York, NY: Random House; 1986.
2. Dunn HL. What high-level wellness means. *Canadian Journal of Public Health.* 1959; November: 447.
3. Ardell DB. *High Level Wellness.* Emmaus, Penn: Rodale Press; 1977.
4. Travis JW, Ryan RS. *Wellness Workbook.* Berkeley, Calif: Ten-Speed Press; 1981.
5. Dunn HL. *High Level Wellness.* Arlington, Va: RW Beatty; 1961.
6. Berg RL, Cassells JS, eds. Institute of Medicine, Division of Health Promotion and Disease Prevention. *The Second Fifty Years: Promoting Health and Preventing Disability.* Washington, DC: National Academy Press; 1990.
7. US Dept of Health and Human Services. *Healthy People 2000: National Health Promotion and Disease Prevention Objectives,* DHHS publication No. (PHS) 91-50212. Washington, DC: US Government Printing Office; 1991.
8. Minkler M, Fullarton J. *Health Promotion, Health Maintenance and Disease Prevention for the Elderly.* Unpublished background paper for the 1981 White House Conference on Aging, prepared for the Office of Health Information, Health Promotion, Physical Fitness and Sports Medicine (USPHS), Washington DC; 1980.
9. US Dept of Health, Education, and Welfare. *Healthy People: The Surgeon General's Report on Health Promotion and Disease Prevention,* DHEW publication No. (PHS) 79-55071. Washington, DC: US Government Printing Office; 1979.
10. American Association of Retired Persons. *A Profile of Older Americans.* Washington, DC: AARP; 1986.
11. Maloney SK, Fallon B, Wittenberg CK. *Aging and Health Promotion: Market Research for Public Education* (Executive summary). Washington, DC: US Public Health Service, Office of Disease Prevention and Health Promotion; May 1984.
12. Smith JA. *The Idea of Health.* New York, NY: Teachers College Press; 1983.
13. Walker SN, Volkan K. *A Model of Health Conception among Older Adults.* Paper presented at the Fourth National Forum on Research in Aging, September 23–24, 1987; Lincoln, Neb.

14. US Department of Health and Human Services, Public Health Service. *Proceedings of the Surgeon General's Workshop, Health Promotion and Aging.* Washington, DC: US Government Printing Office; 1988.
15. American Nurses' Association. *Standards and Scope of Gerontological Nursing Practice.* Kansas City, Mo: ANA; 1987.
16. American Nurses' Association. *Nursing: A Social Policy Statement.* Kansas City, Mo: ANA; 1980.
17. Hall BA, Allan JD. Sharpening nursing's focus by focusing on health. *Nursing and Health Care.* 1986;7(6):315–320.
18. Walker SN, Sechrist KR, Pender NJ. The health-promoting lifestyle profile: development and psychometric characteristics. *Nursing Research.* 1987;36(2):76–81.
19. US Department of Health and Human Services, Public Health Service. *Background Papers for the Surgeon General's Workshop, Health Promotion and Aging.* Washington, DC: US Government Printing Office; 1988.
20. Ardell DB. *High Level Wellness,* ed. 10th ann. Berkeley, Calif: Ten-Speed Press; 1986.
21. US Department of Health and Human Services. *The Surgeon General's Report on Nutrition and Health.* DHHS publication No. (PHS) 88-50210. Washington, DC: US Government Printing Office; 1988.
22. Report on the US Preventive Services Task Force. *Guide to Clinical Preventive Services.* Baltimore, Md: Williams & Wilkins; 1989.
23. Goldberg AP. Health promotion and aging: physical exercise. In: US Department of Health and Human Services, Public Health Service. *Background Papers for the Surgeon General's Workshop, Health Promotion and Aging.* Washington, DC: US Government Printing Office; 1988.
24. Smith EL. Special considerations in developing exercise programs for the older adult. In: Matarazzo JD, Weiss SM, Herd JA, Miller NE, Weiss SM, eds. *Behavioral Health: A Handbook of Health Enhancement and Disease Prevention.* New York, NY: Wiley; 1984.
25. Lazarus RS, Folkman S. *Stress, Appraisal, and Coping.* New York, NY: Springer; 1984.
26. Antonovsky A. *Unraveling the Mystery of Health: How People Manage Stress and Stay Well.* San Francisco, Calif: Josey-Bass; 1987.
27. Holmes TH, Rahe, RH. The social readjustment rating scale. *Journal of Psychosomatic Research.* 1967;11:213–218.
28. Stokes SA, Gordon SE. Development of an instrument to measure stress in the older adult. *Nursing Research.* 1988;37(1):16–19.

Chapter 42

Nurses' Home Health Experience. Part I: The Practice Setting

MARYFRAN McKENZIE STULGINSKY

> This is the first of two chapters on home health nursing written by Maryfran Stulginsky. Both chapters are included in this book because together they give a comprehensive overview of the home health setting and the unique demands of making home visits. In this first part, Ms. Stulginsky focuses on the practice setting through the eyes of nurses who have made the transition from the acute care setting to the home. Although the technical skills may be similar in the home care setting, all else is very different when delivering care in the home. The nurse is *invited* into the home, practice is solitary, intimacy is fostered, shared humanity is built into being in the home, family issues become more visible, and caregiving burdens become evident. Each represents a dramatic "comfort" shift for the nurse in the home setting.

Home care is growing at a phenomenal pace. Although accounting for only a small proportion of our total national health care expenditures, the U.S. Commerce Department has called it one of the fastest growing sectors in the medical market (Weinstein, 1993). The Bureau of Labor Statistics indicates that when most industries experienced decline due to recession, home care employment increased 19.2 percent—almost triple the rate of growth for the health care industry in general (National Association of Home Care, 1992). Predictions for the year 2000 indicate that home health will need 8,000 more registered nurses than employed in 1990 to keep pace with the need (U.S. Department of Health and Human Services, 1991).

Several factors account for this growth. Our population is aging; one half of all home care recipients are over age 65. The use of Diagnostic Related Groups (DRGs) for third-party payment to health care agencies has led to patients being discharged "quicker and sicker" from hospitals. The third-party payer focus on cost effectiveness and the ability to deliver high-tech interventions in the home is changing the face of the industry and its practice (Humphrey, 1988; Lindeman, 1992). With the current political climate and overwhelming consumer preference for home over institu-

From *Nursing & Health Care* 14(8):402–407. Reprinted with permission. Copyright 1993 National League for Nursing.

tional health care, one can only assume that the demand will increase with time.

Home health visits, once exclusively centered around maternal/child health, chronic care, and health promotion, now meet the demands of many populations with a wide variety of problems. Home health care has become synonymous with not only acute care but intensive at-home care (Weinstein, 1993). Third-party payers now consider home health an appropriate, cost-effective point of entry for acute care services (Knollmueller, 1993; National Association of Home Care, 1993). Home health nurses are no longer exclusively strong generalist nurses. Advanced practice nurses are now needed to address the increasing complexity and acuity found in the home (dela Cruz, Jacobs, & McCown, 1991; Weinstein, 1984).

Historically, public health nurses, with a preventive and holistic community focus, made home visits. Today the home health nurse, more likely than not, is a generalist/specialist from an acute care setting where the emphasis is individualized, holistic care and a curative, short-term outcome (Kenyon, Smith, Vig Hefty, Bell, McNeil, & Martaus, 1990).

■ACUTE CARE EXPERIENCE REQUIRED FOR HOME CARE

Current hiring trends of home health agencies reflect a desire for nurses with acute care and high-tech experience. A study by Kalnins in 1989 of 287 home health agency hiring preferences indicated that the staff qualifications most valued were a defined period of medical-surgical experience and physical assessment, venipuncture, intravenous therapy and patient teaching skills. These findings were consistent with those of two other similar studies (Fadden & Stull, 1986; Williams, 1987). Qualifications specifically related to nursing in the community and/or a BSN are frequently preferred but not required by home health employers (Kalnins, 1989; dela Cruz et al., 1992). One has only to peruse a cross-section of classified ads to confirm these findings.

What does this mean? With the attraction of home health's work schedule, the home's presumed less hectic setting, and the industry's increasing need for registered nurses, many nurses are coming to home health assuming they will employ the same set of skills and knowledge base as in their acute care practice (Kenyon, et al., 1990). No assumption could be more naive. While home health nursing does require incorporation of acute care skills, the home health nursing experience is different, and the home visit requires nurses to practice in ways they have seldom, if ever, done before.

It was my first visit, I was nervous. I was covering the weekend and was told this would be easy and quick. The 80-year-old woman living with her daughter had just been discharged after several days in the hospital for recurring congestive heart failure. All I needed to do was physical assessment and check the effectiveness of her meds. Her multiple admissions were starting to get to the daughter, a single working parent. A referral had been made to the social worker, hopefully, the family would be seen next week. I was met at the door by an overwrought daughter who told me her mother was bleeding, she had called the doctor, her young son was upstairs sleeping, and she had to show up at work or be fired. Please, wouldn't I come in and take care of her mom? She would return within an hour, once she had negotiated with her boss for more time off, but it had to be done face-to-face. "I just can't call in one more time over the phone," she told me. I wasn't sure what to do, she seemed so beside herself. I don't think I was even party to the decision, she was gone so fast. I went looking for the patient's room. After introducing myself and performing a quick physical assessment, I noted the presence of blood at the rectum and on the sheets and wondered about how much had been lost. "That smell" led me to the bathroom where a trash can filled with soaked sanitary pads gave me the answer. I knew I was looking at a massive GI bleed. The phone rang, it was the doctor. I reported my findings and he said he would meet the family at the ER. What family? I returned to the patient and spoke to her about the urgent need to rehospitalize her. She was shaking visibly as she flatly refused. I fantasized for a moment about how things would be different if I'd found her like this in a hospital. We would have already started fluids and she'd probably be on the way to the ICU and a host of people would be with me. But here we were, the two of us, blood oozing from her rectum. I wasn't sure what to do. I needed to call 911 but she was refusing treatment. I was with someone else's mother, in someone else's house. I couldn't remove here against her will, and what was I supposed to do with the youngster sleeping upstairs? I had little power here. My advice, which typically carried weight, meant nothing. Although my insides screamed treatment, I found myself quietly sitting on the edge of her bed talking. We held hands. I felt her pain as she told me she had just discovered that her two best friends had died, how she was sure that she'd never return home, how she felt like such a burden to her daughter, how becoming old was one loss after another. I know I blinked back tears. I'll never know what it was that we did or said that made her change her mind. All I know is that the daughter came back as the EMTs arrived. As the daughter and her child got into her car to follow the ambulance, I wondered whether I should be going to the hospital too, should I ride along with this frightened old woman so afraid of dying? We never covered this in orientation. As I drove home from my "simple" first visit, all I could think of was how different this type of nursing was going to be.

A search of the periodical literature reveals minimal comprehensive information dealing with that difference. Unless nurses considering home health care have recent community health content of reasonable quality, how do they prepare for this type of practice? Theoretically, the agency's orientation should help, but orientations often center around logistics, policies and procedures. Community health nursing textbooks and the handful of articles written about home visits offer some advice, but only a few reflect the practical wisdom of nurses who live this experience.

The rediscovery of stories and narrative as tools for teaching and learning has occupied many writers in the humanities and social sciences during the last quarter century, reflecting an acknowledgment of the narrative's contribution to human understanding by an academic world traditionally more logic and science focused. In *Stories Lives Tell*, Witherall and Noddings (1991) advocate for the use of stories in education and propose that choosing to impart a particular tale implies a caring/valuing process. They suggest that stories can help us learn, explain, understand ourselves and others, and make the abstract concrete and accessible.

Within nursing, gaining skilled knowledge from stories of nursing practice has been both inspired and legitimized by the work of Patricia Benner. She believes that we must articulate our level of craft, knowledge and clinical know-how by giving it language and sharing it (Benner, 1992).

Therefore, it is from this frame of reference that I sought an understanding of nurses' home health experience. In an effort to learn how home health care differs from care in formal clinical settings, how skills need to be adapted, and what personal adjustments need to be made by nurses who choose this practice setting, I used a strategy for clinical knowledge development suggested by Benner and Wrubel (1982). My goal was to capture elements of both the art and science of nursing's home health experience. I conducted semistructured interviews with six expert home health nurses in order to solicit knowledge from their lived experience. What follows is a synthesis of their practical wisdom.

▬WHAT IS HOME HEALTH NURSING?

Although both debate and tension over the definition of home health nursing are prominent in the literature (Green & Diggers, 1989; Burbach & Brown, 1988), the nurses I interviewed had little trouble defining their practice. They defined home health nursing as meeting the acute and chronic care needs of patients and their families in the home environment. Inherent in this definition was an appreciation for the family's psychosocial resources, the neighborhood, and the presence or absence of community services. They identified the patient as the controlling center around which the circle of providers took direction. This patient-centered position spoke to each nurse's orientation to ground practice in patient advocacy.

> *Sometimes you have to negotiate with many people in the home—and what the family wants is different from what the patient wants. It's very easy to get caught up in trying to please everyone and you can't do it. Patient advocacy is what you need to fall back on, it sometimes makes you very unpopular, but that's what a nurse is, a patient advocate.*

▬HOW IS HOME HEALTH DIFFERENT?

The answer lies in the word home. For most people, feelings about home are strong. It is one of the richest symbols of Western culture. Basic to the meaning of home are various elements of ownership, control, security, family development, independence, comfort, and protection (Rubenstein,

1990). It is a place where we store our memories, build our dreams, nurse our disappointments, and confront conflict.

Home health nurses are invited into homes. It is not a place they own. They are guests. Entrance is granted, not assumed, as is the case in hospitals. To gain entrance, nurses need to establish trust and rapport quickly. Rapport is not built collectively, on a particular shift for consecutive days. Families often deal with just one home health nurse for approximately a one-hour interval two or three times a week.

Control belongs to clients in the home, a fact that must always be kept in mind. The nurse may be the deliverer of care, but the setting is borrowed and every interaction is negotiated with respect to this. As a result, nursing's power base differs, this piece alone is often nursing's greatest adjustment. On their own turf, families feel freer to question advice, do things their own way, establish their own time schedule, and set their own priorities. Sometimes what they decide is opposite to what is advised.

Practice is solitary in the home. There are no colleagues present for support, assistance, or consultation. It is a practice of total accountability, one that relies heavily on both theoretical and intuitive knowledge. Nurses have to go into the home prepared to use both.

> *Accountability is built into this job—there are people who can't work in home health because they can't stand the feeling of being alone—you can't say here, "Mary, listen to this guy's lungs . . ." You have to function autonomously, you have to accept responsibility for your judgments, and be accountable for what you do in a way that nobody else is. To me, that's the purest type of professional practice.*
>
> *You have to use that inner instinct, that gut feeling, and you have to go with it. If you think something's about to go wrong and you may not see this patient for another two or three days, you really have to follow up even though it's a little early and you might get ridiculed—in home care you can't wait—you might make a mistake and call a physician and it might turn out to be nothing, but you learn to accept the fact. It's better to be safe than sorry. Usually you've developed a rapport with the physician who knows 99 percent of the time you're right.*

▬ SHARED HUMANITY IS BUILT INTO BEING IN THE HOME

Intimacy is fostered in the home. Intimacy implies familiarity, friendship, connection, closeness, and caring. Socializing, an integral part of the home visit (Leahy, Cobb & Jones, 1982), contributes to this. As a result, the boundaries of practice are blurred and that can often be a mixed blessing. Families perceive they are sharing themselves by repeatedly allowing entry to a stranger. Nurses enter at critical points in the life cycle, when families are most vulnerable. Nurses become entrusted, granted privileges extended only to family. They come to know that their visit means more than the skill they offer, providing a myriad of services out of either moral and ethical responsibility, or just plain human caring (Smith, 1987).

Shared humanity is built into being in the home. Although scholars have tended to describe nursing as helper–helped relationship, implying that nurses are somehow elite by virtue of their knowledge and skill, being allowed into someone's home encourages a sharing of self in spite of professional knowledge and skills (Taylor, 1992a). The "ordinariness" of nursing, where the nurse patient relationship is inextricably bound to the humanness of caring cannot be escaped (Taylor, 1992b). Nurses not only do things to create a healing environment, very often they become the healing environment (Quinn, 1992).

What is my greatest strength? My interpersonal skills. I know how to make the best therapeutic use of myself. I become one of the tools.

Family issues become more visible in the home. Behavior is more natural, providing a clearer, but not necessarily total picture of dynamics, ways of coping, and lifestyle choices. Multi-generational patterns of interaction tend to be displayed. Working around scripted relationships becomes a challenge. Visiting nurses have to be realistic about what they can fix. Nurses need to wear many hats while providing care, the least of which have been identified as social worker, friend, spiritual comforter, psychologist, financial counselor, and translator of medical information (Green & Driggers, 1989).

What was I least prepared for when I started? . . . The tremendous psychosocial demands . . . Not that I didn't deal with psychosocial needs before, but nothing like this . . . Intense psychosocial needs are the rule, not the exception.

People can't hide things in the home. You know the expression about dysfunctional families having elephants in their living rooms? I find myself working in a lot of homes with elephants. When you first come to home care you think to yourself "Oh my gosh there's an elephant in the living room! I've got to get it out of here, I've got to move it . . ." Well, you find out soon enough that that's probably not going to happen, no matter what—and about the only thing you're going to be able to do is not feed it and clean up after it, hose it down occasionally so it won't smell so bad. You soon learn that you need to work around it—just the way the family does.

Households of one are a demographic reality in today's homes. In order to survive, these individuals must be supported to be uniquely strong and resourceful (Caserta, 1989). Nurses report finding themselves worrying about patients who have no one else, calling between visits, and keeping in touch after discharge, a responsibility that's both hard to let go and at times a weight to the nurse as a person.

I saw a patient on Tuesday. She wasn't feeling well, really lousy and I told her "I'm going to call you tomorrow just to see how you're doing." Well, I got distracted and didn't call her when I said I would. When I did, there was no answer. I almost went to her house I was so worried. Never do that. I should know better. Just say you'll be in touch and in your own mind say "I'm going to call." In the past, I've said to patients, "I'll call you on the weekend to check on you."

I've stopped doing that because it was always on my mind. It made me very weary, all my energy is tapped out. I've got to find a way to turn it off.

Caregiver burden becomes clearer when visiting the home. In more than seven million U.S. households, families care for disabled relatives and friends (Matthis, 1991). Policy makers, insurers, and providers conceptualize the home as a kind of vacuum into which a wide range of medical services can be transferred; they know little about how care is delivered in households, or how families cope. Few ask if it's even realistic to expect families to deal with the level of care we see today (Gubrium & Sankar, 1990).

Caregiving is now recognized as a complex activity, requiring adjustments in daily schedules, imposing financial burdens and causing individuals to re-evaluate their relationships. For the short term, caregiving can be peripheral to normal living, but when illness persists, household reorganization becomes necessary. In some cases, caregiving demands have been or will be in place for years, placing caregivers (who are not always familymembers) at risk for emotional and physical pathology (Eisdorfer, 1991; Ferrell, Rhiner, Cohen, & Grant, 1991). The success of home care is often built on the supports in place (Hewner, 1986). Often these supports are elderly spouses, relatives, friends, or children who are themselves disabled (Brody, 1985).

I was told the caregiver was angry. I'd be angry too if I'd been living his life. A 75-year-old man who took care of his 70-year-old wife met me at the door. He had a feeding schedule in his hand. She was dying of cancer. He told me that between the q4 hours feedings, which took him an hour to do, and the multiple meds he had to instill, he was getting up at 5 AM and not going to sleep until 12 midnight, and living at the bedside. I asked him where the schedule had come from. He told me the hospital. The first thing I did was call the pharmacist to verify what meds I could mix and give together in order to simplify the schedule.

Care can be inadequate in the home. Nurses enter homes where living conditions, resources, or supports are substandard. Unchanged bandages, under-treated infections, irregular self medication, inadequate nutrition, unclean conditions, and unstable support systems can work against nursing's best efforts. When additional support cannot be obtained and caregivers cannot be prompted to give better care, there are only two choices: withdraw from the case or practice in a substandard environment. Home health nurses rarely withdraw, but what they choose to face is extremely difficult (Collopy, Dubler, & Zuckerman, 1990).

I remember seeing a patient with a nonhealing ulcer on her leg. She lived in this home with an outhouse, no hot running water, a small potbellied stove, dirt floors, roaches everywhere. A filthy dirty house full of sick mangy animals, and this open wound that would not heal. What really made me feel bad was that she was raising her three grandchildren, one of whom was an infant and the grandfather was an alcoholic.

This is the practice setting of home health nursing. No matter what the population, the health problem or task, these are the basic issues that must be faced.

Part II of this article will describe the ways in which home health nurses cope with these and other issues.

■ REFERENCES

Benner, P. (1992). Uncovering the wonders of skilled practice by listening to nurses' stories. *Critical Care Nurse, 12*(6), 83–89.

Benner, P. & Wrubel, J. (1982). Skilled clinical knowledge: The value of perceptual awareness. *Nurse Educator, 7*(3), 11–17.

Brody, E.M. (1985). Parent care as a normative family stress. *Gerontologist, 25*(1), 19–29.

Burbach, C. & Brown, B. (1988). Community health and home health nursing: Keeping the concepts clear. *Nursing & Health Care, 9*(2), 97–100.

Caserta, J.E. (1989). Families. *Home Health Care Nurse, 9(3),* 5.

Collopy, B., Dubler, N., & Zuckerman, C. (1990). The ethics of home care: Autonomy and accommodation. *Hastings Center Report, 20*(2), 1–14.

dela Cruz, F., Jacobs, A., & McCown, D. (1992). Home health care nursing. A clinical speciality in need of graduate education. *Home Healthcare Nurse, 10*(2), 44–50.

Eisdorfer, C. (1991). Caregiving: An emerging risk factor for emotional and physical pathology. *Bulletin of the Menninger Clinic, 55,* 238–247.

Fadden, E. & Stull, J.K. (1986). Unpublished manuscript.

Ferrell, B., Rhiner, M., Cohen, M.Z., & Grant, M. (1991). Pain as a metaphor for illness part I: Impact of cancer pain on family caregivers. *Oncology Nursing Forum, 18*(8), 1303–1308.

Green, J. & Diggers, B. (1989). All visiting nurses are not alike: Home health and community health nursing. *Journal of Community Health Nursing, 6*(2), 83–93.

Gubrium J., & Sankar, A. (1990). Introduction. In Gubrium, J. & Sankar, A. (eds.) *The home care experience, ethnography and policy* (pp. 7–15). Newberry Park, CA: Sage Publications.

Hewner, S. (1986). Bringing home health care. *Journal of Gerontological Nursing, 12*(2), 29–34.

Humphrey, C. (1988). The home as setting for care, clarifying the boundaries of practice. *Nursing Clinics of North America, 23*(2), 305–314.

Kalnins, I. (1989). Home health agency preferences for staff nurse qualifications, and practices in hiring and orientation. *Public Health Nursing, 6*(2), 33–39.

Kenyon, V., Smith, E., Vig Hefty, L., Bell, M.L., McNeil, J., & Martaus, T. (1990). Clinical competencies for community health nursing. *Public Health Nursing, 7*(1), 33–39.

Knollmueller, R. (1993). The role of prevention in home health care nursing practice. *Home Healthcare Nurse, 11*(1), 21–23.

Leahy, K.M., Cobb, M.M., & Jones, M.C. (1982). *Community health nursing.* St. Louis, MO: C.V. Mosby Co.

Linderman, C. (1992). Nursing and technology, moving into the 21st century. *Caring Magazine, 11*(9), 5–10.

Matthis, E. (1991). Family caregivers want education for their caregiving roles. *Home Healthcare Nurse, 10*(4), 19–22.

National Association for Home Care. (1992). Basic statistics about home care, 1992. Washington, DC: National Association for Home Care.

National Association for Home Care. (1993). Toward meaningful reform. *Caring Magazine, 12*(3), 4–10.

Quinn, J. (1992). Holding sacred space: The nurse as healing environment. *Holistic Nursing Practice, 4*(6), 26–36.

Rubenstein, R. (1990). Culture and disorder in the home care experience: The home as sickroom. In Gubrium, J. & Sankar, A. (eds.) *The home care experience, ethnography and policy* (pp. 37–57). Newberry Park, CA: Sage Publications.

Smith, J.B. (1987). Home care is more than Medicare regs. *American Journal of Nursing, 87*(3), 305–306.

Taylor, B. (1992a). Relieving pain through ordinariness in nursing: A phenomenologic account of a comforting nurse-patient encounter. *Advanced Nursing Science, 15*(1), 33–43.

Taylor, B. (1992b). Caring: Being manifested as ordinariness in nursing. In Gaut, D. (ed.), *The presence of caring in nursing* (pp. 181–200). New York: The National League for Nursing Press.

U.S. Department of Health and Human Services. (1991). Health Personnel in the U.S., eighth report to Congress (DHHS no. HRS-P-00-92-1). Rockville, MD: U.S. Government Printing Office.

Weinstein, S. (1984). Speciality teams in home care. *American Journal of Nursing, 84*(3), 342–345.

Weinstein, S. (1993). A coordinated approach to home infusion care. *Home Healthcare Nurse, 11*(1), 15–20.

Williams, S. (1987). Continuing education needs of community health nurses. Unpublished manuscript.

Witherall, C. & Noddings, N. (1991). *Stories lives tell, narrative and dialog in education.* New York: Teacher's College Press.

Chapter 43

Nurses' Home Health Experience.
Part II: The Unique Demands
of Home Visits

MARYFRAN McKENZIE STULGINSKY

The focus of this second home health chapter is on dealing successfully
with the home visit issues presented in Part I. Again, Ms. Stulginsky uses
the words from experienced home health nurses to describe their feelings
working in the home health setting. They report that building trust and rapport is essential. Caregiving in the home involves common sense, imagination, improvising, and at times, "making do." Priorities need to remain fluid
and setting limits encourages self care in an atmosphere where professional
boundaries are rarely secure. The flexibility and autonomy of home health
enables nurses to be the nurse they were taught to be while practicing on
the cutting edge of health care reform.

As noted in part one of this article (Stulginsky, 1993), home care is a growing segment of the nation's health care system. Despite this, nursing literature contains little comprehensive information dealing with the differences between nursing practice in traditional, acute care settings and
practice in the home. In an effort to learn how home health care differs
from care in formal clinical settings, I conducted interviews with six expert
home health nurses in order to solicit their practical wisdom.

Where the first part of this article discussed the issues surrounding
home care's practice setting, part two explores how home care nurses deal
with those issues in their practices.

▬HOME CARE NURSES NEED
TO BUILD TRUST AND RAPPORT

Attitude is essential. The nurse needs to enter the home knowing he or
she is a guest with services to offer that clients are free to accept or reject.
Sensing "where people are" can and must begin immediately—the most
closed family sends signals. Maintaining a respectful distance and not en-

From *Nursing & Health Care* 14(9):476–485. Reprinted with permission. Copyright
1993 National League for Nursing.

tering the family's "space" prematurely is critical. Noticing the family's customs as soon as possible is helpful.

"Oh, you folks don't wear shoes in the house, let me take my shoes off."

I think 90 percent of the communicating I do to build trust is through the physical and only 10 percent is with words.

Demonstrating a willingness to negotiate visit times around family needs indicates flexibility. Honoring that time commitment builds trust. Families need to know when the nurse is coming, even if they say it doesn't matter.

There are so many things people can't count on when they're sick, they need to know that I'm going to be there when I say I'm going to be there. Giving them a range usually works best. For example, I tell families that I'll be at their house between 10 and 11, give or take 15 minutes for traffic. If I'm going to be late, I call. I just think it's the respectful thing to do. I've been on the other side of this, I know how it feels to wait.

Some people you're never going to get to trust [you]. You can do your best, but I would say a 90 percent average is doing well. If you get kicked out of a few homes and some people never bond to you, that's normal. In real life, we don't bond to everyone.

Validating the illness experience sends a message of caring. Often clients need to talk out their health care experiences. They need to sense that someone hears how illness affects their life and is willing to react to it.

To build rapport, I validate everything they say. They can give me all kinds of horror stories about what happened in the hospital, with other nurses, relatives or whatever and I validate it. I'm not going to join them in their attack on the system, but there's a way to do it, to say, "I hear what you're saying."

▬FIRST CONTACT SETS THE TONE

Few families understand why people are sent home from the hospital "still sick." Even fewer understand what home care is. All they know is that the nurse is coming to help and many people have misconceptions about this helping. The first contact sets the tone for what is to follow, and is often crucial in the development of a helping relationship (Berg & Helgeson, 1984). It begins with the initial phone call and follows with the first home visit. Identifying oneself, affiliation, where the referral came from, the purpose of the referral, a brief summary of your knowledge of the situation and negotiating an appointment time all need to be included in that phone call. The conversation should not end until families know how to call back (either the agency or the nurse) should circumstances change (Stanhope & Lancaster, 1988).

There is much to explain and cover on the first visit. People can be in pain, overwhelmed with doubts about how they will manage, and may not be sure if they want to even try—a questionable situation in which to introduce home care's philosophy of empowerment, enablement, and enhancement (Wasik, Bryant, & Lyons, 1990).

Nurses report "hitting the essentials" of the information legally required on first visits in order to give priority to detailed explanations of
home care, the rationale being that the legally required information can
be reviewed during subsequent visits, but that there will be no subsequent
visits if the details of home care are not understood. Carefully defining
what nursing can and cannot do is important, because expectations are
often greater than what the nurse can provide. Mutually acceptable goals,
choice, joint responsibility, and negotiation are emphasized as a part of a
process that nurse and family enter together (Persznecker, Zerwekh, &
Horn, 1989. Speaking slowly and carefully, and allowing processing time
are important. So is offering the pluses and minuses of options.

> *First visit I tell them when I'm going too come and what I'm going to do and then
> let them process it: "That's really lousy, I thought you were going to do more."
> Then I say, "Yes, it is lousy (validating), it is a lot to expect the family to do. We
> can send a home health aide in to help you, but let me tell you about that." Then
> I give them two responses. I tell them about the home health aide and I'll say,
> "Some people feel that's a wonderful help and other people feel it's not worth the
> trouble of having another person in the house, they find it distracting." So they
> don't even have to fish for why they don't want something. . . . People who are
> under a lot of stress like that.*
>
> *Some people go in with the initial assessment and go over every line—that
> takes forever and it can be overwhelming to families. I've learned to go in and lis-
> ten to them talk as I do what I have to do. I've learned the form well enough to
> ask the right questions and recognize answers in their stories.*
>
> *I've learned that trust and rapport take a while to build with older people, but
> once they trust you it is for life! They'll turn down services they can really use just
> because they don't want strangers in the house . . . so I've learned not to offer ser-
> vices until we have a relationship and even then, one at a time. There have been
> times that I've decided to manage myself because having extra people in the home
> was too much for them.*
>
> *There are some people who feel they don't like this new person in the home . . .
> and if I sense that I remind them that I don't have to come, that the choice is
> theirs, no matter what their doctor has said.*

■ ASSESSMENT IN THE HOME INVOLVES COMMON SENSE AND IMAGINATION

Assessing occurs in every patient setting, but getting to the bigger picture
in the home often involves common sense, intuition, and imagination
(Keeling, 1978). In formal clinical settings the physical environment is
often standard, but there's no common baseline from home to home, so
gathering information is often a feat. Sensing (Bayer, 1973; Lentz &
Meyer, 1979; Clark, 1991) must begin with the first phone call and continue until discharge: sights, sounds, smells, tone of words, dress, habits,
body language; how space, time, and touch are used; who visits, who
doesn't, patterns of interaction, availability of social support, what is sacred, what is not, what is in the refrigerator and cabinets; what does the

house, yard, sidewalk, driveway, and street look like, what does that look mean; where is the nearest neighbor and transportation, how available are they; how has illness affected work of the patient and family . . . the list is endless. Nurses report needing giant antennae, fear missing something important, and wonder about where to draw the line. Although our education teaches us to assess by asking questions, we often learn more by listening to stories families tell us.

> *I've learned to stand back and look at the big picture. I don't nit-pick for things. I don't try to address and focus on everything. I try to keep things simple and basic for patients. I focus on safety.*
>
> *We must listen to their stories and listen to their issues. [I knew a diabetic woman.] Her diabetes was just out of control. I said, "Let's just talk." "Talk?" [she replied.] "Don't you want to take my blood sugar?" "No," I told her, "I want to talk." She said, "You probably want to hear what I ate last night." I said, "I doubt very seriously that eating did this to you. What's going on?" She burst into tears: "My grandson got arrested last night . . ." She was under a tremendous amount of stress and had no idea that stress could affect her diabetes.*
>
> *I've learned to listen carefully to off-hand remarks and follow up. Once, someone said something that made me think they weren't eating. So, as I was leaving, I peeked in the refrigerator and a couple of cabinets: Sure enough, there was no food. I went right back upstairs and admitted what I had done and why, and then together, we worked on the problem.*

▬SETTING LIMITS ENCOURAGES SELF CARE

When people are stressed, they often have a tendency to look to others to solve their problems for them. Helping families identify solutions for themselves is of tremendous importance. So too is enabling them to look to their pasts and recognize the strengths that had seen them through earlier difficult times. Home health's interdependent process has as its ultimate goal independence, not dependence—but the lines among the three can be extremely fuzzy. Nurses need to set limits in order to encourage self care, and when exceptions arise, clearly identify them as such.

> *On that first visit, I tell them to picture us as supporting them through the storm. The storm's going to hit and they're going to get wet—it can't be avoided—but they won't be alone. A lot of people want us to handle the storm for them. When families ask me to do something for them [that] I know they should be doing themselves, I'm very clear on telling them, "I think you can do that yourself. You don't need me to do that for you."*
>
> *I've learned to use Family Systems Theory in my home health practice [Klee, 1989]. First visit, I begin a baseline genogram and add to it as time goes by. I ask questions periodically to fill in the gaps. By listening to peoples' stories, its amazing how easy it is to see repeatable patterns and point out connections from the past. I think I'm suggesting more practical solutions this way. Sometimes patients expect things that historically have never been part of the family's operational pattern. They expect that pattern to change simply because they're sick. Pointing out patterns helps them to see how realistic their expectations really are.*

I've learned to plant a lot of seeds by asking how they have handled things like this in the past.

I don't let people use me, but there are always exceptions. I went to a lady's house the other day and her blood pressure was different. I asked if she had been taking her medications and she said no. I said "Why not? The prescriptions were called in last week." She told me she had no one to pick them up. So I asked her why she didn't call me when she knew I was coming to check on how well these medications were working for her. She said, "You don't pick up prescriptions, do you?" I said, "Routinely, no. But in this case I would have made an exception." I made it clear that I was not going to do this on a routine basis.

◼ PRIORITIES NEED TO REMAIN FLUID

Nurses can mentally order their day around timed treatments, clients whose physical difficulties don't do well with early morning visits and geographical locations, only to make daily phone calls and find that plans need to be reworked—sometimes several times a day.

There are several practical guides for setting priorities. While Clark (1991) suggests prioritizing based on:

1. potential threats to health,
2. degree of concern to the client, or
3. ease of solution;

Carr (1989) advises dealing with acute safety needs first, followed by short-term and long-term goals. Regardless of what system nurses choose to adopt, they need to go to front doors with a plan of care that may require reorganization within moments of entering—especially if the nurse's and patient's perceptions don't match.

Shortly after I started in home health, I saw this man who had just moved in with his daughter and her family. We were going in to help manage his uncontrolled diabetes, but the day I saw them no one cared about diabetes. . . . [The whole family] (even the kids) were arguing about Dad: what he should eat, his lack of mobility, his insistence on enemas (a life-long habit). The husband and wife were . . . very exercise and nutrition focused . . . and it was evident that Dad's issue was very troubling to them. Dad was a partially blind 75-year-old widower used to living alone, eating whatever he wanted and handling his episodes of constipation with cathartics and enemas. Now . . . there was extreme family tension because the daughter wanted her father to adopt the family's fitness orientation and give up his past bowel routine. We spent most of the visit talking about bowels, but what we were really talking about was control and autonomy. I spoke to the daughter and her husband about the practicality of expecting a 75-year-old man with this kind of bowel routine to adopt new ways. . . . I spoke to the father about the fact that enemas should not be used to enable a daily BM and why. . . . [W]e worked out a plan whereby Dad would try pushing fluids, eating more roughage, and getting up to walk with the help of the kids (his blindness made him afraid of falling). His daughter agreed to treat his constipation by noon of day 2 if no BM had occurred. . . . Although I assessed the dia-

betes situation as well . . . most of the visit centered around the bowel issue. As I drove away, I felt uncomfortable. I was fairly new to home health and I was still having trouble not being in control. At that time, I saw diabetes as more important than constipation. I felt like I had not stayed on task. . . . Did I miss something that might have been insidiously starting? I knew in my gut that what we spent our time doing had value for the family, but the task-oriented person in me struggled.

SUSPENDING ONE'S VALUES IS DIFFICULT, BUT NECESSARY

Nurses repeatedly enter homes where the value systems or lifestyles are different from their own. The key to making things work lies in accepting things where they are and finding common ground (Price & Braden, 1978). Communicating respect and trust in the family's ability to both determine what is best and make good decisions goes a long way (Carey, 1989). Often, we assume this problem will be more of an issue with the poor and uneducated, but this is not always the case.

I was visiting this family that was quite well off: They lived in a huge house and were used to getting what they wanted out of life. This situation was really throwing them. I had been told that the spouse was extremely well educated, fanatical about detail, and could be very intimidating. Sure enough, the day I visited there were missing supplies and I had to punt. He was so resistive and angry. I felt my stomach clutching just dealing with him. What calmed me down, amazingly enough, was remembering how out of control we all felt when my dad was dying. Somehow recalling that helped me say the right things and the visit went better than I expected.

There will always be scenarios that bother even the least judgmental person. Letting go, choosing to reorder one's view of the world, one's ethnocentric values (Carey, 1989) is difficult, but letting go is what must be done. Each nurse needs to find a way to accomplish that.

If I'm horrified, I don't express that to patients. I don't show it. Many people don't have much to work with. I have to remember I am in their home. After you establish a rapport, you might make suggestions. If it goes against you, you have to look beyond. After you're with them a while, you can ease your way in. Turn it around: If someone was coming into your home, who are they to tell you how to live? When I make suggestions, I say, "I'm not trying to tell you what to do, but I'd like to suggest that this may be a better way." And you know what else? It's so simple, it's not what you say, but how you say it!

SURVIVAL TEACHING IS A MAJOR FOCUS

Nurses in home health are constantly involved in teaching. A "needs to know, wants to know, and ought to know" mentality is central to the patient education process (Carr, 1990). Survival teaching, information that will keep patients safe until the next visit is the major focus. Sometimes the biggest challenge is selling discouraged patients on wanting to know how to survive.

> *You have to prioritize as to what is going to impact survival. I just saw a diabetic woman who had to learn everything. What was the most important thing she needed to know? How to take her insulin. . . . And the second thing she needed to know is how to do the blood glucose monitoring. Then we moved on to signs and symptoms of hypo- and hyperglycemia, then we finally got to diet. What is diabetes wasn't important to her. Once you've taught survival skills, you have a link and then they'll listen to anatomy and physiology.*

Learner readiness is important. Nurses need to be prepared to enable patient education through a variety of strategies—not the least of which involves "non-nursing tasks."

> *I had much to teach and do with this farm lady with diabetes, but her concern was her goats. The mother goat had died delivering twins while [the lady] was in the hospital, and she blamed herself because she wasn't there. She had no motivation to learn anything. She told me if she couldn't take care of her animals and live like she wanted to on her farm, she didn't want to live. This lady was born and raised on her farm. . . . [Except for one vacation, she and her husband had] never been off the farm. We had to go out and bring the baby goats into the house, wash them up, feed them a bottle, and only after that could she concentrate. Her 84-year-old husband and I got the goats. Sometimes you have to do these kinds of things.*

Teaching while doing seems to work best in the home. For example, explaining Lasix while attaching the blood pressure cuff, identifying steps and rationale during treatments, and talking caregivers through a dressing change.

Whatever the method, the goal is to enable and empower others to do for themselves, to get involved in their own learning. Three teaching theories that seem to work well include:

1. relating serious consequences and high chance of recurrence as incentive to learn,
2. identifying major problem areas
3. capitalizing on learner frustration and convincing them that positive benefits can result by initiating a particular behavior (Hellwig, 1990).

> *I teach patients to listen to what their body is telling them and respond to it: "If you find that you would go to the bathroom the other day and you were fine, and today you're huffing and puffing there's something wrong and you need to react."*
>
> *I advise all clients to keep a pad and paper by their bedside. If they don't have one, I take one. I write at the top "Questions to my nurse/doctor." One of the most important things we do is teach people how to be their own advocates because we're with them such a short time. I teach them how to keep a list for when they go to the doctor and to be sure to utilize his or her time to their maximum. This client, who was diabetic, was 68 years old and she had never gone to the*

doctor with a list. She said, "I always get so nervous I forget things." I told her, "I do that too." She said, "You do that too? But you're educated." I said, "Of course. You're under stress, you're trying to remember everything in fifteen minutes or less. Write it down." So before she went to the doctor we made a list. He called me and . . . [said], "That was the most phenomenal appointment I've ever had with her."

▀PROFESSIONAL BOUNDARIES ARE RARELY SECURE

The familiarity created by home visiting generates several practice issues: self disclosure, accepting gifts and hospitality, and maintaining therapeutic distance. As each nurse struggles to find a place of comfort and "rules to live by" rarely are those boundaries secure. One has to learn to live with mixed feelings as part of the practice, to go with what intuitively feels right and know that each situation carries a potential for rewriting the script.

I have what I call a cellophane barrier. It's like Saran Wrap around me. You can see me, feel me, look at me . . . but you can't really touch me. The way you create that barrier is to let them know that you're a professional. . . . We can't be friends because I'm being paid to give a service and be therapeutic and that can't happen if we're trying to be friends. All that said I'll tell you about Tom who was a 37-year-old dying of cancer. There are exceptions to every rule and he's the one. . . . I'll never forget the first time I went to see him [we shook hands and I started asking him about himself] and he said, "So enough about me. Tell me about you." I'm usually pretty comfortable with this, a little bit of self disclosure is a wonderful tool, but eventually I said, "Let's go back to you." But he kept shifting the conversation back to me. I told him, "I'm not comfortable about this. We need to talk about you." "Well," he said, "I'm tired of talking about me. I'm dying and you're here to make sure that this tube runs well and I don't hurt and I trust you're going to do that. I don't want some stuffy professional coming in here. You're going to be with me when I die and I don't want to die with a stranger." It got harder each time I went, we got closer and closer. I told him about my cellophane wrapper and how he poked a hole in it and he said, "If you're allowed to see and touch the real me, why can't I see and touch the real you?" I told him I didn't have an answer for that, all I knew is that I'd been told through my educational process to maintain professionalism. Then he said, "All I'm asking is that you be a real person." He taught me a lot. But when he died it hurt worse than anything. I wonder if we use our professionalism so that we don't feel the hurt so deeply? If I felt the hurt with everybody I'd be completely useless.

I've come to a point in my life where I trust my own decisions. I no longer believe everything I've been taught anymore. I've gotten this personal security and it's such a relief once you can eradicate those old nursing hang-ups.

For many families offering a guest hospitality is part of their upbringing. Nurses need to think carefully about accepting hospitality. In some homes it simply is not safe, while in others it may interfere with the ability to be therapeutic. However, for patients who live alone, the sharing of a cup of tea may well be their only social contact. It comes down to comfort level and often, available time. Most of the nurses interviewed reported that when they accepted hospitality, it occurred after care was given—creating, at least for themselves, a boundary line.

> *People often want to feed me, give me coffee, I always refuse . . . there's something about breaking bread together that makes you cross the boundary, I always say, "Oh how wonderful, but I just ate." Sometimes I do it when I know it's really important, but it's the exception rather than the rule.*
>
> *I have a lady who lives alone and gets a monthly B12 shot. We just got her moved so that she can get meals, she no longer cooks. On the first Monday of the month she doesn't get a meal. So I called the doctor and asked him to write the order to give the shot the first Monday of the month. On that day, I stop at a fast food place, go and give her shot and then we have lunch together. I did it to kill two birds with one stone: It gives her a chance to socialize and a meal she wouldn't have.*

▰ HOMES CAN BE MORE DISTRACTING THAN CLINICAL SETTINGS

Although the home is perceived as being less distracting than formal clinical settings, in reality it can be quite the opposite. Distractions, defined by Pruitt, Keller and Hale (1987) as events or circumstances that divert an individual's attention from the job at hand, can be environmental (cluttered, dirty houses, poor light, noise, smoke), behavioral (manipulative, drug seeking or avoiding behavior), or nurse-initiated (fears of harm, reactions to lifestyle, preoccupations with roles, becoming overwhelmed by the complexity of needs or issue at hand). Although often viewed negatively, distractions can provide useful information.

Distractions are best handled by dealing with them directly or learning to live with them (planning visits around favorite shows that can't be turned off or when children are in school). Debating with families over what's most important, your visit or their issue, doesn't help because for some the visit is secondary. What seems to work well is: carrying a large battery-operated flashlight, asking to lower music or television, requesting telephone conversations be limited during visits, soliciting either time alone or conducting care in a less busy area, leaving and returning another day (if all else fails), and being truthful about allergies to smoke or animals.

Dirty homes, which can be a sign of depression or physical incapacity, may need to be ignored if the nurse carefully concludes that his is how the family chooses to live. When in doubt, asking another nurse to visit the patient helps in the decision process.

> *We had a man who was wheelchair bound and lived alone in a filthy apartment and dangerous apartment house. He'd always say he was in the process of cleaning but it never seemed to happen. Some of us thought that's just the way he wanted to live, but one of our nurses realized he was depressed. He was an intel-*

ligent man, had held a job for years and just felt trapped. She got him transferred to another apartment house with an apartment large enough for his son to move in—a nice place, and now he's a new person. She saw in him things we couldn't see.

■ NURSES NEED TO PROTECT THEMSELVES AS WELL AS THEIR CLIENTS

Threats to safety must be handled realistically. The nurse must keep his or her car locked, not get out if suspicious behavior is occurring, and heed the subtle and not so subtle safety messages offered by family members and neighbors.

When I'm going to a home where I feel physically uncomfortable I make sure my visits are short or I'm careful what time I pick to go there. I occasionally have to go to an apartment house that the police call the Animal House. When I go there I go early in the morning while most people are still sleeping.

Did you ever see the movie Deliverance? Well I've visited families like you see in that movie. I just visited a family like that and there was one son I was very uncomfortable with. The youngest son in the family I think was uncomfortable about my being there with his brother too, so he told me up front to call him prior to visiting so that he could always be present. And I did. Sometimes I was tempted to just go on my own because it was easier but I've learned to pay close attention to things like this.

Protecting can take many forms: keeping the number of caregivers in the home to a minimum, helping manage moments of crisis, notifying appropriate authorities and/or getting patients removed if mistreatment is suspected. Nurses should enlist others in the process of protecting as necessary and be sensitive to situations that may be potentially dangerous both for patients and themselves.

You know how crazy it gets when you call 911? All those emergency medical people come in and despite your being there and identifying yourself as the nurse they take over. So many people respond and they're all asking questions. It's overwhelming. When I call 911 I always stay. I never leave the family to fend for themselves. I puff up and protect my patient.

Remember that lady with the nonhealing ulcer who lived in the house with the pot-belly stove? Well, I stopped at the firehouse and asked them to put a smoke detector in that house because I was afraid for those three little kids. When I was there the firemen . . . told me if ever I pick up that the family is fighting with their neighbors not to go back there. They shoot at each other.

I had a client . . . who was in such pain and the family was stoned all around her, she counted her pills and put her medication under lock and key. Finally as she was getting sicker she said, "I just can't do this." So we put her in an inpatient facility and she died there very comfortably . . . Her daughter was very angry about our removing her from the home because it meant her line to the morphine was gone.

◼MAKING DO—AN ESSENTIAL SKILL

In the hospital, equipment and supplies are standard and generally available. Not so in the home. They are often different from home to home based on the medical equipment house that supplies them. Often the variation is something the nurse hasn't used before. Although nurses are conscientious about ordering supplies, they have no control over use. The house stock can be used by other family members or wasted. Nurses typically carry supplies in the car, but sure enough, they won't have what the patient needs that day. Adapting is both a nursing and caregiver challenge especially if families have been taught to use particular supplies. It may require leaving the home to get supplies elsewhere and returning. Families can feel anxious or angry when routines have to be adapted. The challenge is to make do in a low key manner, and convince the family that although things aren't perfect they are manageable.

What was I least prepared for? The "punting" I had to do going into homes and not having things there. I'm thinking of a gastrostomy patient. The tube fell out I had nothing in the home but I had a foley in my car. I put the foley in, blew up the balloon and called the doctor. I didn't think I'd have to work like that. I went to see this hospice patient who had a colostomy draining right next to a large, deep, gaping abdominal wound. She wasn't getting a good seal and had gone through all the bags in the house because of leakage. It was Sunday, she used an unusually big bag, and all the pharmacies that carried supplies were closed. She desperately wanted to leave the home and attend her child's championship soccer game. So I called the community hospital, pleaded my case to the nursing supervisor, left, went to the hospital and went floor to floor looking through supply carts to try to find something I could make do with. It wasn't perfect but guess what? I found something close and I used a lot of stomahesive paste. She got enough of a seal to go to the game and I found out later the bag lasted several days.

◼TIME IS THE NURSE'S MOST PRECIOUS RESOURCE

Home health nurses' biggest complaint centers around the paperwork involved in making home visits. The volume of paperwork connected with home visiting is extraordinary, because of the need to justify everything for third party reimbursement. Typical of most home health nurses is a car full of supplies and a plethora of charts and forms. Experts offer the following advice to deal with this: avoid writing things twice; either write the complete nursing note in the home or write a detailed sketch so that later you're not spending a lot of time trying to recapture what happened; complete all necessary forms on the day you see patients; fill out all forms as much as possible before approaching the home; use voice mail versus making personal calls; keep a calendar of events due for each patient in their chart to avoid combing notes for due dates; keep an organized list of significant information, i.e. medication changes, resources, referrals in each patient's chart; make arrangement phone calls from the home as much as possible.

▬NURSES NEED TO WORK AND RESPECT THE SYSTEM

Nurses have never gotten paid for all they do and this is especially true in the home. Third party reimbursement has strict regulations about what constitutes skilled care, what gets reimbursed. Much of what arguably qualifies bona fide health care hardly meets the skilled nursing definition. In addition, Medicare's requirement that clients be homebound (and that documentation reflect this) often conflicts with what nurses see as the quality of life needs of their patients (Anderson, 1992). Nurses frequently find themselves in situations where they need to work the system i.e. documenting what needs to be documented or using the "right" language to get reimbursement and client needs met. An ethical dilemma? For some yes, for others no.

> *Home care nurses don't get paid for what they do, neither do agencies—they get reimbursed for some kind of a thing that goes along the medical model, and that's the least of what you do. The most wonderful visit I ever had was down in Baltimore in a row home. He was a brand new diabetic, new to insulin and I went into the house to teach. There was no heat, hot water or electricity, and he didn't know what to do. He gave me the business card of the landlord who was a slum lord, I had heard his name in connection with scandals . . . and there was no phone number on the card, just a post office box . . . the guy had paid his rent . . . so I made a few phone calls to some public agencies, it took about 15 minutes. The next day I came back he had heat, hot water and electricity. (Obviously Medicare would not have reimbursed your agency for what you did on that visit, it wasn't skilled nursing, how did you handle that?) To get reimbursement? I documented that I gave him a list of his medications and instructed the patient regarding frequency and dosage. (Does that bother you in any way?) No, it doesn't bother me at all. What I did was much more valuable than teaching him about diabetes . . . although I probably gave him the list but no teaching occurred, he was too distracted. (What you're saying is that you couldn't have walked out of the home without addressing that issue). No, and we have many situations like this . . . (You mean the way the regs are written we're forced into certain situations out of ethical need?) Exactly right.*

Despite this needing to work the system, it should be respected as well. Adopting or fostering a "Medicare will pay for it" mentality demonstrates little accountability to the greater good. There is no bottomless pit of resources, and practice needs to reflect concern for the most economic way to accomplish goals.

> *I've gotten to the point, I think we all need to, where we've got to think about Medicare and the most economic way to meet people's needs, because we need Medicare for everyone else. I value the system. It's so easy to go in and say, well I need a walker. O.K. I'll call Home Medical Supply. Everyone does that because*

they know Medicare pays for it, it can be taken care of with one phone call, it's delivered to the door and the company takes care of the paperwork. It takes a little bit more time on the nurse's part and it's more inconvenient but most people have access to free walkers by calling the Lions or Kiwanis Club, there's free medical equipment out there if you look. I really do think there is a lot of waste. But you know what? The patients are even becoming more aware. I had a man recently say to me, "That's OK, I don't need that from Medicare, save that for someone who needs it worse than I do." And legitimately he could have had it.

■THE REWARDS OF HOME HEALTH ARE MANY

The rewards of home health are many and on all different levels. The closeness, although a double-edged sword, teaches valuable human lessons. In the home, nurses can see how their interventions made a difference. They report that home health enables them to be the nurse they were taught to be, giving them practice flexibility and autonomy rarely experienced in other settings. They see themselves on the cutting edge of health care reform.

Despite all this, home health nursing is not without liability. Although experienced nurses perceive themselves making a difference, the practice can be a threat to both their physical and emotional well-being (Zerwekh, 1991). Nurses who look to practice in the home must go into it with eyes wide open. Home care is not setting up a hospital in someone's house. Home health nursing is not simply transferring skills from one location to another. Home visit demands are unique.

■REFERENCES

Anderson, K. (1992). Deceptive documentation in home healthcare nursing. *Home Healthcare Nurse, 10*(6), 31–35.

Bayer, M. (1973). Community diagnosis—through sight, sense, and sound. *Nursing Outlook, 21*(11), 712–713.

Berg, C. & Helgeson, D. (1984). That first home visit. *Journal of Community Health Nursing, 1*(3), 207–215.

Carey, R. (1989). How values affect the mutual goal setting process with multiproblem families. *Journal of Community Health Nursing, 6*(1), 7–14.

Carr, P. (1989). Priorities. *Home Healthcare Nurse, 6*(6), 42–44.

Carr, P. (1990). Needs to know, wants to know, ought to know. *Home Healthcare Nurse, 8*(4), 34.

Clark, MJ. (1991). The home visit process. In *Nursing in the community* (pp. 143–159). Norwalk, CT: Appleton & Lange.

Hellwig, K. (1990). Health teaching: The crux of home care nursing. *Home Healthcare Nurse, 8*(4), 35–37.

Keeling, B. (1978). Making the most of the first home visit. *Nursing 78,* March, 24–28.

Klee, M.A.E. (1989). Family influences on home care. In Wimer, A. and Martinson, I. (eds.) *Home health care nursing* (pp. 151–162). Philadelphia, PA: W.B. Saunders.

Lentz, J.R. & Meyer, E.A. (1979). The dirty house. *Nursing Outlook, 27*(9), 590–593.

Pesznecker, Zerwekh, & Horn, (1989). The mutual participation relationship: Key to facilitating self-care practices in clients and families. *Public Health Nursing, 6*(4), 197–203.

Price, J. & Braden, C. (1978). The reality of home visits. *American Journal of Nursing, 78*(9), 1536–1538.

Pruitt, R., Keller, L., & Hale, S. (1987). Mastering distractions that mar home visits. *Nursing & Health Care, 8*(6), 345–347.

Stanhope, M. & Lancaster, J. (1988). *Issues in family health promotion. Community health nursing, process and practice for promoting health care* (pp. 391–397). Washington, DC: C.V. Mosby.

Stulginsky, M.M. (1993) Nurses' home health experience—part I: The practice setting. *Nursing & Health Care, 14*(8), 402–407.

Wasik, B., Bryant, D., & Lyons, C. (1990). Philosophy of home visiting. In *Home visiting, procedures for helping families* (pp. 45–68). Newberry Park CA: Sage Publications.

Zerwekh, J. (1991). At the expense of their souls. *Nursing Outlook, 39*(2), 58–61.

Unit 7
Cultural Influences on Community Health Nursing

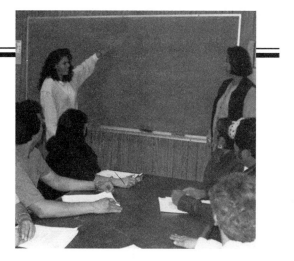

Cultural influences are often an overlooked dimension of health care. The physical aspect of health and illness, as well as the psychological dimension, can easily be identified. In addition, however, all human beings behave in the context of a specific culture that profoundly influences their values, their daily activities, and their reactions to the world around them, such as their response to stress. Culture channels their attitudes toward pain. The way people feel in the face of death, the way they express grief, the way they relate to health care practitioners, the way they raise their children—all are affected by culture.

Culture refers to the beliefs, values, and behavior that are learned by members of social groups. It is a design for living. Culture is more than isolated elements of belief and custom. It is an integrated whole, a pattern of values and behavior that provides people with a map that charts their lives. Although there are some broad cultural values shared by many who live in the United States, groups have retained some aspects of their traditional cultures. Mexican Americans, African Americans, Irish Americans, German Americans, Asian Americans, and many other ethnic groups have their own subcultures. Furthermore, certain customs, values, and ideas are unique to the poor, the rich, the middle class, to you, women, men, and older adults. Regional subcultures also have distinctive ways of defining the world and coping with life. Contrast the relaxed pace of life in rural middle America with the energized pace of urban Americans living in a large coastal city, for example. Other groups, such as the gay community, homeless and migrant populations, the incarcerated, gang members, and substance abusers, have developed their own subcultures. Even occupational or professional groups develop their own special languages and worlds of cultural meanings. How many of us are familiar with the jargon of the computer scientist or the seeming gibberish of a stock broker? Although most people share some features of the larger American culture, many also have learned aspects of one or more subcultures. Even nurses have their own special culture with its unique vocabulary, values, clothes, and customs. And among nurses there are differences. The intensive care nurse uses different jargon, has a different focus of care, and wears different clothing than the community health nurse.

What is making us more aware of the cultural influences? Why does it seem increasingly critical to incorporate cultural sensitivity into community health nursing practice? Advancing waves of immigrants and refugees with markedly contrasting cultures have changed the cultural mix and complexion of the United States and forces all Americans to recognize cultural differences. New research-based knowledge of cultural diversity has enhanced our understanding and has underscored the importance of sensitive transcultural interactions. Greater emphasis on the value of holistic nursing and health care and complementary and/or nontraditional therapies also have sharpened our culturally oriented focus. When health professionals interact only with people of their own culture most problems can be understood in physical and psychological terms. But when seeking to communicate across cultural boundaries, when working with people from different subcultures, it becomes critical to deal with cultural influences on behavior. A missed clinic appointment, for example, may not mean irresponsibility or lack of interest. Instead it might be a highly rational choice in terms of some hidden cultural value, such as a strong orientation to the present. Some women may avoid going to male physicians because of their cultural standards of modesty in the presence of males. A Hmong client may rely on the advice of a shaman instead of consulting with clinic staff. Some mothers may fail to follow recommendations for their children because they believe a condition is actually caused by an "evil eye." If grandmothers or other relatives have authority over the health of children, instructions to mothers alone may be to no avail. If a culture places great emphasis on joint decisions by a group of kinspeople, urging individuals to undergo surgery or other treatments may be a waste of time. Such examples only hint at the many ways in which culture is involved in community health nursing and at the many cultural implications for planning health programs for cross-cultural populations.

One major goal of community health nursing is the prevention of illness. Because prevention involves efforts to change behavior patterns, however, thus changing some aspect of client culture, almost every attempt runs into hidden cultural barriers. Prevention is based on a strong future orientation and a certain degree of optimism about the future. This often contrasts with the present-time orientation and fatalism of many subcultures. Education and teaching for high levels of health may fail because they are based on culture-bound methods of instruction. Some cultures emphasize learning by means of abstract symbols; others stress teaching by active involvement and participation. Unless the community health nurse is aware of how members of different subcultures traditionally learn new things, efforts at teaching are doomed to failure.

In recent years, our awareness of the cultural influences on community health nursing practice has improved considerably. Concomitantly we have developed better tools to assess the needs of culturally diverse groups and to intervene more effectively. The following chapters describe some of these tools and enlarge our understanding of selected cultural practices frequently encountered by community health nurses. They identify ways to enrich nursing practice by identifying and negotiating clients' health care beliefs. Unit VII does not focus on specific cultural groups. It does, however, suggest principles used by community health nurses who have dealt with specific cultural groups and can easily be applied to numerous other subcultures.

Chapter 44

Cultural Assessment: Content and Process

TONI TRIPP-REIMER   PAMELA J. BRINK

JUDITH M. SAUNDERS

> For many years in community health nursing, we have recognized the sig-
> nificance and reality of cultural influences on the health of individuals,
> families, and groups. We have sought to develop an understanding of the
> influence and have attempted to tailor our interventions to the unique cul-
> tural variations of our clients. However, for the most part, a systematic as-
> sessment of clients' cultural beliefs, values, and practices has been ne-
> glected. Too often the community health nurse is pressured by time,
> perhaps unaware of the importance of cultural assessment or possibly un-
> aware of how this is done. As a result, transcultural nursing interventions
> are frequently less than effective. What should the nurse do? Although thor-
> ough study of another cultural system is a major undertaking, the authors of
> this chapter propose that a cultural assessment for nursing purposes is a
> reasonable and manageable task, and they show how it can be done.

Because America is a pluralistic society, nurses need to be prepared to
work with clients from various cultures and to present health care in ways
that are appropriate to each client. Additionally, when nurses understand
specific factors that influence people's health behaviors, they are in a better position to meet their needs. Cultural identification gives a background from which nurses can anticipate client differences in values, religion, dietary practices, lines of authority, family life patterns, and beliefs
and practices related to health and illness. As Affonso points out, cultural
assessments provide meaning to behaviors which might otherwise be
judged in a negative way or continue to be confusing to the nurse.[1] Assessing and understanding cultural variables leads to a better understanding
of patient behavior and the way the patient perceives the illness or health
situation.

Leininger has defined a cultural nursing assessment as a "systematic appraisal or examination of individuals, groups, and communities as to their
cultural beliefs, values, and practices within the cultural context of the

From *Nursing Outlook* 32(2):78–82, 1984. Reprinted by permission of Mosby-Year
Book, Inc.

people being evaluated."[2] Similarly, Tripp-Reimer and brink point out that cultural assessments elicit shared beliefs, values, and customs that have relevance to health behaviors; they are performed to identify patterns that may assist or interfere with a nursing intervention or planned treatment regimen.[3]

The nursing process is heavily dependent on assessment data collection. Yet, what kind of data must be collected for cultural assessment? What does a nurse look for when she is told to "be sure to assess for the cultural variable"?[4] Awareness of and sensitivity to cultural differences among patients and health professionals does not automatically bring clear-cut assessment guidelines.

▬THE CONTENT OF CULTURAL ASSESSMENT

A variety of assessment tools or guides have been devised. They may focus on the individual or the community level; they may be specific to a particular area (e.g., maternal/child health); they may define the areas for cultural assessment narrowly (specific to health/illness concerns) or broadly (encompassing major cultural subsystems).

The most comprehensive tool used for cultural assessment is George Murdock's *Outline of Cultural Materials.*[5] Devised primarily for anthropologists concerned with ethnographic description of a culture group, the *Outline* was originally developed as a tool for the Cross-Cultural Survey, an organization established in 1937 by the Institute of Human Relations at Yale University as part of its program of interdisciplinary research in the social sciences. The *Outline* is divided into 88 categories, each of which contains up to nine major subdivisions (which are similarly divisible). Examples of the 88 major categories include interpersonal relations, marriage, family, kinship, property, finance, fine arts, recreation, law, health and welfare, sickness, death, religious beliefs, and old age. This *Outline* includes the major cultural domains and allows the option of adding additional ones for specific study needs. While not devised as an assessment tool for health professionals, the *Outline of Cultural Materials* provides the most readily available comprehensive treatment for identifying cultural categories.

A second source, Brownlee's *Community, Culture and Care: A Cross-Cultural Guide for Health Workers,* is devoted to the process of practical assessment of a community with specific attention to areas most relevant for health.[6] Each chapter deals with three aspects of assessment: what to find out, why it is important, and how to do it.

However, both the Murdock and Brownlee guides were developed for group assessment and are so comprehensive that they are difficult to use in a clinical setting with individual clients. They do, however, serve as good guides for curriculum planning and community assessments.

In addition to these highly comprehensive sources, a number of cultural assessment guides for nurses have recently become available.[7–14] These guides identify the content areas for assessment. This information is crucial, since one must know what to look for before one can assess it.

These guides were selected for review because they identify major cultural areas that may be important in a variety of clinical settings, Additionally, a number of good assessment tools are available for assessing clients in specific clinical areas, particularly maternal–child health.

The general cultural assessment guides are similar in that they identify major cultural domains that may be important variables in working with culturally distinct clients. Table 44-1 identifies the topical content in each cultural assessment guide, and thus may be used as a reference for nurses wishing to address specific cultural domains. As indicated in Table 44-1, the authors identify many of the same content areas for cultural assessment. In addition, the same two limitations are present in each guide: they are both concerned with obtaining content for cultural assessment, rather than with the process of performing the assessment; and client-specific data are not separated from normative data.

For many clients, a thorough cultural assessment is not necessary; most clients do not need complete assessments in all areas. Complete assessments of all systems (biological, psychological, environmental, and sociocultural) are not routinely performed on all clients because they would be too time consuming and costly for both the practitioner and the client. The point is that cultural data are embedded in many good nursing assessment tools. Basic cultural data include: ethnic affiliation, religious preference, family patterns, food patterns, and ethnic health care practices. For many clients, this will give sufficient information to determine if further, more in-depth assessment of cultural factors is needed. If the client is not adhering to a prescribed or recommended treatment plan, cultural factors may be important. In these cases, a more thorough cultural assessment is warranted.

▬THE PROCESS OF CULTURAL ASSESSMENT

Cultural assessment does not require information on every element of the culture. Nurses need to identify the major values, beliefs, and behaviors as they influence and relate to a particular clinical setting or health problem. Various cultural factors will differ in relative importance depending upon the specific client health problem and nursing intervention. Cultural assessment involves a shared negotiation or contract between client and professional in which each is treated as an equal bringing important and relevant materials to the interview.

Phase I: Data Collection

Phase I is a three-stage data collection process. In stage one, the nurse performs a general assessment that gives an overview of the characteristics of the client and identifies areas of potential need for more in-depth assessment. The nurse treats the client as a cultural informant during the assessment interview making no judgments or conclusions. The nurse attempts to collect the subjective data in the client's own words as much as possible. Objective data are collected as usual without conclusions or generaliza-

TABLE 44-1 Comparison of Cultural Assessment Guides

	BROWNLEE	ORQUE	BLOCH	RUND & KRAUSE	TRIPP-REIMER	LEININGER	KAY	AAMODT	BRANCH & PAXTON
I. Values									
General	X	X	X		X	X		X	X
A. Health	X		X		X	X		X	X
B. Human nature	X	X		X	X	X			
C. Man-nature	X	X			X	X			
D. Time	X	X	X		X				
E. Activity	X	X			X				
F. Relational	X	X	X	X	X				
G. Other	X	X	X	X	X	X		X	
II. Beliefs									
A. Health									
1. Health Maintenance	X	X	X	X	X	X	X	X	X
2. Illness	X	X	X	X	X		X	X	X
a. Cause of Illness	X	X	X	X	X		X	X	X
b. Diagnosis	X	X	X	X	X		X	X	X
c. Treatment	X	X	X	X	X		X	X	X
B. Religious	X	X	X		X	X		X	X
C. Other	X	X	X		X	X		X	X
III. Customs									
A. Communication	X	X	X		X	X		X	
1. Verbal	X	X	X		X			X	
a. Language	X	X	X		X				
b. Tempo	X	X	X		X				
c. Styles of Persuasion	X				X				
d. Other	X	X	X		X			X	
2. Nonverbal	X	X	X		X				
a. Eye Contact	X	X	X		X				
b. Touching	X	X	X		X				
c. Silence	X	X	X		X				
d. Other	X	X	X		X			X	

Component									
B. Decision-making	X	X	X	X		X		X X	X
C. Religious	X	X	X	X		X		X X	X X X
D. Food	X	X	X	X		X			X X
1. Standard Diet	X	X	X			X			X
2. Health Related (Illness/ Developmental)	X	X	X			X			X
E. Family interactions	X	X	X	X		X		X	X X X
1. Roles	X	X	X	X		X			X X X
2. Other	X	X		X		X			X X
F. Grief/dying	X	X	X	X		X			X X
G. Sick role (patient role)	X	X	X	X		X			X
H. Other	X	X	X	X		X		X	X
IV. Social Structure Components									
A. Family structure	X	X	X	X		X		X	X X
B. Religion	X	X	X	X		X		X	X X
C. Politics	X	X	X	X					
D. Economic	X	X	X	X		X			X
E. Education	X	X	X	X		X			X
F. Available health systems	X	X	X	X		X		X	X
1. Orthodox	X		X	X		X		X	X X
2. Alternative	X	X	X	X		X		X	X X
a. Practitioners	X	X	X	X		X		X	X
b. Facilities	X	X	X	X		X		X	X X
G. Ethnic affiliation	X	X	X	X		X			
H. Art	X	X	X	X					
I. History	X	X		X					X
J. Physical environment	X	X		X				X	
K. Culture change	X	X	X		X	X			
L. Other	X	X		X		X			X

tions. In stage one, data should be collected about the client's background (e.g., ethnicity, degree of affiliation with ethnic group, religion, and patterns of decision making). Data should also be collected about content that may influence the interaction between the client and the nurse (e.g., language, styles of communication—verbal and nonverbal—and norms of etiquette).

In stage two, the nurse elicits problem-specific cultural information. Here the nurse is interested in content associated with a particular health area, such as prenatal classes, diabetic diet teaching, mental health counseling, or preschool immunizations. During this stage the nurse elicits the client's subjective reason for seeking the health professional and ideas about the problem as well as the client's previous and anticipated treatment. In this step, the nurse may find the following questions helpful:

1. What do you think has caused your problem?
2. Why do you think it started when it did?
3. What does your sickness do to you; how does it work?
4. How severe is your sickness? Will it have a long or short duration?
5. What kind of treatment do you think you should receive?
6. What are the most important results you hope to receive from this treatment?
7. What are the chief problems your sickness had caused you?
8. What do you fear about your sickness?[15]

Stage three takes place after a nursing diagnosis has been made and is directed at cultural factors that may influence intervention strategies. For example, the nurse may ask about the client's traditional diet when planning nutritional education.

The following set of questions may be used to elicit the necessary information:

1. Is this condition (e.g., pregnancy) good or bad?
2. What have you been doing for this problem/condition in the past and presently?
3. What do you plan to do?
4. How should a person who has this condition/problem act?
5. How should one who has this condition/problem be treated by family members?

Phase II: Data Organization

In this phase, the cultural content material is placed in context; it is a process of data organization. This may occur concurrently with the steps in Phase I. A thorough cultural assessment differs from assessments of systems that have generally accepted standards. The purpose of assessing biological and psychological domains is to determine where deviations occur from normal, and then to bring the client into alignment with the "standards." For cultural assessments, the purpose is different. Here, the assessment is done to identify deviations in cultural parameters with the goal of modifying the client's system *or* modifying the health care professional's system in order to increase congruence between them.

Phase II is more complex than biological or psychological assessments. The nurse is interested in the extent to which the client's beliefs, values, and customs are congruent with a trifold set of standards.

- standards of the client's identified culture or ethnic group;
- standards of the nurse's own culture;
- standards of the health care facility that serves as the setting for the interaction.

If areas of incongruence are identified, the nurse needs to find out if the client's system is adaptive (beneficial), neutral, or maladaptive (harmful) in relation to possible interventions. If the client's system is adaptive or neutral, it can be incorporated into the plan for intervention. For example, parenting practices, food preferences, pain expression, or adherence to fixed time schedules may vary from those of the nurse's culture or those of the health care facility, but would still fit into the treatment plan. In this case, they can be directly incorporated into the plan, making it more congruent for the client. If, on the other hand, the nurse determines that the client's beliefs, values, and customs are detrimental to achieving the desired health outcomes, the nurse needs to determine: a) ways of persuasion that aid alteration of the client system if the client is amenable to change; or b) ways of understanding the client and the rationale for not altering the client's system, if the client will not change.

Cultural assessment differs from other assessment areas in that the health professional must obtain normative data from the client as well as the client's individual problem focus. Behavioral norms and concomitant beliefs and values, unlike physiological norms, are not readily available for all the possible ethnic or cultural groups in the world. All norms for all groups related to health and illness have not been collected and conveniently made available to nurses.

Also, cultural assessment is reflexive. First, data are obtained on how the client perceives the values, customs, and beliefs for the identified cultural or ethnic group. Second, data are collected on how the particular client fits within those normative patterns. This latter assessment, however, occurs *after* the initial assessment and nursing diagnosis and during the planning phase of the intervention. Table 44-2 illustrates how data from Phase I can be recorded in each of the three stages. This table further illustrates how data from Phase I are organized in Phase II according to congruence with the client's identified group, the nurse, and the health care facility.

Cultural assessments are both content and process. They begin with awareness of cultural richness and diversity and lead to culturally relevant nursing diagnoses that give direction to nursing intervention. Each part of cultural assessment requires basic data collection and data processing to arrive at a tentative nursing diagnosis and intervention plan. Further, each part requires processing this data before and after the nursing diagnosis is made. However, it is the initial assessment that leads to judgments about

TABLE 44-2   The Process of Cultural Assessment

PHASE I: ASSESSING CULTURE CONTENT OF CLIENT'S SYSTEM

	Stage 1: Background Assessment Variables	Stage 2: Problem Specific Variables	Stage 3: Intervention Specific Variables
VALUES	V^1	V^2	V^3
BELIEFS	B^1	B^2	B^3
CUSTOMS	C^1	C^2	C^3

PHASE II: PLACING CULTURE CONTENT IN CONTEXT

		Client's Identified Group's System	Nurse's System	Health Care Facility System
VALUES	V^1			
	V^2			
	V^3			
BELIEFS	B^1			
	B^2			
	B^3			
CUSTOMS	C^1			
	C^2			
	C^3			

$\approx$ = congruent $\neq$ = incongruent

the nature and context of the problem and thus shapes the process that follows.

REFERENCES

1. Affonso, D. Framework for cultural assessment. In *Childbearing: A Nursing Perspective,* 2nd edition edited by A. L. Clark. Philadelphia, F. A. Davis Co., 1979, pp. 107–119.
2. Leininger, M. Culturological assessment domains for nursing practices. In *Transcultural Nursing: Concepts, Theories and Practices,* ed. by M. Leininger. New York, John Wiley & Sons, 1977, pp. 86–87.

3. Tripp-Reimer, T., and Brink, P. Cultural brokerage. In *Nursing Interventions: Treatments for Nursing Diagnoses,* ed. by G. Bulechek and J. McCloskey. Philadelphia, W. B. Saunders Co., 1985.

4. Brink, P. J., ed. *Transcultural Nursing: A Book of Readings.* Englewood Cliffs, N.J., Prentice-Hall, 1976.

5. Murdock, G., and others. *Outline of Cultural Materials.* 4th rev. ed. New Haven, Conn., Human Relations Area Files, 1971.

6. Brownlee, A. T. *Community, Culture, and Care: A Cross-Cultural Guide for Health Workers.* St. Louis, The C. V. Mosby Co., 1978.

7. Leininger, *op. cit.,* pp. 85–106.

8. Aamodt, A. Culture. In *Culture, Childbearing, Health Professionals,* ed. by A. L. Clark, Philadelphia, F. A. Davis Co., 1978, pp. 2–9.

9. Branch, M. F., and Paxton, P. P., eds. *Providing Safe Nursing Care for Ethnic People of Color.* Englewood Cliffs, N.J., Prentice-Hall, 1976.

10. Bloch, B. Bloch's assessment guide for ethnic/culture variations. In *Ethnic Nursing Care: A Multi-Cultural Approach,* ed. by M. S. Orque and B. Bloch. St. Louis, The C. V. Mosby Co., 1983, pp. 49–75.

11. Orque, M. Orque's ethnic/cultural system: a framework for ethnic nursing care. In *Ethnic Nursing Care: A Multi-Cultural Approach,* ed. by M. S. Orque and B. Bloch. St. Louis, The C. V. Mosby Co., 1983, pp. 5–48.

12. Kay, M. Clinical anthropology. In *The Anthropology of Health,* ed. by E. E. Bauwens. St. Louis, The C. V. Mosby Co., 1978, pp. 3–11.

13. Rund, N. and Krause, L. Health attitudes and your health program. In *The Anthropology of Health,* ed. by E. E. Bauwens. St. Louis, The C. V. Mosby Co., 1978, pp. 73–78.

14. Tripp-Reimer, T. Cultural assessment. In *Nursing Assessment,* ed. by J. Bellack and P. Bamford. North Scituate, Mass., Duxbury Press, in press.

15. Kleinman, A., and others. Culture, illness and care: clinical lessons from anthropologic and cross-cultural research. *Ann. Intern. Med.* 88:251–258, February 1978.

Chapter 45

An Empowerment Approach to Community Health Education

MAUREEN E. BRAGG

The author of this chapter describes an innovative approach to health education among a group of Native Americans. The process can work as effectively with any group in the community; success lies within the skills of the group facilitator. Here is a unique opportunity for the community health nurse to use her or his skills in group dynamics along with concepts of group empowerment. Maureen Bragg takes the reader through a step-by-step approach to group work which focuses on group ownership and control; change comes from within and not from values which are externally assumed and applied by the health care provider, a mistake frequently made by caregivers. Application of the process is demonstrated through an ongoing project within the author's agency, and the results are shared here.

Community health nurses use the tool of health education with many culturally diverse populations. The goal of community-based health education is to help people acquire the knowledge and skills which will enable them to practice healthy lifestyles. This cannot be accomplished by merely distributing brochures, viewing videos, or providing presentations or lectures. Health education is empowering people to understand who they are, where they come from, and what they and their community can be.

An empowerment model for health education programs is defined as a social-action process that promotes the participation of people, organizations, and communities in gaining control within the larger society (Wallerstein and Bernstein, 1988).

Because we live in a culturally diverse society it is imperative that these programs be culturally relevant. Health educators or public health nurses (PHNs) need to design programs that build on the strengths of the values, beliefs, and attitudes of the communities where they work. This requires extensive research involving meetings with community leaders and including the leaders in the design and implementation of the program. There is no "one size fits all" community-health strategy or program.

This chapter was especially written for this edition of this book.

504

Prevention and education activities must be consistent with the priorities and values of each community (Green, 1988). Programs should include cultural activities that provide an alternative to dysfunctional behavior, increase community awareness of the benefits of a healthy lifestyle, and strengthen social interchange within the community.

An emerging trend among community-based health programs is the increase in program ownership—both perceived and actual—by community organizations, rather than by outside delivery systems. This orientation (Thomas, 1990) establishes community partnerships composed of institutions, organizations, and interest groups that collaborate on each aspect of program planning and implementation.

There are five basic steps in designing and implementing effective community health programs:

1. Identify barriers
2. Obtain community input
3. Create community support
4. Acknowledge community ownership
5. Provide technical assistance

▬STEP ONE: IDENTIFY BARRIERS

Barriers can be geographical, socioeconomic, cultural, and/or educational. When working with minority populations the most common barriers are:

- Language
- Limited transportation
- Low literacy levels
- Lack of child care
- Low self esteem
- Poverty and unemployment

Orlandi (1986) identifies the complicated and complicating factors in the two final barriers:

- Entropy: the tendency for community members to perceive themselves as powerless when confronted with enormous economic and sociocultural barriers and to express a lack of motivation to engage in self-improvement activities.
- Relevance of health promotion: the belief that more pressing concerns such as poverty and unemployment should be addressed prior to the health promotion campaign.

In meetings with community leaders, other obstacles specific to the individual community may emerge, preventing community participation and interest. That these barriers be recognized and addressed before pursuing a program is imperative. Failure to take this step may jeopardize the future of any intervention.

▬STEP TWO: OBTAIN COMMUNITY INPUT

There are many ways to accomplish community input, including:

- Holding one-on-one meetings with community leaders.
- Conducting community needs assessments. Needs assessment is a process by which information and data are collected and analyzed to identify the needs and problems (perceived or actual) within the community. This process must be inclusive and collaborative and ultimately build concensus on how best to meet community education needs (McKay, 1986).
- Attending community meetings, gatherings, events.
- Conducting focus groups. Focus groups are a research tool that enable you to ask the people you want to reach—your target audience— what they think and how they feel about a particular subject (HIV, brochures, etc.). Groups are small, usually 8–12 people who meet with a moderator for 1–2 hours (Greenbaum, 1987).

When obtaining community input, focus on barriers to the program and solutions to those barriers, as well as the community's perceived health needs or priorities. These needs and priorities may determine the level of future participation in the program.

For example, poverty and unemployment may be a top concern. One solution would be to incorporate job-training skills within the program. Another obstacle could be child care. Establishing a room or section at the meeting location where trained teens care for and entertain the children may provide a solution.

Other basic community input might include dates, times, and meeting locations convenient for the majority; and, for political reasons, which local leaders should be contacted.

▬STEP THREE: CREATE COMMUNITY SUPPORT

Find out what will motivate people to participate in the program. For some it could be incentives: baseball caps or t-shirts. A contest could be held to give a culturally relevant name to the program as well as a contest to design its logo. Place the winning name and logo on the incentives, and honor the winners at a community event by presenting them with framed certificates of recognition.

▬STEP FOUR: ACKNOWLEDGE COMMUNITY OWNERSHIP

Community involvement is the backbone of health programs. The community must be involved in every aspect of program planning and implementation. There must be shared decision-making, mutual respect, and trust. The health educator or PHN must become a facilitator–consultant and not be perceived by the community as an outside, self-aggrandizing authority figure. The community must feel it is an integral part of the process.

The PHN or health educator must work with the community to develop collaborative programs and activities that meet their mutual goals and priorities.

▬STEP FIVE: PROVIDE TECHNICAL ASSISTANCE

To ensure the program will continue long after initial funding is exhausted, training should be included as part of the program. This training can consist of grant writing and fundraising, important tools the community can use to obtain funds from private foundations and public agencies.

Another important aspect of training should be incorporated throughout the program: leadership development. This will create a pool of community leaders who are trained and motivated to keep the program operative.

▬SAMPLE PROGRAM

The following example is based on the above five-step process for creating effective community health programs.

Central Valley Indian Health (CVIH), a comprehensive Indian Health Service program in Central California, was awarded in July 1995 a grant for a project: "Health Education Through the Arts." Two years of preparation went into this program.

1. Identify Barriers

Initially, the CVIH Outreach Department identified community leaders in its six service areas. Next, formal and informal meetings were held with them, the core topic being the lack of participation by a large percentage of the community in self-help programs past and present. The causal factors identified were common to most of the six areas:

Limited Transportation. Most of the population lived in isolated rural areas. Public transportation didn't service their area, and few members of the community owned or had access to a private vehicle. In turn, they couldn't attend activities held outside their immediate territory.

Poverty/Unemployment. The jobless rate topped 34% in most of these communities. The high-school dropout rate surged past 30%.

Relevance of the Activities. With people up against pressing, primal concerns like food, shelter, jobs and the like, a program regarding the health risks of tobacco or substance abuse didn't exactly command center stage.

Entropy. The despairing and pervasive worldview among most of the target population was that no matter what programs or activities they support, no change will come: They will remain poor, unemployed, and powerless.

Ageism. Past programs have targeted youths ages six to 14—ignoring all other age groups.

2. Obtain Community Input

Community input has made clear that future programs and activities must address the aforementioned issues to garner support and participation. Indeed, a successful program would have to:

- hold activities in or near the six communities.
- provide job-skill training.
- develop cultural and economic autonomy and strength.
- build individual and communal self-esteem.
- involve community members of all ages.

Given these findings, the Outreach Department subsequently set up health-information booths at community gatherings, pow-wows, and events sponsored by related agencies.

Along with brochures and posters dealing with diabetes, substance abuse, cancer, and other health related topics, a community-needs assessment form was offered to attendees; to encourage their completing the form, staff members gave them free raffle tickets for prizes that included t-shirts, baseball caps, and tote bags.

The key results of the needs assessment were as follows: A successful new program will:

- promote traditional Native American values of love, honor, and respect.
- include Native American stories, myths, and legends.
- allow the community to participate in the design and execution of the activities.
- offer a life-nurturing alternative to corrosive behavior like substance abuse.

Based on these results, the Outreach Department held more meetings with the community: tribal chairs, spiritual leaders, elders, youth leaders, tribal councils, and community-health representatives.

The meetings spurred the design of a new program anchored to the use of the arts to encourage healthy behavior.

3. Create Community Support

A community-wide contest was subsequently held to design the new program's logo and to give it a culturally relevant name. Entries came from all over the service area.

The winners received a cash award and, more importantly, were honored at the agency's New Year's Eve Pow-Wow. In addition, the winning logo and name were affixed to incentives: t-shirts, tote bags, baseball caps, and coffee mugs.

The winning name, *Quara Mia-weh,* is Mono Indian for "Going Far." Members chose it because they felt they'd be going far on two levels: the spiritual and the physical.

The winning design is two lines of Indian people of all ages holding hands. This was picked because members believed that working together would spark their growing together in spirit.

4. Acknowledge Community Ownership

Theater troupes were formed in three of the service areas, the members ranging in age from four to 67 years old. The three areas were determined by community interest and commitment. Each troupe elected a chair, secretary, and treasurer, and determined meeting dates, times, and places.

All troupes were taught basic fundraising techniques (bake sales, raffles, and so on), and all controlled money they raised. Routine expenditures include gasoline and food for meetings; but a big fundraiser is being planned to buy renowned Sioux-designed tepees, which will be used for camping when the troupes travel to other parts of the state to perform.

The health educator, meanwhile, is the agency program director for this grant. This role is nontraditional in that the educator is a consultive facilitator—not an authority figure—and is perceived as such.

The troupes meet one to two times weekly; the health educator attends one to two times monthly. All meetings are held in or near the service area where members live.

Troupe decisions result from the democratic process, during which members learn group dynamics: communication and negotiation techniques, peaceful conflict resolution, decision-making, goal formulation, planning, and organizing.

All of these skills play a critical role in boosting each individual's positive self-esteem and in giving each a fighting chance in the job market.

In concert with the positive effects of this dynamic, invitations to perform are being received from tribes in three states. Each troupe meets and decides which invitations it wants to accept.

The plays themselves are based on traditional American Indian values: love, honor, respect. Each play, in turn, focuses on a healthy community behavior common to American Indians prior to the European invasion—a behavior that enabled individuals and tribes to survive and flourish.

Those behaviors, gleaned from local storytellers, myths, legends and histories (written and oral) are then shown to be just as vital to existence and self-fulfillment in today's world.

All plays are written and directed by the members with assistance from the health educator.

5. Provide Technical Assistance

A local cable-television company provides technical training in video camera operating and tape editing. A local high school drama department teaches the troupes theater lighting, sound, and staging. And a local university holds workshops in grant writing, thus ensuring the program has the ability to continue long after the initial funding is exhausted.

▬ RESULTS/FINDINGS

The members of the theater group learned the basics of fundraising. Their first two raffles raised almost $3000. This money covered travel expenses (eg, gas and food) during their statewide performances. In addition, the money went for food serviced at meetings and rehearsals.

Participants also learned important life and job skills:

- self expression and communication
- the art of compromise
- negotiating skills
- planning and organizing techniques
- peaceful conflict resolution

Some unplanned, unexpected outcomes occurred with the teen participants. Their overall reading aptitude showed dramatic improvement. Also, because their scriptwriting involved research, they became more familiar with how to use their school and public libraries, including the reference desk and computerized card catalogue.

In the meantime, the most important outcome of the program was expressed by a 13-year-old participant: "Now I really believe I can become whatever I want to be—and I want to be a nurse."

Successful community health programs, then, can be a critical education tool. Moreover, launching such programs doesn't require superhuman talent; however it does require finding out what community members want—and then giving it to them.

To do so, the nurse must meet with the community and listen carefully to what members perceive as both their needs and the barriers to fulfilling them. Next, the nurse must work with members to develop solutions to their problems and then connect them to competent and sympathetic resources in their area.

Finally, this: If a community perceives it genuinely "owns" a program, it is, quite logically, more apt to strive for the program's success.

▬ REFERENCES

Green, L.W. (1988). Bridging the Gap Between Community Health and School Health. *American Journal of Public Health 78*:1149.

Greenbaum, Thomas L. (1987). *The Practical Handbook and Guide to Focus Group Research.* Lexington, MA: Lexington Books.

McKay, Emily G. (1986). *Developing a Community Needs Assessment.* National Council of La Raza, Washington, D.C.

Orlandi, Mario A. (1986). Community-based Substance Abuse Prevention: A Multicultural Perspective. *Journal of School Health 56*(9): 394–401.

Thomas, S.B. (1990). Community Health Advocacy for Racial and Ethnic Minorities in the United States: Issues and Challenges for Health Education. *Health Education Quarterly 7*(1): 13–19.

Wallerstein, N., and E. Bernstein. (1988). Empowerment Education: Freire's Ideas Adapted to Health Education. *Health Education Quarterly 15*(4):379–394.

Chapter 46

Cultural Relativity and Poverty

MIRIAM E. MARTIN   MARSHELLE HENRY

People living in poverty are a population of concern to community health nurses. Often though, poverty is the only characteristic the poor share, for their cultural orientations, values, beliefs, practices, and needs vary. In order to avoid ethnocentric judgments and provide the most effective nursing services to the poor, nurses must maintain a culturally relativistic perspective. Miriam Martin and Marshelle Henry discuss the importance of understanding clients' behaviors within the context of their own cultures. They suggest ways in which nurses can do this, using a helpful case study to illustrate culturally relative practice.

Although Lewis (1971) referred to the culture of poverty in describing the lifestyles of poor people a number of years ago, current viewpoints do not support the notion that social class connotes a cultural group (Tripp-Reimer, 1984). In fact, misconceptions about the poor can be reinforced by using a culture of poverty model (Mason, 1981; Moccia & Mason, 1986; Stumpf, 1983). These misconceptions can lead to incomplete assessment for health care needs because behaviors are prejudged. Cultural categories can be used, however, to outline and describe lifestyle and health behaviors of individuals and families living in poverty. Furthermore, a culturally relativistic approach to understanding clients who are "different" from health professionals can improve the quality of care and clients' receptiveness to it. Excessive emphasis on developing trust and rapport (Stumpf, 1983, p. 230) would be less necessary if care providers were culturally relativistic in interacting with clients from other cultures, socioeconomic groups, or value systems.

Tripp-Reimer (1984) stated, "From a culturally relativistic perspective the caregiver would attempt to understand the behavior of transcultural clients within the context of the clients' own culture." Such an approach is essential if health professionals do not judge client behavior from their own cultural standards, and if effective communication with clients is to be achieved. Too often health behaviors and family interactions are observed and interpreted from care providers' viewpoints (Mason, 1981; Pesz-

From *Public Health Nursing* 6(1):28–34, 1989. Reprinted by permission of Blackwell Scientific Publications, Inc.

necker, 1984; Stumpf, 1983). When clients' perspectives are not valued or sought, ethnocentric judgments and actions often follow.

Community nurses often work with families that have been intergenerationally dependent on the social and economic resources of the community. The ethnic characteristics of these clients vary from community to community (Bullough & Bullough, 1972), however, the pattern often includes several generations within the same household, who receive public assistance for food, shelter, and health care. Nurses and other health care providers sometimes stereotype these families as "freeloaders," lacking initiative, and being unwilling or unable to learn a "better way of life" (Bullough & Bullough, 1972; Mason, 1981). In any case, the label of poverty often accompanies these families.

■ VALUES, BELIEFS, AND CUSTOMS

Tripp-Reimer's model of cultural strata (Fig. 46-1) shows that customs are based on beliefs, and beliefs are rooted in values. Values are the most elusive of these three concepts. Often persons are unaware of their values even when they can articulate their beliefs and customs. Past, present, or future time orientation; the issue of valuing doing versus being; and relational patterns are value areas that influence health behaviors of individu-

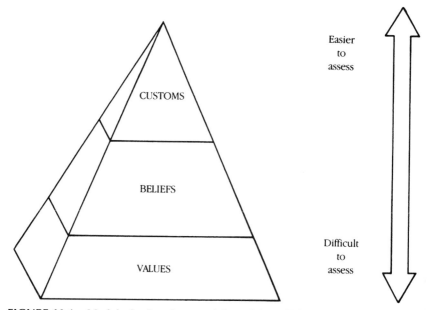

FIGURE 46-1   Model of cultural strata. Adapted from Tripp-Reimer, T. (1984). Cultural assessment. In J. Bellack & P. Bamford (Eds.), *Nursing assessment: A multidimensional approach*. Monterey: Wadsworth Health Sciences. Reproduced by permission of the publisher.

als, families, and groups. Beliefs about illness causation and one's own control over health care outcomes are important to the lifestyle associated with poverty. Although beliefs can be verbalized by many, they are not objectively observable. Therefore, open, judgment-free dialogue between the clients and nurses is essential if client perception of health needs and problems is to be ascertained.

On the other hand, customs (or behaviors) can be observed and described by an objective outsider. For example, they can be observed and recorded by the nurse when making a health assessment and can contribute to the data base used in planning nursing action. It is important also to validate the meaning of observed behaviors in communicating with clients. The nurse working with a family in poverty can approach the relationship from a culturally relativistic perspective by obtaining information about family customs such as dietary practices, communication patterns, kinship relations, religious practices, and health care behaviors.

▬ CASE STUDY

The A family was a rural, midwestern family that had few resources with which to break the intergenerational cycle of poverty. Although they had been involved with social service and nursing agencies for several years, this case study describes them while they were assisted for several months by a nursing student working in a community nursing agency for part of her clinical experience.

Mr. and Mrs. A and their six children lived in a two-bedroom trailer on the edge of a small town. Mr. A was a laborer at a local feed store and Mrs. A received AFDC for the two youngest children. The community nursing agency had been working with the family for two years, since the birth of the youngest child. When the community nurse visited, concerns about parenting behaviors and questions of child neglect were raised because the family had experienced lack of food, many moribund and active cockroaches were present in the trailer, and the children were often scantily dressed, even in winter.

The student's goal in working with the family was to learn the family's perception of their health status and needs. Her observations are outlined using the custom categories mentioned above.

Dietary Practices

Portions and types of food available for family consumption were dependent on the time of the month. At the beginning of the month, the refrigerator was full. Milk and meat were plentiful. Carbohydrates were abundant; many loaves of bread and boxes of pancake mix were on the kitchen counter. Although fresh fruits and vegetables were not present during the home visits, canned vegetables and fruits were usually available. Toward the middle of the month the food availability decreased. Pancakes, macaroni and cheese, and canned vegetables became the dietary mainstays. At the end of the month the refrigerator, cupboards, and counter were empty.

Throughout the month, the only meal of the day that was at a regular time was lunch, which was prepared to coincide with Mr. A's break from work. He sat down for the meal, and the children ate after he returned to work. The family rarely sat at the table for a meal, and food was often eaten while standing or sitting in the living room area. Many times the children would skip meals. Later, they would go to the store an buy candy with change given them by Mrs. A. Sometimes the children would find food for themselves when the parents were absent from the home. For example, one afternoon the 5-year-old pierced a can of peas with a can opener, and he and the 2-year-old drank the juice.

Communication Patterns

A hierarchy existed in the communication patterns. Mr. A talked very little to visitors. He gave directions to others through Mrs. A. She then talked to visitors and to the teenage daughter. The daughter, who was responsible for the younger children when both parents were away, in turn gave instructions to the younger children. She also was allowed to deal with guests, such as the nurse, when the mother was absent. The younger children's communications were directed upward through their older siblings. No family member gave personal or family information to outsiders. Indeed, they related very cautiously to the nursing student.

Family and Kinship Relations

Most of the extended family lived within the county, and the oldest daughter often babysat for her many cousins. Mrs. A frequently visited her mother-in-law, and cousins often stopped by. Occasionally, relatives would stay for days or weeks at a time. Social events took place within the bounds of the extended family—birthday parties, watching television, or excursions to the tavern. When problems arose, family members were the first, and usually the only, resources to be consulted. On those occasions when it was perceived that a family member had been insulted by an outsider, the whole family would consider the outsider as an enemy.

Religious Practices

The A family did not attend church but occasionally made reference to an ultimate plan or order. While discussing a death in the community, Mrs. A and her daughter both agreed that "when it's your time to go, it's your time to go." If asked to explain the cause of certain events, the reply was often, "That's just the way it is."

Health Behaviors

One or more of the children had a runny nose most of the time. Colds and fevers were routinely ignored. When the symptoms of an ailment became severe enough to cause unpleasant behavior changes in a child, medical attention was sought. Most often, the child was taken to the local family practice physician.

▬BELIEFS

Observation of the approach of those in poverty to the health care system reveals that there are beliefs specific to the poor. These beliefs make the strongest case for the nurse's need to be culturally relativistic. It is important to recognize that the poor are often treated differently by health care providers than their middle-class or affluent counterparts.

> *Professional health workers are themselves middle class and represent and defend its values, and show its biases. They assume that the poor (like themselves) have regular meals, lead regular lives, try to support families, keep healthy, plan for the future. They prescribe the same treatment for the same diseases to all, not realizing that their words do not mean the same things at all. (What does "take with each meal" mean to a family that eats irregularly, seldom together and usually less than three times a day?) (Strauss, 1979, pp. 17–18)*

It is not surprising that the poor seek care less often than others and that they distrust health care workers. They often see helping professionals as ". . . meddle-some, interfering with the individual's ability and right to decide on his/her own how to handle problems, set priorities, make compromises and devise substitutes. A related and commonly held perception is that many agencies employ threats—of cutting off financial support, of reporting disapproved behavior to other agencies or of removing children from their parents" (Fitchner, 1981, p. 174). The poor often see the world as a we-they duality. "In this dualistic view, 'we' or 'us' is defined as 'our neighbors, relatives and friends who are struggling as we are' or succinctly, 'the people at the bottom'" (Fitchner, 1981, p. 169). "They" are everyone else, the outside world, including health professionals who wish to help.

The A family was no exception to these beliefs. The teenage daughter took her role as the family's "secret keeper" very seriously in the absence of her parents. She talked freely about impersonal things; however, if family-centered questions arose she would answer. "I don't know." Until later in the relationship with the student, Mrs. A did not reveal feelings about her involvement with the health care agency. Later, she expressed fear that her children could be removed from the home. She said that her usual nurse did not understand being poor or having such a large family. She once talked of moving to the next county. Although she knew that eventually the new county could insist on social service and nursing involvement, she felt a reprieve from "interference" from health professionals would be good for her family.

▬VALUES

Although values are the most difficult of the cultural components to assess, many of those specific to the impoverished in society have been documented.

Time Orientation

Whereas mainstream middle-class Americans have a future orientation and are willing to put off gratification, the poor are often present oriented and see no plausible reason for delaying gratification (Fitchner, 1981; Gladwin, 1967; Jaco & Palgreen, 1975; Seward, 1872). Seward (1972) explained, "The chief concern is with living now—getting the daily bread and enjoying the satisfaction the moment yields" (p. 45). This was true in the A family. Even when little money was available, the children were allowed to buy candy and potato chips. At the beginning of the month the family would make a trip to the next town for pizza and ice cream. Middle-class observers might argue that the money would have been better used to provide more nutritious food at the end of the month. That simply was not how this family functioned. The pizza and ice cream were enjoyable experiences that brought immediate gratification.

Activity Orientation
The poor are generally more oriented toward the importance of being rather than the importance of doing (Centers, 1949; Irelan & Besner, 1967; Kahl, 1959). Just getting by or making it is an accomplishment in itself. Even though this family was living in what many would consider substandard conditions, their view was that they had a home and food, in whatever shape or form, and that was a significant accomplishment. Their assessment was that they were making it, which was in conflict with the assessment of the health care professionals working with them.

Relational Orientation
The middle class tends to emphasize the importance of the individual, while the poor often place greater importance on the family. The extended family also is more evident in poor families (Reul, 1974). The A family functioned as a unit to fight the outside system. This approach is often referred to as an inflexible family boundary system. For example, when the teenage daughter felt that the pressure she received at school about her attire and hygiene was no longer tolerable, she dropped out after the eighth grade. The family supported her decision, viewing it as an appropriate response to not being one of "them."

Another aspect of relational orientation is the perceived importance of children versus that of the parents. In the middle-class nuclear family, children are usually the pivotal focus. Parents, especially mothers, schedule work days around the children's schedules. With the poor, the focus is often on the adults, and the children learn to accommodate to the adult schedules (Reul, 1974; Waxman, 1977). For example, in the A family, lunch was served because the father was home then. He received the first helpings of food and sat at the table to eat. The children were given the food that was left over and usually ate in front of the television.

▄APPLYING CULTURAL THEORY
Hasty moral decisions can be made when interacting with persons who are impoverished. Indeed, Lewis (1971, p. 22) pointed out that middle-class people often focus on the negative aspects of poverty:

They tend to have negative feelings about traits such as an emphasis on the present and a neglect of the future, or on concrete as against abstract orientations. I do not intend to idealize or romanticize the culture of poverty. As someone has said, "It is easier to praise poverty than to live it." However, we must not overlook some of the positive aspects that may flow from these traits.

The A family had strengths. The mother and older daughter spent a major portion of their day playing with the younger children, the children interacted happily, and, once she was considered "safe," the nursing student was accepted as being "one of us." For example, she was invited to watch the husband compete in an arm-wrestling match, was drawn into conversations about friends and neighbors, and was given a bead bracelet that had been made by the teenage daughter.

It is essential that nurses recognize that families in poverty have strengths in spite of their hardships. Furthermore, the impersonal approach sometimes present in bureaucratic systems is not effective when working with poor clients. Several authors keyed in on the importance of the client identifying with the health professional as "my" worker.

The client may place emphasis on the relationship between himself and the professional worker as an individual, not as an interchangeable member of the agency staff. A client who feels comfortable with a particular agency worker may feel that the worker in some sense belongs to him, and may be particularly upset by being switched to another caseworker within the same agency. (Fitchner, 1981, p. 175)

Fitchner (1981) also explained that the 9-to-5 Monday-through-Friday work week, with its 50-minute hours, can have deleterious effects on the clients. "The client may also feel, perhaps unconsciously, that whenever he needs help, the worker should be available to him, rather than being available only during business hours and by appointment" (p. 175).

In accordance with the doing orientation of the middle class, of which most health professionals are members, nurses tend to judge progress with the clients in terms of the number of interventions implemented. With the A family, the community health nurse and the social worker had collaborated to develop a lengthy plan to eradicate the problems they had identified in this family: nutritional deficit, impaired home maintenance, alteration in parenting, and potential for cognitive impairment in the children. The interventions included homemaker visits twice weekly, nutritional and child care teaching by the nurse, and social worker follow-up visits every month. This family was given goals to accomplish: cockroaches were to be exterminated, clothes were to be washed and put away every Monday, and counters were to be free of dirty dishes and garbage at each visit by a health professional. Although this plan was action oriented, it served to compound further the we-they duality that already existed with the A family; it is another case of "us" getting directives from "them." It was clear that the family was only involved minimally, if at all, in determining what the problems and interventions were.

The nursing student believed that working to alter behaviors was less of a priority than establishing a working relationship with this family, which could later be used to mobilize existing strengths. The student derived her interventions from the nursing diagnosis: ineffective nurse–client relationship. Communication strategies were employed to deal with this diagnosis.

■ COMMUNICATION STRATEGIES

As mentioned, different groups have distinct communication customs. The culturally relativistic nurse uses the knowledge about the customs of a specific client to enhance communication with that client. With the A family, the nursing student understood the importance of silence and minimal verbalization concerning certain topics, and the use of nonverbal communication with the family. She also ascertained that a certain amount of self-disclosure might be appropriate.

Silence or Minimal Verbalization

In a study of a white, blue-collar neighborhood on Chicago's south side, it was found that speech is not valued equally in all social contexts or among all cultural groups. "In Teamsterville, talk is negatively valued in many of the very situations for which other American communities most highly prize speaking strategies" (Philipsen, 1975). As an example, a white-collar man who talks things through with a boss, wife, or child is culturally supported for this behavior. For the Teamsterville man, however, talking things through was not acceptable behavior. Furthermore, the poor prefer action to philosophizing, and give little credence or respect to intellectualization (Bernstein, 1960; Irelan & Besner, 1967; Miller & Riessman, 1961).

The impoverished often find little meaning in the spoken word; they hear too many false promises. In addition, although they may be spoken to politely, they believe that those same polite people will later gossip about them (Fitchner, 1981; Reul, 1974). For these reasons, many of those nursing care plans that recommend helping the client verbalize feelings may be inappropriate. A clear example of this was Mrs. A's resistance to talking about how she felt about the plan the social worker and the nurse had established for her. She agreed with whoever was making the home visit, promising to comply with the plan, but did nothing to achieve its goals. Her nonverbal message was clear, "I don't like your plan," at the same time that her verbal message was polite and compliant. Instead of expecting this client to verbalize feelings and wishes in the traditional middle-class therapeutic model, professionals must hear the unspoken message.

Nonverbal Communication

Related to the perception that the outside world sees them as less than human, the poor often are skilled at picking up on nonverbal signals that communicate this message, intentionally or not. For example, the student's first inclination in this home was to not sit on the sofa and not to hold the children because of the unclean conditions. This could have been a nonverbal communication to the family that they were unacceptable. In allowing the 2- and 5-year-olds to sit in the same chair with her, the student made friends. Later the teenage daughter told visitors that the student was "O.K." because "she likes kids." This small nonverbal gesture went a long way in helping to minimize the we-they duality. Daniel (1982, p. 148) explained the impact of other nonverbal messages:

> *When a professional makes a poor person wait for six hours in order to obtain a food order for hungry children, when a professional fiddles with papers on his desk while the poor person is talking to him, when the professional works in the poor neighborhood but lives in the suburbs, and when the professional comes to the poor person's home wearing a facial expression of fear and disgust, the translation of these messages, by the poor person, may lead to a break in the communication relationship between the poor and the professional person.*

Need for Disclosure

How is it that health professionals can expect clients to share the intimate details of life with them, details the clients fear may be repulsive to listeners, while they, the professionals, remain strangers? "The thought of permitting access to private data, without any kind of reciprocity . . . is a direct assault on a person's conception of himself" (Coe & Wesson, 1976, pp. 109–110). Consistent with the student's goal of breaking down barriers that reinforced the we-they duality, it was decided that a high level of self-disclosure would be used in the first visit. The family's response to this approach was positive. After the student stated where she was from, what her parents did, and a little about where she had worked and gone to school, the teenager asked her the following questions in the course of the conversation: How old are you? Do you have a boyfriend? Do you like school? Do you have to pay a lot of tuition? Do you have kids? and Are you going to have kids? Answering the questions with yes, no, or short answer was adequate and provided little threat to the student. It was important for the family to find those things in the student's life that related to experiences with which they had some familiarity. Not only does self-disclosure serve to make the professional more accessible, it communicates that the professional does not distrust or fear the family.

The student was able to establish a relationship with this family. She was able to join, although perhaps only partially, their inner circle. She abandoned the immediate interventions to change the family behaviors in relation to sanitation and dietary habits. This may have been frustrating for the agency staff; however, with enough time, the student felt confident that she could use the relationship she had established to maximize the strengths of this family to facilitate the desired changes eventually.

■ CONCLUSION

As is illustrated in this case study, it is essential that nurses and other health professionals practice cultural relativity if disenfranchised and impoverished clients are to be dissuaded from we-they beliefs. The interaction approaches that were used effectively with this family are easily and appropriately transferable to other clients with whom community nurses practice.

At the same time that the United States economy is viewed by many as improving, increasing numbers of people who were employed for most of their adult lives are now unemployed and/or homeless. These "different" clients may well share middle-class values and lifestyle preferences with the health care providers who are intervening for them. Ethnocentric approaches to these people might even be seen as horizontal violence within one's own group. Accurate, compassionate assessment and intervention are based on active involvement of the client in the process, using their insights and perspective to define problems and solutions. This kind of client participation can contribute to decreasing the alienation and powerlessness associated with the cycle of poverty (Bullough & Bullough, 1972; Mason, 1981; Moccia & Mason, 1986).

A culturally relative approach to all clients perceived by nurses as "different" can enhance the effectiveness of nurse-client interaction and increase the likelihood that nurses can make a difference in the lives of clients. For example, relating to the person with chronic mental illness from a culturally relative perspective communicates respect for the individual rather than fear and dismay about the disease. It almost goes without saying that cultural relativity also applies when nurses work with clients from other ethnic, racial, or cultural backgrounds.

Nursing's primary task is to help clients cope with the health problems they face. This task can be accomplished when nurses are perceived by clients as helping persons who respect the clients and sincerely wish to understand, as much as possible, the distress they are experiencing. A culturally relative perspective establishes a framework for effective nurse–client interaction.

■ REFERENCES

Bernstein, B. (1960, September). Language and social class. *British Journal of Sociology, 11,* 217–276.

Bullough, B., & Bullough, V.C. (1972). *Poverty, ethnic identity, and health care.* New York: Appleton-Century-Crofts.

Centers, R. (1949). *The psychology of social classes.* Princeton: Princeton University Press.

Coe, R., & Wesson, A. (1976). Factors influencing the use of communicating health resources. In R. Kane (Ed.), *The health gap: Medical services and the poor.* New York: Springer.

Daniel, J. (1982). The poor: Aliens in an affluent society: Cross-cultural communication. In L.A. Samovar & R.E. Belmont (Eds.). *Intercultural communication: A reader* (3rd ed.). Belmont, CA: Wadsworth.

Fitchner, J. (1981). *Poverty in rural America: A case study.* Boulder, CO: Westview Press.

Gladwin, T. (1967). *Poverty USA.* Boston: Little, Brown.

Harrington, M. (1971). *The other America: Poverty in the United States.* New York: Penguin Books.

Irelan, L., & Besner, A. (1967). Low-income outlook on life. In Irelan, L. (Ed.), *Low-income lifestyles.* Washington, D.C. USDHEW, Welfare Administration, Division of Research.

Jaco, D., & Palgreen, P. (1975). Communication and modernization in Appalachia. In J. Wilber (Ed.), *Poverty: A new perspective.* Lexington, KY: University of Kentucky Press.

Kahl, J.A. (1959). *The American class structure.* New York: Rinehart.

Lewis, O. (1971). The culture of poverty. In M. Pilisuk & P. Pilisuk (Eds.), *Poor Americans: How the white poor live.* New Brunswick, NJ: Transaction.

Mason, D.J.(1981). Perspectives on poverty. *Image, 13,* 82–85.

Miller, S.M., & Riessman, F. (1961). The working class subculture: A new view. *Social Problems, 9,* 86–97, Summer.

Moccia, P., & Mason, D.J. (1986). Poverty trends: Implications for nursing. *Nursing Outlook, 34*(1), 20–24.

Pesznecker, B. L. (1984). The poor: A population at risk. *Public Health Nursing, 1*(4), 237–249.

Philipsen, G. (1975). Speaking "like a man" in Teamsterville: Cultural patterns of role enactment in an urban neighborhood. *Quarterly Journal of Speech, 61,* 13–22.

Reul, M. (1974). *Territorial boundaries of rural poverty.* Lansing, Michigan State University Press.

Seward, G. (1972). *Psychotherapy and culture conflicts in community mental health* (2nd ed.). New York: Ronald Press.

Strauss, A. (1979). Medical ghettos. In A. Strauss (Ed.), *Where medicine fails* (3rd ed.). New Brunswick, NJ: Transaction.

Stumpf, P.S. (1983). The culture of poverty: An overused conceptual model. In P.L. Chinn (Ed.), *Advances in nursing theory development.* Rockville, MD: Aspen.

Tripp-Reimer, T. (1984). Cultural assessment. In J. Bellack & P. Bamford (Eds.), *Nursing-assessment: A multi-dimensional approach.* Monterey: Wadsworth Health Sciences.

Waxman, C. (1977). *The stigma of poverty: A critique of poverty theories and policies.* New York: Pergamon Press.

Chapter 47

Ethics and Transcultural Nursing Care

MICHELE J. ELIASON

Nursing ethics is an emerging concept of interest and differs from biomedical ethics. Its focus is more on care than cure and emphasizes the ethical dilemmas included in everyday practical problems, as well as more philosophic issues. Combining this with nursing care across cultures, Michele Eliason suggests ways to overcome ethnocentrism and prejudice to deliver care within a cultural context. Several case examples of disparity in health beliefs are offered. Nurses respond to clients with their own cultural beliefs and values that are different from the clients and the author provides *ethnorelative* solutions that are free of bias and demonstrate ethical nursing care. Guidelines for culturally sensitive and ethical nursing practice conclude this chapter.

A review of current scholarship in nursing reveals an increase in the appearance of articles concerning two seemingly unrelated topics: nursing ethics and transcultural nursing. By *nursing ethics,* I mean the moral guidelines used to select or justify nursing practices. Nursing ethics, a relatively new topic of interest, promises to be different from biomedical ethics in much the same ways as nursing practice differs from medical practice. That is, the emphasis is more on care than cure and the ethical dilemmas include everyday practical problems, as well as more philosophic issues.[1-5] *Transcultural nursing* refers to nursing care across cultures. For purposes of this article, the definition of culture by Strauss[6] will be used: "the shared patterns, knowledge, meanings, and behaviors of a social group. Culture is the basic road map for comprehending the world and it provides the unwritten rules for living." Of course, these unwritten rules include ethical guidelines and values so that culture and ethics are inextricably entwined. Transcultural care has sometimes been considered in a narrow sense, such as comparing the health beliefs and practices of people from different countries or geographic regions. However, culture can be more broadly construed to include differences in health beliefs/practices by gender, race, ethnicity, economic class, sexual identity, age, and so on.

I argue that nursing practice and theory cannot be ethical unless cultural factors are taken into consideration, and that ethical/transcultural

From *Nursing Outlook* 41:221–228, 1993. Reprinted by permission of Mosby-Year Book, Inc.

nursing is not an esoteric speciality area, but central to the philosophy and practice of nursing. Leininger[7-9] has long advocated the position that culture care is necessary for nursing practice, and she set out a theoretical framework and methodologies for guiding research on cultural health beliefs, as well as establishing guidelines for nursing practice.

Although ethics has informed nursing practice since the beginning, nursing ethics as a unique field is a relatively new endeavor.[5] In the past, nursing was strongly influenced by biomedical ethics, which in turn was developed from the modernist movement in Western philosophy. This powerful modern approach proposed that all human beings have an essential core of being, an authentic self that transcends the body. Individual rights are supreme, and because of a common essential core, all human beings are deserving of the same rights. This type of reasoning allowed for the development of universal principles to govern human conduct. The result for medicine and nursing is the belief, still commonly held, that we should treat every patient equally. Alternatively, there is a belief that we base care on individual needs. This belief assumes that nurses can recognize culturally different needs and address them effectively.

As the postmodern movement gains momentum in nearly every discipline of the academy, there is growing recognition that to treat all clients equally means to treat some of them poorly. The postmodern movement challenges the possibility of an essential human core and instead stresses the importance of the particular historical and social context in which each individual grows.[10-12] Therefore examining the social context and knowing the influence of the historical context is crucial to providing relevant health care. In many ways, nursing has always been attuned to sociohistorical context, in that changes in medicine, environmental factors, and resulting changes in the types of clients nurses see are reflected in ever-evolving nursing practices. Nursing has been, however, somewhat slow to accept the need for culturally sensitive care on an individual level. For example, students in my nursing class have given the following responses regarding cultural diversity training:

- "I don't think it is necessary to study other cultures. All we need to know is how to care for specific diseases. People are people."
- "I was raised with high morals that accept all humans as equal. I will care for all of my patients in the same way, regardless of any personal differences."
- "Anyone living in the U.S. has an obligation to learn the ways and language of the U.S. It is not the nurse's responsibility to learn about other cultures."

This article examines some of the ramifications of an ethics that incorporates transcultural nursing guidelines. In the first part, two interrelated barriers to culturally sensitive health care, ethnocentrism and prejudice, are discussed. Next, the use of nursing diagnoses in a culturally sensitive nursing practice is examined. Then several examples of disparity between health care provider and client health beliefs are discussed. Finally, a brief discussion of guidelines for conducting ethical, culturally sensitive nursing practice is presented.

▬ BARRIERS TO CULTURALLY SENSITIVE NURSING CARE

Ethnocentrism

Ethnocentrism generally refers to an individual's belief that his or her own cultural group's beliefs and values are the best or the only acceptable beliefs. It includes an inability to understand the worldview or beliefs of another culture.[8] Ethnocentrism may stem from a lack of exposure or knowledge about other cultures. Most people are gradually exposed to the beliefs, customs, and values of their own culture over a long period of time, starting at birth. This acculturation process, known as socialization, involves both cognitive components, such as formal education, some types of religious education, and reading, and affective components, such as being punished for misbehavior or silenced for expressing "unacceptable" views. The affective component of socialization, although largely invisible, is much stronger and more emotionally charged than the cognitive component. The result is that most people have internalized the values of their culture well, but cannot always articulate them readily, and if they examine the beliefs carefully, do not always agree with them. A first step in developing cultural sensitivity is to examine one's own culture carefully and become aware that alternative viewpoints are possible.

Ethnorelativity is the ability to conceive of alternative viewpoints and to respect the beliefs of another culture even though they are different from one's own. Ethnorelativity should be a goal of nursing education.

Health care itself may be construed as a culture, and nurses have been socialized into the health care systems values, customs, and practices. Since the health care system is primarily (and historically) made up of white people from the middle-class, the health care system and the dominant culture are interrelated and overlapping.

Prejudice

Prejudice can be defined as strongly held opinions about some topic or group of people. Prejudices may be positive or negative. Positive prejudices often stem from a strong sense of ethnocentrism ("my culture is superior to others"). Prejudice may also stem from ignorance, misinformation, past experiences, or fear, and comes in many interrelated forms. For example, negative attitudes about people of other skin colors is called *racism*, negative attitudes about older people is *ageism*, about women, *sexism*, and about lesbians and gay men, *homophobia*. The belief that heterosexuality is the only acceptable form of relationship is *heterosexism*. When prejudice is the result of ignorance or misinformation alone, the negative attitudes may be easily overcome by education. When prejudice is deeply rooted in the affective components of socialization, the process of overcoming prejudice is much more difficult. All people have prejudices. The danger arises when people in power allow prejudices to affect their relationships with culturally different clients.

Nursing Diagnosis Within a Cultural Context

Some nurses who work with culturally diverse clients have been critical of the use of nursing diagnoses. For example, Geissler[14] found that many nurses were concerned that nursing diagnoses put the emphasis on the client being wrong and the health provider being right, present a danger of perpetuating stereotypes, and have a high risk for mislabeling problems. One good example of the danger of nursing diagnosis with culturally different clients is the use of the diagnosis "altered communication." A client who is fluent in her own language, but who does not speak English, may receive such a diagnosis. Would it not be equally correct to diagnose the nurse as having altered communication for a deficiency in the client's native language? When a client fails to follow instructions because she or he does not understand them, should the client receive a diagnosis of noncompliance? What if the instructions (say, for a particular diet) are in conflict with the client's religion?

▀EXAMPLES OF DISPARITY IN HEALTH BELIEFS

Several examples of situations in which a nurse and a client have different cultural values or beliefs about some aspect of health care are listed below. In some instances, a nurse may conclude that the client's belief threatens the client's recovery or health and attempts to challenge the belief. In other instances, the client's belief is compatible with health and may be respected. In other examples, the nurse has certain prejudices or ethnocentric beliefs that influence the care the nurse gives.

Example #1

Carlos is a 15 year old from a poor urban area where drugs proliferate and many young men trade sex for drugs or money. You are fairly certain that Carlos does not use IV drugs, but know that he often has sex with men for money. Carlos believes that only homosexual men are at risk for AIDS. Because he considers his prostitution a job, not a sexual identity, he does not think of himself as being at risk for AIDS.

Ethnocentric Solutions:
1. Convince Carlos that he is gay because he has sex with men; therefore he is at risk for AIDS.
2. Diagnose Carlos as "noncompliant" because he does not alter his behavior after you inform him of the risks.

Ethnorelative Solutions:
3. Respect Carlo's beliefs and try to teach him about risky behaviors without discussing sexual identities or applying a label to his behavior.

Example #2

Harold and Sarah are expecting their first child. Sarah comes to a prenatal clinic for her first visit. The nurse notes that Sarah is 26 years old, well-educated, and healthy. Sarah is informed that she has no unusual risks for her pregnancy. The baby is born healthy, but 10 months later, the clinic is being sued because the baby has Tay-Sachs disease and Harold and Sarah were not told that they, as Ashkenazi Jews, were at risk.

Ethnocentric Solutions:
1. Blame Sarah for not informing the clinic, because she did not "look Jewish."
2. Blame the clinic administrators, who did not include "Jewish" as a racial identity as well as a religion.

Ethnorelative Solutions
3. Alter clinic health assessment records to ensure reporting of racial/ethnic identity. Educate staff on health and risk for illness factors that differ by race or ethnicity.

Example #3

June, a 35-year-old surgical nurse, grew up in a fundamentalist religion, although she rarely attends church now. June admits a middle-aged female patient who is to undergo major surgery the next day. The patient, Barbara, insists that her companion, Alicia, be present for the preop teaching and any discussions of her health. June explains that only spouses or biologic family members will be allowed to visit Barbara in the recovery room or the ICU after surgery. When Barbara explains that she considers Alicia her spouse, June leaves the room. Later she comments to coworkers, "It wouldn't be so bad if she didn't throw her homosexuality in my face like that! It really bothers me when those people flaunt their sexuality!" She avoids Barbara's room for the rest of the shift.

Ethnocentric Solutions:
1. Uphold hospital policy and do not allow Alicia to visit or make decisions with Barbara.
2. Refuse to care for Barbara, or if giving her care, avoid any discussion of her sexual identity.

Ethnorelative Solutions:
3. Reconsider hospital policies. Must "significant others" be so narrowly defined? What are the purposes of the restrictions?
4. Examine personal beliefs. How did June come to be so negative about lesbians? Does her religious background—much of which she has already rejected—affect her current views?
5. Find out more information about the health care needs of lesbians. Ask Barbara about her wishes and include Alicia in her care.

Example #4

Tammi is a 75-year-old woman who was born in China and immigrated to the United States when she was 40. She lives in a predominantly Chinese neighborhood and maintains her traditional values and customs. Although the nurse introduced himself as Tony several times and has asked Tammi to call him by his first name, she continues to call him "doctor." Whenever Tony calls her Tammi, she looks away, but does not say anything about it. Tony is finding it increasingly difficult to communicate with Tammi. Later Tony learns from Tammi's daughter that it is not proper to call strangers by their first name, and it is disrespectful for 25-year-old Tony to call an elder by her first name. It is also not considered polite to make demands upon authority figures, but to take what they offer.

Ethnocentric Solutions:

1. Diagnose an alteration in communication or lack of assertiveness because Tammi failed to inform Tony of her wishes.
2. Tell Tammi that in this country, we call people by their first names.

Ethnorelative Solutions:

3. Ask her how she would like to be addressed. Offer your whole name and she can choose how to address you.
4. Offer her choices instead of asking open-ended questions.

Example #5

Clara is an 82-year-old African-American woman from a small rural community. She has arthritis and congestive heart failure. She has experienced considerable knee pain recently, and Ruth is following up on her prescription for an antiinflammatory. Ruth, a community health nurse, discovers that Clara never filled the prescription, but is using a "mustard plaster" made of various greens from her garden. She states that the pain is gone and she has no need for expensive pills.

Ethnocentric Solution:

1. Label her as "noncompliant" and encourage her to fill the prescription.
2. Try to persuade her that the greens have no therapeutic value. She should use "real" medicine.

Ethnorelative Solutions:

3. Try to determine whether there are other reasons for her rejecting the medication, such as not being able to afford the prescription.
4. Believe her when she says she has no pain and encourage her to continue the mustard plaster treatments.

▬GUIDELINES FOR CULTURALLY SENSITIVE (ETHICAL) NURSING PRACTICE

An ethical, transcultural nursing approach cannot result in a set of prescriptions or universal principles, unless respect for others' beliefs may be considered a universal principle. However, nurses can be provided with a set of tools for solving transcultural nursing problems that contribute to more ethical practice.

1. Perhaps the most important tool is self-examination. Nurses need to critically and continually examine their own beliefs. As these beliefs are scrutinized, some may be rejected, some transformed, and others celebrated. Only by knowing one's own cultural beliefs well can one be ready to learn about another culture. After examination of personal cultural beliefs, reading about health beliefs and customs of other cultures can be very helpful. There are a growing number of texts on transcultural nursing available, although at this point they are primarily limited to racial/ethnic cultural groups.[15–17]

2. Use language that is sensitive and inclusive. For example: say *gay, lesbian, bisexual,* not "homosexual"; do not say *man* or *mankind* when you mean to include women. *African-American* and *Latino* are now more well-accepted terms than black or Hispanic. *Asian* is more acceptable than "Oriental." Pay attention to the changing trends in language and incorporate them into your spoken and written language.

3. Do not make assumptions about anything. If in doubt, ask.

4. Listen carefully.

5. Do not say "I understand" if you do not. That is patronizing.

6. Ask clients how they wish to be addressed.

7. Find out who (if anyone) clients wish to include in their care and include that person(s) in all discussion of health status and in decision making.

8. Find out what the client knows and expects about the illness and its treatments. Evaluate whether the client's health beliefs are congruent with your own or the dominant health care system. If they are not congruent, determine whether there will be negative consequences for the client's health.

Leininger[9] noted that "human beings of any culture in the world have a right to have their cultural care values known, respected, and appropriately used in nursing and other health care services." Randall-Davis[18] offered several practical models of interviewing culturally diverse clients that allow nurses to discover and discuss cultural health beliefs. These articles can serve as guidelines for ethical/transcultural nursing practice. The most important fact that nurses need to keep in mind is to respect and listen to their clients. Clients are the experts on their own bodies and health, but their health beliefs are shaped by the cultures in which they were raised or currently live. Cultural beliefs are not necessarily right or wrong, good or bad; they are a fact of our multicultural world.

■ REFERENCES

1. Watson J. Nursing: human science and human care: a theory of nursing. New York: NLN, 1988.
2. Cooper MC. Gilligan's different voice: a perspective for nursing. *J Prof Nurs* 1989;5:10–16.

3. Fisher B, Tronto J. Toward a feminist theory of caring. In: Abel E, Nelson M. eds. Circles of care. Albany, New York: State University of New York Press, 1990.
4. Cooper MC. Principle-oriented ethics and the ethic of care: a creative tension. Adv Nurs Sci 1991;14:22–31.
5. Fry ST. Toward a theory of nursing ethics. *Adv Nurs Sci* 1989;11:9–22.
6. Strauss R. Culture, healthcare, and birth defects in the United States: an introduction. Cleft Palate J 1990;27:275–8.
7. Leininger M. Transcultural health care issues and conditions. Philadelphia: FA Davis, 1976.
8. Leininger M. Ethical and moral dimensions of care. Detroit: Wayne State Press, 1990.
9. Leininger M. Transcultural care principles, human rights, and ethical considerations. J Transcult Nurs 1991;3:21–23.
10. Dzurec L. The necessity for and evolution of multiple paradigms for nursing research: a poststructuralist perspective. Adv Nurs Sci 1989;11:69–77.
11. Weedon C. Feminist practice and poststructuralism. London: Basil, 1987.
12. Eliason MJ, Macy NM. A classroom activity to introduce cultural diversity. Nurs Ed 1992;17:32–6.
13. Geissler E. Transcultural nursing and nursing diagnoses. Nurs Health Care 1991, 12:190–2, 203.
14. Leininger MM, ed. Culture care diversity and universality: a theory of nursing. New York: National League for Nursing Press, 1991.
15. Spector RE. Cultural diversity in health and illness. Norwalk, Connecticut: Appleton and Lange, 1991.
16. Gigler JN, Davidhizar RE. Transcultural nursing, St. Louis: Mosby, 1991.
17. Randall-Davis E. Strategies for working with culturally diverse communities and clients. Bethesda: Association for the Care of Children's Health, 1989.

Chapter 48

Understanding, Eliciting, and Negotiating Clients' Multicultural Health Beliefs

LAURIE E. JACKSON

Clients from many cultural groups explain and treat illness in ways that are different from and may be in conflict with the biomedical beliefs and practices that are the basis of the American health care delivery system. Eliciting clients' health beliefs and self-care practices and negotiating treatment plans with them can help avoid problems caused by discrepancies in belief systems. Laurie Jackson presents three major categories of belief systems (biomedical, personalistic, and naturalistic) commonly found in the United States as well as in other countries. Questions designed to discover clients' health beliefs are included, along with guidelines for arriving at plans of care that accommodate those beliefs and case studies that illustrate the process of negotiation.

People of various cultures have different beliefs about causes, diagnosis and treatment of illness. Curing behavior based on different beliefs often appears irrational or bizarre to an outsider, but such behavior can usually be understood by examining the belief system on which particular actions are based. The health beliefs and practices of some ethnic groups can be quite distinct from and may conflict with those of most American health care providers. The discrepancies in beliefs between clients and providers can lead to treatment failure and frustration on both sides, and can cause clients to drop out of care. It is possible, however, for health professionals to prevent extreme client frustration by openly discussing both cultures' belief systems and by negotiating treatment plans.[1]

Health care providers cannot be experts on every culture with which they are likely to come into contact. However, in general terms, systems of health belief can be divided into three major categories: biomedical, personalistic and naturalistic.[2] While not all diseases fit neatly into these three categories, they provide a useful framework for understanding many health beliefs.

Reprinted/adapted with permission from 18(4):30–43, April 1993 *The Nurse Practitioner*. Reprinted with permission from Springhouse Corporation.

BIOMEDICINE

Biomedicine is sometimes called Western medicine because it was developed in and is the dominant belief system of the United States and other Western countries. According to the health-belief category of biomedicine, disease is the result of abnormalities in the structure and function of body organs and systems.[1] These abnormalities are due to processes that conform to the basic patterns of cause and effect, as seen in physics, chemistry and the sciences of the mind.[2] Of the three health-belief categories, only biomedicine provides an explanation of contagion.[2] In Western medicine, processes believed to cause disease include pathogens such as bacteria and viruses; biochemical alterations in the body due to conditions or events, such as nutritional deficiencies, the aging process, injury or stress; and environmental factors such as alcohol, cigarette smoke and other chemicals.

Diagnosis in biomedical systems involves identifying the pathogen or process responsible for a particular physical abnormality. This is accomplished through physical examination of the patient as well as the use of sophisticated laboratory procedures. The purpose of treatment is to destroy or remove the entity causing a disease or, when that is not possible, to repair, modify or control the affected body systems or functions. Curers in Western medicine are highly trained clinicians—experts in both diagnosis and treatment who are accomplished in such disciplines as anatomy, physiology, pathology, pharmacology and surgery. According to this belief system, prevention of disease involves avoiding pathogens, chemicals, activities or dietary agents known to cause body malfunction.

See Box 48-1 for an example of how the biomedical methods of diagnosing and treating a disease process compare with those of other health-belief systems.

PERSONALISTIC SYSTEMS

The second category of health beliefs is called personalistic. A personalistic medical system can be defined as one in which illness is believed to be caused by the active, purposeful intervention of a sensate agent that may be a supernatural being (e.g., a deity or god), a nonhuman being (e.g., a ghost, ancestor or evil spirit) or a human being (e.g., a witch or sorcerer).[2] In such a system, the "sick person literally is a victim, the object of aggression or punishment directed specifically against him, for reasons that concern him alone."[3] In personalistic systems the agent—witch, ghost, ancestor, deity—causes disease by using techniques such as theft of soul, witchcraft, possession, poison or intrusion of a disease object. For example, an ancestor, angry that proper rituals of respect have not been observed, might send a snake to bite a person, cause a tumor to grow or render a woman infertile. An irritated neighbor could ask a person skilled in witchcraft to cast a spell, perhaps to make someone unable to digest food or ill with a high fever.

BOX 48-1   *Diagnosis and Treatment of a Disease Process in Biomedical, Personalistic, and Naturalistic Health Belief Systems*

BIOMEDICINE
A woman presents to a physician with fever and chills, rapid breathing, painful cough and general malaise. The physician takes her temperature, listens to her lungs with a stethoscope, sends blood and sputum samples to the laboratory and orders a chest X-ray. The diagnosis of pneumococcal pneumonia is made, and an antibiotic is prescribed to eradicate the offending organism. Other people try to prevent catching this disease by avoiding contact with the patient's sputum.

PERSONALISTIC SYSTEMS
(Navajo Indian approach)
    A woman experiences several days of fever and chills, rapid breathing, painful cough and general malaise. When her condition continues to worsen, the family asks a singer (the term for a Navajo healer) to visit the woman. He consults with her about possible causes of the sickness, and discovers that she accidentally ran over a snake with her car several days before the sickness began. The singer decides that this violation of the taboo on killing snakes has caused the Holy People to send evil spirits to make the woman ill. He selects a curing chant appropriate to the cause of the illness, and schedules a full two-night ceremony.
    Preparations are carried out by the woman's kinsmen: Arrangements are made to pay the singer and secure gifts for his assistants; food is gathered and prepared to feed all who come; the patient's hogan (dwelling), where the ceremony will take place, is cleaned; and people gather ritual material. When all is ready, the singer and his assistants arrive. Using clean riverbed sand and colored pigments, they make a sandpainting on the floor of the hogan. The painting consists of symbolic representations of powerful supernatural beings and takes about four hours to complete. The beings depicted in the sandpaintings will be summoned by their pictures and impregnate the painting with their power and strength. They will then cure the patient in exchange for the offerings of the patient and the singer.
    After the painting is finished, the singer intones a protecting prayer and sprinkles the painting with sacred pollen. The sick woman then enters the room and sits on the painting. The singer gives her an infusion of herbs to drink. Then, while praying and singing, he applies sand from the sand figures to matching parts of the patient's body. This procedure is repeated four times, along with other prescribed acts. Through this ritual the patient absorbs the powers of the beings whose likenesses appear in the picture. Their supernatural strength and goodness is transferred from the sand to the patient via the singer. The evil within the woman is then neutralized by the power of the deities.

NATURALISTIC SYSTEMS
(Chinese traditional medicine approach)
    A woman experiences several days of fever and chills, rapid breathing, painful cough and general malaise. She goes to see a physician, who asks many questions, examines her tongue and takes her pulse. Findings include

> **BOX 48-1   *Diagnosis and Treatment of a Disease Process
> In Biomedical, Personalistic, and Naturalistic Health
> Belief Systems (continued)***
>
> a red tongue with dry, yellow coating, a superficial rapid pulse, thirst,
> constipation, dark urine and yellow sputum. A diagnosis of heat clogging the
> lungs is made. The woman's father had recently died, and her grief has
> weakened the vital energy of her lungs. Thus when she sat close to a heater for
> a long period of time the heat was able to invade her lungs. The physician
> treats the woman at the clinic with acupuncture, selecting points from the lung
> and large intestine channels that will activate the dispersing function of the
> lung and relieve the exterior symptoms. He then sends her home with a
> prescription for herbs that will reduce heat. He tells her to return to the clinic
> for daily acupuncture treatments for the next week and otherwise to stay in
> bed.

Treatment within a personalistic system involves identifying the agent
behind the act and rendering it harmless, as well as lifting the spell or otherwise reversing the technique used by the agent. Curers are thus required
to have supernatural or magical powers since they must use trances or
other divinatory techniques to find out who caused the disease, why, and
how it may be cured.

Once the cause of a sickness is known, either the curer or the patient
can take the steps necessary to correct the problem. Treatment of the
physical symptoms affecting a patient is of secondary concern, since the
patient's condition will not improve without addressing the cause of
the disease. In fact, there may be two levels of curers: a diviner to make the
diagnosis and possibly perform the curing ritual, and a lesser curer, such
as an herbalist, to implement the cure or treat the physical symptoms.[4]

Prevention of illness in a personalistic system involves making certain
that social networks with fellow humans, ancestors and deities are in good
working order. This involves avoiding acts known to arouse resentment
among neighbors and fellow villagers, as well as paying careful attention to
propitiatory rituals that are a god's or ancestor's due.[4] In addition, a person may wear amulets, tattoo sacred texts on parts of the body or have protective spells cast to mitigate malevolent powers.

Personalistic medical etiologies are usually components of broader explanatory systems and may be entwined with religious beliefs. The same
deities, ghosts, witches and sorcerers who send sickness may also be seen as
responsible for other kinds of misfortunes, such as blighted crops, personal quarrels, financial reversals, lost articles and accidents resulting in
injury or death.[4] Personalistic beliefs are predominantly found among
groups that are, or were, relatively small, isolated, nonliterate and lacking
contact with ancient high civilizations. These include indigenous inhabitants of the Americas, of Africa south of the Sahara Desert and of Oceania,
as well as the tribal peoples of Asia.[2]

An example of a disease process treated using a personalistic system is presented in Box 48-1. The personalistic system employed is that of the Navajo Indians.[5-6]

▬ NATURALISTIC SYSTEMS

The third category of beliefs is called naturalistic. Unlike personalistic beliefs, naturalistic ones explain sickness in impersonal, systemic terms. Health is believed to result from the equilibrium of insensate elements in the body, especially heat and cold. For health to prevail, these elements must be in a balance appropriate to the age, condition, and natural and social environment of an individual. When this equilibrium is disturbed, illness results.[2]

Contemporary naturalistic systems all developed from the Great Tradition medicine of ancient classical civilizations, particularly those of China, India and Greece.[2] Chinese traditional medicine today forms the basis of the traditional health-belief systems of several Asian countries, including Japan, Vietnam, Korea, Taiwan, Singapore, Hong Kong and China.

Another naturalistic system, Ayurvedic medicine, arose in ancient India, and is still widely practiced there and in neighboring countries.

The medical system of ancient Greece, also a naturalistic one, was called humoral pathology. It traveled both east and west, first with Moslem culture, then with Spanish and Italian explorers. As a result, variants of humoral pathology are today the most important explanatory elements in the medical systems of rural and some urban people in Latin America. Variants are also found in the Philippines, survive among low-income blacks and poor white Southerners in the United States, and are still found at both sophisticated and folk levels in Iran, Pakistan, Malaysia and Java.[2] (In the United States and Europe, medical beliefs and practices that are not part of orthodox, scientific medicine are called folk medicine. Particular folk medicines can be described as having either naturalistic or personalistic disease etiologies.[2])

In spite of their diverse origins and widespread distribution, contemporary naturalistic systems all explain illness as being caused by excessive heat or cold entering the body and causing an imbalance. Sometimes actual temperature is involved, but more often heat and cold are viewed metaphorically. Thus, foods, medicines, conditions (e.g., menses, pregnancy and childbirth), environmental conditions and emotions are ascribed hot and cold qualities.

For example, in Chinese traditional medicine anger is believed to be a hot (yang) emotion. A person who becomes intensely angry or is angry over a long period of time exposes his or her body to excessive heat and risks becoming ill with a hot disease. Liver-fire blazing upward, comparable to essential hypertension in biomedicine, is an example of a hot disease. Similarly, a person who eats too much melon, a cold (yin) food, could be expected to experience a cold disease, such as what Western medicine calls diarrhea. Whether an illness occurs after excessive exposure to heat or cold depends on the condition of a person's body at the time of the exposure.

Diagnosis in a naturalistic system is concerned with identifying the cause of a disease as being excess heat or excess cold. Some systems, such as Chinese traditional medicine, have precise and well-defined procedures to do this. Once the cause is identified, treatment attempts to restore proper balance. Remedies are divided into those with hot properties and those with cold ones, so illnesses believed to have hot causes are treated with cold remedies, and illnesses believed to arise from cold causes are treated with hot remedies. Treatments may include herbs, foods, dietary restrictions, medications from Western medicine (antibiotics are often attributed with hot or cold properties), massage, poultices, enemas, acupuncture, cupping or coining. Cupping is the practice of heating the inside of a glass jar to create suction, then attaching it to the skin over a painful area; coining involves rubbing the skin vigorously with a coin, causing bruising, to expel the invading element.

Curers in naturalistic systems are usually doctors in the full sense of the word: They are physicians or herbalists who are specialists in symptomatic treatment and who know the medicines and other treatments that will restore the body's equilibrium.

Prevention of sickness in a naturalistic system involves striving to maintain a balance of the hot and cold forces in one's mind, body and environment. This is accomplished by avoiding or protecting oneself from extremes of heat and cold, in both literal and metaphorical terms. For example, in Latin American humoral systems, childbirth is considered to be a cold condition. Postpartum complications, including what Western medicine would diagnose as infections, could be caused by further exposure to cold. Thus, women who have recently given birth are expected to avoid such actions as touching a cold floor with bare feet, bathing, undressing in a cold room, going outside on a cold day or eating foods considered to be cold in nature. Instead, these women are advised to seek heat in the form of a warm environment or protective clothing, as well as through specific foods and herbs known to provide heat.

Box 48-1 illustrates how a disease process is managed using a naturalistic system, in this case Chinese traditional medicine.

▬COEXISTENCE OF BELIEF SYSTEMS

The three categories of belief systems are rarely mutually exclusive within an individual or a society. A person or group that uses one system to account for a majority of sickness may nevertheless explain some diseases according to another system.[4] Indeed, some countries have parallel medical institutions, including medical schools, clinics and hospitals, based on different belief structures. Clients choose where they wish to seek care based on a personal assessment of their disease, or a referral between the systems by providers. This is true in China, where Chinese traditional medicine and biomedicine are both formally recognized, and in India, where Ayurvedic medicine and biomedicine coexist in the health care system. In other countries, including the United States and much of the developing world, institutionalized health care is based primarily on biomedicine, with a variety of other beliefs and practices found outside the formal institutions. In such countries patients may seek care outside the formal health care system instead of, or in addition to, entering that system.

▬ELICITATION OF HEALTH BELIEFS

Familiarity with a particular culture facilitates the elicitation of health beliefs, but is not essential. Information about distinct ethnic groups is readily available from the literature. A number of sociocultural assessment guides have been developed to assist practitioners caring for clients of different ethnic groups.[7]

The following questions are designed to elicit information about a client's health beliefs:[1]

- What do you think caused your problem?
- Why do you think it started when it did?
- What do you think your sickness does to you?
- How does it work?
- How severe is your sickness?
- Will it have a short or long course?
- What kind of treatment should you receive?
- What are the most important results you hope to receive from this treatment?
- What are the chief problems your sickness has caused you?
- What do you fear most about your sickness?

Difficulties may be expected in obtaining answers to these questions from clients who do not subscribe to biomedicine. Fearing ridicule, they will most likely hesitate to reveal unorthodox beliefs to health professionals. Practitioners will therefore need to act in ways that are unhurried, sensitive yet persistent, and respectful of the client. It may take more than one visit before these clients feel comfortable enough to reveal their true beliefs.

Elicitation of health beliefs is often further complicated by the fact that the client and provider either do not speak the same language or do not speak the other's language well enough to discuss complicated concepts. In such cases every effort should be made to find competent interpreters. Whenever possible, interpreters should be of the same sex as the client because the client may not reveal some symptoms to members of the opposite sex.

To provide patients with interpreters, hospitals frequently enlist employees of the client's ethnic background who are working in nonprofessional positions in the institution. Such employees are often unfamiliar with English medical terms and may not be able to translate accurately. Using clients' children or other family members to interpret may also lead to problems. For example, a Hispanic woman being seen for a vaginal discharge in a migrant clinic was so embarrassed when her teenage son was asked to interpret that she left.

In addition to asking interpreters to translate questions and responses, practitioners can also, when appropriate, ask them to provide information about relevant cultural beliefs and practices. A word of caution is necessary, however: Interpreters who are members of the client's culture may be of a different social class than the client, or may be more acculturated and anxious to appear part of the dominant culture. In some cases, interpreters may be disdainful or dismissive of the client's belief system. Care must be taken to insure that the client's words are translated accurately and completely.

When speaking through an interpreter, practitioners should look at and talk directly to the client, and attempt to use the simplest words possible. They should stop after every sentence or two and wait for the translation before proceeding. Sentences should be rephrased if the interpreter appears hesitant.

NEGOTIATION OF TREATMENT PLANS

Once the client's beliefs are known, health professionals can focus on negotiating a treatment plan acceptable to both parties. Providers should not attempt to change client's beliefs. Changing beliefs is a difficult, if not impossible, task, and the effort usually proves to be counterproductive. Instead, clients can be involved in making decisions about their care in a way that does not threaten their beliefs and that increases the likelihood that they will carry out prescribed treatments.

In general, clients who do not believe in biomedicine seem willing to cooperate with treatment from that system as long as it makes sense to them and does not conflict with their own belief systems. Studies have shown that clients and their families know what to expect from different types of healers and thus enter the biomedical health care system wanting and expecting Western medicine.[1] They most likely already will have tried treatments from their own belief structures without finding relief, and will be open to receiving the care offered by mainstream health institutions. They may, in fact, have strong expectations about the kinds of treatments they want. Western medicine, especially antibiotics, injections and intravenous infusions, is considered powerful by many who do not necessarily subscribe to its underlying theories. Clients may even have a particular form of treatment in mind and, if this expectation is not elicited and discussed, may be disappointed and uncooperative if they do not receive it.

In order to negotiate a plan of care, practitioners should first explain relevant points of biomedicine in simple and direct terms understandable to the client. Five major issues of clinical concern should be included in the explanation: etiology, onset of symptoms, pathophysiology, course of illness (including type of sick role—acute, chronic, impaired—and severity of the disorder) and treatment.[1] It is extremely important to use interpreters if language is a problem.

The practitioner should then openly compare the client's belief system with biomedicine, pointing out discrepancies and giving the client opportunities to ask questions or raise objections.[1] Familiarity with the client's culture can be helpful to this process because it may give the practitioner clues about possible problems. If the client raises objections to the plan of care, the practitioner can encourage the client to think of ways to circumvent the problem. Suggestions can be discussed until a plan that meets the expectations and treatment goals of both is agreed upon.

Most clients will not raise objections to a proposed treatment. Many cultures consider direct questioning or confrontation to be rude, and clients may not feel comfortable with this kind of behavior even when given encouragement. It may not be until a client returns and admits lack of adherence to the plan that problems will be revealed. Questioning at this point is often more fruitful.

The problems that can be encountered by failing to take the client's health beliefs and expectations into account or to negotiate a treatment plan are illustrated in the following example.

A Vietnamese refugee was seen at a clinic in the United States complaining of fatigue. Physical examination and laboratory tests revealed no obvious organic cause for the fatigue, while the client's history provided many reasons to suspect depression as the cause. The clinician told the woman she could find nothing wrong with her, informed her of the diagnosis of depression and tried to engage her in conversation about her emotional state. The client gave minimal responses to the questions and became increasingly hostile. Finally she jumped up and left. She did not return to see the clinician again.

While the clinician's diagnosis of depression in this case was most likely correct within the framework of Western medicine, from the client's perspective the provider made two grave errors. The first was in telling her that nothing could be found wrong with her. The health beliefs of Vietnam are based upon Chinese traditional medicine. According to this system, even complaints that biomedicine considers trivial, such as restlessness, excessive dreaming or becoming easily angered, are considered significant and treatable signs of imbalance. The client probably had never before failed to have a symptom explained or treated, and quite likely thought her case was not being given serious consideration.

The second error was immediately telling the woman she was depressed and using a discussion about her emotions as the only form of treatment. Asian cultures attach severe stigma to mental illness and discourage the direct expression of emotional distress. Instead, clients from Asian cultures tend to somatize their problems by expressing emotional problems through physical complaints. Assuming a sick role is a way to mobilize social support and gain relief from routine responsibilities while avoiding stigma.[8]

Had the clinician elicited the client's beliefs and expectations and explained those of biomedicine, a treatment that would have validated the client's sick role could have been found. This might have been something as simple as prescribing vitamins. Then, during subsequent visits, the clinician could either have attempted to discuss emotional concerns as part of treatment or casually encouraged such conversation. This course of action could have prevented the client from dropping out of care and could have provided her with an important source of emotional support.

GUIDELINES FOR NEGOTIATION

It is impossible to provide detailed outlines for negotiating plans of care with clients, as each case will differ depending on where discrepancies between beliefs lie and whether or not the discrepancies affect care. However, in negotiating treatment options with clients, practitioners should generally seek to preserve helpful beliefs and practices, accommodate beliefs that are neither helpful nor harmful from the viewpoint of Western medicine, or repattern harmful beliefs or practices. If there is insufficient knowledge about the effects of a given practice, the practice should be studied and evaluated to determine its relative helpfulness or harmfulness.[9]

PRESERVATION OF HELPFUL BELIEFS OR PRACTICES

Many of the beliefs and practices of non-Western systems have proven to be efficacious when studied by Western medicine. For example, acupuncture has been shown to be effective in treating certain types of problems.[10] Many medications commonly used today in biomedicine, including digoxin and quinine, were originally herbal medicines used by traditional healers. Major research projects have recently been undertaken to identify the active ingredients and potential clinical applications of other herbal medicines used in a variety of cultures.[11] Traditional childbirth practices, such as remaining active throughout labor and giving birth in nonrecumbent positions, are now being encouraged by some practitioners of Western medicine. Vigorous mouthwashing after meals is a Hindu custom which has been shown to prevent dental caries.

There are many other practices that have not been studied or approved by Western medicine. Nevertheless, in many cases they can provide physical or psychological relief for clients, sometimes even when Western medicine fails to do so. Practitioners should be open to learning about such practices and encourage their use when it seems they might be beneficial and cause no harm. Box 48-2 provides such an example.

ACCOMMODATION OF NEUTRAL BELIEFS AND PRACTICES

Most of the beliefs and practices of other health-belief systems are neither helpful nor harmful from a biomedical viewpoint. Nevertheless, they may sometimes interfere with treatment dictated by biomedicine. If there is no conflict with a proposed plan of care, practitioners should respect the significance and meaning of the belief or practice. In other instances they

---

BOX 48-2   *Preserving Healthful Beliefs and Practices*

A Cambodian teenager who had been living in the United States for several years with a non-Asian family began to experience severe interruptions of sleep and consequent fatigue due to nightly visitations by ghosts. He had lost most of his family under the Khmer Rouge regime and had experienced many horrors in the regime's work camps. When counseling did not alleviate the problem, the boy's physician prescribed antidepressant medication. After several weeks on the medication the boy was sleeping better but was still quite agitated; he blamed this agitation on the ghosts. At this point, the boy told his family that Buddhist monks could perform a special ceremony to get rid of ghosts. The family arranged to have this done by local Cambodian monks. Several weeks after the ceremony the boy said he had had no further visits from ghosts and felt much calmer. He continued to take the antidepressant medication.

---

may be called upon to facilitate them. Examples of such neutral practices include the postpartum diets prescribed for Chinese and Mexican-American women, the ritual disposal of the placenta and cord practiced in some societies, consultation with other curers in conjunction with Western medical treatment, the wearing of amulets and various culturally prescribed hygiene practices.

BOX 48-3   *Accomodating Neutral Beliefs and Practices*

A Chinese infant was seen in a New York clinic on several occasions over a two-month period for recurrent diarrhea. Stool cultures revealed no unusual organisms and changes in the infant's formula did not alleviate the problem. The clinic staff was puzzled as to the cause of the diarrhea and decided to make a home visit.

It was summer and the family's apartment was extremely hot. When the visiting nurse entered the kitchen she found several bottles of home-prepared formula lined up on the windowsill. Several other bottles were in the refrigerator. When asked by the nurse why some of the formula was in the refrigerator and the rest was out, the mother responded that, because she had recently given birth, she had to avoid cold. In order to avoid exposure to the cold of the refrigerator, she would have her husband remove the bottles she needed for the day before he left for work in the morning.

The nurse explained that when the formula sat out in the heat all day organisms would grow that could cause diarrhea. She asked if there was a way that the bottles could be kept cold until they were needed. After giving the matter some thought, the mother said that she could put on a coat, hat, and gloves before removing bottles from the refrigerator. The nurse agreed with this plan of action. Following the nurse's visit the baby had no further problems with recurrent diarrhea.

In cases where beliefs and practices do not interfere with treatment or cause other problems, practitioners can help clients find a way to resolve the contradictions. For example, some Puerto Ricans regard penicillin as a hot remedy inappropriate for a hot disease.[1] If in such a case a practitioner believes that penicillin is the most effective treatment, she can explain this to the client and identify ways to neutralize the hot properties of penicillin. Box 48-3 illustrates this process of negotiation.

REPATTERNING OF HARMFUL PRACTICES

Most cultures, including Western ones, have practices that are dysfunctional or harmful to health from a biomedical viewpoint. Attempts should be made to change them, but whenever possible, without trying simultaneously to modify underlying belief systems. Examples of harmful practices from Western culture include sedentary lifestyles, smoking, and excessive consumption of alcohol, fat and refined sugar. Examples from other cultures include the Cambodian practice of putting mud on the umbilicus of newborns, which results in a high incidence of tetanus; not allowing infants to drink colostrum in Vietnam and Laos; the clitoral circumcision and infibulation (excision of the clitoris and stitching together of the sides of the vulva) practiced in some African countries; use of pepper enemas in

---

BOX 48-4   *Repatterning of Harmful Practices*

A Vietnamese toddler with pneumonia was admitted to a large children's hospital in the United States. During examination the child was found to have what appeared to be cigarette burns on his back. Child Protective Services (CPS) was notified immediately. A nurse then noticed that the burns were in a symmetrical pattern and became curious about them. She arranged to have an interpreter come to the ward and asked the mother to explain the burns.

The mother said that when the child became very ill, she did not know what to do. She called an older Vietnamese woman good at curing illness, who burned his back with herbs. This practice is common in Asia and is known as scarring moxibustion. Moxibustion involves applying heat to acupuncture points. It is usually done by attaching burning mugwort leaves wrapped in paper to the end of acupuncture needles. In cases of severe illness, however, the burning mugwort may be applied directly to the skin, resulting in burns. This is believed to release the bad elements causing the illness.

When the child's condition worsened, friends helped the mother get him to the hospital.

The nursing staff and CPS caseworker agreed that what the mother needed was information about how to use the American medical system and an explanation of why scarring moxibustion was seen as unacceptable in this country. Before discharge the mother was given a tour of the hospital's outpatient clinic and introduced to the staff. She kept a followup appointment, and thereafter the child was seen regularly in the clinic. No further burns were noted.

West Africa; and extreme dietary restrictions imposed during pregnancy in Burma.

It is difficult to change cultural practices. They are generally deeply ingrained, and tradition often carries more weight than the word of newly met practitioners of Western medicine. Nevertheless, practitioners should clearly and respectfully explain their opposition to harmful practices and offer alternatives. Box 48-4 presents a situation where health care professionals attempted to repattern a harmful traditional practice.

▀CONCLUSION

Elicitation of health beliefs and negotiation of treatment plans with clients is unquestionably a time-consuming and sometimes difficult process. It requires that practitioners be openminded, flexible, creative and persistent. The results, however, can justify the time and energy expended. Fewer clients are likely to be dissatisfied and drop out of care if their beliefs are taken into account. Practitioners will be able to provide more effective care to clients who understand, agree with and follow their prescribed treatment regimen.

▀REFERENCES

1. Kleinman, A. et al.: "Culture, Illness and Care: Clinical Lessons from Anthropologic and Cross-cultural Research," **Annals of Internal Medicine,** 1978, 88, pp. 251–8.
2. Foster, G.M.: **Medical Anthropology,** New York, John Wiley and Sons, 1978.
3. Ibid., p. 53.
4. Foster, G.M.: "Disease Etiologies in Non-Western Medical Systems," **American Anthropologist,** 1976, 78, pp. 773–82.
5. Kluckhorn, C. and Leighton, D.: **The Navajo, Revised Ed.,** Cambridge, Mass., Harvard University Press, 1974.
6. Perezo, N.J.: **Navajo Sandpainting: From Religious Act to Commercial Art,** Tucson, Ariz., University of Arizona Press, 1983.
7. Tripp-Reimer, T. et al.: "Cultural Assessment: Content and Process," **Nursing Outlook,** March/April 1984, 32:2, pp. 78–82.
8. Lin, H.B. et al.: "An Exploration of Somatization among Asian Refugees and Immigrants in Primary Care," **The American Journal of Public Health,** September 1985, 75:9, pp. 1,080–4.
9. Jelliffe, D.: **Mother and Child Health: Delivering the Services, 2nd Ed.,** New York, Oxford University Press, 1985.
10. Jackson, L.: "Acupuncture: An Important Treatment Option," **The Nurse Practitioner: The American Journal of Primary Health Care,** 13:9, pp. 55–66.
11. Stevens, W.K.: "Shamans and Scientists seek Cures in Plants," **The New York Times,** Jan. 28, 1992, pp. B5, B9.

Chapter 49

Cactus Juice, Copper Bracelets, and Garlic: Self-Care Issues Facing Community Health Nurses

MARLENE A. DEHN

Cultural differences among groups of clients in community health nursing are often recognized through their self-care practices. What do nurses do with this information shared by clients? Is it important enough for the nurses to explore in depth or is the information just interesting and perhaps entertaining? Marlene Dehn describes a community, rich in cultural diversity, and a variety of cultural practices shared by clients. Because all of the agency's nurses were having similar experiences, an inservice program was suggested so the nurses could be informed of the nature and value of self-care practices within their community. More importantly, the nurses could learn how to integrate self-care practices with traditional health care practices and clients could benefit from both approaches. It is suggested that other community health nurses adopt a similar approach in their agencies.

Sandy Jones, a young community health nurse, came back into the health department office from a home visit with Mrs. Johnson, an elderly client. She chuckled to no one in particular, "Do you know what she told me she does to cure an earache? She has someone roll up a cone of paper and blow cigarette smoke into her ear." Joann, an older nurse, responded, "That reminds me of the day that Mrs. Ortega was holding Jose upside down to cure his 'fallen fontanel.' My assessment was that the baby was dehydrated. I had to negotiate pretty carefully to get some rehydration treatment. Later we taught baby care classes in the neighborhood and were able to teach mothers more about dehydration. Eventually, as they started to trust us, more and more mothers starting asking the community health nurses for advice."

The conversation continued with several experienced nurses offering anecdotes about self-care practices they had encountered with their clients. Jane related her discomfort with the high doses of vitamin C that some of her clients use. Not to be left out, Carla recounted some anec-

This chapter was especially written for this edition of this book.

dotes about the health care practices of her Hmong clients. The nurses agreed that most of the time they could combine their own nursing approach with the client's preferences, but it was sometimes tough going because they didn't always know what to anticipate. Eventually the staff decided that they could offer new staff nurses information on unique self-care practices existing in their community. They decided to organize all the information they could locate about their clients' self-care and share it at a staff workshop. A self-care inservice series was initiated and used as a forum to celebrate the rich cultural diversity and unique approaches to self-care that exist in the community where the staff practices nursing.

The series strengthened the nurses' appreciation for health practices encountered within a culturally diverse population. They practice in a community in the San Joaquin Valley of California that is growing quickly as a result of immigration. One-third of the residents are Latino, a population that continues to grow through further legal and undocumented migration from Mexico and Central America. Almost 20 percent of the residents are refugees who immigrated from Southeast Asia as a result of the war in Vietnam. For decades Central California has attracted people from all over the United States and many countries to work in agriculture.

At times the nurses feel frustrated because the families they see have such different points of view from their own, and the only way an effective solution is reached is to work within the clients' own belief systems, skills, and motives. The nurses sometimes wonder if anything works. Some clients avoid doctors and clinics altogether, treating their own symptoms even when the nurse would consider it unwise.

■OUTSIDE THE "SYSTEM"

The evidence that people do not depend on doctors and nurses for most of their care is substantial. The majority of symptoms experienced by the layman are largely self treated. Zola (1983) determined after extensive examination of international studies that approximately two-thirds of people with symptoms do not consult their physician. They may feel that they have sufficient knowledge or resources within their own family or lay community. Moreover, self-care meets specific social needs. The person getting care from the family is the recipient of nurturing from loved ones. In addition to social convenience, some people do not seek care simply because they do not have access to medical care due to financial reasons. They may seek alternatives that are less expensive or more trusted.

Health care services account for only a minor percentage of the factors that influence health. Major determinants of health promotion are lifestyle and environmental factors (Department of Health and Human Services, 1990). The media is a pervasive source of health information, more so than direct contact with a health care provider. Television communicates the latest fad diet or quotes from a fitness guru faster than health professionals can by using other means.

▬ DESIGNING STAFF WORKSHOPS

In spite of busy schedules, a staff workshop can be organized around information to which nurses have easy access. The first step is to meet and agree on what elements of self-care are likely to be important in their community; over-the-counter medicines, culture-based remedies, nutritional treatments, physical treatments and exercise, or religious practices. The second step is to review the elements of a self-care assessment interview, as discussed below, to determine what information is useful to collect. The assessment is incorporated into the nurses's regular communication with the client. When information is collected in this manner, the workload is not increased significantly.

A single workshop or a series of short seminars can be conducted by the staff once anecdotes are collected. They can be arranged into themes that can be presented at a session, for example, the self-care practices of a specific ethnic group. Topics such as prevention of colds or "laying on of hands" can be used for other workshops. Samples of remedies are shared when possible. Staff enthusiasm about the anecdotes from field experiences always carries the day and humor gives the stories zest.

▬ SELF-CARE ASSESSMENTS

As a part of nurses' everyday communication with clients, a self-care assessment should be included. A good place to start is to determine the self-care practices of a single family or a group.

Understanding clients' points of view is essential. Spector (1996) offers a model of "facets of health" which proposes that clients maintain a healthy state by staying in balance with forces around them. Health in this model refers to physical, mental, and spiritual health. Spector writes that people use traditional methods from their own heritage to maintain, to protect, and to restore their health. Traditional self-care occurs in addition to use of the medical care system. A health care assessment includes information about spiritual and mental health, as well as physical health. Actions that clients take to protect their health (health promotion) are as important as treatment of illness.

Generally, asking clients what they do to stay well is a good way to start the inquiry. Do they feel that they do anything to stay healthy? Do they take vitamins? What foods do they consider to be beneficial? What do they do to handle stress or sadness or anxiety? Do they get any spiritual assistance?

The conversation can then lead to discussion of what clients believe generates wellness or causes illness. There may be explanations such as staying warm, leading a good life in the eyes of God, eating well. Later the nurse can inquire about what methods the client uses to care for specific symptoms such as "the blues," headache, diarrhea, colds, fever, earache, backache, toothache, colic, and other illness. What treatments were handed down from parents and grandparents? What treatments are used in addition to what the doctor recommends?

Discussion with clients also can be organized by inquiring whether they use specific substances such as teas, salves, herbs, or over-the-counter medications. It is useful to determine what properties these substances are believed to have, curative or preventative. Clients may use spiritual practices or rituals such as prayer or laying on of hands. Special nurturing such as letting children have special games in bed or their favorite foods is common practice. Families may use a wide variety of over-the-counter treatments.

After the nurse understands a health practice in detail using observation, experience, and information from the client, the next step is to trace the cultural, ethnic, religious, or geographic antecedents of the practice, and to determine whether the process is considered preventative or curative. It is also important to be able to explain what action must be taken to complete the care and whether any rituals or recipes are involved.

The nurse can refer to literature from anthropology, folklore, nutrition, religion, history, agriculture, and botany as well as public health nursing, pharmacology, and medicine to see if explanations are offered from other sources. Eventually it is important to reach a conclusion about efficacy and safety of the self-care practice and determine a way to incorporate it into the plan of care for the family.

▬COMMON AND UNCOMMON SELF-CARE STRATEGIES

Nurses are likely to learn about many types of teas, herbs, and simple nutritional approaches to self-care. There is an amazing variety of substances that clients use such as chamomile for ulcers, asafetida to ward off colds, grapefruit for arthritis, pineapple or peppermint for stomach problems, whiskey with salt for toothache, eucalyptus spray for backache, bagbalm for cracked skin, and carrots to improve eyesight. Garlic and its properties is very popular: garlic as a poultice, garlic as a cold preventative, garlic to lower cholesterol. Usually, in the case of foods and herbs, a nurse can locate historical or folklore sources in the literature that describe similar practices in other populations or parts of the world. Borrowing treatments from the past may account for much of the resurgent popularity of natural and herbal foods used for health promotion and minor illness treatment.

Nurses have collected an amazing variety of home remedies from families in their care (Dehn, 1990). Frequently beneficial properties are attributed to foods. One nurse found the use of onions to relieve nasal congestion and found similar practices among the Cheyenne. Many people keep salves, lotions, poultices, or other products on hand to use in case of injury or rash. One of the most common is aloe vera, a plant that relieves the pain from burns.

In addition to topical substances nurses have examined other treatments such as the use of copper bracelets as a cure for arthritis. Because copper bracelets are common, nurses should be aware of client beliefs about their efficacy. Tracing the history of this practice might remind a nurse to consider the therapeutic value of faith.

Reflexology, or foot massage, and acupressure are frequently used as alternatives or complements to medical care. Origins of these practices can be traced around the world. For example, shiatsu and other forms of massage have been borrowed from the Japanese and incorporated into family self-care practices. Shiatsu is commonly taught to students taking massage courses.

Laying on of hands and anointing of an ill person accompanied by prayer is practiced by people of various faiths and many cultures. As a form of nurturing and respite it can be an important resource for patients and assistance to the nurse. Other therapies such as visualization, aroma therapy, color therapy, and color imaging also can be explored.

When working with clients in the home setting, the client's motivation is a primary factor. Any practice that has been confirmed in the literature to be safe and that will cement client cooperation should be incorporated into the health care plan.

▄CULTURE SPECIFIC SELF-CARE PRACTICES

In a region like the San Joaquin Valley of California where immigration is ongoing, nurses deal with a large variety of culture-specific self-care practices. In California there are numerous undocumented aliens. For them, obtaining health care is a severe problem because they fear deportation. A referendum in 1994 created barriers to health care for aliens that will take many years to resolve in the courts. As a result, alternatives are sought out even more so within the immigrant community. For many immigrants, *curanderos* or shamans were common health care providers in their countries of birth, and many continue to use them in their new country.

Nurses find instances of illnesses known to the Latino population that should be understood so that established treatment methods can be planned to incorporate basic beliefs about these illnesses. *Susto* (fright) or *empacho* (digestive disturbance) or *caida de la mollera* (fallen fontanel) are seen. Nurses find instances when patients consider certain foods useful for the purpose of correcting imbalances in the body. They also see self-treatment of diabetes with cactus juice and self-treatment of arthritis by methods not accepted by the medical establishment. At times their clients employ religious practices for health benefits.

A case in point is a home visit that was made recently by a nurse when she noticed what appeared to be an altar in the living room. The altar consisted of dirt molded with honey and formed into the shape of a "giant Hershey's Kiss." It had nose, eyes, and mouth fashioned from white shells. The daughter of the family related that her mother had the "saint" made and the house cleansed by a woman in another town for the cost of $300. The family felt that their health and fortunes had improved since "Eleggua" had been constructed. Headaches disappeared, colds had been prevented. As long as the family kept the saint happy by offering it Bacardi, cigarettes, food, and money, they would be protected. The nurse was familiar with comparable practices in another context. After some consultation she traced the saint to the practice of Santeria (Guizar, 1996). Santeria, as a religion, is not prominent in this region of California.

According to Gonzalez-Wippler (1992), Santeria is the outgrowth of religious practices imported from Nigeria and adapted to the Hispanic–Catholic context in Latin American countries, especially Cuba and Puerto Rico. Eleggua also is interpreted as Saint Anthony. Eleggua provides access to other deities, so keeping him happy is of utmost importance. Understanding the meaning of the family altar in the above instance allowed the nurse to incorporate the family's existing system of health beliefs into her plan for health services.

Nurses working with Southeast Asian clients frequently report on specific nutritional preferences, especially as they are related to pregnancy and childbirth. Especially important are foods and beverages that must be provided after delivery to ensure a healthful outcome.

Also important is client distrust of certain aspects of the American health care system. Hmong belief in spirits as sources of disease has been an important factor. Nurses often describe the common experience of finding thin strings around each wrist of a sick Hmong patient, or those undergoing a major life change. Each string represents a prayer of wellness or good fortune from loved ones. To remove them is as significant to the Hmong as stopping an antibiotic prematurely is among practitioners of Western medicine.

Nurses also have been involved in difficult situations where Hmong families have had severe reservations about surgery and preferred to follow the advice of a shaman rather than American physicians. One family's choice was to refuse surgery for their son's club foot due to the belief that other family members would be affected negatively if an operation were performed. The amount of alienation between health care providers, the family, and the community were so divisive that the child's best interests were forgotten (Kirby, 1990; Pulaski, 1990).

▬ UNIQUE VIEWPOINTS

One nurse carefully examined the common practice of relating physical symptoms to the weather. She traced the development of biometeorology, the study of weather as it affects humans. She found sufficient information to convince her that there is scientific support for those who are concerned about how the weather affects their allergies, heart disease, or arthritis (Barney, 1996).

▬ INSIGHTS

The most important effect of the self-care assessment is that nurses take the time to examine everyday habits that they might otherwise ignore, and to contemplate their value for health promotion. If they analyze their own self-care habits they realize how many of their own health habits stem not from professional sources, but from remedies or preventatives handed down for generations.

Respect for clients is a result of the self-care assessment. Discovering a client's home remedies and prevention strategies allows the nurse to see the client as an expert on a particular practice. Informants represent their own tradition and knowledge instead of being dependent. While the nurse may not agree with a practice, it is the preserve of the client. New respect is developed for the capabilities of clients and the basis for peoples' motivations and theories about health care are discovered.

▬SUMMARY

The self-care workshop is an excellent vehicle for community health nurses to gain experience with the rich variety of health care as it is practiced by the lay public. Throughout history there have been alternatives to Western medicine as we know it. Most actions that influence health, for better or worse, are taken by people themselves. In this context it is useful for nurses to gain a sense of reality about what impact they do or do not have over the welfare of their clients and what alternatives people seek when they assume control over their own health. People in every community are resources for information on self-care. Simply asking clients what they do for self-care produces a vast array of practices to promote health, allay symptoms, and treat minor illnesses. This sharing of experiences is an excellent way to build respect for clients.

▬REFERENCES

Barney, C. (1996), Personal communication.

Dehn, M. (1990). Vitamin C, chicken soup and amulets; Students view self-care practices. *Nurse Educator 15* (4), 12–15.

Gonzalez-Wippler, M. (1992). *The Santeria experience.* (Rev. ed.). St. Paul, MN: Llewellyn Publications.

Guizar, C. (1996). Personal communication.

Kirby, K. (1990). Personal communication.

Pulaski, A. (1990, Jan 4). Judge will decide fate of Hmong child caught in cultural vise. *The Fresno Bee*, pp A1, A10.

Spector, R.E. (4th ed.). (1996). *Cultural diversity in health & illness.* Stamford, CT: Appleton & Lange.

U.S. Department of Health and Human Services. (1990). *Healthy people 2000: National health promotion & disease prevention objectives.* (DHHS Publication No. PHS 91-50212), Washington, D.C.: U.S. Government Printing Office.

Zola, I.K. *Socio-medical inquiries.* (1983). Philadelphia: Temple University Press.

Unit 8

Community Health Nursing Leadership and Effecting Change

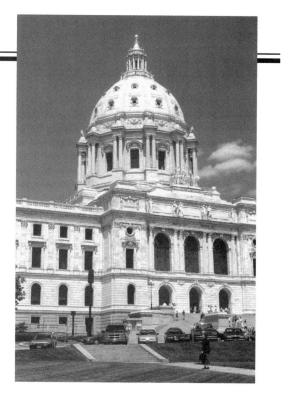

The health system today, as we read in the first section of this text, faces tremendous changes and challenges. No longer can government programs solve the health system's problems. Instead, there is an emphasis on self-reliance and private enterprise. An endless array of health needs, formerly subsidized by government funding, have come face to face with limited resources. Costs now drive much of the decision-making in health system reform, quality of health services is in jeopardy, and rationing (making services available to some but not to others) is a reality. But there is reason for hope. Global economics, privatization, individual impact, and concern for quality and social justice are exerting pressure—and providing enablement—to design a more equitable and accessible system of health services. Already new patterns of health services delivery and changing roles for health care providers, especially for community health nurses, are evident, as described in earlier sections.

A number of chapters in this text have explored the ways in which community health nursing is responding to changes in the health system. But what additional actions do community health nurses need to take? How can nurses help to promote healthier communities and influence change in the system rather than simply reacting to it? Should health and health care be a right for all? If so, nurses have a powerful reason to redefine the boundaries of their responsibility. Nurses who are committed to promoting the public's health cannot be reactive and wait for health problems to bring people into the system. Rather, they must be proactive, seeking out aggregates with real or potential health needs, identifying populations at risk, designing protective, preventive, and health promotive community interventions, and helping to shape public policy. In short, they need to become agents of change and leaders in community health.

A leadership role for nurses in the health system is not a new concept. Nurses have never lacked the opportunity for leadership. The challenge for nursing, rather, is to seize it, as did Florence Nightingale and Lillian Wald, who were early role models of community health nursing leadership and influence. Independent nursing judgment, decision-making, needs assessment, and client diagnosis have been hallmarks of public health nursing practice. However, as the health system changes in response to shifting social, political, and economic forces, so must the role of the community health nurse. If this field of nursing's mandate is to address the health needs of populations and communities, nurses must influence change at the macro level. They can accomplish this by assuming leadership roles in community health, as is forcefully illustrated in this unit.

Concomitant with nurses exerting leadership influence in community health is the need for political activism and involvement in health policy formation. Community health nurses can no longer be content only to carry caseloads of clients, intervene with families, and promote the health of selected community groups. They have a responsibility to look beyond the individual or group and influence the health of society in general. Public health is the only health discipline with this perspective and the only field that, by means of collaborative teamwork, addresses the needs of whole communities. It is public health professionals who watchdog environmental safety for the public. It is public health professionals who lobby for money to establish programs for the homeless, who create awareness of the need to stop family violence, and who work to reduce teen pregnancy. It is a public health orientation that reminds city planners about underserved areas in a community or that makes lawmakers aware of the health implications of proposed legislation. Nurses in community health must provide leadership and influence change for the betterment of the public, building on this public health legacy.

Effective leadership and management of change in community health require a number of important skills. One of the most critical is the ability to envision possibilities for the future. Leadership combines vision and the ability to communicate that vision to others. The community health nurse as leader must be able to first paint a picture of what could be and then create enthusiasm for and commitment to that goal. The nurse-leader learns how to be personally powerful and how to empower others. The nurse-leader learns how to integrate ethical decision-making into her or his efforts for change. Community health nurses must network to gain the information required for decision-making and to build stronger support systems in the profession and with other professional groups. They must become politically astute and learn political advocacy. They must develop skill and experience in health policy analysis, formation, and evaluation. To succeed in influencing change they must get involved. This unit provides many excellent examples of community health nursing's potential to influence the health of populations and communities. In reading these, one is reminded of what can be done and of the challenge nurses face to expand their sphere of influence.

Chapter 50

Nursing Leadership in Health Policy Decision Making

NORMA J. MURPHY

> The need for health system reform continues and so too does the need for support of health promotive and preventive health services. If nurses are going to help address the needs of populations at risk and promote healthy communities, they must assume an active leadership role in health policy decision making. How can this be done? In this chapter Norma Murphy describes a theoretical framework for this role. She then discusses a variety of practical ways that nurses can be involved in health policy formation. She challenges nurses to participate in the policy-making process and become leaders in promoting primary health care for all.

Because nurses believe in the principles of primary health care,[1] their participation in the policy-making process is critical to the reform of the health care system. Through their perspective on the development of health-promotive, community programs, nurses can bring a balance to the decision-making process about the use of health care resources. As members of committees within institutions and governments, nurses communicate their nursing perspective to influence policy. In this article I offer a theoretical framework and practical methods for nurses to become participants in the formation of primary health care policies. By learning how to participate in policy formation, nurses will become involved in decision making and thereby bring the benefits of primary health care to the client.

THEORETICAL FRAMEWORK

As society strives for conditions that allow citizens opportunities to pursue goals and live with dignity, health is seen as a resource to make this possible. Health, however, is influenced by environmental circumstances often beyond one's control. In a 1986 discussion paper, "Achieving Health For All," by Jake Epp, health is envisaged as a resource enabling people to manage or change their surroundings as they strive to achieve satisfaction in their lives.[2] The article emphasizes the role of individuals and commu-

From *Nursing Outlook* 40(4):158–161, 1992. Reprinted by permission of Mosby-Year Book, Inc.

nities in defining their meanings of health. As environmental circumstances become increasingly linked to health care needs, consumers, health professionals, and health policymakers face new responsibilities in making social conditions optimal for health. As Butterfield[3] points out, the modification of socioeconomic conditions such as poverty, unemployment, and isolation becomes a priority in health care planning because these conditions are "the precursors to poor health throughout the world."

The principles of primary health care are encompassed in the holistic perspective prominent in nursing theory; therefore nurses could make a distinct contribution to the implementation of primary health care. Holism directs nurses to recognize the client's central position in decision making about health and health care issues.[4-7] Therefore in practice, nurses focus on assisting clients in changing their circumstances or in accepting what cannot be changed at the time.

In this respect they assume an advocacy role—imparting information, providing consultation and support, educating, and counseling. Some believe that, with advocacy, there is a maximum transfer of information to the client, a prominent client participation in the decision, and a freedom felt by the client to implement the decision.[8] Advocacy helps clients make informed and knowledgeable decisions affecting both health and the satisfaction of their needs; the client becomes an active participant in defining health needs and the appropriate use of resources, as well as a recipient of care. Using a holistic approach, nurses respond not only to biologic needs, but also to the socioeconomic circumstances that affect well-being.

As policymakers redirect health care delivery, nurses' distinct philosophy enables them to fulfill innovative roles in nursing practice, such as serving as a point of access to the health care system. With the trend toward self-care, clients increasingly require support services. Working from their holistic perspective, nurses can respond directly to clients' needs by focusing on health promotion and by supporting clients as they learn new ways to work and live.

The services available to clients through nurses include health screening; education in prevention, crisis intervention and rehabilitation; counseling; and the assumption of an advocacy role for clients needing to change socioeconomic circumstances. Expansion of these services is important in assisting clients with mental health problems and chronic illnesses. As clients learn to manage the circumstances in their environment and to have meaning in their life, stress, dependence, and disease frequently are reduced.

The implementation of primary health care, through intervention that affects the socioeconomic circumstances, may foster the development of communities. For some time, community health nurses have recognized the impact of social factors on well-being and have developed community interventions. These interventions have focused on educational programs, such as stress management for clients experiencing abuse.

The implementation of primary health care, however, requires that community health nurses apply this principle in new ways. For example, using a client-centered approach to research, nurses are able to study the variables that cause widespread drug use within particular communities. On the basis of their information, health policies and programs may be tailored to respond to causative factors and specific needs. Solutions may involve teaching constructive use of leisure time, creating opportunities for socialization, or supporting members of the community who lobby the government for improved employment opportunities. Through programs such as these, nurses assist clients in taking responsibility for their life-style and quality of life, even though the clients are thwarted by unemployment.

Community health nurses need to coordinate care between many professionals. The implementation of primary health care would require nurses to participate in planning between professionals and representatives of various governmental sectors such as health education, manpower, and community groups. By participating in planning, community health nurses, committed to an equitable distribution of health resources, would not only initiate collaboration on behalf of the client but participate in the formation of policies to address the client situation and health problems. Through participation in policy-making, nurses assist in altering the socioeconomic factors that affect the client's health. These interventions offer a distinct example of the implementation of primary health care and define a new role for community health nurses in which practice is guided by a holistic perspective.

As the concept of primary health care emphasizing client responsibility for health becomes more influential in the formation of health policies, health professionals must participate in decisions concerning the use of health care resources to ensure clients have access to the resources to meet their needs. This professional responsibility is particularly important at a time when proposals to health policymakers for the allocation of health care resources to primary health care programs compete with the demand for high technologic care in acute care institutions. Indeed, clients and health professionals may favor a balance in the allocation of resources allowing the development of primary health care programs simultaneously with the continuing support of acute client care.

But as Anderson,[9] citing Navarro, points out, "Decisions in health policy are not controlled by health care professionals." In his study Navarro finds that boards of institutions are frequently composed of people from the business sector. He emphasizes that it is misleading to believe that administrators and physicians are the primary policy decision makers. With nonhealthcare professionals shaping health policy, decisions are made, as Anderson demonstrates, according to sociopolitical and economic variables, and not by health professionals advocating for client needs. Although policymakers recognize the economic need to establish primary health care programs, funding for highly technologic hospital services remains a priority.

If the health care system is to respond to the country's social and economic well-being, as well as the public's health care needs, health-promotive and illness-preventive programs must be established in conjunction with up-to-date technologic care. Because the prosperity of the country is determined in part by the health of its citizens, policymakers need to understand that the preventive emphasis of primary health care contributes directly to the social and economic well-being of the country. By understanding the long-term benefits of primary health care, the decision makers should recognize the need to set new priorities in the use of health care resources favoring a balance between technologic and primary health care.

To advocate for clients needing primary health care, nurses and associate health professionals must become active in the decision-making process. Nurses, however, may be reluctant to promote a change in health care because, traditionally, they have not had a recognized role in the use and the distribution of health care resources. A perceived lack of knowledge about the decision-making process may underlie their concerns.

Forester[10] offers a framework for understanding the planning of a policy change by policy analysts. He emphasizes the importance of clear and accurate communication as the means to assist others in understanding an alternate way of viewing a problem or an issue. His framework offers direction for nurses hoping to influence policy change within a complex health care system—at the level of government, institutions, or community agencies. For many nurses a barrier to client advocacy is the lack of opportunities to communicate with associate health professionals, administrators, and politicians about the role professional nurses can play in a system founded on the principles of primary health care. Equally prohibitive to nurses' ability to affect policy is their lack of access to the information needed to influence a change process. In addition, the health system has failed to recognize nurses as professionals with expert knowledge useful in creating solutions to complex problems. Forester's communication guidelines offer nurses assistance in developing their communication skills in an advocacy role.

As analysts use communication networks or structures, Forester[10] argues, they are able to reformulate problems so that strategy and action are possible. Through direct and open communication, analysts are able to interpret the context of problems and direct the attention of decision makers to alternative solutions. Forester emphasizes that, to gain a position of influence, analysts must have adequate contact with the decision makers, to access and interpret information critical to the problems, as well as to influence acceptance of alternate solutions. Both the use of the analysts' expert knowledge and organization of structurally and politically relevant information is critical to influencing the decision-making process. Forester also adds that as the decision makers communicate with the analysts, substantive relationships develop that encourage greater participation of those involved in the decision-making process.

■ PRACTICAL METHODS
Government Organizations

Through government organizations, some nurses are already influencing the health care decision-making process. Through the lobbying efforts of the Canadian Nurses' Association and the American Nurses' Association, nurses in both countries have affected decisions at the national levels of government. In the association the nurses' appreciation for the principles of primary health care provides motivation in complex discussions with policymakers. In the CNA's 1984 lobby of the Federal Ministry of Health and Welfare for the inclusion of the "health care practitioner" amendment,[11] the profession demonstrated an ability to influence policymakers.

While the CNA Board has lobbied at the national level, similar activities have taken place provincially. For example, in Nova Scotia nurses are members of a government committee studying the recommendations of a Royal Commission on Health Care. Because of government inclusion of nurses on this committee, it could be argued that these nurses are seen by politicians as professionals with expert knowledge and an ability to contribute models and theories for alternative approaches in health care and health care delivery.

Nursing Associations

If primary health care, with its emphasis on client advocacy, is to be incorporated effectively into our health care system, nurses must independently face the challenge of influencing the health care decision-making process.

As members of the national nursing association, nurses collaborate in establishing standards for health care and nursing practice that then become a consistent communication or lobby for change within the health care system. Because the national associations' recommendations for change are sensitive to the socioeconomic circumstances of the clients, the nursing associations' proposals speak directly to the concerns policymakers wish to address. The value and effectiveness of the professional association directly relates to its consistency on issues and the number of nurses who are able to communicate on professional issues in a socially responsible and knowledgeable manner.

As nurses recognize their ability to effect change, the professional association may be used more frequently by nurses, as well as nursing administrators, educators, researchers, and theorists.

Committees Within Institutions

Through participation on committees within institutions, community agencies, or government, nurses are able individually to implement the guidelines of Forester. Although nurses may be under the impression that their experience is insufficient for effective participation, the organization and processes of nursing practice offer a framework for decision making and problem solving. In their positions as health professionals working within the organizational structure, nurses can access the information needed to develop health issues and communicate to associate health professionals and administrators knowledge that is relevant to quality client care and to community health issues. As nurses begin to take part in decision making by developing and using networks of professional relationships, they can encourage decision makers to consider solutions guided by the principles of primary health care and emphasize the role professional nurses play in primary health care practice. With increasing success, nurses will gain the professional recognition they deserve.

Interest Groups

Through participation in interest groups, nurses together can examine and take positions on important professional issues. Their recommendations guide the professional association and serve an educative function, enabling nurses to focus and clarify their positions. As a result, nurses address the perceptions and decisions of policymakers practically in hospital, community, and governmental settings.

The Media

Nursing journals and newspapers, and the mass media, provide other means for nurses to promote holistic alternatives to current health care policies. The mass media may be used to educate the public, associate professionals, administrators, and politicians about professional nursing practice. Education serves as an important tool or an instrument in shaping a change in perceptions about the role of professional nurses in primary health care. Nurses' ideas, experiences, and research findings, thereby, may become an instrumental aspect of the nurses' role as a client advocate.

▬CONCLUSION

Although nurses' equal participation in policy formation is a long-term goal, it immediately requires the development of a network of professional relationships as well as the education of nurses in the policy process and in organizational and communication skills. The university preparation of nurses, particularly at the graduate level and in continuing education programs, should include a component examining the processes of policy change. Having been educated to understand the policy-making process, nurses would then be better prepared to be equal partners with associate professionals in decision making.

Primary health care offers clients opportunities to develop resources enabling them to achieve personal satisfaction. As more people realize that the health of citizens is central to the prosperity of a country, the establishment of primary health care will become a priority. If nurses value the principles of primary health care as integral to responsive and flexible health care services, then they must assume a leadership role in health policy decision making.

Through membership in the professional associations, committees, and interest groups, and through the use of the media, nurses can communicate that primary health care is a viable alternative to the public's health care needs. Through nurses' participation in policy decision making, not only will the likelihood of establishing primary health care be improved, new standards for the decision-making process will be set. As health professionals who believe in advocating for clients, nurses can do no less than strive toward achieving a leadership role in implementing the principles of primary health care in the health care system.

▬ REFERENCES

1. World Health Organization. Primary health care. Geneva: World Health Organization, 1978:2–3.
2. Health and Welfare Canada. Achieving health for all: a framework for health promotion. Ottawa: Ministry of Supply and Services, 1986:3.
3. Butterfield P. Thinking upstream: nurturing a conceptual understanding of the societal context of health behaviour. Adv Nurs Sci 1990;12(2):1–8.
4. Phillips JR. Research and the riddle of change. Nurs Sci Q 1990;3(2):55–6.
5. Benner P. Quality of life: a phenomenological perspective on explanation, predication, and understanding in nursing science. Adv Nurs Sci 1985;8:1–14.
6. King IJ. A theory for nursing: systems, concepts, process. New York: John Wiley and Sons, 1981.
7. Rogers M. An introduction to the theoretical basis of nursing. Philadelphia: FA Davis, 1970.
8. Bramlet M, Geuldner S, Sowell R. Consumer-centric advocacy: its connection to nursing frameworks. Nurs Sci Q 1990;3(4):156–61.
9. Anderson J. Home care management of chronic illness and the self-care movement: an analysis of ideologies and economic processes influencing policy decisions. Adv Nurs Sci 1990;12(2):71–83.
10. Forester J. What do planning analysts do? Planning and policy analysis as organizing. Policy Studies J 1980;9(1):595–604.
11. Canadian Nurses' Association. Canada health act we've won. Can Nurse 1984;8:5.

Chapter 51

Nursing's Past, Present, and Future Political Experiences

BETHANY A. HALL-LONG

For community health nurses to be leaders and effect change in the health system and in community health requires political expertise and involvement. In this chapter, Dr. Hall-Long demonstrates nursing's long history as a political force and yet cites research showing that nurses today need to be far more active in influencing public policy. She proposes strategies that promote improved public policy education, socialization, and participation for nurses. She also challenges nursing to become politically proactive in the early stages of policy formation and to unite on public policy issues.

Contemporary public policy shifts and political opportunities make it important for the nursing profession to revisit the efforts of its political pioneers. Such historical inquiry can reveal "old truths about nursing's past and shed light on its emergence, helping to determine whether as a profession it has grown up or just grown older" (Church, 1985, p. 188) in the public policy arena. In addition to reviewing some of nursing's political roots, an examination of nursing's policy research and political activities can offer insight to the profession for improved political transformations.

Since the nursing profession is 97 percent female, much of the battle that nurses have had to fight to gain recognition in the policy process has been for women's rights. Among the many women's groups and female dominated professions, nursing has been one of the premiere political forces. "Nurses organized the first major professional association for women, edited and published the first professional magazine by women, and were the first major professional group to integrate black and white members" (Bullough & Bullough, 1984, pp. 41–42). Despite the profession's earlier organizational capabilities, the female profession of nursing "represents 67 percent of the health care providers in the United States, and very few are in positions where they can influence health policy making" (Sohier, 1992, p. 63).

The small cadre of contemporary nurse leaders in politics (De Back, 1990; Milio, 1989) continue to face extensions of public health and nurs-

From *N&HC: Perspectives on Community* 16(1):24–28. Reprinted with permission. Copyright 1995 National League for Nursing.

ing practice policy issues that their earlier predecessors also encountered. Although not exhaustive of all politically astute nurse leaders, critical players in nursing's political establishment and American Women's History can be traced to such leaders as Nightingale, Barton, Dock, Wald, and Sanger.

Florence Nightingale is known as the wealthy young British woman who founded the nursing profession during the Crimean War era. Her efforts have earned her the title, "consummate political nurse" (Goldwater & Zusy, 1990, p. 6). She was influential in the reformation of hospitals and in crafting and implementing public health policies for the British Sanitary System (Kalisch & Kalisch, 1982). Florence Nightingale was the first nurse to exert political pressure on government and remains among a small cadre of politically renowned nurses.

During the American Civil War, the school teacher who volunteered as a nurse, Clara Barton, was responsible for organizing the nursing services. She is not only known for her role in improving battlefield health care, but also for establishing the American Red Cross. Barton's persuasion of Congress in 1882 to ratify the Treaty of Geneva so that the Red Cross could perform humanitarian efforts in times of peace has had lasting impressions on national and international policies (Kelly, 1991).

By the turn of the 19th century, America was influenced by such politically skilled nurses as Margaret Sanger, Lillian Wald, and Lavinia Dock. Margaret Higgins Sanger, a public health nurse in the Lower East Side of New York, was instrumental in addressing health issues of factory workers, especially women. Her experience with a large number of unwanted pregnancies among the working poor facilitated her role in promoting public birth control education and accessibility. Despite the legal and social ramifications, she opened the first birth control clinic in America in Brooklyn. Her political activism has had a lasting impact on women's health care policies (Kelly, 1991).

Like Nightingale, Wald was a wealthy young woman who took a different path from most women in her social class. The path she chose led to the improvement of the welfare and health of women and children in the United States. She cofounded the Henry Street Settlement House in New York, which was devoted to providing health care, social services, and education to the sick poor. One of Wald's greatest contributions came with her political ingenuity and pressure to see the creation of the United States Children's Bureau. The Bureau was established by Congress in 1912 to oversee fair child labor laws that facilitated the well being of the country's children (Kelly, 1991).

Wald's friend, Lavinia Dock, was a prolific writer and political activist who was among the early feminists. She was a devoted suffragette who eagerly participated in protests and demonstrations until the 1920 passage of the Nineteenth Amendment to the U.S. Constitution which allowed women to vote. In addition, she waged a campaign for legislation to allow nurses versus physicians to control the profession. In 1893, with the assistance of Isabel Hampton Robb and Mary Adelaide Nutting, she founded the very politically active organization, the American Society of Superintendents of Training Schools for Nurses of the United States and Canada, a precursor to the current National League for Nursing (NLN) (Goldwater & Zusy, 1990; Kelly, 1991).

▬NURSING ORGANIZATIONS MANIFEST
THE CYCLICAL NATURE OF INTEREST GROUPS

The value of organized efforts among nurses was recognized during the late 19th century. The National Associated Alumnae of the U.S. and Canada and American Society of Superintendents of Training Schools of the U.S. and Canada were formed in the 1890s. These groups were the precursors of the current American Nurses Association and National League for Nursing respectively. Nursing alumnae groups were formulated mostly in response to state licensure requirements, standards of education, and welfare issues of nurses (Kelly, 1991). The leaders of the groups, typical of other female occupations of that time, were mostly older and unmarried. These dedicated women actively tried to gain influence in the male-dominated hospitals and colleges.

Over the years, the number of nursing organizations have dramatically increased. Expository works reflect how nursing associations or interest groups have played a positive role in influencing and promoting nursing practice and public health policies (American Academy of Nursing, 1987; Bullough & Bullough, 1984; Kelly, 1991). Political effectiveness of organizations is influenced by organizational skills, resources, and incentives. Divisiveness and turf battles have been known inhibitors of the nursing interest groups' political capabilities for years (American Academy of Nursing, 1987; Raymond Rich Associates, 1946). However, nursing associations have become increasingly aware of the need for intraprofessional interaction and consensus on public policy positions.

"Nursing organizations have not remained static. They have arisen in many forms; they have competed for members, powers . . . they have differentiated and diversified; they have merged; some have declined and died. . . . Changes happened in response to a multitude of variables within and external to the profession" (American Academy of Nursing, 1987, p. 1). Thus, nursing shares with other disciplines and professions the cyclical nature and central role of interest groups. Some are national and international organizations, while others are regional, state, local, or specialty-focused. Despite their differences, all organizations are in a dynamic relationship with their legal, economic, social, technological, and political environments.

An example of this progressive involvement in the political arena was displayed by the organizational steps leading to the ANA's Political Action Committee (ANA-PAC). In 1971, a small group of nurses in New York State formed the Nurses' For Political Action (NPA), a nonpartisan, nonprofit association of registered and practical nurses. The NPA was set up to influence state and national policy makers, to educate other health care professionals and the public about nurses and health policy, and to recognize nurses' role in the health care delivery (*American Journal of Nursing*, 1972). The NPA was appointed as an ad hoc committee of the ANA's Board of Directors in 1973 to investigate the establishment of a policy arm for the ANA. In conjunction with state political action groups and the NPA, an independent arm of ANA, the National Coalition for Action in Politics (N-CAP) was formed. The N-CAP's focus was on educating, assisting, and stimulating political education and participation of nurses as well as nonpartisan fund raising (*American Nurse*, 1974; *American Journal of Nursing*, 1971). In 1986, the N-CAP became part of the ANA and was renamed the ANA-PAC.

Effective alliances among nursing associations have been formed and include such entities as the Tri-Council For Nursing, the National Federation of Specialty Nursing Organizations (NFSNO), and the Nursing Organization Liaison Forum (NOLF).

The Tri-Council For Nursing originated in 1981 and was composed of the American Nurses' Association (ANA), the National League for Nursing (NLN), and the American Association of Colleges of Nursing (AACN). In 1985, the American Organization of Nurse Executives (AONE) joined the alliance without any change in title. The collective efforts of these groups such as the Tri-Council for Nursing have played an important role in advancing the profession and the nations' health in the policy arena (Carty & Cherry, 1989). According to the American Academy of Nursing (1987), the Tri-Council for Nursing "grew out of a succession of efforts to respond to the multiple interdependencies and the need for a more unified approach by the nursing profession to its publics" (p. 22). A major intent of the alliance is to facilitate coordination and communication on key professional issues and activities as well as to assist with promoting concordance on federal legislation of mutual concern.

Similarly, NFSNO is a loosely structured alliance of nursing specialty organizations. Its members range from large national organizations (e.g., the American Association of Critical-Care Nurses) to very small groups (e.g., National Intravenous Therapy Association). Since its origins in 1981, NFSNO's focus has been on coordinating efforts of practice, education, and other areas of mutual concern among nursing organizations. In 1985, NFSNO decided to include only clinical specialty organizations as members and to exclude large multipurpose nursing organizations such as the ANA or NLN.

NOLF is another coalition of nursing organizations that attempts to give a unified approach to national policy issues and nursing interests. ANA, in collaboration with representatives from a number of other nursing organizations, established NOLF in the early 1980s. NOLF, a diverse forum within the ANA, meets at least annually to promote concerted actions by national nursing organizations. Its members can include organizations that are also part of the NFSNO alliance such as the American Critical Care Nurses Association.

▬ RESEARCH ON NURSING'S POLITICAL SOCIALIZATION STILL IN ITS INFANCY

The nursing profession, like other female professions, is using a number of political efforts to influence policy development while attempting to eliminate sexist images. Women in society are becoming more and more actively involved in local, state, and national politics and the 1990s have been deemed the decade of women in politics.

Despite such progress, women's deliverance from apolitical images and behavior has been slow. Whicker, Jewell, and Lovelace (1989) describe how women have made some inroads in obtaining elected political office at the state (13.9 percent of positions) and local (17.1 percent of positions) levels. The authors discuss women's political paradox of constituting 53 percent of the population, yet possessing only a small fraction of elected offices at all levels of government. With the 1992 elections, U.S. Congressional records were broken in regard to the number of women winning elections. Women comprised 11 percent of the 435 members of the U.S. House of Representatives and seven percent of the 100 members of the U.S. Senate. Most significantly, 1992 saw the election of the first African-American woman to the U.S. Senate (Carol Moseley Braun, D-Illinois), and the first nurse to the U.S. House of Representatives (Eddie Bernice Johnson, D-Texas).

An increased number of anecdotal articles on public policy education, socialization, participation, and research (Batra, 1992; Buerhaus, 1992; Sharp, Biggs, & Wakefield, 1991) have appeared in the nursing literature. However, actual policy studies in nursing have minimally increased since Milio's (1984) comprehensive literature review which found sparse nursing policy research in nursing and no nursing policy analysis research by nurses. Research on nursing's political socialization, education, and participation levels is in its infancy. In developing nursing administration curriculum, Scalzi and Wilson (1990) surveyed 184 top-level, U.S. nurse executives in home health, acute care, long-term care, and occupational health settings. They found that law and health care policy were ranked as the most time consuming and most important by nurse executives regardless of the practice setting. The role of education and socialization in health policy and politics was deemed essential for future nurse administrators.

Barry's (1989) descriptive research study of the political socialization processes of 33 nurses in specialized policy-making roles in the state and federal governments found that nurses involved in policy making were not "typical" of employed nurses. They, like other political pioneers in nursing, tended to be older, not married, childless, and had higher levels of formal education. In addition, Barry found that formal nursing education had not been a major factor in socializing these nurses for their political roles. The majority of the nurses had acquired an interest in the public policy process after they had completed basic nursing education as a result of interactions with non-nurses immersed in the public policy process.

Hanley (1983) underscored the need for political education in all generic and continuing education nurses programs to enhance the influence of education and political behaviors. Her exploratory study found that nurses with baccalaureate-level education were as active as teachers and engineers in such political behaviors as voting, campaigning, communal activity, and protest. Building on Hanley's work, Gesse (1989) examined education as a predictor of the political participation of nurse-midwives who belonged to the American College of Nurse-Midwives. She found that the members' political behaviors, particularly voting, increased after involvement with the political activities of the American College of Nurse-Midwives. However, contrary to Hanley's study, education was not identified as a predictor of political participation.

Hayes and Fritsch (1988) found a significant relationship between nurses' political attitudes and the amount of their political activity. Their descriptive correlational study of 250 registered nurses in Massachusetts revealed that the early political socialization and education of nurses boosted nurses' political attitudes and eventual political participation. In addition, higher levels of education and professional organizational membership were associated with greater participation.

In 1988, Daffin examined the political expectations and participation of registered nurses (n = 447) in Alabama who were employed in clinical practice, academia, and administration. Of her sample, 91 percent expected politically active nurses to participate in the nine political roles of voter, monitor, negotiator, networker, leader, spokesperson, campaigner, lobbyist, and player. However, only 26 percent of the sample indicated that they actually participated in these roles. Nurse administrators had the highest political expectations and participation, and were trailed by the nurse educators who were followed by the nurse clinicians. Daffin concluded that although nurses have high political expectations, they primarily are limited to their political role of voting.

Archer (1983) explored the political participation activities of over 500 nurse administrators in home health, hospitals, and schools of nursing. The three political activities observed most frequently among her the subjects were voting, writing letters to legislators, and belonging to and/or serving on community or nursing organizations or boards. Ninety-four percent of Archer's participants felt that nurses were not as active politically as they should be. In turn, they listed potential reasons for their low political participation which included inadequate political socialization and education, apathy, divisiveness among nursing's associations, and the lack of knowledge of and skills in the political process.

To fill the void of political frameworks in nursing, Hall-Long (1993) devised a public policy process model. The Tri-Council for Nursing's political efforts with the 1991–1992 Nurse Education Act's reauthorization was used as the exemplary case to test the model. Analysis of the data gathered from interviews and questionnaires collected from 15 participants, representing the Federal Government and the Tri-Council for Nursing, supported the utility of the model in analyzing the political process at the national level. Ancillary findings of this case study furthermore revealed that organized nursing often perceived its effectiveness and frequency of select political strategies in a more favorable rating than did governmental respondents.

▬A UNITED VOICE IS MORE POLITICALLY POWERFUL THAN FRAGMENTED ECHOES AND DIVERSE APPEALS

A number of political implications can be extracted from nursing's political pioneers, organized efforts, and policy studies. Nurses at the bedside, in academia, and administration are affected on a daily basis by public policy. Thus, the inclusion in such debates demands that all nurses be proactive in the earliest stages of policy development. Individual nurses can influence policy decisions at all intergovernmental levels, and organized nursing's unified efforts such as with *Nursing's Agenda For Health Care Reform* (Tri-Council for Nursing, 1991) will be critical to exerting nursing's influence early on in the political process. In addition to these policy development efforts, nurses need to strive to promote better political strategies. As previously discussed, these strategies entail improved public policy education, socialization, and general participation.

Specific strategies can include: integration of public policy courses and/or content into nursing curriculum; active socialization and recognition of nurse educators, administrators, and clinicians for public policy participation; taking part in organizational or professional legislative networks and/or grassroots initiatives; establishing educational or work experiences in diverse public policy-making settings at the local, state, and federal levels; conducting public policy research; giving testimony at public hearings; assisting with campaign efforts, and running for public office. Nurses have direct experience and a thorough knowledge of the health care needs of individuals, families, and communities. The profession represents experts in addressing the diverse health care needs of the country's underserved and most vulnerable groups. Nurses need to now collaborate with the public and media in engineering policy positions that promote the nation's health as well as the public policy-making role of the nursing profession.

In turn, organized nursing needs to unite on the public policy front. A united, central voice is much more politically powerful than fragmented echoes and diverse appeals. Coalitions among nursing organizations and professional and consumer groups can provide many opportunities to advance nursing's policy agenda and "victories."

Obviously, the implications for positive political change are enumerable. Following the lead of our political pioneers risk-taking behavior, contemporary nurses need to face the political challenges of the 21st century to guarantee representation around the public policy-making tables. Once around these tables, political voices and power will be welded to the nursing profession and to the consumers they represent.

▬REFERENCES

American Academy of Nursing (AAN). (1987). *The evaluation of nursing professional organizations: Alternative models for the future.* Washington, DC: American Academy of Nursing.

American Journal of Nursing. (1972). Nurses political action group formed. *American Journal of Nursing, 71*(10), 1784.

American Nurse (1974). N-CAP: Nursing's political action arm. *American Nurse, 6*(6), 1, 12.

Archer, S. (1983). A study of nurse administrator's political participation. *Western Journal of Nursing Research, 5*(1), 65–75.

Barry, C. (1989). *A descriptive study of the political socialization processes of nurses in specialized roles in federal and state governments.* Dissertation Abstracts International (University Microfilms No. 89-19002).

Batra, C. (1992). Empowering for professional, political, and health policy involvement. *Nursing Outlook, 40*(4), 170–176.

Buerhaus, P. (1992). Teaching health care public policy. *Nursing & Health Care, 13*(6), 304–309.

Bullough, V., & Bullough, B. (1984). *History, trends, and politics of nursing.* Norwalk, CT: Appleton-Century-Crofts.

Carty, R., & Cherry, B. (1989). National Center For Nursing Research. In C.E. Lambert & V.A. Lambert (eds.), *Perspectives in nursing: The impacts on the nurse, consumer, and society* (pp. 254–277). Norwalk, CT: Appleton & Lange.

Church, O. (1985). New knowledge from old truths: Problems and promises of historical inquiry of nursing. In J. McCloskey & H. Grace (eds.), *Current issues in nursing* (2nd ed., pp. 182–189). Boston, MA: Blackwell.

Daffin, P. (1988). *Similarities and differences in political expectations and participation among nurses in clinical practice, education, and administration.* Dissertation Abstracts International (University Microfilms No. 89-09780).

De Back, V. (1990). Nursing needs health policy leaders. *Journal of Professional Nursing, 6*(2), 69.

Gesse, T. (1989). *Education as a determinant of political participation of nurse-midwives.* Dissertation Abstracts International (University Microfilms No. 89-09780).

Goldwater, M., & Zusy, M. (1990). *Prescription for nurses effective political action.* Philadelphia, PA: Mosby.

Hall-Long, B. (1993). *A policy process model: Analysis of the Nurse Education Act of 1991–1992* (doctoral dissertation). George Mason University, Fairfax, VA.

Hanley, B. (1983). *Nurse political participation: An in-depth view and comparison with women teachers and engineers* (doctoral dissertation). The University of Michigan, Ann Arbor.

Hayes, E., & Fritsch, R. (1988). An untapped resource: The political potential of nurses. *Nursing Administration Quarterly, 13*(1), 33–39.

Kalisch, P. & Kalisch, B. (1982). *Politics of Nursing.* Philadelphia, PA: Lippincott.

Kelly, L. (1991). *Dimensions of professional nursing* (6th ed., pp. 423–426). New York, NY: Pergaman Press.

Kessler, T. (1989). Research and policy formation: Is there a fit? *Journal of Professional Nursing, 5*(5), 246.

Milio, N. (1984). Nursing research and the study of health policy. In *Annals of Nursing Research,* New York, NY: Springer.

Milio, N. (1989). Developing nursing leadership in health policy. *Journal of Professional Nursing, 5,* 315–321.

Raymond Rich Associates. (1946). Report on the structure of organized nursing. *American Journal of Nursing, 46*(10), 648–661.

Scalzi, C., & Wilson, D. (1990). Empirically based recommendations for content of graduate nursing administration programs. *Nursing & Health Care, 11*(10), 522–525.

Sharp, N., Biggs, S., & Wakefield, M. (1991). Public policy: New opportunities for nurses. *Nursing & Health Care, 12*(1), 16–22.

Sohier, R. (1992). Feminism and nursing knowledge: The power of the weak. *Nursing Outlook, 40*(2), 62–93.

Tri-Council for Nursing. (1991). *Nursing's agenda for health care reform.* Washington, DC: American Nurses Association.

Whicker, M., Jewell, M., & Lovelace, L. (1989). *Women in Congress.* Unpublished study, Virginia Commonwealth University, Richmond, VA.

Chapter 52

Leadership For Expanding Nursing Influence On Health Policy

CAROLYNE K. DAVIS   DEBORAH OAKLEY

JULIE A. SOCHALSKI

Community health nursing's mandate to be concerned for the health of ag-gregates clearly requires an enlarged role in health policymaking. How can this be done? For many nurses, this appears to be a formal, formidable, and impossible task. But it is not. It can be done if nurses increase their political expertise and their activity in the political arena. Practical suggestions for accomplishing both these tasks are offered by the authors of this chapter. They discuss three major principles for nurses to practice, and they de-scribe a set of guidelines for gathering political support and for effectively intervening in the policymaking process at state and national levels. Enlarg-ing on this discussion, the authors present a set of practical checklists for political activity and an example of nurses who became effectively in-volved in the political process in Michigan.

Health policy development at the federal level has become highly political, with billions of federal dollars awarded for health care and health man-power. Influence in shaping U.S. health policy requires a knowledge of the political process and a commitment to working with the various levels of health policy decision makers. Until recently, the nursing profession has relied on a small cadre of people to influence federal or state legislative policy development. To increase nursing's effectiveness in competing for scarce resources, the number of politically active nurses will have to in-crease as well.

Traditionally, physicians and other health care professionals have domi-nated in shaping health policies. By learning the art of politics, nurses can exert political influence and have a major effect on such health policy areas as nurses' training, research, medicaid and medicare, and other leg-

From *Journal of Nursing Administration*, Vol. XII, No. 1:15–21, January 1982. Reprinted by per-mission of J. B. Lippincott Company.

islation and regulations that affect both acute and long-term care agencies. At the federal level, about 2,500 health-related bills and resolutions are introduced during every two-year congressional session. While only two percent of these are enacted into law, many have the potential to affect nursing. Thus, it is essential that nurses make their views known to influence the outcome of these policies.

▬LEADERSHIP

In this article, a brief presentation of the nature of the leadership role prepares the way for a discussion of principles and specific strategies nursing leaders can use to develop their own and others' political influence, with the goal of advancing nursing's concerns for better health care.

According to Blau, as well as Claus and Bailey, leadership should be viewed as multidimensional, encompassing the wise use of power, managerial functions, and human relations processes.[1,2] When combined, these characteristics can influence members of a group to move toward goal setting and goal attainment. The concepts of leadership and power have an active orientation, identifying leaders not only by the power they possess, but also by their responsible use of it. Power is the resource by which leaders coordinate activities and effect change.

In working with groups, powerful nursing leaders who understand and are committed to group goals make the most of the resources of group members, and encourage appropriate actions that yield desired results.[3] Successful leadership requires a well-developed reciprocal relationship between the leader and the group members. Nursing leaders need to establish those reciprocal relationships locally with other nurses and nursing groups to augment nursing's ongoing policy-influencing activities.

▬INITIATING ACTIONS

There are three major principles of action for nursing leaders to follow for effective policy intervention at local, state, and national levels. They are: 1) obtain and maintain current and accurate information on policies affecting nursing; 2) disseminate that information to build support; and 3) direct activity to affect targeted policy issues.

Stay Informed

Obtain and maintain current and accurate information. Identify all formal sources and channels for collecting, translating or digesting, and disseminating information. The most prominent examples of formal channels are professional nursing organizations, especially their legislative offices. Frequent personal contacts with these offices can help you become a part of the formal communication network.

A second, equally important step is to monitor informal channels. Many informal channels for communication exist among nursing leaders, and usually complement formal channels.

It is important to recognize that information obtained through formal and informal channels is always flavored by the sender. This is not to suggest that the information is inaccurate or distorted; rather it means that the emphasis will vary according to the interests of the source. For example, the rescission of Nurse Training Act funding would result in reductions within several areas for nursing. Some information sources would focus on the effects on capitation, while others would emphasize the devastating effect on nursing research efforts. Each is important, but the primary interest of the message originator would lead to differing emphasis. Thus, it is wise to evaluate the tone and emphasis of the information you receive by taking the source of that information into account.

Build a Support Base

Disseminate the information to recruit support, as well as to inform. Your first contacts should be key persons who have access to larger numbers and can build a base of support. Previous activists for nursing causes are a good starting point since they usually are persons who have mobilized groups and can identify other previous or potential supporters.

Identifying these key persons and maintaining communication with them is essential to the development and expansion of an informed support group. Data sent to the support group should be well coordinated to ensure their accuracy, currency, and consistency.

Provide Direction

Supporters need direction, and will look to their leaders for it. A concise plan of action, including specifically identified activities for workers at all levels and appropriate methods of feedback, is particularly effective. The checklist in Box 52-1 serves as a guide for organizing such activities.

Strength does come from numbers, so it is critical to present a unified front on the issues. However, internal strife is to be expected as a part of the politicizing process, and is usually directly proportional to the number of groups or personal interests involved. One way to minimize its effects is to maintain an orientation toward group goals rather than personal need satisfaction.

▬ GUIDELINES FOR INTERVENTIONS

Based on the experiences of our own group of politically active nurses in Michigan's Second Congressional District, we can provide some specific suggestions for influencing members of the legislative and executive branches of government. Since few nursing administrators have an established routine for visiting with legislators—local or national—and other governmental decision makers, two checklists are presented. Box 52-2 is a checklist for meeting with legislators; Box 52-3 is a checklist for meeting with administrative decision makers and aides. Keeping in mind that successful policy-making participation is more than episodic, construct a "decision tree," showing key actors and the timetable for their annual budget-making deci-

---

BOX 52–1   *Checklist for Organizing and Directing a Political Action Group.*

1. Organize a steering committee responsible for coordinating the dissemination of information as well as directing the activities of supporters. It is important to include persons with experience in mobilizing support for policy intervention, and key leaders from each group you are trying to recruit for support.
2. Develop a briefing sheet to inform supporters about the issue. This should be a concise description that presents all pertinent facts related to the central issue and its impact on them and the profession. Dissemination of the briefing sheets to their respective groups is the responsibility of each member of the steering committee.
3. Include with the briefing sheet a list of activities that all supporters can undertake in response to the issue. Names, addresses, and phone numbers of legislators to call or write should be included. List proper forms of address and provide suggestions that workers can use in their messages. Phone numbers for mailgrams and other Western Union services are very important to include, especially when time is short. Provide directions for use of these services (for example, cost, allowable number of words, how long it takes for the message to be sent, and sample messages).
4. Assemble phone lists of all other key leaders locally, statewide, or nationally who should be informed of the issue and the activities being initiated. A good way to organize these lists to insure completeness and eliminate duplication is to use index cards with names, addresses, phone number, position, and other relevant information.
5. Use of the telephone is effective for contacting supporters when time is limited, and also as an introduction to or reinforcement of materials being sent by mail. The message to be given in each contact should be determined by the steering committee to insure uniformity. Each contact should be recorded, noting the message given, the individual's response, and the activities he or she will undertake.
6. Identify for all contacts and supporters one central phone as the "headquarters" reference point. A central number will help coordinate information dissemination and facilitate effective feedback.
7. Frequent steering committee meetings are essential so that members can report the results of their activities and plan new strategies. Coordination is the unequivocal basis for success. Once the communication channels are under control, the committee can divert some attention toward developing strategies for influencing targeted legislative groups.

---

sions. In many cases, the most effective interventions are made to affect decisions one or two fiscal years in the future. As a general rule, emergency organizing is useful to limit threatened damage, but action to *improve* budgetary allocations for nursing requires considerable advance planning.

Working Effectively with Legislators

Of particular importance in working with legislators is a clear statement of what you actually want. A one- or two-page briefing sheet should present

---

BOX 52–2   *Checklist for an Effective Visit with a Legislator.*

1. Know your legislator. Send someone to the city newspaper or local library to do research. Even if you know a lot, you may find out more.
2. Make an appointment. Be satisfied to see a staff member who specializes in health, or sometimes education, depending on the specific reason for your visit. Often the aide knows more about details and is important to have on your side in any case. Getting ten minutes of a legislator's or an aide's time is good; getting half an hour should be considered a marked success.
3. Take along a briefing sheet to discuss and leave with the legislator or aide. It should not be longer than two pages (or both sides of one page). Make it neat and attractive, but not "cute." Be professional. Use ANA and NLN material when appropriate.
4. Ask the legislator to do something that is within his or her power to do. Be specific and reasonable about what you want and include it prominently in the briefing sheet.
5. It is helpful to append a list of organizations or people known to the legislator who support your position. Letters, Xeroxed copies of newspaper articles, copies of resolutions, or a simple list will do.
6. State arguments in terms the decision maker uses and values. Cost savings and cost effectiveness are central concerns for most legislators these days. Nurses may be primarily concerned about the quality of care, but legislators care about tradeoffs in expenditures. *Emphasize the impact on the legislator's local constituency.*
7. Follow up. Establish a continuing dialogue. Write to express gratitude for time and thought spent in your meeting. Write when important new information is available. If you and the legislator or aide disagree, keep writing, but be understanding of their position.

---

the basic facts. With hundreds of actions pending, it is impossible for legislators to remember details about each one. Thus, it is helpful to review the actual amounts of money in question, the regulations being discussed, and other particulars. Remember that the power of legislators is limited. Members of Congress cannot single-handedly change policy, but they can help by contacting colleagues, helping set up meetings with other important people, telephoning or writing members of the administration, working with other interest groups, speaking to constituent groups, and so on.

When asking for help beyond a single vote on a particular issue, it is most effective to ask legislators to do something that suits their style, philosophy of government, and general political orientation. For instance, party-goers are more likely to agree to attend a party while serious speech-givers will usually address a convention. The goal is to recruit the legislators' active involvement, so it is important to find *some* action(s) they will actually take.

It is equally important to discuss nursing concerns with a legislator's top aide. If there is no chance for a brief conversation, simply leaving a business card is a significant step toward being perceived as a person with needed information and relevant involvement. If an aide continues to be inaccessible

---

**BOX 52–3   *Checklist for an Effective Meeting with Members
of the Executive Branch.***

1. Learn as much as you can about the participants. Talk to others who may
   know more about them; check the newspaper and library files; read *Who's
   Who*. Keep your own files on important people.
2. Organize a coalition of top people. Expertise and interest are strengthened
   by the contributions of people from other organizations and institutions.
   The coalition may dissolve after a single meeting, or after a series. It does
   not need to be permanent; its goal is to arrange for an effective contact.
3. Prepare briefing material, including two to five pages stating exactly what
   you want and why. Use data, but summarize research results.
4. Practice making the presentations and fielding potential questions from the
   participants. Agreement within the coalition group is extremely important.
   A professional, but not highly polished presentation is a necessity.
5. Evaluate the effectiveness of the presentations and the meeting. Keep notes
   and circulate some record of the meeting to other leaders.

---

to you, find another staff member with a different temperament, appearance, or background to do the job. Be goal-oriented, not ego-sensitive.

It is useful at this point to mention some specific "don'ts." In conversations with legislators, do not get sidetracked. Conversation about trivial topics consumes time. It is a healthy ice-breaker, but you can keep it brief by moving on to say something like, "We are really deeply concerned about nursing, and we came to talk with you about. . . ."

Do not use jargon or too much technical language. Your language should convey your highly professional status and expertise, but not distance or parochialism. Enhance mutual respect and always try to emphasize the relationship of your issues to the legislator's constituency.

Contacting the Executive Branch

Often the executive branch of government is harder to affect than the legislature, but don't neglect it since many proposals originate with state and national administrative offices. Prevention is more effective than cure. Work with the executive branch can be frustrating, though, since bureaucratic priorities are often difficult to diagnose.

Despite these difficulties, nursing leaders need to know who is most influential in making decisions that affect the profession. Contacts should be maintained with budget offices, planning units, or other divisions of government that initiate, monitor, or evaluate nursing activities. In the federal government, the Office of Management and Budget is particularly important. An arm of the Governor's office or a small staff close to a departmental director is frequently most influential at the state level. Regardless of how power is distributed, a number of offices, each with its own authority, are sure to be involved. The focal point of contacts depends on the particular proposal, and much of the work will involve government administrators outside the nursing office. Once identified, educate these contacts about nursing, and influence their opinion by discussing and clarifying other points of view. Formal as well as informal channels of communication can be used to accomplish these goals.

Building Long-Term Political Involvement

In the long run, effective lobbying for nursing concerns requires local political movement. Enough nurses must become politically active to make nursing a local political force that can strengthen the existing national presence. The case presentation that follows is one example of successful local organization. Readers who find it useful should be careful to adapt it to the existing situation in their own community.

In Michigan's Second Congressional District, we wanted to build long-term political participation by nurses. The first step was to create a group as representative as possible of all nursing interests. Two briefing sessions were held with our local congressman to open a dialogue that we hoped would increase his commitment to act on nursing issues. This, in fact, is what happened. Because of an earlier lobbying effort, a small nursing group from the University of Michigan already had access to the congressional office. But we recognized that, although our particular interests might be diluted somewhat by expanding, long-term influence would depend on a large and diverse interest group. A congressperson may favor narrow issues, but his or her decisions are always made within the wider context of tradeoffs. Muting a small group's self-interest from time to time may maximize long-term gains. In other words, through solidarity the gains are greater for nursing.

CREATING AN INTEREST GROUP.   Lists were particularly helpful in building a representative group. We built our list in a tree-like fashion, including all nursing organizations and agencies with large nursing staffs in our congressional district. We also made note of key members and their political interests.

Selected representatives were invited to form a steering committee for the first briefing meeting with our congressman. At a planning meeting, each member made index cards for all the local people they thought might be interested in attending the meeting. This list was later augmented to include the entire leadership of the local Michigan Nurses' Association District, leading nurse administrators, bargaining agents, and faculty members. The purpose was to build an inclusive, not an exclusive, group.

The planning group selected a local community college as the site for two meetings with the congressman. It also approved the invitation letter and established subcommittees for invitations to others, parking, hospitality, and preparation of background materials for all invitees. Invitations were duplicated on a copying machine and sent out two to three weeks in advance. An R.S.V.P. was requested to monitor the numbers planning to attend. If the number had been small, a telephone follow-up would have been initiated.

ACCOMPLISHING YOUR GOALS.   Both meetings were well attended by 70 to 85 of the nearly 150 persons invited, a high attendance rate for a political event. A small percentage who said they would come but did not was offset by nonrespondents and spontaneous arrivals of people missed on the invitation list. An agenda and background materials were distributed to focus attention on relevant issues. We were careful to avoid internally divisive issues as entry into practice, since Congress has no formal role to play in this area.

In the first meeting considerable time was spent circulating informally and conversing in small groups. This kind of activity is good for coalition-building, particularly if the "greeters" are good at directing conversation. It also allows a more human view of the legislator, as nurses individually exchange thoughts with him or her. This informal period should not take too long, however, since the main purpose is serious business. The agenda for this meeting was to establish contact with an expanded group of nurses and to have the congressman and others involved with the legislative process provide an update on current legislation affecting nursing. This plan provided a forum for participants to raise their concerns about specific pieces of legislation.

The agenda for the second meeting included very brief presentations from a number of major interest groups within nursing, including the nurse anesthetists, the State nurses' association, academic units, the black nurses' association, and nurse researchers. In both meetings, the congressman presented updates and exchanged questions and opinions with the audience as a whole.

Box 52-4 provides steps for organizing a meeting with a legislator. In our experience, it was most effective to have an informal, but well structured format. Be sure to provide the legislator in advance with information from national or state nursing organizations so that he or she will understand the issues and be prepared to make commitments for real action. It is too easy for legislators to say they will "study" an issue; meetings should be times when public commitments are firmly made. Assign a member of your group to drive the legislator to the meeting, or to meet him or her at the door and talk briefly, armed with a few ready facts and figures.

Meetings are only one way to involve legislators in nursing issues. Our local ANA district legislative committee has regularly scheduled legislative breakfasts with a rotating list of state and local political leaders. Whatever method is used, nurses need to remember that, ultimately, legislators are interested in votes. If a legislator is generally supportive of nursing, then it is in the nurses' best interest to keep him or her in office. When a legislator is not generally supportive, it is a nursing leadership responsibility to help organize on behalf of an opposition candidate who *is* supportive. '

Remember, however, that an elected official can only help nursing causes. He or she cannot do our job in policy intervention. The nursing profession must be responsible for the daily work required to identify problems, formulate viable legislative proposals, and work for their adoption.

BOX 52–4   *Steps in Organizing a Political Meeting.*

1. Take the initiative. If other groups are not ready to organize a meeting, set up an ad hoc coalition for the purpose. Meet first with a very small group chosen for their political and organizing experience.
2. Include all the organizations and important people who are willing to be involved. To compile names, turn to lists of officers and members of organizations, friendly colleagues, your own rolodex, agency directories, nurses mentioned in newspaper articles, or letters to the editor. Include important nursing leaders from outside your politician's district if they might have an interest.
3. Spend some money. The biggest expenditure will probably be for postage. Influence often requires a moderate investment of some personal resources, especially time, money, and prestige. The budget may include items for typing, copying, and mailing the invitations; for refreshments, room rental, and photographs; supplies (name tags, pens, registration pads, agendas, and other relevant material); and follow-up correspondence. Some or all of these items can be donated, but remember that recruiting donations often takes precious time in a professional life. Do not make contributing money a prerequisite for membership on the planning committee. Do not ask for donations at the meeting. Political fund raisers come later. Of course, if participants volunteer contributions, do not turn them down.
4. Choose a neutral meeting site and include a map in the invitation.
5. Convey a sense of personal commitment in the invitations. Address each clearly and neatly; do not use labels. Use commemorative stamps for the outside envelope, but choose stamps representing a cause that all of your invitees will respond to favorably.
6. With your invitation, include a self-addressed, stamped postcard or a similarly prepared envelope and R.S.V.P. letter so that invitees need only sign their name and send it back. Request correction of addresses and telephone numbers even if they cannot attend. It is helpful to use a ready-made stamp for the return address.
7. Prepare name tags and kits or handouts in advance. Make handouts brief, but to the point. Colored paper helps.
8. Serve a minimum of food. Every aspect of the meeting should convey its importance. Nursing is concerned with serious issues, and should not get distracted by potlucks or other elements of a social event. The atmosphere should be comfortable, but organized and professional.

In our congressional district, a group of nurses has worked in the election campaign of a supportive congressman. As part of our organizing effort, we obtained a list of registered nurses in the congressional district. A similar list can be obtained from most State Boards of Nursing for a nominal fee; although the list is not arranged by voting districts, a close approximation can be obtained by sorting the list by zip codes. This ad hoc group of nurses has worked closely with the congressman's campaign staff—a requirement for effective political activity—to perform various grassroots organizing tasks. As a result, nursing has become an active force within the

---

BOX 52–5 The Basic Activities of an Effective Government Relations Operation.

1. Know the territory. Know who the actors are, where the power is, and who is making the decisions. Keep that information current.
2. Be thoroughly grounded and familiar with legislative processes, particularly the appropriations process.
3. Maintain effective contact with legislative and agency staff.
4. Develop an effective monitoring and response mechanism.
5. Know who and what your resources are and how and when to use them.
6. Be clear and concise in your request for assistance from officials. Learn to be patient. Results sometimes come slowly.
7. Know your competition and colleagues in the lobbying business. Know how and when to work with them on mutual problems.
8. Demonstrate an understanding of and appreciation for current economic constraints on public financing.
9. Develop an effective constituent relations program that builds public support for your group and provides constituent support for legislators sympathetic to your interest.
10. Know how and when to say thanks. There are an infinite number of ways to do this. Don't forget to do it.

Source: Adapted from Remarks by R. Kennedy, Vice President for State Relations, University of Michigan. Used with permission.

2nd Congressional District. This is evidenced by the congressman's willingness to solicit opinions for nursing leaders on health-related legislation.

WORKING COOPERATIVELY. Throughout, there has also been careful, and increasingly close, liaison with local and state leaders of organized nursing. Since the long-term strength of nursing rests with its organizations, ad hoc efforts should be designed to supplement, not compete with, district and state legislative committees. Early tensions, which may be an inevitable accompaniment to new organizational forms, have been replaced by mutually beneficial, respectful working relationships.

Maintaining Contacts
When working at the national level, contacts need to be developed at all levels within the administration, from the Division of Nursing all the way through the Office of Management and Budget. These contacts supplement the ongoing relationships already established by such groups as the ANA, NLN, and other nursing organizations. The major tools in this effort are information and persistence, strengthened by ad hoc coalitions within nursing and frequently aided by assistance from local congressional representatives.

Such contacts, which may include formal meetings and individual interviews, can often be made in conjunction with other trips to Washington, including those to seek grant monies, to conduct research interviews, for national board and other meetings of nursing and non-nursing organizations, to testify before Congress on nursing and other issues, and vacation visits. Position papers, graphic documentation, and short briefing sheets may be prepared for each contact, with each especially tailored to the particular needs and opportunities of the meeting.

▬ CONCLUSION

Box 52-5 provides a brief summary of the basic activities designed to develop effective programs for participating in state or national policy making. Political power can best be generated by leadership within nursing. The use of our political power to attain nursing's goals for better health care is an important dimension of our professional responsibilities. The 1990s can be a decade when the nursing profession gains an important role in health policy making if nurses will invest the time and energy necessary to develop their political expertise and influence.

▬ REFERENCES

1. P. M. Blau, *Exchange and Power in Social Life* (New York: John Wiley, 1964).
2. K. E. Claus, and J. T. Bailey, *Power and Influence in Health Care: A New Approach to Leadership* (St. Louis: C. V. Mosby, 1977).
3. G. L. Lippitt, *Organizational Renewal: Achieving Viability in a Changing World* (New York: Appleton-Century-Crofts, 1969).

Chapter 53

Politics and Practice: Introducing Norplant Into a School-Based Health Center in Baltimore

PETER L. BIELENSON   ELIZABETH S. MIOLA

MYCHELLE FARMER

As community health nurses seek to become involved politically, it is help-ful to learn from others' experiences in this arena. This chapter describes a case study in developing and implementing public policy. To combat the serious public health problem of a high number of adolescent pregnancies, the Baltimore City Health Department in Baltimore, MD instituted a policy to offer contraceptives on site in selected schools. The program was the first of its kind in the nation. The authors of this chapter who are with that health department outline the steps they took, the problems they encoun-tered, and the strategies they employed to implement the policy success-fully. They provide important insights into how to gain community accep-tance and involve communities in the development of public health policies.

▬ INTRODUCTION

The city of Baltimore has long had one of the nation's highest adolescent birth rates. The emotional, social, and economic costs of this problem are significant. In 1990, 10% of all 15- to 17-year-olds living in Baltimore gave birth, with direct costs of teenage births to the government (through Aid to Families with Dependent Children [AFDC]; the special supplemental food program for Women, Infants, and Children [WIC]; food stamps; and medicaid) of $222 million.[1] Health risks to adolescent mothers and their children are well documented, ranging from pregnancy complications such as preeclampsia to low-birthweight babies.[2] In addition, there are the long-term consequences of lower levels of educational and job attainment for the mothers and higher rates of living in poverty for their offspring.[3,4]

Over the past decade, many different approaches have been attempted to combat the problem of adolescent pregnancy and birth in Baltimore.

From *American Journal of Public Health* 85(3):309–311, 1995. Reprinted by permis-sion of American Public Health Association.

These approaches include 1) the development of an inner-city, mall-based comprehensive health clinic that provides a host of services, including family planning, to over 5000 adolescents each year; 2) a citywide media campaign promoting abstinence; 3) school-based efforts, including peer-taught and teacher-taught abstinence curricula in middle schools, male outreach activities, and sex education; and 4) the development of family planning services in two middle and six high school-based comprehensive primary care centers. These activities have resulted in some success. After several years of increasing rates, Baltimore's adolescent birth rate has stabilized (Baltimore City Health Department, unpublished natality statistics, 1992). However, it remains among the highest in the country, and further approaches are being considered.

One widely discussed approach is making the implantable contraceptive Norplant more readily accessible to adolescents. Norplant has been available to adolescents in Baltimore City Health Department family planning clinics since the summer of 1992. However, clinicians working in the health department's school-based health centers, after hearing requests for Norplant from students and parents, felt that these centers would be the best setting for adolescent Norplant insertions and would provide the best access to this contraceptive.

The Baltimore City Health Department operates school-based health centers that provide comprehensive primary and preventive health care to enrolled students at eight secondary schools.[5] These schools are all in locations where there is a particular need for accessible adolescent health care.

Family planning counseling and exams have been available on site at the school-based health centers since their inception in 1985. Vouchers for contraceptives, to be redeemed at off-site locations, were given to students who desired them. However, this voucher system did not work well because students rarely followed up to obtain contraceptives. To alleviate this problem, the health department decided to make oral contraceptives, foam, and condoms available in the health centers at the start of the 1990/91 school year. The decision became policy only after an extensive survey of parents of students enrolled in the clinics demonstrated strong support (75% in favor) for offering contraceptives on site.[6] The contraceptive availability policy has been very well accepted by students, staff, and parents. A follow-up survey in the second year of this policy revealed no parental complaints about the availability of contraceptives on site (P. Beilenson, unpublished data, 1991).

▬THE DECISION AND THE REACTION

As Norplant began to be discussed in the general media, health care professionals in the school-based health centers were asked by students and parents about its availability in these sites. These requests, combined with the fact that the current contraceptive policy was so well accepted by parents, led the commissioner of health to decide to make Norplant available on a pilot basis at one of the health department's school-based health centers in the 1992/93 school year.

The school chosen as the pilot site, a combined middle and high school for pregnant and parenting teens, was selected for two reasons. first, adolescents who have already given birth are at even higher risk of pregnancy than other adolescents.[7] Second, the principal of this school was very supportive of the program.

In December 1992, as the health department's Bureau of School Health began to develop the structure for this pilot program, the media learned that Baltimore would be the first city in the nation offering Norplant at a school-based health center. The media coverage—local, national, and international—was almost universally favorable and plans for implementing the pilot program were finalized.

However, in late January 1993, shortly after the first Norplant was inserted at the school, a small but vocal group of citizens spoke out in opposition to the program. This group contended that the Norplant policy targeted inner-city African-American teenagers (some argued that this amounted to "genocide"); that Norplant had not been tested in this population; that Norplant users would be less likely to practice safer sex and therefore would be at higher risk for human immunodeficiency virus (HIV) and other sexually transmitted infections; that the health department was promoting the use of this contraceptive over abstinence; that Norplant had dangerous side effects; and that the program excluded families from the decision-making process of their adolescents.[8,9]

The strategies used by the opposition were similar to those used nationally against other school health programs instituting reproductive care. These strategies included misinformation, manipulation of public meetings, preying on fears of parents, intimidation and pressure tactics, and accusations of racism.[10]

To ensure that these concerns got a public airing, a city councilman introduced legislation calling for a hearing on the health department's policy of offering Norplant in the schools. The hearing, held in early February 1993, was contentious. The opponents' claims were refuted (Box 53–1) and their public opposition to the program subsided as it became obvious that the general public was in favor of making Norplant available as long as it was not promoted and no coercion was involved. The Norplant program continued during the hearing process and Norplant continues to be available to students in the school-based health center.

▬OUTCOMES

In the first semester after the new policy was implemented, 11 of the approximately 100 nonpregnant students in the school received Norplant from the school-based health center. Before receiving Norplant, each of these 11 students attended a counseling session at the school, accompanied by a parent or guardian; in most instances, a relative was also present during the insertion procedure. All of the students have tolerated Nor-

BOX 53–1   *Opposition Claims and Baltimore City Health Department Responses About the Health Department's School-Based Norplant Policy*

OPPOSITION CLAIM	HEALTH DEPARTMENT RESPONSE
Targeting inner-city African-American teens is genocide.	The policy is simply one of equity: making all contraceptives available in school-based health centers to those who would not otherwise be able to get them.
Insufficient testing of Norplant has been done on African-American adolescents.	(1) Food and Drug Administration trials of Norplant did include similar populations in Newark and San Francisco. (2) Norgestrel (the hormone found in Norplant) has been used in oral contraceptives by hundreds of thousands of African-American adolescents over the past 25 years, with no known differences in efficacy or side effects from those experienced by the rest of the population.
The new policy will lead to higher rates of sexually transmitted diseases and HIV infections in teenaged Norplant users because they will feel protected against pregnancy and will thus neglect to use condoms.	(1) The students will receive extensive counseling on the importance of condom use in conjunction with Norplant. (2) Norplant recipients in the first school-based site will be evaluated to ascertain the efficacy of this counseling.
The health department is promoting Norplant and sexual promiscuity over abstinence.	Abstinence is the only method of contraception that the health department promotes; the school system also has an abstinence curriculum. Norplant is simply another contraceptive option available to sexually active teenagers in the school-based health centers.
Norplant has dangerous side effects.	Norplant's side effects are primarily "nuisance" side effects; a stringent follow-up protocol will be observed to identify patients who need to have the implant removed or who need further counseling about side effects.
The program excludes families from adolescents' decisions about contraception.	Families are strongly encouraged to be present both for counseling sessions and for the actual insertion procedure.

plant well; there have been no requests for removal and no students have exhibited any but minor side effects. All of these students reported using condoms at least as frequently as they did before receiving Norplant (with follow-up of 5 to 12 months), and most reported using condoms significantly more frequently since getting the implant. As support for these students' self-reports on condom use, we know of only a single case of a sexually transmitted disease among these Norplant recipients. One possible explanation for this increased use of condoms is the intensive counseling on condom use all students receive before getting the implant, combined with extensive follow-up counseling.

▀PLANS FOR THE FUTURE

With the successful implementation of this policy, the health department has expanded the availability of Norplant to three more high schools, with plans to expand to the remaining two high schools that have school-based health centers over the next year. (The implant will not be available in the two middle school health centers.) In light of the controversy the initial proposal generated, however, the health department educated various segments of the community about Norplant before this expansion. The health department 1) discussed the issue with religious groups and a city-wide community health advisory group; 2) discussed the issue with interested parents in each school; 3) educated the teaching and administrative staffs of the schools; and 4) made presentations to student groups about postponing parenting, including a discussion of abstinence, Norplant, and other contraceptive methods.

▀DISCUSSION

If community acceptance can be obtained, school-based health centers are ideal places to offer contraceptive services. They are readily accessible to students, a well-recognized advantage in delivering any kind of health care to adolescents. This accessibility is also important for the health care staff, who can locate the students easily when follow-up and compliance are important. In addition, the close, trusting relationship that typically develops between school-based health center staff and individual adolescents is critical to the success of efforts to provide effective health care to teens.

One important lesson our experience teaches is that the community may not immediately accept measures that make good public health sense. Extensive education of all involved, including community members, elected officials, and religious groups as well as all pertinent staff (who might not be knowledgeable about the proposed intervention), is essential to the successful and smooth implementation of controversial policies. The lead time necessary for doing this important groundwork is rarely appreciated by funders or program managers as a sound investment.

There is a real need for affected communities to be in on the development of public health policies from the beginning, playing a major role in identifying the community's important health problems, suggesting inter-

586 *Readings in Community Health Nursing*

vention strategies, and working with health experts to implement them. However, any progressive public health initiative, from family planning to violence and substance abuse prevention, is likely to arouse opposition; fear and anger may make rational discourse difficult. If progress is ever to be made against the major public health and social problems affecting us, public health leaders must be willing to stand up to confrontation and to point out ignorance and misconceptions.

Although some public health advances in the past were controversial (e.g., fluoridation of public water supplies), many were less so, in part because they primarily dealt strictly with health issues. For example, many of the epidemic diseases of the past were curtailed or eradicated either by simple changes in hygiene or by the introduction of effective antibiotics. In contrast, many of today's public health initiatives are controversial because they attempt to address issues that are both social and medical in nature. As an example, the Norplant issue touches on adolescent sexuality and the social and ethical questions of coercion vs choice.

In addition, Norplant raises concerns in some about genocide or selective use. Because some minority communities distrust the health care system, they view Norplant as a means of controlling certain populations. The negative consequences of the infamous Tuskeegee syphilis study on the practice of public health cannot be overestimated; the study's strong repercussions in the Black community continue today.

Consequently, with any public health initiative that might be perceived as having a disproportionate impact on minorities (another example would be needle exchange programs for intravenous drug users), public health practitioners must educate the affected community about the scope of the problem and about the specific initiative as a potential solution. How this is done depends on the specific locale. First, local public health practitioners need to know their community and which community leaders must be involved. In Baltimore, for example, religious leaders and their organizations are very influential forces in the city. With the Norplant issue, the opinions of teachers and principals of the affected schools must be considered. Obviously, parents of adolescents in the schools must also be involved. In addition, formal and informal leaders should be sought out and involved: recreation center directors, school volunteers, neighborhood librarians—all those who have grassroots knowledge of the needs and perceptions of the community. It is with the involvement of all these members of a community that the likelihood of successful implementation of progressive, controversial public health policies will be the greatest.

1. *Teenage Pregnancy and Too-Early Childbearing: Public Costs, Personal Consequences.* 5th ed. Washington, DC: Center for Population Options; 1990.
2. Strobino DM. The health and medical consequences of adolescent sexuality and pregnancy: a review of the literature. In: Hofferth S, Hayes CD, eds. *Risking the Future.* Vol. 2. Washington, DC: National Academy Press, 1987:93–122.

3. Nord CW, Moore KA, Morrison DR, Brown B, Meyers DE. Consequences of teen-age parenting. *J Sch Health.* 1992;62:310–318.
4. McAnarney ER, Hendee WR. Adolescent pregnancy and its consequences. *JAMA.* 1989;262:74–77.
5. Feroli MS, Hobson SK, Miola ES, Scott PN, Waterfield GD. School-based clinics: the Baltimore experience. *J Pediatr Health Care.* 1992;6:127–131.
6. Santelli JS, Alexander M, Farmer M, Papa P, Johnson T, Rosenthal B, Hotra D. Bringing parents into school clinics: parent attitudes towards school clinics and contraception. *J Adolesc Health.* 1992;13:269–274.
7. Mott F. The pace of repeated childbearing among young American mothers. *Fam Plann Perspect.* 1986;18:5–12.
8. Hopkins T, Marshall T. Norplant faces rising opposition. *Baltimore Afro-American.* January 30, 1993:A1.
9. Fletcher M. City's contraceptive plan is attacked. *Baltimore Sun.* February 10, 1993:1A.
10. Rienzo BA, Button JW. The politics of school-based clinics: a community-level analysis. *J Sch Health.* 1993;63:266–272.

Chapter 54

Policy as Intervention: Environmental and Policy Approaches to the Prevention of Cardiovascular Disease

THOMAS L. SCHMID   MICHAEL PRATT   ELIZABETH HOWZE

To prevent cardiovascular disease, the leading cause of death in the United States, the authors of this chapter propose two major strategies for intervention. One is to enact policy changes at both legislative and organizational levels to regulate against factors harmful to cardiovascular health. The other is to modify the social environment to enhance heart-healthy behavior. They state that previous interventions targeting individual behavior change have been mostly disappointing and they advocate a population perspective. They describe practical ways to implement policy and environmental strategies and show their value for addressing other health problems in addition to cardiovascular disease.

■ INTRODUCTION

Policy and environmental interventions account for much of the success of the first public health revolution.[1] Sanitarians contributed to the nation's health through improved environmental conditions fostered by rules (policies) that required cleaner food preparation facilities in slaughterhouses, factories, and restaurants; better technologies (environmental changes), such as refrigeration; better sanitation, including garbage collection, sewage treatment, and water purification; and significant changes in norms, attitudes, and behaviors (e.g., washing hands and not spitting in public).[1-3]

■ STRATEGIES TO ADDRESS CHRONIC DISEASES

A contemporary public health revolution must respond to chronic diseases such as cardiovascular disease and cancer that have complex and multiple causes. It is now generally accepted in the more developed world that people's behaviors and the environments that elicit and maintain them, rather than inadvertent exposure to infectious disease agents, are the primary

From *American Journal of Public Health* 85(9):1207–1211, 1995. Reprinted by permission of American Public Health Association.

causes of today's major health problems.[4] Risk factors for cardiovascular disease, the leading cause of death, are primarily behavioral and include tobacco use, inadequate physical activity, and poor diet.[5-7]

POLICY AND ENVIRONMENTAL CHANGE

Societal-level changes necessary to address endemic chronic diseases successfully will include changes in policy and the environment to foster and maintain individual-level behavior change.[4,8] The need for such an approach is recognized in the Victoria Declaration on Heart Health, a consensus statement drafted by leading scientists and experts in public health. The Victoria declaration calls for those in public health "to join forces in eliminating this modern epidemic [cardiovascular disease] by adopting new policies, making regulatory changes, and implementing health promotion and disease prevention programs directed at entire populations."[8] The declaration strongly advocates combining health education efforts with environmental and policy measures, because neither can be as effective alone.

It is unreasonable to expect large proportions of the population to make individual behavior changes that are discouraged by the environment and existing social norms. It is equally unrealistic to expect communities or organizations to enact policy changes for which there is no broad-based understanding and support.[3,9] To be effective, a public health approach to cardiovascular disease prevention must incorporate environmental and policy measures as well as education and skills development for each of the sectors of individuals and organizations involved.

Policy Strategies

Policies can be defined as "those laws, regulations, formal, and informal rules and understandings that are adopted on a collective basis to guide individual and collective behavior."[10] For this paper, we have subdivided policy into two areas: legislation or regulation and organizational policy. Legislation and regulation include formal policies written into or having the effect of laws enacted by appropriate governing bodies. Examples of public health-based legislation and regulation abound and include seat belt laws, restaurant codes, and clean indoor air laws.

Organizational policies are policies instituted within specific organizations (e.g., corporations, schools, or health departments) that define appropriate behavior within the confines of the organization (e.g., a prohibition against smoking). Although they do not affect the public as a whole, organizational policies on public health can have a considerable cumulative impact; smoke-free schools, hospitals, work sites, and public places are examples.

Environmental Strategies

Environmental strategies are a second major category of intervention. We define environmental interventions as measures that alter or control the physical or social environment. Environmental measures may address availability, accessibility, or social norms. A successful environmental intervention has involved changing the food supply to make low-fat milk available.[11-14] Opening school gymnasiums and opening shopping malls before or after business hours can increase physical activity by increasing access. Modifications of the social environment include normative changes in attitudes and behaviors such as expectations for routine condom use or shifts in student peer group expectations about drinking and driving. Other examples include passengers using seat belts or asking permission to smoke. The demarcation between policy and environmental efforts is not always clear; policies may be used to effect environmental change. For instance, a city government may pass ordinances requiring that public housing projects include recreational facilities, that new subdivisions include sidewalks, or that office complexes provide walking paths.

As in national and international movements such as the Healthy Cities and Healthy Communities projects,[15] new community-focused efforts in the United States are beginning to take this broader perspective. These programs recognize the need to facilitate behavior change by removing policy and environmental barriers to healthy behavior as well as fostering those policies, rules, procedures, and conditions that encourage health-promotive behaviors.

Another rationale for expanding community-based programs to include more environmental- and policy-level activities comes from behavioral science theory (e.g., the theory of diffusion of innovations).[3,9] Green suggests that individual-centered efforts were appropriate for the first generation of community-based cardiovascular disease programs because the nation was then in the early stages of the diffusion process.[3,9] In this stage, "early adopters" make positive health choices based mainly on new information. As we move to later generations of community-based programs, the target groups may include more "late adopters," and therefore the programs may need to focus more on health-fostering policies and environments.

Individual Behavior Change

Over the last two decades, efforts to reduce chronic diseases have grown, especially efforts to prevent cardiovascular disease. For most programs in the United States, from the large research and demonstration trials sponsored by the National Heart, Lung and Blood Institute[16-18] to smaller state[19-22] and locally sponsored community projects,[23,24] the primary focus has been on interventions to encourage individual behavior change. These first- and second-generation community-based trials recognize the multifactorial nature of cardiovascular disease and consistently advocate approaches involving multiple strategies across multiple channels and across all sectors of the population. However, the main focus has been on information and skill building. Results from most of these comprehensive cardiovascular disease prevention programs, as well as risk-factor-specific efforts such as the COMMIT smoking cessation program, have, on the whole, been disappointing.[25-29] Although the newer programs are becoming more inclusive, environmental and policy approaches have not received much attention in the United States.

The individual, high-risk approach has been supplanted by a population perspective that recognizes the value of reducing risk for selected groups of high-risk individuals but also recognizes the substantial number of additional lives that can be saved by even slightly reducing the mean population level of risk.[30–32] The traditional focus on enhancing knowledge and attitudes may be, in part, a result of a historical and philosophical reluctance of some behavioral scientists to participate in actions that reduce an individual's free will and choice.[3] However, while initial efforts often result in moderate short-term success, the level of success for behaviorally focused interventions generally dissipates over time.[3] Most smokers relapse,[33] and most dieters regain lost weight.[34]

An effective public health response to chronic disease must take a broad, communitywide perspective that focuses on prevention over treatment and avoids "blaming the victim" by recognizing the pervasive control that the environment has over behavior. Supportive environmental changes may be as important as or more important than individual behavior change efforts.[8,9,32,35]

■ NEED FOR POLICY
AND ENVIRONMENTAL APPROACHES

Behavioral psychologists have long recognized that the conditions necessary to maintain behavior may not be those required for acquisition. They note that once behaviors have been learned, conditions or stimuli sufficient for them to reoccur, even at a much later time, may be minimal. For instance, environmental cues sufficient to elicit relapse in an ex-smoker, alcoholic, or overeater may be below the threshold level of individuals who have not regularly engaged in these behaviors.[36] Lack of will, self-control, and attitudes have less to do with the prevalence of smoking or obesity than do cheap cigarettes and vending machines.

The transition to the next generation of public health diseases with a basis in personal behavior has spawned many behaviorally focused interventions. However, in some cases, the pendulum may have swung too far toward individual behavior change and away from the passive public health strategies that have been so instrumental in the public health advances of the last century. Passive public health strategies do not require individuals to take action on an individual basis or to make specific behavioral changes. Rather, an action such as a change in environment or policy is taken on the societal level to reduce exposure to health risks or to lead to healthy behavior.[18] The likelihood of success for a preventive measure varies inversely with the frequency and complexity of the behavior change required for persons to be protected.[37] For example, public drinking water is chlorinated, thus eliminating the need to increase awareness of waterborne pathogens and to teach people to assess water quality and appropriately treat their personal water supply.

Most public health problems are best approached through a combination of active and passive strategies. The 50% reduction in motor vehicle fatality rates per mile driven over the past 25 years is an excellent example of the synergy between active and passive public health strategies. Improved roadways, better designed automobiles, speed limits, seat belts, air bags, seat belt and drunk driving legislation and the enforcement of those laws, driver education, and campaigns promoting seat belt use and safer driving have all contributed to the reduction in mortality.[37] Similar applications to the behavioral risks for cardiovascular disease must be developed.

SUCCESS IN OTHER HEALTH CARE SYSTEMS

Finland's North Karelia Project is an example of a comprehensive public health program to prevent heart disease that incorporates policy and environmental interventions in an effective, community-focused manner.[12] Recent results from this national effort indicate that changes in the risk factors targeted by the program can explain most of the decline in ischemic heart disease observed over the last 20 years.[38] Incentives for producing healthier food have also been incorporated into Norway's nutrition and food policy,[11] and an important strategy of the Heartbeat Wales project was "to achieve environmental, organizational, structural, and policy changes to support healthy choices by individuals."[39]

SUCCESS IN OTHER FIELDS

Experiences from areas outside cardiovascular disease are also instructive. Policy and environmental strategies have long been used to control the sale and consumption of alcohol. Here, policy-level interventions make good public health sense because there is abundant evidence that government policies on alcohol can directly affect per capita consumption, type of alcohol used, age of use, distribution of use, and probability of alcohol problems.[40–42] These effects can be produced by local, state, and national policies.[42,43] Approaches can be grouped into three broad categories: price, promotion (conditions of sale), and the product itself.

Price

Alcohol consumption is sensitive to price, and in many countries taxes have been used to moderate consumption. In the United Kingdom, taxes on alcohol have been associated with a shift not only in consumption patterns but also in disease rates; cirrhosis of the liver, formerly a disease of the lower class, is now more common in the upper class.[42] Because young people are especially price sensitive, taxes can be very effective in delaying the onset, as well as the frequency, of abuse.

Promotion

Controlling the conditions of sale is an effective mechanism for regulating use. Variables used to control alcohol sales include age and proximity to schools or churches; other controls involve requiring concurrent purchases of food in restaurants, prohibiting sale of single cans or premixed drinks in convenience stores, and holding the licensee responsible for violations. Limiting promotions of alcohol beverages and requiring counter-advertising have analogues for food, tobacco, and physical activity.

Product

Changing the product to make it less harmful is a common public health strategy but one not always well received. For example, proposals to add vitamins to wine to prevent alcoholic nutritional deficiencies and attempts to develop "safer" cigarettes have been resisted under the presumption that their net effect would be to condone use and increase consumption.

■ GENERALIZING TO MODIFIABLE CARDIOVASCULAR DISEASE RISK FACTORS: PHYSICAL ACTIVITY, NUTRITION, AND TOBACCO

Generalizing these strategies to other areas seems appropriate. The tobacco control community has used these strategies for several years. Price relates directly to tobacco use, and taxes have been shown to be an effective method of discouraging sales, especially to minors.[44] Limitations on promotion of tobacco through direct and indirect advertising appear to be gaining support. Restrictions on conditions of sale, including prohibiting vending machines or the sale of individual cigarettes, prohibiting marketing or promotion around young people, and making retailers responsible for violations, have proven to be effective tobacco control strategies. Increased public acceptance of these policy and environmental efforts has evolved over the last two decades.

Strategies used in health care systems of other countries and those used to control other health risks can also be appropriately applied to rules and conditions that inhibit physical activity and encourage poor dietary behaviors. Support for such approaches is limited but perhaps growing. For instance, taxes on high-fat foods have been suggested as a way to help finance health care reform and as a "user" fee to offset the additional health care costs associated with increased heart disease.[45] A survey of six midwestern communities suggests that there is public support for additional public health efforts to regulate the sale and consumption of high-fat foods and tobacco through policy and environmental change.[46,47] The potential synergy between policy and other health education actions is suggested by the observation that the three survey communities that had been exposed to a community-based cardiovascular disease prevention program were the most supportive of policy and environmental change.[46,48]

■ STATE HEALTH AGENCIES: SETTING THE AGENDA AND ESTABLISHING A NEW FOCUS

Advantages

Environmental- and policy-level activities can make efficient use of limited public health budgets. In the era of health care reform, these activities serve a strategic function by helping agencies move from a direct service role to one of guidance, agenda setting, and coordination of community-based efforts. Environmental and policy interventions use the force of law and regulation to change behavior and social norms rather than trying to achieve change through the more clinical and less efficient model of individual remediation.

Behavioral science theory also supports the value of environmental- and policy-level efforts. For instance, in terms of diffusion of innovations theory, the focus may be on "later adopters"[3]; from a transtheoretical approach, "precontemplators"[49] may be targeted; and, in the argot of smoking cessation practitioners, "hardcore" smokers may be the focus. Policy and environmental efforts help create the supportive environments these groups need to initiate and sustain long-term behavior change.

Barriers

Reluctance to promote environmental- and policy-level interventions stems from a variety of sources, including inadequate training for health educators and others in the philosophy and application of policy and environmental change, lack of institutional permission for such activities within a state health agency's scope of work, resistance to change, and concern that individual freedoms may be reduced. When policy and environmental choices are considered, the health agency's responsibilities might include fostering public discussion and providing balanced empirical data. Public antipathy toward additional intrusions on freedom may, in part, represent concern about where to draw the line. For instance, some people see each step toward the control of firearms in order to reduce violence as a step further down the slippery slope of prohibition and abridgment of freedom.

How policies and environmental changes are adopted may be as important as their functional outcome. Ensuring informed public participation in such discussions and decisions may also make rational intermediate steps appealing. Getting schools to provide healthy menu choices or discouraging them from selling soft drinks and candy is more acceptable when it comes as a result of parental choice rather than government mandate. Although policy and environmental strategies should not be used as a vehicle for a moral message (e.g., that those who do not maintain a healthy life-style lack will or moral substance), providing assistance in framing public debate may be appropriate.

The climate for policy and environmental interventions in many areas, such as tobacco and firearms control, has changed dramatically over the last few years. Activities and actions previously considered revolutionary or inappropriate for a state agency are now common and expected. Advocacy for clean air regulation, restrictions on the sale and promotion of tobacco, and increased taxes on tobacco and counteradvertising are becoming regular components of state and local health agency programs.

The normative changes that have occurred for tobacco control can be traced, in part, to the cutting-edge efforts of earlier advocacy organizations such as "Doctors Ought to Care." Social scientists have suggested that changes in attitudes are, in part, facilitated by expanding the boundaries of behavior.[50] The civil rights movement purposefully pushed the boundaries of acceptable public behavior to shift the norm in the same direction. Health departments may not be the sole agents for such activities, but they can help define the logical boundaries for discussion. These efforts make it clear that, if policies are to be adopted and to be successful, changes in the social environment are as important as changes in the physical environment.

CONCLUSION

As health agencies move further from a direct service role to one that helps empower communities to address the underlying conditions that promote cardiovascular disease, they will be called upon to make significant changes in what they do and in how they interact with their constituents. Setting the public health agenda so that policy and environmental options are included in public discourse and expanding the focus from the individual or consumer to include others such as the manufacturer or retailer are appropriate goals for state health agencies. The focus should also be expanded to include the wide variety of policy and environmental conditions that influence cardiovascular disease risk behaviors.

Many government and private agencies, such as zoning boards, parks and recreation associations, licensing boards, and boards of education, make decisions that have important implications for cardiovascular health. Through their "assurance" role, health departments have a responsibility to see that public health is represented in these decisions. Also, from our perspective, focusing on policy and environmental change does not mean using the government to increase the power of centralized decision makers; rather, it means using these strategies to work with the community to address barriers to heart-healthy living. Health departments that support disincentives for high-fat foods, tax breaks for cafeterias that offer healthy food choices, policies that require zoning ordinances to include sidewalks, or school facilities open to the public might be labeled radical or experimental today; tomorrow, however, they may be considered prudent stewards of the public health.

Acknowledgment

An original draft of this paper was developed for the Environmental and Policy Approaches to Cardiovascular Disease Prevention workshop, September 1993, Atlanta, Ga.

REFERENCES

1. Rosen G. *A History of Public Health.* Baltimore, Md: Johns Hopkins University Press; 1993.
2. Breslow L. Foreword. In: Bracht N, ed. *Health Promotion at the Community Level.* Newbury Park, Calif: Sage Publications; 1990:11–13.
3. Green LW, Richard L. The need to combine health education and health promotion: the case of cardiovascular disease prevention. *Int J Health Promotion Educ.* 1993;1:11–17.
4. Farquhar JW. *The American Way of Life Need Not Be Hazardous to Your Health.* New York, NY: WW Norton & Co; 1978.

5. Smith C, Pratt M. Cardiovascular disease. In: Brownson RC, Remington PL, Davis JR, eds. *Chronic Disease Epidemiology and Control.* Washington, DC: American Public Health Association; 1993:83–95.
6. Remington R. From preventive policy to preventive practice. *Prev Med.* 1990;19:105–113.
7. McGinnis JM, Foege WH. Actual causes of death in the United States. *JAMA.* 1993;270:2207–2212.
8. Advisory Board International Heart Health Conference. *The Victoria Declaration on Heart Health.* Victoria, British Columbia, Canada: British Columbia Ministry of Health; 1992.
9. Green LW, McAlister AL. Macro-intervention to support health behavior: some theoretical perspectives and practical reflections. *Health Educ.* 1984;11:322–339.
10. Wallack L. Media advocacy: promoting health through mass communication. In: Glanz K, Lewis FM, Rimer BK, eds. *Health Behavior and Health Education: Theory, Research and Practice.* San Francisco, Calif: Jossey-Bass; 1990:370–386.
11. Klepp K-I, Forster JL. The Norwegian nutrition and food policy: an integrated policy approach to a public health problem. *J Public Health Policy.* 1985;6:447–463.
12. Puska P. Community-based prevention of cardiovascular disease: the North Karelia project. In: Martarazzo JD, Weiss SM, Herd JA, Miller NE, Weiss SM, eds. *Behavioral Health: A Handbook of Health Enhancement and Disease Prevention.* New York, NY: John Wiley & Sons Inc; 1984: 1140–1147.
13. Wechsler H, Wernick SM. A social marketing campaign to promote low-fat milk consumption in an inner-city Latino community. *Public Health Rep.* 1992;107:202–207.
14. Milio N. *Nutrition Policy for Food-Rich Countries: A Strategic Analysis.* Baltimore, Md: Johns Hopkins University Press; 1990.
15. Hancock T. The evolution, impact and significnace of the healthy cities/healthy communities movement. *J Public Health Policy.* 1993;14:5–18.
16. Farquhar JW, Fortmann SP, Flora JA, et al. Effects of community wide education on cardiovascular disease risk factors: the Stanford Five-City Project. *JAMA.* 1990;264:359–365.
17. Carleton RA, Lasater TM, Assaf AR, Feldman HA, McKinlay SM. The Pawtucket Heart Health Program: cross-sectional results from a community intervention trial. *Circulation.* 1994;89:922. Abstract.
18. Shea S, Basch CE. A review of five major community-based cardiovascular prevention programs. Part I. Rationale, design and theoretical framework. *Am J Prev Med.* 1990;4:203–213.
19. Mittelmark MB, Hunt MK, Health GW, Schmid TL. Realistic outcomes: lessons from community-based research and demonstration programs for the prevention of cardiovascular diseases. *J Public Health Policy.* 1993;14:437–462.
20. Schwartz R, Smith C, Speers MA, et al. Capacity building and resource needs of state health agencies to implement community-based cardiovascular disease programs. *J Public Health Policy.* 1993;4:480–494.
21. Elder JP, Schmid TL, Dower P, Hedlund S. Community health health programs: components, rationale, and strategies for effective interventions. *J Public Health Policy.* 1993;14:463–479.
22. Wheeler FC, Lackland DT, Mace ML, Reddick A, Hogelin G, Remington RD. Evaluating South Carolina's community cardiovascular disease prevention project. *Public Health Rep.* 1991;106:536–543.
23. Cook TJ, Schmid TL, Braddy BA, Orenstein D. Evaluating community based program impacts. *J Health Educ.* 1992;23:183–186.
24. Kreuter MW. PATCH: its origin, basic concepts, and links to contemporary public health policy. *J Health Educ.* 1992;23:135–139.
25. COMMIT Research Group. Community Intervention for Smoking Cessation (COMMIT): I. Cohort results from a four-year community intervention. *Am J Public Health.* 1995;85:183–192.
26. COMMIT Research Group. Community Intervention for Smoking Cessation (COMMIT): II. Changes in adult cigarette smoking prevalence. *Am J Public Health.* 1995;85:193–200.
27. Susser M. The tribulations of trials—intervention in communities. *Am J Public Health.* 1995;85:156–158. Editorial.

28. Fisher EB. The results of the COMMIT trial. *Am J Public Health.* 1995;85:159–160. Editorial.
29. Luepker RV, Murray DM, Jacobs DR, et al. Community education for cardiovascular disease prevention: risk factor changes in the Minnesota Heart Health Program. *Am J Public Health.* 1994;84:1383–1393.
30. McAlister AL. Population behavior change: a theory-based approach. *J Public Health Policy.* 1991;12:345–361.
31. Blackburn H. The public health view of diet and mass hyperlipidemia. *Cardiovasc Rev Rep.* 1980;1:361–442.
32. Bracht N. Introduction. In: Bracht N, ed. *Health Promotion at the Community Level.* Newbury Park, Calif: Sage Publications; 1990:19–25.
33. Smoking cessation during previous years among adults—United States, 1990–91. *MMWR Morb Mortal Wkly Rep.* 1993;42:404–406.
34. Jeffery RW. Population perspectives on the prevention and treatment of obesity in minority populations. *Am J Clin Nutr.* 1991;53:1621S–1624S.
35. Wallerstein N, Bernstein E. Introduction to community empowerment, participation, participatory education and health. *Health Educ Q.* 1994;21:141–148.
36. McGinnies E, Ferster EB. *The Reinforcement of Social Behavior.* Boston, Mass: Houghton Mifflin Co; 1971.
37. Wintemute GJ. From research to public policy: the prevention of motor vehicle injuries, childhood drowning, and firearm violence. *Am J Health Promotion.* 1992;6:451–464.
38. Vartiainen E, Puska P, Pekkanen J, Tumilehtro J, Jousilahti P. Changes in risk factors explain changes in mortality from ischemic heart disease in Finland. *BMJ.* 1994;309:23–27.
39. Corson J. Heartbeat Wales: a challenge for change. *World Health Forum.* 1990;11:405–411.
40. Adrian M. International trends in alcohol production, trade and consumption, and their relationship to alcohol-related problems. *J Public Health Policy.* 1984;5:344–367.
41. Single E. International perspectives on alcohol as a public health issue. *J Public Health Policy.* 1984;5:238–254.
42. Smith CJ, Hanham RQ. *Alcohol Abuse: Geographical Perspectives.* Washington, DC: Association of American Geographers; 1982:chap 3.
43. Room R. Alcohol control and public health. *Annu Rev Public Health.* 1984;5:982–986.
44. Breslow L, Johnson M. California's Proposition 99 on tobacco, and its impact. *Annu Rev Public Health.* 1993;14:585–604.
45. Terris M. Public health policy for the 1990s. *J Public Health Policy.* 1990;11:281–295.
46. Schmid TL, Jeffery RW, Forster JL, Rooney B, Klepp K-I, McBride C. Public support for policy initiatives regulating alcohol use in Minnesota: a multi-community survey. *J Stud Alcohol.* 1990;51:438–442.
47. Schmid TL, Jeffery RW, Forster JL, Rooney B, McBride C. Public support for policy initiatives regulating high-fat food use in Minnesota: a multicommunity survey. *Prev Med.* 1989;18:791–805.
48. Jeffery RW, Forster JL, Schmid TL, McBride C, Rooney B, Pirie PL. Community attitudes toward public policies to control alcohol, tobacco, and high-fat food consumption. *Am J Prev Med.* 1990;6:12–19.
49. Prochaska JO, DiClemente CC. Stages and processes of self-change of smoking: toward an integrative model of change. *J Consult Clin Psychol.* 1983;51:390–395.
50. Freedman JL, Carlsmith JM, Sears DO. *Social Psychology.* Englewood Cliffs, NJ: Prentice-Hall; 1974.

Chapter 55

Returning to Work After Childbirth: Considerations for Health Policy

MARCIA GRUIS KILLIEN

> Social and health policies provide guiding principles for societal action and influence quality of life. Many times such policies, while perhaps well intended, have a deleterious effect on certain populations. One example is the impact of social policies on women working during pregnancy, seeking parental leave, and returning to work after childbirth. In this chapter, Dr. Killien discusses changes in the American family, describes perinatal employment patterns and problems, and shows how social policies have not addressed the needs of working women. Using policy research data like that generated by Dr. Killien, community health nurses can help to shape public policy changes to improve the health of populations at risk.

The profiles of both the American family and the workplace are changing. The "traditional" American family—including a father who is employed full time as the sole family wage earner, and a mother who stays home to care for the children—represented about 70% of families 50 years ago; today, this model describes fewer than 10% of American families.[1] Women are working in the paid labor force in unprecedented numbers. In 1990, 57.9% of all women aged 20 years and over were employed outside the home, with black women (60%) being slightly more likely than white women (58%) or Hispanic women (55%) to be involved in paid work. These women account for nearly half (45%) of all workers, including 41% of all full-time workers.[2]

Nowhere are these changes so apparent as during the childbearing period of the family life cycle. It has been estimated that about 85% of the female labor force will be pregnant at some point during their working lives. Among women who work during their first pregnancy, 78% work continuously for at least 6 months of their pregnancy and 47% are still employed less than 1 month before delivery.[3] Over half (53%) of women return to work during the first year following childbirth.[2,4] Whereas in the 1960s only 17% of first-time mothers were employed by their baby's first birth-

From *Nursing Outlook* 41(2):73–78, 1993. Reprinted by permission of Mosby-Year Book, Inc.

day, during the 1980s the figure had risen to 53%.[3] Most mothers have returned to work by 4 to 6 months postpartum, with 85% of mothers in one recent study employed by 3 months postpartum.[5]

Most women work because of the economic needs of their families. In 1960, 42% of families were solely supported by a male; in 1988 this figure had dropped to 15%.[6] In two-parent households, working women were estimated to have contributed 26% to 39% of the family income; 41% of married working women have husbands who earn less than $15,000 a year.[7] One out of four mothers is single.[8] It is likely that the single mother's family depends heavily on her income. However, in 1986, 60% of all single working mothers with children under 14 earned less than $15,000 annually and only 15% made more than $25,000.[1] The burden of childcare costs is heaviest for women who earn low wages, with 22% of the average monthly income of working mothers below the poverty line going to pay for childcare.[9] Thus the earnings of female workers are critically important to the well being of their families.

Contributions of women to the workplace are equally vital. Increasing proportions of executive, managerial, and professional workers are women, with women representing 11% of managers and 15% of professionals in 1990. However, women continue to be overrepresented in traditionally female occupations and among part-time, lower-paying jobs. In 1990, 59% of employed women held positions in sales, administrative support, or the service industries.[2] Part-time and temporary employment continues to be especially prevalent among women with young children.[8] While this choice allows many women to benefit from work outside the home and still care for their children, it often pays relatively little, rarely provides fringe benefits, and offers limited opportunities for advancement.[10] In addition, interruptions in labor force participation have been found to limit women's access to and advancement in higher status occupations, such as professional and managerial jobs.[11] Thus women often try to limit their time away from work for childbearing and childrearing.

Past research on maternal employment has largely focused on the relationship between the mother's employment status and the child's development and behavior.[12] Such work has been based on the implicit, if not explicit, assumption that maternal absence is harmful to children. Many child health experts advocate that mothers remain at home for varying periods after birth, ranging from 4 months to 5 years (e.g., Koester,[13] and Bowlby[14a]). However, such recommendations contrast with reports of the actual behaviors of women returning to work. Little research has examined the reasons mothers return to work when they do, or the impact of these decisions on their own health, the well-being of the family, and the workplace. This article should help to bridge these gaps; its purposes are 1) to describe employment patterns of women during the perinatal period and their decisions about returning to work after childbirth within the context of current policies; and 2) to discuss the implications of these data for future social and health policy.

■SOCIAL AND HEALTH POLICIES

Social policies have been defined as "guiding principles or courses of action adopted and pursued by societies and their governments as well as by various groups or units within societies."[14] Social policies address the "intra-societal relationships among individuals, groups, and society as a whole."[14] MacPherson[15] subscribed to this definition and elaborated, "Social policies tend to, but do not need to, be codified in formal legal documents and address life in a society. . . . Health policy is one type of social policy. . . . [that] influence[s] the quality of life and human relations in a society." Examples of social policies affecting the relationships between families and work include pregnancy leave, parental leave, flexible work schedules, and childcare benefits.

Perhaps the most explicit social policy addressing childbearing families and employment is embodied in the Pregnancy Discrimination Act of 1978. Historically, social norms and workplace policies forced U.S. women to leave their jobs when they became pregnant or "started to show." American legislation was "protectionist," restricting prenatal and postpartum employment, yet offering little protection of income, benefits, or job security.

In 1964 the passage of Title VII of the Federal Civil Rights Act disallowed employment discrimination on the basis of gender. But various interpretations of this law effectively circumvented full protection of many of the rights of pregnant workers. Additional protection was provided in 1978 by an amendment to Title VII, the Pregnancy Discrimination Act. This amendment formed the legal basis for ensuring that benefits from health insurance plans for sickness or temporary physical disability must be extended to female employees disabled by pregnancy, miscarriage, abortion, childbirth, or recovery from these conditions. The Pregnancy Discrimination Act also prohibits refusing to hire or promote pregnant women, arbitrarily terminating employment or requiring mandatory leaves due to pregnancy, refusing to reinstate employees on pregnancy leaves, or failing to accrue retirement benefits for pregnant employees. The limitations to this amendment are that the law is applicable to employers with 15 or more employees and that "disability" refers only to medical disability, estimated at 6 weeks or less for normal pregnancies, and requiring medical certification.[7]

These laws offer women the choice to continue working throughout pregnancy, and provide protection for the woman during the period of "physical recovery from childbirth," usually considered to be 4 to 6 weeks postpartum (e.g., Pritchard[16]). These laws, however, do not provide protection for the parent who chooses to remain at home to care for a child, commonly called *parental leave*.[17] A 1989 bureau of Labor Statistics national survey of businesses that employed 100 or more workers indicated that 37% of female employees and 18% of male employees could take unpaid parental leave, with the maximum duration averaging 20 weeks.[18] Paid leave for either mothers or fathers was found to be rare. The increased prevalence of parental leave—albeit unpaid leave—for women, versus men, reinforces the belief that it is the mother, not the father, who should be at home to care for children. Class differences are also evident from the national survey information. The availability of parental leave declined for workers in less prestigious occupations; leave was most available for professional and administrative employees and least available for workers in technical, production, and clerical jobs.

Two other policies that may influence employment decisions of new mothers are the availability of flexible work schedules and childcare benefits. Flexible work arrangements are those that give employees the opportunity to begin and end work within a range of hours, thereby helping to accommodate family commitments. In 1989 only 11% of all workers in medium and large firms had formal flexible work arrangements available to them; the percentage of white-collar workers with this benefit was nearly double that of blue-collar workers. Generally employees were expected to work during the middle of the work day, with limited flexibility for non-daytime work hours.

Only 5% of employees were found to be eligible for employer-subsidized childcare benefits. These benefits included both on-site or near-site childcare facilities, as well as reimbursement accounts funded to some degree by employer contributions. The availability of non-employer subsidized reimbursement accounts for dependent care nearly doubled between 1988 and 1989, with 23% of workers eligible for this benefit in 1989. Such accounts allow employees to obtain federal income tax advantages through salary-reduction arrangements with their employers. The proportion of employees eligible for reimbursement accounts also varied among occupational categories. While 36% of professional and administrative employees were eligible, only 11% of production and service employees had such plans available.[18]

■ METHODS

How does this context of social policy influence employment decisions of mothers? This article describes employment patterns of employed women during the perinatal period, their reasons for returning to work, and the implications for health policy, using data gathered as part of a 5-year study of health outcomes of working mothers.[19]

Data for the larger study were gathered from women who met the following criteria at the time of study enrollment: married, or in a committed relationship with a male partner; pregnant with their first child; employed 20 hr/week or more; and planning to return to work within 1 year of the child's birth. Participants were recruited through advertisements in local media and prenatal clinics. This article is based on data available from 85 women who completed data through the 4-month postpartum visit.

Data were gathered on three occasions: during mid-pregnancy, and at 1 and 4 months postpartum. Multiple data collection methods were used, including a mailed questionnaire and a personal interview.

Employment patterns and participant characteristics were measured through self-report on single-item questions on written questionnaires, which were completed prenatally and then at 1 and 4 months postpartum.

Data on reasons for returning to work were gathered through participants' responses to the question, "Why did you return to work when you did?" asked by a research assistant during interviews conducted after each woman's return to work. Responses were audiotaped and transcribed, then coded into categories developed through content analysis during a pilot study on a similar population.[20] A subsample of 20% of participant interviews were coded by two members of the research team; interrater agreement on coding was 98%.

The participants ranged in age from 22 to 41 years, with a mean age of 31. All of the women reported some education beyond high school; 44.7% had earned a bachelor's degree and 36.5% held graduate or professional degrees. The majority of participants (94%) were white (Table 55-1).

Over 50% of the new mothers studied were employed in professional and managerial occupations, with the next largest occupational group (17.6%) composed of clerical workers. Participants reported working 20 to 55 hours/week at the time of study enrollment, which was during pregnancy; 70.6% worked 40 hours/week or more.

TABLE 55-1   Personal and Employment Characteristics of Participants

CHARACTERISTIC	%
Personal	
Ethnicity	
White	94.1
Asian	4.7
Black	1.2
Family income	
$10,000–29,000	12.0
$30,000–49,000	26.5
$50,000–69,000	25.5
$79,000 or more	36.1
Employment	
Occupation	
Professional	55.3
Clerical	17.6
Technical	7.1
Service/sales	7.1
Managerial	5.9
Hours worked per week in pregnancy	
20–29 hours	9.4
30–39 hours	20.0
40 hours	35.3
41–55 hours	35.3

The majority of participants were members of two-earner families. The total family income reported ranged from $10,000 to over $70,000; over a third reported total annual family incomes over $70,000.

RESULTS
Perinatal Employment Patterns
Over 70% of the study participants worked to within 1 week of delivery, with over a third taking no leave before childbirth (Table 55-2). By 4 months postpartum, nearly 80% had returned to paid employment (Table 55-3). Five women returned to work within the first month following delivery. By 6 weeks postpartum, the duration commonly recommended for physical restoration (e.g., Pritchard et al.[16]), 15% of the new mothers had returned to work. The median time of returning to work was 12 weeks postpartum. At 4 months postpartum, of the women who had returned to work, nearly half (48.5%) were employed 40 hours/week or more (Table 55-4).

Reasons for Returning to Work
Participants were asked during an interview conducted after their return to work why they had returned when they did. Their responses were coded into five categories. *Financial* reasons included needing money/income and needing health care and other benefits. *Self-fulfilling* reasons included responses that indicated benefits to the woman herself (e.g., to enhance her physical or mental health, to obtain social support, or to regain a sense of identity, and personal readiness). *Workplace policy* reasons were those that included mentioning specific policies that the participant perceived as "mandating" her return to work (e.g., "My leave was up"). *Work-motivated* reasons were those opportunities or demands (not policy related) the respondent perceived as originating from her employment setting, including perceived pressure or desire from her employer or co-workers to return, work deadlines that needed to be met, to fulfill commitments made at a prior date, or to take advantage of a unique opportunity for advancement at work. *Family/baby-motivated* reasons were those originating from a family member (i.e., spouse or infant) and included statements

TABLE 55-2 Duration of Pregnancy Leave

DAYS LEAVE PRIOR TO DELIVERY	%
None	34.2
1–7	38.2
8–14	13.1
15–84	15.5

TABLE 55-3   Week of Return to Employment Following Childbirth

POSTPARTUM WEEK	%
2–4	5.9
5–6	9.4
7–8	13.0
9–12	25.8
13–16	24.8
After 16	21.1

such as "My husband wanted me to return" and "My baby was ready." It was possible to categorize all participant responses into these five categories, many women gave more than one reason for their returning to work. The majority (76.3%) indicated that their decision was motivated by financial reasons. While the need for money was expressed, the need to obtain employer-supported health care benefits was also apparent. Other important reasons for returning to work included adherence to workplace leave policies (30.5%), because work provided the women with personal fulfillment (30.5%), or because of workplace opportunities, demands, or commitments (25.4%). Relatively few women (1.7%) cited family reasons for returning to paid employment (Table 55-5).

The strong influence of economics on the decision to return to work is supported by additional data on the availability to study participants of paid postpartum leave. Participants were asked to identify all sources of paid leave used to support their time away from work following childbirth; sources included sick leave/"maternity" leave, vacation time, personal leave, and paid parental leave (Table 55-6). Many participants combined several types of employee benefits to support their leave. While nearly half (46%) of the participants remained off work for more than 12 weeks postpartum, fewer than 5% had paid leave to support this extended time with

TABLE 55-4   Hours Worked at 4 Months Postpartum

HOURS PER WEEK	%
Under 20	7.1
20–29	21.5
30–39	22.8
40	37.1
41–50	11.4

TABLE 55-5 Reasons for Returning to Work

REASON	%
Financial	76.3
Self-fulfilling	30.5
Workplace policy	30.5
Work motivated	25.4
Family/baby motivated	1.7

Percentages sum to more than 100% because respondents could provide more than one reason for returning to work.

their infants. Nearly a third had no paid leave available to use postpartum. When leave was available, it was most often identified as either sick leave or vacation time. When asked at 4 months about their perceptions of adequacy of their leaves from work, 47.1% indicated their leave was too short; none indicated their leave had been too long, but a third perceived their leave to be adequate in length.

Health Impact

Returning to work too soon may have an impact on women's health and their ability to fulfill work and family responsibilities. At 4 months postpartum, half the participants indicated they were currently working "too many" hours (Table 55-7). Additional indicators of participants' health at the 4-month data collection point included assessments of the impact of health on work. Of the women who had returned to work by this time, 23.9% had been absent from work due to their own illness during the past month; 28.4% had been absent from work due to the child's illness. A larger proportion of women (61.2%) had come late to work or left work early for health-related reasons. Over a third (38%) reported that while they were not absent from work, they believed that poor health interfered with their ability to perform on the job.

TABLE 55-6 Postpartum Use of Paid Leave

TYPE OF LEAVE BENEFIT USED	LENGTH (WEEKS)	%
Sick leave/disability	1–8	46.3
Vacation	1–7	46.3
Personal leave	1–16	7.5
Parental leave	1–13	7.5

TABLE 55-7   Indicators of Health at 4 Months Postpartum

INDICATOR	%
Current work hours	
Too few	4.7
Right amount	25.9
Too many	50.6
Not working	18.8
Work interference	
Illness days	23.9
Child's illness days	28.4
Shorter work day due to health problem	61.2
Work interference due to health problem	38.1

IMPLICATIONS

Employed mothers face a fundamental dilemma.[21] It is a pervasive societal assumption that it is in the best interest of the child to be cared for within their families, primarily by the mother, during early infancy, if not longer. Simultaneously, economic realities demand that women need to provide a share of the family income and have access to health care benefits to provide for their children's well-being. The dilemma is further compounded by the assumption that in order for women to gain equality with men, they must participate in work in the same way men do, with little accommodation to the demands of family life. This assumption seems to provide the basis for social and workplace policies that restrict time away from work and options such as flexible work schedules or childcare located near the worksite. All too often, commitment to work (and therefore job security and advancement) is defined as the ability to put all other life activities aside. In this environment, coupled with the limited availability of high-quality and affordable childcare, children become a barrier to women's equal participation in society.

The data presented here were from a sample of women with many educational and economic resources. Workplace policies and options are even more restrictive for women who are single, less well educated, or employed in traditionally blue collar occupations. Professional women have greater access to leave than do women employed in service industries, they have twice the availability of work time flexibility, and more availability of employer-supported childcare.[18]

Social policies are changing, albeit slowly, in response to the increasing recognition of the importance of women as part of the labor force. Employers are recognizing that family-supportive benefits are necessary to recruit and retain employees (e.g., Shellenbarger[22]). Employers who have restructured to accommodate family-related issues report higher employee retention rates, fewer absences, less tardiness, higher morale, and higher productivity.[23] As health care benefits become a major, if not *the* major, industry expenditure, employers realize that it is to their advantage to be concerned about the health and well-being of their female, as well as their male, employees.

Within this context, what is the responsibility of the nursing scientific community? Our scientific work in the future must provide data that can facilitate the creation of "informed" public policy about the impact of existing policies on the health of women, families, and the workplace. Our research questions need to be more relevant to policy-makers and our studies more focused to be usable by legislators and corporate policy setters. Questions remaining to be answered include, "What is the relationship between timing of return to work and postpartum mother's health and work productivity? What is the effect on women's health of differing workplace policies? What is the effect on the workplace of differing family supportive policies? What characteristics can be used to identify those women who would benefit the most from which workplace options?"

The United States is the only Western industrialized nation without a national family leave policy.[24] The Family and Medical Leave Act, debated by Congress in 1990 and 1991 and vetoed repeatedly by President Bush, indicates that policy-makers are beginning to consider family-supportive policies. However, even if the current family leave proposals were to be enacted, there still would be the need to move further in addressing issues suggested in this article, for example, 1) the provision of leave options for childbearing women and men employed in small businesses; and 2) providing job security and paid leave to employees to care for needy family members.

As a society we are faced with a major public policy decision. What are the limits of our expectations of what the individual family is capable of and responsible for in meeting the needs of its members? What should be expected of both public and private sectors of society in meeting these needs? Who is responsible for creating and maintaining the balance between family and workplace priorities? Is the study of these issues and policies a high priority for nursing research? None of these questions have easy answers. Answers depend on the extent to which we claim the problem as one shared by society as a whole and by the discipline of nursing, not only the families who must juggle work and family on a daily basis.

Acknowledgment

I gratefully acknowledge the contributions of Dr. Monica Jarrett, Dorothy Pattison, Karen D'Apolito, Charlene Martin, Ann Fetrick, and Margaret Savage to this article.
The research was funded by the National Center for Nursing Research , #NR01-1920.

■ REFERENCES

1. Fernandez J. The politics and reality of family care in corporate America. Lexington, Massachusetts: Lexington Books, 1990:5–20.
2. US Department of Labor, Bureau of Labor Statistics. Working women: a chartbook. Bulletin 2385. Washington: US Government Printing Office, 1991.

3. O'Connell M. Work and family patterns of American women, maternity leave arrangements: 1961–1985. Current Population reports, Special Studies Series P-23, No. 165. US Bureau of the Census. Washington: US Government Printing Office, 1990:11–57.
4. Bachu A. Fertility of American women: July 1990. Current Population Reports, Population Characteristics Series P-20, No. 454. US Bureau of the Census, Economics and Statistics Administration. Washington: US Government Printing Office, 1990.
5. Tulman L, Fawcett J. Maternal employment following childbirth. Res Nurs Health 1990;13:181–8.
6. Wilkie J. The decline in men's labor force participation and income and the changing structure of family economic support. J Marriage Family 1991;53:111–22.
7. Gardin S, Richwald G. Pregnancy and employment leave: legal precedents and future policy. J Pub Health Policy 7, 458–469.
8. US Department of Labor, Women's Bureau. Working mothers and their children. Facts on working women, No. 89-3. Washington: US Government Printing Office, 1989.
9. US Bureau of the Census. Child care costs hit the poor harder. Census and You 1989; 26(7):7.
10. Callaghan P, Hartmann H. Contingent work: a chart book on part-time and temporary employment. Washington: Economic Policy Institute, 1991.
11. Wolf W, Fligstein N. Sex and authority in the workplace. Am Soc Rev 1979;44:235–52.
12. Gottfried A, Gottfried A. Maternal employment and children's development: longitudinal research. New York: Plenum Press, 1988.
13. Koester L. Supporting optimal parenting behaviours during infancy. In: Hyde J, Essex M, eds. Parental leave and child care: setting a research and policy agency. Philadelphia: Temple University Press, 1991:323–6.
14. Gil D. Unravelling social policy: theory, analysis, and political action. 2nd ed. Cambridge, Massachusetts: Schenkman. 1976: 13, 14.
14a. Bowlby J. Attachment and loss, Volume II: Separating: anxiety and anger. New York: Basic Books, 1973.
15. MacPherson K. Health care policy, values, and nursing. Adv Nurs Sci 1987;9(3):1–11.
16. Pritchard J, MacDonald P, Gant N. Williams obstetrics. 17th ed. Norwalk, Connecticut: Appleton-Century-Crofts, 1985.
17. Wisensale S, Allison M. Family leave legislation: state and federal initiatives. Family Relations 1989;38:182–9.
18. Buraff Publications. The national report on work and family. 1990;3(9):3.
19. Killien M. Returning to work: impact on postpartum mothers' health [Unpublished grant porposal.] University of Washington, Seattle.
20. Krippendorff K. Content analysis: an introduction to its methodology. Newbury Park, California: Sage, 1980.
21. Skold K. The interests of feminists and children in child care. In: Dornbusch S, Strober M, eds. Feminism, children, and the new families. New York: Guilford Press, 1988:113–35.
22. Shellenbarger S. More job seekers put family needs first. Wall Street Journal 1991 Nov 15:B1, B10.
23. Allen K, Baber K. Starting a revolution in family life education: a feminist vision. Family Relations 1992;41:378–84.
24. Kamerman S, Kahn A, eds. Child care, parental leave, and the under 3s: policy innovation in Europe. New York: Auburn House, 1991:1–22.

Chapter 56

The Nurse as Change Agent: Task Force—Genesis of a Change

MARGARET MILLER

> Community health nursing practice requires that the nurse understand and manage change. It is one thing to recognize a need for change, and another to initiate and carry through a change project, acting in the role of change agent. One must carefully assess the situation, work effectively with the client system, and recognize the many variables, such as resistant community officials or scarce funds that could affect the change process and outcomes. In this chapter, Margaret Miller describes her role as a successful change agent in a community project to reduce young people's alcohol consumption.

While this author was a student of nursing at Western Connecticut State College, she became aware of what appeared to be an alcohol abuse problem in the community's teenage population. This awareness was due in part to the emphasis placed by the nursing program on the expanded role of the nurse within the community.[1] Her concern about adolescent alcohol abuse became more acute as her own teenaged son approached the legal driving age. She had also witnessed many instances of public drinking among the community's youngsters. More and more news media coverage of the national increase in teenage drinkers and the attendant problems had been noticed. It was decided that a survey should be made in an attempt to document the amount of alcohol use and abuse within the adolescent community.

The community survey was patterned after a similar, but much more extensive, one conducted for the National Institute on Alcohol Abuse and Alcoholism. Using the criteria developed for the national survey, it was found that within the local adolescent population, approximately 50 percent of the males and 33 percent of the females could be classified as problem drinkers (those reporting to have been drunk four or more times in the past year, and/or two or more negative consequences of drinking be-

From *Nursing Clinics of North America* 14(2):347–356, June 1979. Reprinted by permission of W. B. Saunders Company.

havior).[2,3] In addition, there was a sharp increase in adolescent drinking at age sixteen. The survey also indicated that the 3 D's—drinking, driving, and drunkenness—were prevalent among area teenagers.[2]

Other statistics from the area report indicated:

1. There was *no* direct correlation between adolescent alcohol use and parental drinking levels.[4]
2. There *was* a direct correlation between peer group alcohol use and respondents' use.[2]
3. More teenagers felt that a very important reason for drinking was in association with activities of a sociable nature. However, those categorized as heavy drinkers were more inclined than others to view drinking to relieve personal pressures as a very important reason to drink.[2]
4. Approximately 82 percent of those studied felt that they had no problem with alcohol, and none reported feeling that they had a considerable or serious problem.[2]

▄IDENTIFICATION OF PLANNED CHANGE

There appeared to be no correlated effort to deal with adolescent alcohol abuse among the various groups interacting with teenagers. It was felt that the attention of authorities in the community should be drawn to what the investigator had perceived to be a serious problem. It was hoped that these authorities could be motivated to formulate a plan of action to help adolescents, parents, educators, and other community members identify and deal with the role alcohol appeared to play in the lives of these young people. The author decided to make the development of this action plan her change project for her Leadership and Change course.

Specifically, the desired change would involve the collaboration of education, health, law enforcement, and religious communities with the local alcohol council, parks and recreation officials, and youth-aid groups officials, parents' groups, and *adolescents* in the development of a comprehensive plan to aid and guide young people in mature, responsible decision-making regarding the use or nonuse of alcoholic beverages. It was felt that this multifaceted approach was necessary in view of the varied aspects and the broad scope of the problem.

▄DESCRIPTION OF CHANGE PROCESS

The situation facing the change agent was one of a dual client system. One client system, the community adolescents, would be the beneficiaries of the hoped-for change. However, it was felt that this system's power to effect any meaningful change was negligible because of its relative powerlessness in city government. On the other hand, the other client system, the city administration, had the power to support and effect change, and thus was chosen by the change agent as the primary client system with which to work.

Briefly, the organizational structure of the community in which this change was to be attempted is as follows:

1. The electors (voters) are the ultimate decision-makers.
2. The mayor, board of education, city treasurer, city clerks, common council, town clerk, board of selectmen, and voter registrars are elected officials who enact legislation, collect and appropriate monies, and administer city business.
3. Reporting directly to the mayor are 33 boards, agencies, commissions, and departments who are the functional units of the city government.

▄ APPROACHES TO CHANGE

Two basic approaches were utilized during this change process: Reinkemeyer's theory of planned change, and an element of the traditional approach. The utilized element of the latter was the "circulation of ideas to the elite" (presenting ideas to people in power, or to people who can influence those in power).[4]

The Reinkemeyer theory of change was utilized throughout the change project. Phase I of this theory is "the development of a felt need and desire for changes."[4] Reinkemeyer elaborates on this phase by stating that one of the elements of this phase could be helping the client system perceive a discrepancy between what is and what could be.[4]

Working Through Educational System

It was decided to attempt to initiate the desired change through the educational system. Since the board of education in this city is theoretically as powerful as the mayor's office, it was felt that recruiting allies within the educational system would be the logical starting point. It was hoped that awareness of the problem of adolescent alcohol abuse within the community could be developed in school officials, who would then become motivating forces in developing that awareness at the board of education level.

A copy of the area's adolescent alcohol-use report was submitted to the high school principal for his review. Several attempts were made by the change agent to meet with the principal, school psychologist, and teachers. Repeatedly, scheduling difficulties were given as the reason for not holding the meeting, and the change agent began to feel that the principal was not actually interested in discussing the survey results or ideas to alleviate the problem of teenage alcohol abuse. Finally, a meeting of the social psychology teacher, the school psychologist, and the change agent was held. The principal, however, did not attend.

During the meeting, the alcohol-use survey results were discussed, and all participants agreed that a problem did exist. However, resistance to the change idea was again encountered. There was a considerable amount of disagreement on the part of one school official regarding the seriousness of the problem. Both school officials expressed a great deal of skepticism about the ability or feasibility of the educational system's playing a large role in the proposed change. The school officials agreed that an approach to the superintendent of schools or board of education at that time would be met with a considerable amount of resistance. Since school budgets were being cut, the school system's administration was not being very receptive to any ideas for new projects. The change agent truly felt that she was facing passive indifference, at best, and possibly active resistance in dealing with the educational system. She was dissuaded from approaching the superintendent or the board of education because she had found no real ally within the system.

Working Through Community Action

It was decided to move back to the drawing board with Phase I. Because the change agent felt that she needed outside assistance to motivate community officials, a meeting was held with the newly appointed executive director of the Midwestern Connecticut Council on Alcoholism (MCCA). The alcohol-use survey results were discussed, and a great deal of interest was expressed by the MCCA director. Because alcohol abuse in juveniles and the elderly was a problem that he had placed at the top of his priority list, he was eager to have a community awareness program instituted. The change agent felt that she had finally found a strong ally to help promote the change idea.

At this point, the change agent and the MCCA director utilized Phase 4 of Reinkemeyer's theory. In this phase, "the change agent with the client system examines alternative routes and tentative goals and then establishes actual goals and intentions of actions."[4] Several plans to initiate the desired public awareness and change process were discussed.

1. Meeting with various religious and educational leaders, mental health workers, youth aid group officials, and parents' group leaders to encourage development and coordination of alcohol abuse control programs.
2. Use of the news media to generate and promote generalized public awareness and support of alcohol abuse control programs.
3. Requesting the mayor to appoint a task force consisting of leaders from the education and health fields along with private citizens, alcohol abuse experts, and teenagers to study the problem of adolescent alcohol abuse and possibly formulate a viable program to deal with the problem.

Regarding Plan 1, it was decided that this approach would be extremely fragmented and time- and energy-consuming. It was also felt that because most of these organizations are privately funded or depend on governmental grants for their support, this could possibly prohibit alcohol abuse control programs from being given high priority.

Inasmuch as no well-thought-out public awareness program had actually been formulated, Plan 2 was felt to be inadvisable. It was also thought that those involved in city government and fund allocation could possibly be negatively affected if they first learned about the desired change through the newspaper rather than having it brought to their attention through the ordinary chain of command.

Plan 3, asking the mayor to appoint a task force, was felt to be the most logical and expedient first-line approach. Several factors led to this decision.

1. The mayor was a newly elected official—a member of a political party in opposition to the party that had historically been in power in city government—who was interested in making innovations and moving the community in a different direction.
2. The governor had declared March as Alcohol Month, thus generating statewide interest.
3. The state Alcohol Council had approached the alcohol abuse program via a task force, and had already presented several plans to the state legislature.

A meeting of the mayor, the executive director of MCCA, and the change agent was held to discuss the results of the area's adolescent alcohol-use survey as well as the idea of a task force assigned to study the problem and make recommendations for solutions. Phases 1, 2, and 3 of Reinkemeyer's theory were used. Phase 1 was explained previously. Phase 2 of the theory is the establishment of a change relationship between the change agent and client system.[4] Phase 3 is stated to be "clarification or diagnosis of the client system's problem, need or objective," in which the "client system is helped and encouraged to define the true nature and extent of the problem."[4]

At this time, the alcohol-survey results were again discussed. Both the MCCA director and the change agent presented themselves as resource persons on whom the client system could rely. They jointly assisted the client system (the mayor) in defining the true nature of the problem. For instance, the mayor was given definitions of terms such as "alcohol abuse" and "problem drinkers," and was helped and encouraged to view teenage alcohol abuse as a contributor to problems in many areas of life. The mayor expressed concern about the statistics of the survey as well as an interest in a plan to deal with the problem. After the mayor had agreed that alcohol abuse was a multifaceted problem for teenagers, he was able, with little assistance, to discern that a multidisciplinary approach to the problem was necessary if there was to be any hope for success.

He agreed to appoint a task force to study the problem and make recommendations for a program to aid area adolescents in making decisions about use or nonuse of alcohol. However, he suggested that the task force be addressed to the study of alcohol and drug abuse. This alteration in the planned change was readily accepted by the MCCA director and the change agent.

Appointment of Task Force

The mayor suggested that a committee of no more than seven persons be formed so that meetings could be scheduled more easily and work could progress more efficiently. Committee appointees were discussed, and it was decided that an alcohol expert, an educational professional, a health professional, an adolescent, and two or three private citizens would be appropriate task force members. The mayor also volunteered the use of a conference room in City Hall for meetings of the task force. At that time, he appointed the MCCA director and the change agent to the committee, and gave his verbal promise to appoint other members within two or three weeks.

It was approximately four months before all the committee appointees were selected. When this task was accomplished, Phase 5 of Reinkemeyer's theory, the transformation of intentional into actual change behavior, had been completed.[4] The committee grew from the proposed seven persons to fifteen. The mayor had carefully selected the appointees. The committee now consists of an alcohol expert (the MCCA director), a high school teacher, the director of a drug abuse center and one of his volunteer counselors, three adolescents, *two* nurses (one of which is the change agent), and seven private citizens who had been active in youth work and government in the past. The mayor has given the committee six months, with an optional additional six months, to conduct a study and make recommendations for solutions to the teenage alcohol/drug abuse problem.

Phase 6 of Reinkemeyer's theory is permanent adoption of a change, and Phase 7 is termination of the change agent/client system relationship.[4] These phases have not yet been worked through during this change process. Work on a comprehensive anti-alcohol/drug abuse program cannot begin until the task force report has been submitted to the mayor, and termination of the change agent/client system relationship will not be possible until the task force has been disbanded. However, the change process has been firmly set into motion. Reinkemeyer states, "Theories of planned change do not assume that the change agent possesses a ready made solution which he must 'sell' to a client system. Rather, he is someone with a clear mandate and special competence to help plan and effect change."[4]

At this point, there is a great deal of optimism about the eventual realization of the planned change; that is, that a multidisciplinary program to aid teenagers in making mature, responsible decisions regarding drug and alcohol use will be instituted in the community.

ROLES OF CHANGE PROCESS PARTICIPANTS
Change Agent

The change agent kept the momentum for change by initiating each of the meetings with key personnel involved in the process. As information provider, the change agent supplied copies of the adolescent alcohol-use survey (the result of which had initially shown the need for change), explained pertinent points of the report, and gave additional information when necessary. She also assumed the role of information-seeker, gathering additional data from school officials and the executive director of MCAA before meeting with the mayor. As a motivator, the change agent was able, by getting to the right people at the right time, to capitalize on pre-existing interest in the problem of alcohol and drug abuse in community teenagers. The change agent's enthusiasm and dedication to her change idea was an important factor in motivating the city power structure to act.

A democratic style of leadership was employed by the change agent throughout the process.[2] Participation of other persons involved in the change was actively sought and encouraged. The change agent was receptive to the ideas of the other participants and readily agreed to alterations in the original plan (i.e., having the task force address itself to alcohol and drug abuse). This type of leadership was effective because after the initial resistance from school officials, the progression from planned to actual change was rather rapid and resistance-free.

MCCA Executive Director

The executive director of MCCA was of tremendous assistance in transforming the change idea into a reality. As an expert in the field of alcohol abuse, he was a powerful ally during the meeting with the mayor, and was an effective coleader at that time. He provided information that was far beyond the change agent's area of expertise. He also provided the extra motivating force that was necessary to convince the mayor to appoint a task force. The MCCA director also utilized the democratic leadership style by seeking and encouraging the participation of the mayor during the proceedings. It is felt that the coleadership system worked extremely well in this instance, and that the leaders supported and complemented each other in the effort.

City Mayor

The mayor played many roles. In his role as representative of the primary client system—city government—he was an interested and receptive information-receiver. It is felt that this, coupled with his concern about drug use among the community's teenagers, helped motivate him to assume his second role—that of cochange agent. Through his position in the city hierarchy, the mayor was able to take action by appointing a task force to study the problem more fully and make recommendations for problem-solving.

▬EVALUATION OF CHANGE PROCESS

It is felt that the combination of the traditional approach and the Reinkemeyer theory worked very well during this change process. By interacting with the city administration, the change agent expedited the establishment of actual goals and intentions of actions. Circumvention of the educational system freed a stalled change process and led to working with a much more diversified city administration agency. Thus, the process started moving again, and a more comprehensive change idea could be presented and acted upon.

Working with a city administration actually means that one is working from an organizational center outward, rather than through a top-to-bottom or bottom-to-top chain of command. In other words, planned change can be sabotaged from either end. It is possible that city and private agencies may not be receptive to the idea, or the electorate could veto it even if it is accepted by the other segments of the organization.

Modification of the change process might have been directed at working through a straight-line chain of command rather than through the hub-and-spoke method. In this way, perhaps a firmer foundation or a clearer mandate for the change could have been provided. However, it is believed that this modification would have involved a much more lengthy, cumbersome, and perhaps ineffective approach. For example, it is entirely possible that had the idea been presented to city and/or private agencies (e.g., Parks and Recreation, Boy Scout Council, etc.), it might have been shelved and might never have reached the attention of the mayor. Budget, staffing, and other problems could have prevented these agencies from taking an active interest in the change idea. By the same token, had the change agent presented the idea directly to the public via the news media (assuming, of course, that the media would cooperate), sufficient interest might not have been generated to effect any change at all. It is hoped that by going to the organizational center, the motivating forces will be increased and the resisting forces decreased so that real change can be attained.

The task force is composed of individuals who are very interested in the problem of adolescent drug and alcohol abuse and possible solutions. Subcommittees have already been formed to study in depth various aspects of the problem and to make recommendations. There is a plan to complete a comprehensive report for the mayor by the end of six months, or at least to have done enough work to earn an extension. The participants are optimistic that after comprehensive recommendations have been made, they will be accepted and acted upon. There is hope that ultimately a multifaceted, coordinated approach to guiding young people in the responsible use of alcohol and other drugs will be possible through heightened public awareness, education, and improved recreational opportunities and health care. Of course, actual evaluation of the success of any project concerned with averting human tragedy is subject to individual interpretations and value systems. This author feels that if only one young person is guided away from substance abuse, or one youthful abuser is rehabilitated, the effort will have been well spent.

■SUMMARY

After alcohol-use patterns in a community's teenage population were researched, a change idea was conceived. This idea was, in essence, a multidisciplinary approach to the development of a comprehensive plan to aid young people in making responsible decisions regarding the use or nonuse of alcoholic beverages. Reinkemeyer's theory of planned change was utilized throughout the change process. A community-wide task force has now been appointed and is actively studying the adolescent drug and alcohol abuse problem. Within the next few months, comprehensive recommendations for solution of the problem will be made. The task force is optimistic that an effective program will be initiated to combat alcohol and drug abuse within the community's adolescent population.

▬REFERENCES

1. Merton, R. K. The Social Nature of Leadership. *Am. J. Nurs.* 69:2614, 1969.
2. Miller, M. An Evaluative Survey of Alcohol Use in High School Students, Grades Ten through Twelve. Unpublished research study, Western Connecticut State College, 1977.
3. Rachal, J. V., et al. *A National Study of Adolescent Drinking Behavior, Attitudes and Correlates.* Springfield, VA: National Technical Information Service, 1975.
4. Reinkemeyer, A. M. Commitment to an Ideology of Change. *Nurs. Forum.* 9:341, 1970.

Chapter 57

Healthy Cities: A Model of Community Change

BEVERLY C. FLYNN

An example of community health nursing leadership and effecting change is evident in the Healthy Cities movement. Dr. Beverly Flynn, who is Head of the World Health Organization Collaborating Center in Healthy Cities as well as Director of Healthy Cities Indiana, describes the Indiana Healthy Cities project in this chapter. She presents case studies of six participating cities in Indiana who through a process of community leadership development and social change took action locally to create healthy cities. She applies Etzioni's four levers of social change as a framework for analysis of community change and gives examples of short-term actions and long-range strategies used by the cities to promote healthy public policy and community health.

There can be no health without community.[1(p291)]

The Healthy Cities movement grew out of the realization that more than half of the world's population lives in cities, where the problems are most concentrated and the resources are most plentiful. It is the cities that hold the future of the world, yet they face some of the most complex problems in human history. The city is viewed as an appropriate context for community health, because it is the closest level of government to the people and capable of developing the economic, social, and political resources needed to address local concerns.

The Healthy Cities movement began as an initiative of the World Health Organization (WHO) in Europe in 1986.[2] Three world documents provide the background for the Healthy Cities project: the WHO Constitution, the Global Strategy for Health for All, and the Ottawa Charter for Health Promotion.[3–5] These documents recognize that a person's health is determined by a broad range of social, economic, environmental, and po-

The author thanks Melinda Rider, Associate Project Director, Healthy Cities Indiana, for her comments and suggestions on this article.

From *Family and Community Health* 15(1):13–23, 1992., Reprinted by permission of Aspen Publishers, Inc.

litical factors. Intersectoral action, therefore, was recognized in these documents as a key strategy to achieve health for all. However, putting the concept into practice was found to be the most challenging and difficult aspect of implementation.[6] In the Ottawa Charter for Health Promotion, five broad action areas were identified that provided the framework for the Healthy Cities project: the development of healthy public policies, the creation of supportive environments, the strengthening of community action, the development of personal skills, and the reorientation of health services.[5] The WHO began the development of the Healthy Cities program in Europe as a means to implement the goal of health for all based on these action areas within the context of equity and social justice. The WHO Healthy Cities project in Europe currently is being implemented in 30 European project cities and 17 national networks involving hundreds of cities (some working on multicity action) through a process of political commitment, visibility for health, institutional change, and innovative action for health.[6] Healthy Cities currently is becoming a means to the democratization of Central and Eastern Europe, with cities in Western Europe providing the technical assistance and support for the infrastructure needed by cities in these countries. There are now more than 400 Healthy City initiatives throughout the world (in addition to Europe) in North America, Australia, and in developing countries of the Americas, the Eastern Mediterranean region, and now beginning in Africa.

This article presents case studies of six cities participating in Healthy Cities Indiana, which began in 1988 with a grant from the W.K. Kellogg Foundation. The Indiana program was one of the first Healthy Cities programs in the United States and was modeled after the European Healthy Cities project. Healthy Cities Indiana is a collaborative effort between Indiana University School of Nursing Department of Community Health Nursing, Indiana Public Health Association (IPHA), and six Indiana cities (Fort Wayne, Gary, Indianapolis, Jeffersonville, New Castle, and Seymour). Three of the cities are large urban cities, and three are small rural cities, all with populations ranging from 15,000 to more than 700,000.

▬THE CONTEXT FOR COMMUNITY CHANGE

As successful as Healthy Cities has been in Europe, there are differences between the United States and Europe that make adaptation difficult. In the United States, political authority is highly fractionalized and decentralized. Public health, according to the Institute of Medicine's report on the future of public health, is in disarray and lacks the power needed to pursue essential programs.[7] Although the government funds some services, in general it subsidizes the private health care delivery system. There is little funding for community health. Although the United States has people who are willing and accustomed to taking local action to solve problems, these people frequently do not realize their potential in community health promotion.

Healthy Cities Indiana builds on the strengths of people in the United States and Indiana. These strengths include values of self-reliance, the work ethic, pluralism, and a strong affinity for self-government. Healthy Cities Indiana seeks to promote a public-private partnership in public health through a process of community leadership development and social change.

■THE HEALTHY CITIES INDIANA PROCESS

Although the specifics of the Healthy Cities Indiana process are reported elsewhere, it will be useful to provide a brief summary of the process.[8, 9] Initially 16 cities were targeted by project staff and IPHA leadership to participate in the Healthy Cities Indiana program. Local forums about the Healthy Cities Indiana program were held with city leaders in seven cities before the complement of six cities was finalized. The forums were conducted by program staff, and once local support for participation was evident, the mayor and local health officer signed a memorandum of understanding for placing health on the political agenda of the city, for broad-based (intersectoral) participation in the Healthy City process, and for the formation of public policies that promote health (healthy public policies).

Once the six cities were identified, program staff and city leaders discussed whether a broad-based committee existed in the city or a new Healthy City committee needed to be organized. In each case, the city leaders decided that either a broad-based committee did not exist or, if one did exist, the focus was too narrow to incorporate the Healthy City concept. As a result each of the cities formed a new Healthy City committee consisting of community leaders from different city sectors and population groups. The categories of committee membership were generated by staff, but the mayor, local health officer, and other community leaders decided who would best represent those categories.

The Healthy City committee is the structure within which the Healthy Cities process occurs. Healthy Cities Indiana emphasizes a community leadership development approach in Healthy Cities. This is accomplished through a number of methods including consultation, analysis of information, conferences and statewide workshops, network sessions, staff technical support, and viewing videotapes and reading Healthy City and related materials.

Each committee is expected to conduct a community assessment to identify the city's strengths and needs, set its own priorities and goals, secure resources, establish steering groups, and take action that will work locally. The ultimate goal of Healthy Cities Indiana is to provide data-based information to policy makers and to promote healthy public policies.

■SOCIAL CHANGE AT THE COMMUNITY LEVEL

Selected concepts of social change can be applied to Healthy Cities Indiana and bear further elucidation. Although various theories and conceptual models have been used to explain and predict changes in health behavior, most emphasize factors that influence change in individual health behavior. The increasing focus on community health is based on the recognition that behavior is greatly influenced by the environment in which people live. It has been suggested that the best measure of community change needs to incorporate analysis 1) at the *individual level,* to determine how much individuals are influenced by a community project; 2) at the *subsystem level,* to elicit changes within community organizations and groups; 3) at the *level of interrelationships among various subsystems,* to detect the importance of "social connectedness" in the community; and 4) at the *entire community level,* to assess changes in norms and values such as policy changes.[10] The presentation of case studies in this article includes selected aspects of the subsystem level (ie, description of the structure and activities of the Healthy City committees) and the level of interrelationships among various subsystems (ie, description of the Healthy City projects developed by these committees). It is too early in the history of Healthy Cities Indiana to assess changes at the individual or entire community levels. Such changes need considerably more time for the projects to reach all people in the community, for an impact on policy to occur, and for evaluation to be completed.

To facilitate the presentation of these studies on the two levels that can be assessed, Etzioni's four levers of social change provide a useful framework for analysis.[11] These four levers are as follows:

1. Knowledge of the community: the problem, its causes, and consequences;
2. Development of effective goals and organization;
3. Provision of power bases to support the needed changes; and
4. Development of community participation and consensus.

None of the four levers of change exist in isolation. They are interdependent and interactive in nature. All four levers need to be addressed for effective social change. Selected indicators of each lever of social change are presented later, and the progress of each of the six cities on these levers is indicated.

It should be noted that the cities involved in Healthy Cities Indiana are at various stages of social or community change. Etzioni's levers of social change can be applied to Healthy Cities Indiana to determine which cities are most effective in the Healthy Cities process. The other cities also can benefit from this analysis by adjusting their efforts toward those levers needing attention.

Knowledge of the Community

Etzioni's first lever of social change is related to acquisition of knowledge.[11] As indicated before, Healthy Cities Indiana emphasizes community leadership development, and considerable attention is given to knowledge development about the city and the surrounding county. All members of the six Healthy City committees were given a data set about their city and county that was prepared by project staff. Included were data from the US Bureau of the Census, Vital Statistics, and from the Indiana State Board of Health. Project staff discussed the data with committee members, and community strengths and problems were delineated by the committees. Based on these discussions, the committees were able to determine gaps in information about their cities and, with staff support, conducted local surveys to augment the existing information. Table 57-1 summarizes the ways each of the cities obtained further information about their city.

Each of the Healthy City committees was concerned about obtaining community input into the Healthy City process. They conducted the more traditional household surveys as well as special surveys aimed at children, youth, the elderly, and other hard-to-reach populations. Another technique found useful was vision workshops to identify what community people of all ages saw as being the future of their healthy city, as well as to identify strengths and weaknesses in their community. Interestingly, most community groups had a vision of a healthy city that included a green and clean environment that supported equality among residents and promoted positive family and intergenerational relationships. (Almost no one mentioned a good health care system.) One city used a poster competition in grades 4 through 12. The children and youth reported a similar vision of the future, one that included a healthy and safe environment, recreation for kids, broad-based support for health in the community, good relationships among people, and an absence of drugs and violence. Project staff assisted the committees in the identification or development of survey

TABLE 57-1   Knowledge of the Community

CITY	METHOD OF OBTAINING KNOWLEDGE
A	Health survey Drug survey Service agency survey
B	Health survey KidsPlace survey* PRIDE survey†
C	Health survey KidsPlace survey* Neighborhood vision workshops Service agency survey
D	KidsPlace survey* Neighborhood vision workshops Household health survey
E	Poster competition Neighborhood vision workshops
F	KidsPlace survey* Health survey

*Office of the Mayor (1984). KidsPlace Survey, Seattle, Washington.
†PRIDE = Parent Resource Institute for Drug Education. National Parents Resource Institute for Drug Education, Suite 210, 50 Hurt Plaza, The Hurt Building, Atlanta, GA 30303.

instruments, provided committee member training in the conduct of the vision workshops, and analyzed and summarized the data for review of the committee.

Development of Effective Goals and Organization

Etzioni's second lever of social change is related to developing effective goals and organization.[11] Table 57-2 summarizes the progress of the Healthy City committees according to their priorities, the effectiveness of their committees, and their ability to establish a formal structure. Based on the previously mentioned surveys, all of the cities have identified priorities for action. However, they vary in committee functioning, which leads to effective development and implementation of solutions. Each of the members of the six Healthy City committees completed a Healthy City Committee Effectiveness Inventory that assessed five components of group dynamics: maintenance of morale, sharing, leadership, maturity or self-readiness, and task or work accomplishment. The mean scores of the committees' effectiveness are summarized in Table 57-2. Each item was marked from 1 to 4, with 4 being the rating for high effectiveness and 1 for low effectiveness. Only two of the committees indicated that their overall functioning was below 3.

The committees also are at different stages in formalizing their structure. Two of the committees have established bylaws, have incorporated, and have tax-exempt status, which permits them to receive funding for their Healthy City projects. All but one committee had organizational rules, and one did not commit its rules to writing. Two other committees are beginning to look at their structure; one of these has decided it will incorporate and apply for tax-exempt status.

Provision of Power Bases to Support Change

Etzioni's third lever of social change is developing power bases.[11] The Healthy City committees vary in how effective they have been in establishing their power bases to support their action plans. Three indicators of power are summarized in Table 57-3. The first relates to the extent to which the Healthy City committee is broad based. Although committee members were selected to represent the community broadly, attrition and turnover have occurred. Based on a review of minutes of committee meetings, two of the committees have not been functionally broad based. They have recognized this and are taking steps to remedy this narrow focus among committee members, which has been a limitation to the Healthy City process. A broad-based committee provides not only intersectoral input into decision making but also serves to balance the committee's decisions in terms of protecting the best interest of the total community. The second indicator of power relates to the committee's ability to develop proposals and receive funding for their Healthy City projects. Proposals have been prepared by five of the cities, and three cities have received funding. The third indicator of power relates to the extent to which the mayor and local health officer are strongly represented on the Healthy City committee. All of the cities have been able to elicit this support.

TABLE 57-2   Development of Effective Goals and Organization

CITY	PRIORITIES	HEALTHY CITIES COMMITTEE EFFECTIVENESS INVENTORY (MEANS)	FORMAL STRUCTURE
A	Environmental health Physical and mental health Economic health	3.06	Organizational rules Beginning to look at bylaws Will incorporate Will become tax exempt
B	Teenage pregnancy Child care Recycling/environment Affordable health care Drug abuse Health	3.12	Organizational rules Bylaws Incorporating
C	Community safety Indigent health care Organ donor Homelessness Economic development Infant mortality	2.73	Organizational rules Beginning to look at bylaws
D	Health Youth Recreation Recycling Community pride City clean-up	3.13	Unwritten organizational rules
E	Health Environment Equity/equality Family issues	2.79	None
F	Health Poor housing Traffic problems Child and adult abuse Health education Literacy and health	3.08	Organizational rules Bylaws Subcommittee on housing Incorporated and tax exempt

Development of Community Participation and Consensus

Etzioni's fourth and final lever of social change is the development of community participation and consensus.[11] Table 57-4 summarizes each city's progress in developing active participation and action programs. Each of the cities has identified steering groups that further develop the action planned by the Healthy City committee and monitor progress. The steering groups consist of members of the Healthy City committees and

TABLE 57-3   Provision of Power Bases to Support Change

CITY	BROAD-BASED HEALTHY CITY COMMITTEE	FUNDING	MAYOR/LHO* REPRESENTED
A	High	1 Proposal, funding received	Yes/Yes
B	High	1 Proposal, funding received 1 Proposal under review	Yes/Yes
C	Moderate	1 Proposal under review	Yes/Yes
D	High	No	Yes/Yes
E	Low	2 Proposals, funding received for 1	Yes/Yes
F	High	1 Proposal, funding received 1 Proposal being developed	Yes/Yes

*LHO = local health officer.

additional community members, thus broadening the scope of community participation in Healthy Cities.

Local action programs (the Healthy City projects) represent both short-term action and long-range strategies aimed at promoting healthy public policy. Some examples of short-term action are the Healthy Moments Public Service Announcements (PSAs). These 2-minute radio messages were prepared by one of the cities and shared with the other cities. They addressed a wide range of health topics such as immunizations, leaf burning, humor and healing, fever, common cold, water conservation, smoking, and walking. Members of the Healthy City committee volunteered to announce these messages, which were presented over the radio by the city's Healthy City committee. Some of the short-term projects have become long-range strategies. For example, one city decided that to address the problem of physical fitness, a community walk would be held in conjunction with a midsummer art fair. The hospital, parks and recreation department, and other committee members organized the walk. The response from the community was very positive, resulting in a request to continue the family walking program on a monthly basis. Members of the program meet at the hospital for breakfast and continue with a walk. The program has been so successful that the Healthy City committee had requests from other communities to help them develop a similar community walking program. These projects have empowered the committee members to apply their skills and resources in taking further action in addressing their community's problems.

Some examples of long-range strategies include the establishment of an in-school teen parenting program that combines education and health. This program received state educational funding and has affected the

---

TABLE 57-4   Development of Community Participation and Consensus

CITY	NUMBER OF ACTIVE STEERING GROUPS	ACTION PROGRAMS
A	4	Impact guidelines for new businesses Stepping Out Against Drugs walk for health Service directory Recycling/environment
B	4	Curbside recycling In-school teen parenting program Healthy Moments radio PSAs* Health promotion pamphlets Indigent care clinic
C	6	In-school teen parenting program Homeless health Service directory Trash hauler crime watch Indigent health care
D	2	Recycling Teen recreation
E	4	Environmentalist forum Youth network Human equity and equality Physical health Neighborhood action
F	5	Low-income housing Family walking program Healthy Moments radio PSAs* County wide coalition on abuse Mouthguard campaign for youth

*PSAs = public service announcements.

---

city's educational policy such that teen parents are encouraged to continue their education. Another example is recycling of solid wastes, which was started in three cities. One city has expanded its project of a recycling day to the development of recycling drop-off areas throughout the city. Plans are under way to develop a city-wide recycling center that can manage solid wastes and reduce the need for landfill dumping. Another innovative program, still in the planning stages, involves the trash haulers and the city police. This city discovered that most crime occurs between 5 AM and 7 AM, when the city trash haulers are collecting. The Healthy City committee decided to institute a crime watch program that involves the trash haulers and links them with the city police through their truck radios. Through this program, the Healthy City committee envisions that the trash haulers will be able to report crime early and be a haven for children who may be victims of crime.

CONCLUSIONS

This article has presented the results of participation by six cities in Healthy Cities Indiana on selected indicators of Etzioni's[11] four levers of social change, focusing on the subsystem level and the interrelationships among various subsystems as suggested by Bracht.[10] A complete analysis of social change within these cities would require validation with other indicators of the four levers and would include the measurement of change at the individual and entire community levels of analysis. Because Healthy Cities Indiana only began working with these cities less than 3 years ago, the Healthy Cities process needs considerably more time before such analyses can occur.

Variations among the cities occurred on two levers of social change: goal setting and organization and providing power bases to support community change. According to this analysis, all cities have addressed two of the four levers of social change. The cities most effective in the Healthy Cities process are cities A, B, and F, which have addressed selected indicators of all four of the levers. Although the remaining three cities are less effective in social change, they are in the process of improving their potential in the Healthy Cities process by making adjustments in those levers on which they rated low.

Although the Healthy Cities committees have identified priorities for action, they vary on their ability to organize themselves effectively. These are issues of concern to the committees and are guiding their current actions. Four of the cities have formalized or are involved in formalizing their structure, and the other two have decided to delay action in this area. One committee decided it was in a transition stage of involving city neighborhoods in the Healthy Cities process and it was too early to formalize a structure that was still emerging. In the other case the committee has decided that it has been able to reach consensus on the rules of operation without formalizing them in writing. Although these decisions are understandable, they limit the committees' abilities to receive external funding directly for their projects and activities. Most funding agencies require tax-exempt status prior to application for external funding. Stable funding for committee activities will need to be "in kind" (ie, indirect, by placing external funds in another organization with tax-exempt status) or come from the city government. There are limitations to each of these approaches. In-kind services can be unstable, affected by cutbacks in organizations' budgets, and the placement of funds in another organization can dilute the visibility of the Healthy City committee. Dependence on city funding can "politicize" the Healthy City process, as funding is subject to change in the short run, with the potential turnover of mayors and city councilors who support the process. The Healthy City committee needs to be aware of these limitations so that members can establish a plan of action to address them.

In addition to the struggle for effective committee functioning, two of the Healthy City committees have had difficulty maintaining broad-based committees, causing unnecessary delay in proceeding with the Healthy

City process. Efforts are under way by these committees to correct the problem. The Healthy city committees' members realize that a broad-based committee is needed as a power base to support change. All but one of the Healthy City committees have applied for external funding for their activities. Interestingly, this committee has made the decision not to formalize its structure in terms of bylaws, become incorporated, and apply for tax-exempt status. All of its efforts have been supported by in-kind services throughout the community. A counterbalance to this indicator of power in the city has been the development of a broad-based Healthy City committee that has had stable membership. All of the Healthy City committees have had consistent membership representation by the mayor and local health officer, which has lent considerable support to their projects.

Clearly, social change, as exemplified by Healthy Cities Indiana, takes time and is a dynamic and ongoing process. In spite of this, the Healthy City committees have been very successful in acquiring knowledge of their communities' strengths and problems. In addition to analyzing existing census and health data, the committees conducted population surveys to help clarify their understanding of the community. They also have developed a level of community participation and reached consensus on programs of action. These activities require a high level of community leadership skill that is important in social change and to the Healthy Cities process.

It is evident from this analysis that the six cities participating in Healthy Cities Indiana are involved in a complex process of social change aimed at the health of the community. The cities' efforts and perseverance exemplify that there is health with community.

▬ REFERENCES

1. Milio N. Healthy Cities: the new public health and supportive research. *Health Promotion Int.* 1990;5(4):291–297.
2. Tsouros AD. *World Health Organization Healthy Cities Project: A Project Becomes a Movement.* Copenhagen, Denmark: FADL Publishers; 1990.
3. *Basic Documents.* 38th ed. Geneva, Switzerland: World Health Organization; 1990.
4. *Global Strategy for Health for All by the Year 2000.* "Health for All" Series; No 3. Geneva, Switzerland: World Health Organization; 1991.
5. Ottawa Charter for Health Promotion. *Health Promotion.* 1986;1(4):ii-v.
6. *City Networks for Health. Technical Discussions on Strategies for Health for All in the Face of Rapid Urbanization.* Geneva, Switzerland: World Health Organization; May 1991.
7. Institute of Medicine. *The Future of Public Health.* Washington, DC: National Academy Press; 1988.
8. Flynn BC, Rider MS. Healthy Cities Indiana: mainstreaming community health in the United States. *Am J Public Health.* 1991;81(4):510–511.
9. Flynn BC, Rider MS, Ray DW. Healthy Cities: the Indiana model of community development in public health. *Health Educ Q.* 1991;18(3):331–347.
10. Bracht N. *Health Promotion at the Community Level.* Newbury Park, Calif: Sage Publications; 1990.
11. Etzioni A. *Social Problems.* Englewood Cliffs, NJ: Prentice Hall; 1976.

Index

Page numbers followed by *f* indicate figures; those followed by *t* indicate tables; those followed by *d* indicate displays.

A

Access to care
  definition of, 204
  direct payment and, 300
  ethics and, 214
  failure of in U.S., 213–214
  health care reform and, 199t, 204–205
  for homeless families, 452
  market-driven, 217
  nurse as advocate and spokesperson for, 217–218
  policy and, 11–12
  1960's public programs for, 301
  of underserved populations, 10–11
Accountability
  for child abuse, 359
  in family nursing, 382–383
Acid-fast bacillus isolation
  of individuals with active tuberculosis, 77–78, 78d
Activity orientation, culture and, 516
Acute care nursing
  community health nursing versus, 136–137
  nurse practitioners in, 308, 309t
Adolescent Family Life Act of 1981, 418
Adolescent Health, Services, and Pregnancy Prevention Act of 1978, 412–413, 417
Adolescent pregnancy
  contexts of problem
    economic, 416
    historical, 413–414
    international, 414–416
  costs of, 411–412
  historical perspective on, 410–411
  prevention of
    primary and secondary strategies for, 419–420
    school-based program for, 581–587
  public policy and, 416–418
  reduction of, 180, 181, 183
  scope of, 411–412

Adolescents
  alcohol abuse program for, 609–617
  alcohol and drug use by, 62
  obese, 234
  prenatal and postnatal home-based care for, 123
  public health—social service partnerships for, 129–130
  teen parenting program for, 625–626
  violence among, 51, 53
Advanced practice nursing, American Nurses' Association definition of, 303
Advocacy
  in HIV control, 442–443
  in home care, 471
  as nursing role, 556, 558
  for prevention
    of homelessness, 456
  for single-parent family, 367–368
Affirmation of strengths, in family nursing, 354
African-Americans
  health care for, 214
  tuberculosis in, 72
Agency for Toxic Substances and Disease Registry, The (ATSDR), 144–145
Agent, epidemiologic, 258–259, 259t
Aggregates
  at-risk, 105–107
  community health nursing for, 107–108
  definition of, 103–105, 136–137
Aid to Families with Dependent Children (AFDC), 411–412, 416, 418
Alcohol
  adverse effects of, 60–61
  advertising and, 259
Alcohol abuse
  adolescent
    nurse-initiated task force for, 609–619
  detection of, 64
  interventions for, 61–62, 64, 65, 67, 68
  policy and environmental strategies for, 592–593
  treatment programs for, 66
Alcohol and drug prevention education
  kindergarten through grade 12, 399d–400d

Medical education, 102
Medical management, 307–308, 308t
Medicare
  home nurse attitude toward, 488–489
  payment reform and, 301–302
Medicine, versus nursing, 102
Mental development, of infants and young
    children, 405
Mental health
  healthy people 2000 objectives and,
    394d
  of homeless children, 449–450
  of homeless mothers, 451, 452
Mental illness, in homeless, 449–450, 451,
    452
Minority groups
  ethics and, 522–529
  health beliefs of, 530–542
  public health initiatives and, 586
Mission, quality care and, 283
Mission statement
  for community health improvement,
    179–180
  in program development, 235–236
Mobile outreach health services, for home-
    less families, 453–455
Mothers, homeless, 450–452
Murdock, George, *Outline of Cultural Mate-
    rials,* 496

N
National health insurance, 9, 11–12, 212
National Institute of Occupational Safety
    and Health (NIOSH), 161
Native Americans
  community health program for,
    507–510
  personalistic health beliefs of, 532d, 534
  tuberculosis in, 72
Needs
  family-supported
    physical, 334
    psychosocial, 334–335
Needs assessment
  community, 226, 227
  in program development, 236–237
  for self-help groups, 426–427
Nightingale, Florence
  on aboriginal races, 274–275
  on army medical care and sanitation,
    276–278
  environmental health and, 21
  on hospital construction, organization,
    management, 270–271
  on nursing education, 111, 112
  on public health nursing, 110–120
  as reformer, 110–111
  reforms of
    British Army, 268–269, 275–278
    workhouse infirmaries, 111–114

as statistician, 266–278
Nurse-client relationship
  in case management, 290, 292–293
  power issue in, 381–382
  for quality care, 286–287
Nurse practitioners
  case managers and, 302
  community health nurses and, 299–310
  comparison with community health
    nurses
    scope of practice, 303t
  home care nurses and, 306–307
  in primary care, 306–308
  reimbursement for Medicare services,
    302
  role of, 299
  in schools, 168
Nurses
  as change agents, 609–617
  public health role of, 381–382
Nursing
  American Nurses' Association definition
    of, 461
  future of
    trends affecting, 90–92
  philosophy of, 556
  roles in, 556–557, 558
  vision statement of, 91–92, 96
Nursing center
  clients of, 165–166
  community support for, 165
  as primary care provider, 305–306, 306t
Nursing diagnosis
  within cultural context, 525
  in environmental health, 148
Nursing education
  for aggregate decision making, 108
  for case management, 296–297
  for community-based practice, 35
  for community health nursing, 35,
    107–108
  for HIV/AIDS population, 33
  improvements needed in, 34–36
  individualistic versus patient group-
    directed, 102–103
  new approaches in, 95–96
  Nightingale on, 115–116
  for occupational health nursing,
    160–161
  for primary health care, 207–208
  in public health policy, 208
Nursing faculty, in community organiza-
    tion, 35–38
Nursing home care, 307
Nursing practice
  culturally sensitive
    barriers to, 524–525
    guidelines for, 527–528
  justice versus caring in, 214–216
Nursing process, in family health, 343–350

Tuberculosis (*continued*)
  employment activity risks for, 79d
  incidence of, 67–68
  infection with, 74
  isolation protocols for, 77–78, 78d
  multidrug-resistant, 83–84
  personal respiratory protection, 79
  personal respiratory protection for,
    79–80
  populations at risk for, 75–76, 76d
  prevention of, 79–80
  prevention of active disease, 80–83, 82d
  prophylaxis for, 82, 82d
  prophylaxis fpr, 71–72
  risk for nurses, 72–73, 79d, 86, 86d
  screening for, 80–81, 86d
  signs and symptoms of, 75d
  transmission
    prevention of, 75–79
  transmission of, 73
  treatment of, 82–83
Twelve-step programs, for chemical dependency, 66

U
Uninsured population, 213, 214
Universal health insurance, access to care
    and, 9, 11–12
Utilitarian approach, to ethical dilemmas,
    139, 142–143

V
Value
  exchange through public health nursing, 245–246, 246f
  perceived, 243
Values
  assessment of, 512–513, 515–516
  in home care, 482
  quality care and, 283
Victimization
  nursing research on, 47

of women and children
  nursing response to, 50–51, 52t, 53
Violent and abusive behavior
  healthy people 2000 objectives
    nursing response to, 50–51, 52t, 53
  healthy people 2000 objectives and, 40,
    42t–44t, 394d, 400d
  homeless mothers and, 451
  incidence and prevalence of, 40
  as nursing priority, 40–56
  nursing role in, 44–46
  policy changes and, 41–44
Visiting Nurse Service, founding of, 212

W
Wald, Lillian, 163, 164
  health care reform and, 211, 212, 213
  legacy of, 219
  public health nursing and, 222, 225
Wellness
  definition of, 459
  for elders, 459–467
  family, 343–350
  in occupational health, 162
  promotion of, 18
Wellness programs, 161–162
Women
  abused, 41, 44, 45
  access to care and, 214
  alcoholism in, 60
  victimization of
    nursing response to, 50–51, 52t, 53
  working
    postpartum health of, 605, 606t
    pregnancy and social health policy,
      600–601
Worker assessment
  in occupational health, 156
  in occupational health and safety, 156
Workhouse infirmaries, Nightingale's reforms for, 111–114

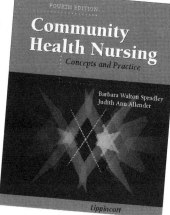
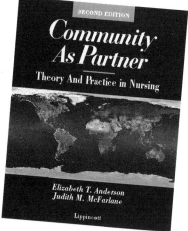
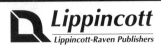